D1573238

Gastrointestinal Surgery

Springer
New York
Berlin
Heidelberg
Hong Kong
London
Milan
Paris
Tokyo

Gastrointestinal Surgery

Pathophysiology and Management

HAILE T. DEBAS, MD

Maurice Galante Distinguished Professor of Surgery
Former Dean, School of Medicine
University of California, San Francisco

With 262 Illustrations

Illustrations by Christine Gralapp

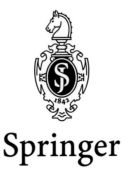

Springer

Haile T. Debas, MD
Maurice Galante Distinguished Professor of Surgery and
  Former Dean, School of Medicine
University of California, San Francisco
San Francisco, CA 94143-0410
USA

Library of Congress Cataloging-in-Publication Data
Debas, Haile T.
    Gastrointestinal surgery : pathophysiology and management / Haile T. Debas.
      p. ; cm.
    Includes bibliographical references and index.
    ISBN 0-387-00721-0 (h/c : alk. paper)
    1. Gastrointestinal system—Surgery.   2. Gastrointestinal system—Pathophysiology.
  I. Debas, Haile T.   II. Title.
    [DNLM: 1. Digestive System Diseases—surgery.   2. Digestive Physiology.   3. Digestive
  System Diseases—physiopathology.   4. Digestive System Surgical Procedures—methods.
  WI 900 D286g 2003]
  RD540.D23 2003
  617.4′3—dc21
                                                                          2003042830

ISBN 0-387-00721-0   Printed on acid-free paper.

Printed in the United States of America.

9 8 7 6 5 4 3 2 1   SPIN 10918890

www.springer-ny.com

Springer-Verlag New York Berlin Heidelberg
A member of BertelsmannSpringer Science+Business Media GmbH

To my wife Kim,
for her unconditional love and support
and for all the sacrifices she has made over the last 35 years
to allow me to enjoy a career in academic surgery and administration.

Contents

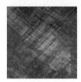

Preface

Many excellent textbooks of surgery exist. Most of these are large, multiauthored, and have the distinct advantage of drawing on the experience of many surgeons with expertise in specific areas. The advantage, however, is often obtained at the expense of a unified approach and style that a book written by a single author can provide.

In writing this book about gastrointestinal surgery, I use an integrated approach to discuss fundamental anatomy and physiology; then examine how normal function is altered by disease, i.e., pathophysiology; and finally, provide the clinical correlates. Based on these three pillars of understanding particular disease processes, I then discuss surgical treatment as a means of correcting the abnormal physiology to restore health. I hope this approach will provide the reader a coordinated understanding that minimizes the need for rote memorization.

I believe that, when the student understands normal physiology, how disease disturbs that physiology, and how surgical treatment might restore normalcy, one need not remember too many extraneous facts. Instead, a foundation of understanding is established that stays with the student even after the details are forgotten. The Jesuits have an attractive definition of *culture* as "that which remains after you have forgotten all you have learnt." While I hope that the readers of this book will not totally forget all the facts they have *learnt*, the concept of a *culture of understanding* is, nevertheless, valid.

The previous discussion applies to clinical conditions in which surgical strategies exist to correct the abnormal physiology. Unfortunately, in many surgical diseases, extirpation of the diseased organ is possible while correction of the pathophysiology is not. But, even here, the *physiologic approach* to surgical therapy has relevance. It enables the reader to better understand not only the cause of clinical symptoms and signs but also the physiologic insult that invariably results when organs or portions of them are removed. I have also attempted, therefore, to discuss the altered pathophysiology imposed by certain surgical procedures and the adaptive physiologic processes that are brought into play postoperatively.

I have not intended that this book provide the comprehensive information that multiauthored texts can provide. Rather, I attempt to offer a clinical and therapeutic approach to surgical diseases of the gastrointestinal tract based on how diseases and surgical procedures alter normal physiology. In this way, again, I hope that understanding will replace rote memorization of details. While the book should primarily serve the needs of medical students and surgical residents and fellows, I hope that surgeons in practice and academic environments will also find it useful.

HAILE T. DEBAS, MD, FRCS (C), FACS
San Francisco, California

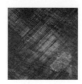

Acknowledgments

I wish to express my deepest gratitude and appreciation to Ms. Patricia Meagher, without whose commitment to the project, hard work, perseverance, organization, and sense of editorial perfection, this book would not have been possible. To her, the book has been a labor of love. I just hope that the final product is worthy of her Herculean effort to see this ambitious book to the finish.

Ms. Christine Gralapp provided the illustrations. Her beautifully simple drawings have enlivened the pages of the book and will, undoubtedly, simplify the reader's task in understanding concepts of pathophysiology and treatment of surgical diseases.

Dr. Henry I. Goldberg, Clinical Professor of Radiology at the University of California, San Francisco (UCSF), provided the radiological images for the book. I am most appreciative of his indispensable contribution to the book and grateful for the privilege of tapping into his enormous experience and expertise in gastrointestinal radiology. I am also grateful to Dr. Vincent McCormick, Clinical Professor of Radiology at UCSF, for providing the radiological images for abdominal trauma.

Dr. Linda Ferrell, Professor of Pathology at UCSF, contributed most of the figures depicting gross and microscopic surgical pathology. Dr. Ferrell's vast case collection and enormous experience and expertise in gastrointestinal pathology adds an important dimension to the book. I am very indebted to her.

I am also grateful to three other colleagues at UCSF: Dr. James Ostroff, Professor of Medicine, and Dr. John Cello, Professor of Medicine and Surgery, who contributed the endoscopic images; and Dr. Theodore Schrock, Professor of Surgery, who contributed several photographs of surgical specimens.

Finally, I wish to thank Ms. Daisy Leo, my Senior Executive Assistant, who somehow juggled my busy schedule to enable me to spend the time necessary to write the book.

Finally, I would like to acknowledge the contributions of generations of surgical residents with whom I have had the privilege to associate and from whom I have learnt so much in an enjoyable 30-year career in academic surgery.

HAILE T. DEBAS, MD, FRCS (C), FACS
San Francisco, California

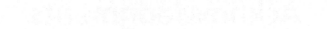

Esophagus

The esophagus is a simple muscular tube closed at each end with a sphincter. It begins where the pharynx ends at the level of the C-6 vertebra and ends at the cardia of the stomach, some 3 to 5 cm below the diaphragm, after passing through the diaphragmatic hiatus. The esophagus is approximately 40 cm in length and, for the sake of convenience and clarity in discussion, it is distinguished by three sections: cervical, thoracic, and abdominal. Anatomic relationships of the esophagus are detailed in Figure 1.1 and Table 1.1.

The major function of the esophagus is to transport food from the pharynx into the stomach in a coordinated fashion. Although its mucosal lining secretes mucus, secretion is not considered an important part of esophageal function.

UPPER ESOPHAGEAL SPHINCTER

Located at the upper end of the esophagus, the upper esophageal sphincter (UES) is composed of striated muscle condensation covering 2 to 3 cm, reinforced by the transverse fibers of the cricopharyngeus muscle (Figure 1.2). The UES remains closed except during swallowing, when it relaxes in response to pharyngeal contraction. In the resting state, the UES maintains a pressure of approximately 40 mm Hg. This pressure is essential to prevent aspiration of esophageal contents during gastroesophageal reflux or when swallowed food empties poorly. Failure of the UES to relax in response to swallowing may result in upper esophageal dysphagia and aspiration.

BODY OF THE ESOPHAGUS

The muscular coat of the upper third of the body of the esophagus (i.e., the cervical esophagus) is composed of striated muscle, while that of the lower two thirds is smooth muscle. The smooth-muscle coat consists of an inner circular and an outer longitudinal layer. The esophagus has no serosal layer.

The mean resting pressure in the body of the esophagus varies from −8 to +5 mm Hg, depending on the respiratory cycle. In response to swallowing, however, a coordinated peristalsis sweeps from the upper to the lower end of the esophagus. The mean amplitude of contractions during esophageal peristalsis is 60 ± 5 mm Hg. When the lumen of the esophagus is acidified, strong peristaltic waves are initiated that serve to rid the esophagus of acid. This "esophageal pump" mechanism is important in the overall health of the gastrointestinal system.

LOWER ESOPHAGEAL SPHINCTER

The lower esophageal sphincter (LES) is located at the terminal end of the esophagus and represents the distal 3 to 5 cm of the organ (see Figure 1.2). Most of the LES lies within the abdominal cavity, but a short segment often extends above the diaphragm. A small condensation of circular smooth-muscle fibers resides in this region, too indefinite to constitute an anatomical sphincter. The specialized nature and unique innervation of the smooth muscle of the terminal esophagus provide the basis for a physiological sphincter. These specialized smooth-muscled fibers contain receptors for a number of peptide (e.g., vasoactive intestinal peptide, substance P) and nonpeptide neurotransmitters that are released locally from peptidergic and nonpeptidergic neurons.

The LES is a high-pressure zone interposed between the body of the esophagus and the cardia of the stomach (Figure 1.3). Normally, a mean pressure of 20 ± 5 mm Hg is maintained at all times except during swallowing, when the pressure falls to 0 mm Hg, allowing esophageal peristalsis to empty the swallowed food into the stomach. In its resting state, therefore, the high pressure of the LES prevents reflux of gastric contents into the esophagus.

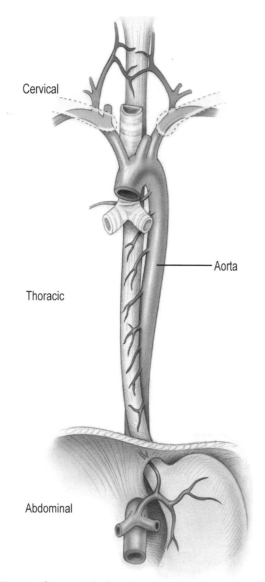

Cervical

Thoracic

Aorta

Abdominal

FIGURE 1.1. The cervical, thoracic, and abdominal esophagus, its blood supply and anatomic relationships.

TABLE 1.1. Essentials: Esophageal Anatomy
Muscular tube, 40-cm long
■ Closed at proximal end by UES
■ Closed at distal end by LES
■ Inner circular muscle coat
■ Outer longitudinal muscle coat
■ Striated muscle at upper one third
■ Smooth muscle at distal two thirds
No serosa
Nerve supply
■ Vagus nerve
Blood supply
■ Cervical: Inferior thyroid
■ Thoracic: Aortic branches
■ Abdominal: Left gastric, inferior phrenic
Abbreviations: LES, lower esophageal sphincter; UES, upper esophageal sphincter.

coordinated contraction of the body of the esophagus and carrying the food past the LES—which remains in a state of relaxation—and into the stomach. The LES then contracts in sequence with esophageal peristalsis. By the time the bolus reaches it, the stomach is in a state of receptive relaxation brought about by esophagogastric vagal reflexes and activated by increases in luminal pressure due to esophageal contraction. This process of stomach relaxation is mediated by release of VIP and NO from nerve terminals within the fundus and body of the stomach. This normal swallowing mechanism is depicted in Figure 1.4.

ESOPHAGEAL MUCOSA

The innermost lining of the esophagus is composed of nonkeratinized squamous cell epithelium, except for the distal 3 to 5 cm, where the lining progresses from squamous epithelium to columnar mucosa, similar to that in the upper cardia of the stomach.

BLOOD AND NERVE SUPPLY AND LYMPHATICS

The cervical esophagus receives its blood supply from the inferior thyroid arteries; the thoracic esophagus from the bronchial arteries, from direct branches of the thoracic aorta, and from the intercostal arteries; and the abdominal esophagus from ascending branches of the left gastric artery and the inferior phrenic arteries (see Figure 1.1). Venous drainage accumulates in the periesophageal venous plexus, which empties into the inferior thyroid veins in the neck, into bronchial azygous and hemiazygous veins in the thorax, and into the coronary vein in the abdomen. The coronary vein drains into the portal vein, and hence, in portal hypertension, the venous plexus at the distal esophagus dilates to form esophageal varices.

The LES contracts and increases its pressure in response to sudden increases in abdominal pressure and to alkalinization of the gastric lumen. As mentioned above, the LES relaxes in response to swallowing, a function mediated by local release from neurons in the LES musculature of vasoactive intestinal peptide (VIP) and nitric oxide (NO). Other factors contributing to the lowering of LES pressure are nicotine, gastric acidification, ingestion of fats, and release of cholecystokinin (CCK). Essential features of LES anatomy are summarized in Table 1.2.

SWALLOWING MECHANISM

When food or fluid enter the pharynx, pharyngeal contractions are initiated. At the very beginning of swallowing, both the UES and LES relax. Pharyngeal contractions deliver the food into the upper esophagus, initiating a

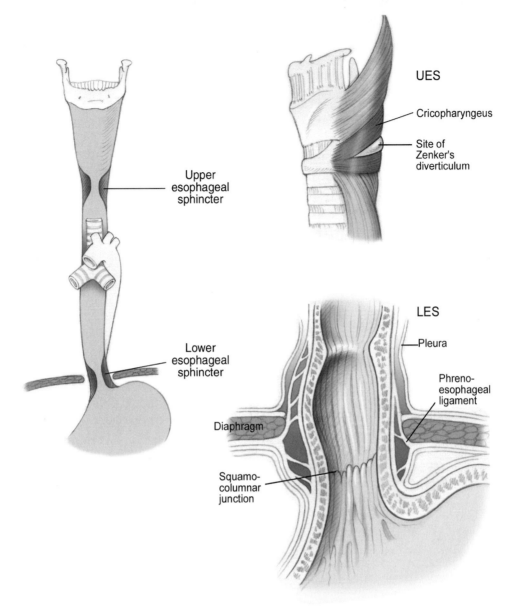

FIGURE 1.2. The upper esophageal sphincter (UES) and lower esophageal sphincter (LES) govern the swallowing mechanism to prevent aspiration and reflux of food. The UES is at the level of the cricoid, of which the cricopharyngeus muscle is an important component. The LES straddles the diaphragmatic hiatus and is more a physiological than an anatomical sphincter. The squamo-columnar junction between esophageal and gastric mucosa lies within the LES. (Adapted from Rothberg M, DeMeester TR. Surgical anatomy of the esophagus. In: Shields TW, editor. General Thoracic Surgery, 3rd ed. Philadephia: Lea & Febiger; 1989:78; and Feldman M, Sleisenger MH, Scharschmidt BF, eds. Sleisenger & Fordtran's Gastrointestinal and Liver Disease: Pathophysiology, Diagnosis, Management. Philadelphia: WB Saunders; 1998.)

The nerve supply of the esophagus (Figure 1.5) derives from the vagus and the cervical sympathetic trunk. The vagus provides the essential innervation of the body and sphincters of the esophagus. The cervical esophagus is innervated by branches of the recurrent laryngeal nerves, while the thoracic and abdominal portions are innervated directly from the vagal neural plexus surrounding the organ. At the hiatus, considerable variation exists from individual to individual. In about 60% of human subjects, the anterior vagus is a single strand at the hiatus, while the posterior vagus is single in more than 90% (Figure 1.6). Sensory innervation is provided by C-fibers that contain substance P and calcitonin generelated peptide (CGRP), two neuropeptides that mediate sensation.

Lymphatic drainage of the cervical esophagus goes to deep cervical and paratracheal nodes (Figure 1.7). The thoracic esophagus drains into the pulmonary hilar and subcarinal nodes. The lower thoracic esophagus drains into inferior paraesophageal and parahiatal nodes, while the abdominal esophagus drains primarily into nodes along the left gastric artery.

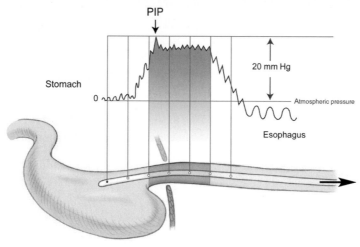

FIGURE 1.3. The lower esophageal sphincter (LES) can be identified by measuring the resting pressure of the distal esophagus at various points. It is 3.0–5.0 cm in length, with a mean resting pressure of 20 ± 5 mm Hg. When the sensing device is below the diaphragm, inspiration causes a positive pressure inflection. The opposite is true above the diaphragm. The pressure inversion point (PIP) indicates the level of the diaphragm.

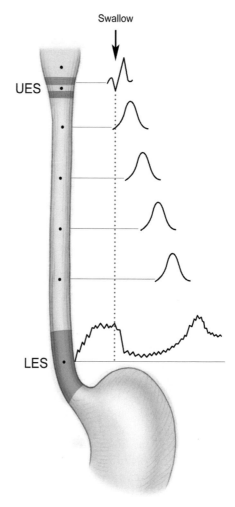

TABLE 1.2. Essentials: Lower Esophageal Sphincter (LES)
Length: 3–5 cm
Mean resting pressure (LESP): 20 ± 5 mm Hg
Factors that increase LES pressure   ▪ Increased abdominal pressure   ▪ Alkalinization of stomach   ▪ Hypergastrinemia
Neurotransmitters   ▪ Relaxation: Vasoactive intestinal peptide, nitric oxide   ▪ Contraction: Acetylcholine
Factors that lower LES pressure   ▪ Gastric acidification   ▪ Ingestion of fat   ▪ Cholecystokinin   ▪ Nicotine

FIGURE 1.4. Normal swallowing mechanism: At the initiation of swallowing, the pharynx contracts and the upper esophageal sphincter (UES) relaxes. At the same time, the lower esophageal sphincter (LES) relaxes and stays relaxed until the peristaltic wave of contraction sweeps down the esophagus and arrives at the LES. The LES then contracts in sequence with the peristalsis, by which time the swallowed bolus has entered the stomach.

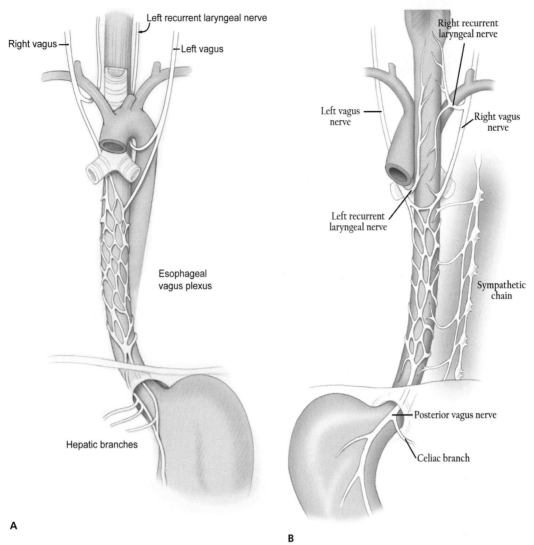

FIGURE 1.5. Nerve supply of the esophagus: The nerve supply, shown (A) anteriorly and (B) posteriorly, derives from the vagus and the cervical sympathetic trunk.

PATHOPHYSIOLOGY

Normal function of the esophagus and its sphincters is impaired in a number of clinical conditions. Motility impairments are summarized in Table 1.3.

ABNORMALITIES OF THE UPPER ESOPHAGEAL SPHINCTER

Increased UES and/or Failure of Relaxation

Sometimes seen in elderly patients who have sustained a cerebrovascular accident, failure of normal relaxation of the UES causes an inability to swallow. These patients may drool saliva or suffer from intermittent aspiration. Failure of UES relaxation is considered a primary defect in the etiology of pharyngoesophageal, or Zenker's, diverticulum.

Hypotensive UES

Occasionally seen in patients with severe gastroesophageal reflux, hypotensive UES causes a susceptibility to pulmonary aspiration. Whether hypotensive UES occurs as an isolated phenomenon unrelated to gastroesophageal reflux is unknown.

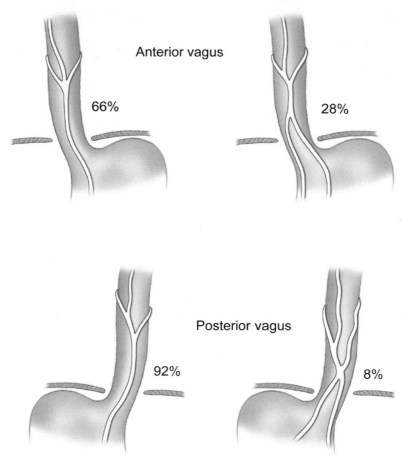

Anterior vagus

66%

28%

Posterior vagus

92%

8%

FIGURE 1.6. Configurations of the anterior and posterior vagus at the level of the diaphragm can vary from individual to individual and may be important in performing surgical procedures.

ABNORMALITIES OF THE BODY OF THE ESOPHAGUS

Diffuse Esophageal Spasm

In diffuse esophageal spasm (DES), coordinated esophageal peristalsis is lost. Instead, a large segment of the esophagus contracts at once, generating very high luminal pressures. The distal half of the esophagus is often affected. The patient experiences squeezing retrosternal pain accompanied by difficulty in swallowing. In DES, both upper and lower sphincters function normally and relax appropriately in response to swallowing. The motility abnormalities of DES are depicted in Figure 1.8. A significant association exists between DES and epiphrenic diverticulum, suggesting that high intraluminal pressures may contribute to the development of this pulsion-type diverticulum.

Achalasia

In classic achalasia, esophageal peristalsis is lost (Figure 1.9). Instead, in response to swallowing, the body of the esophagus exhibits feeble, uncoordinated contractions. In advanced cases, the esophagus may show little, if any, contractile function. Because failure of the LES to relax is a dominant feature of achalasia, the condition is described again later under Abnormalities of the Lower Esophageal Sphincter.

Scleroderma

When scleroderma affects the esophagus, it spares the sphincters. The abnormality is in the body of the esophagus, where peristalsis is lost and contractions in response to swallowing are uncoordinated. While DES causes high-amplitude contractions, in scleroderma the contractions are often feeble. The condition is distinguishable from achalasia because LES function is normal, both in its pressure profile and in its normal relaxation response to swallowing. The patient might also exhibit other manifestations of scleroderma, such as Raynaud's phenomenon.

When esophageal scleroderma coexists with abnormal gastroesophageal reflux, severe esophagitis and esophageal shortening are apt to occur due to loss of the protective "esophageal pump," favoring stasis of acid refluxate in the distal esophagus.

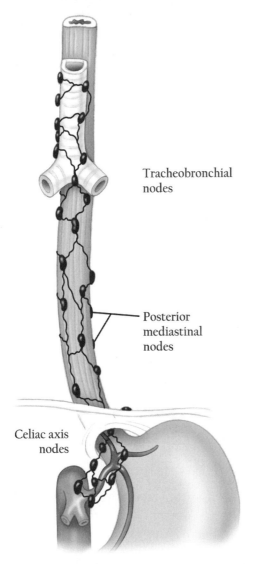

FIGURE 1.7. Lymphatic drainage of the esophagus: The three major groups of nodes that drain the esophagus are the tracheobronchial, posterior mediastinal, and celiac axis nodes.

Other Conditions

Loss of normal esophageal peristalsis that cannot be categorized under any diagnosis may be seen. Patients with severe gastroesophageal reflux disease sometimes demonstrate abnormal motility in the body of the esophagus. This abnormality typically reverses when reflux is corrected and the esophagitis disappears.

ABNORMALITIES OF THE LOWER ESOPHAGEAL SPHINCTER

Hypotensive LES

Hypotensive LES is often seen in patients with sliding hiatal hernia and reflux esophagitis. Typically, patients

TABLE 1.3. Essentials: Motility Disorders of the Esophagus

Upper esophageal sphincter
- Failure of UES relaxation (e.g., stroke)
- Zenker's diverticulum

Body of the esophagus
- Diffuse esophageal spasm
  High-amplitude aperistaltic contractions
  Loss of peristalsis
  Normal LES
- Scleroderma
  Loss of peristalsis
  Low-amplitude contractions
  Normal LES

Lower esophageal sphincter
- Achalasia
  Failure of LES relaxation
  Increased LESP (not always)
  Feeble aperistaltic contractions of esophageal body
- Hypertensive LES
  High resting body pressure
  Normal LES relaxation
- Hypotensive LES
  LESP < 15 mm Hg
  Normal LES relaxation

Abbreviations: LES, lower esophageal sphincter; LESP, lower esophageal sphincter pressure; UES, upper esophageal sphincter.

with reflux esophagitis have LES pressures far lower than 15 mm Hg.

Chronic Gastroesophageal Reflux

Chronic reflux of acid peptic contents of the stomach into the lower esophagus may manifest in different ways: heartburn, chest pain, esophagitis, Barrett's esophagus, and Barrett's ulcer.

Heartburn

Heartburn is the classic substernal burning pain of reflux described earlier.

Chest Pain

The chest pain characteristic of gastroesophageal reflux is substernal or left chest pain that might mimic myocardial infarction. This symptom can occur even in the absence of gross esophagitis. Once cardiac causes are eliminated, the esophagus as the source of the pain must be investigated, either by the Bernstein test or, better still, through 24-h pH monitoring of the esophagus in the ambulatory setting. This procedure is described below.

Esophagitis

Chronic reflux of acid induces inflammatory injury of the esophageal mucosa, particularly if the esophageal pump

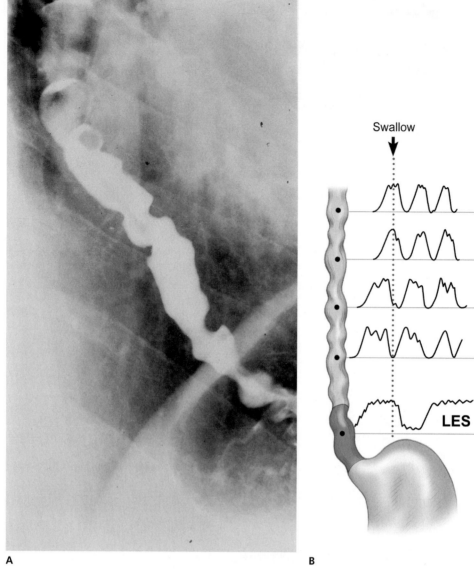

A   B

FIGURE 1.8. In diffuse esophageal spasm (DES), a large segment of the esophagus contracts at once, generating high luminal pressure and resulting in a corkscrew-shaped esophagus. (A) The distal half of the esophagus is often affected by multiple indentations, indicating local contractions, as demonstrated in the x-ray. (B) As shown in motility studies, the lower esophageal sphincter (LES) is usually normal and relaxes normally. Contractions are uncoordinated and esophageal peristalsis is lost. (Courtesy of Henry I. Goldberg, MD.)

mechanism is defective. The result is development of a low-grade esophagitis, seen histologically as expansion of the basal zone to more than 15% of the epithelium and lengthening of the papillae toward the surface (Figure 1.10). Vascular lakes and balloon cells may be present, but polymorphonuclear (PMN) and eosinophilic cell infiltration is absent. When destruction of the epithelium is severe, high-grade esophagitis may be present and is often associated with ulcerated lesions and PMN infiltration (Figure 1.11). Ulcerative esophagitis can cause upper gastrointestinal bleeding. The continuous process of inflammation, ulceration, and repair eventually causes stricture of the distal esophagus and may lead to esophageal shortening.

Barrett's Esophagus

The metaplasia from squamous to columnar epithelium represents the development of Barrett's esophagus. Typically, Barrett's mucosa appears as a circumferential sheet or discontinuous islands of pinkish mucosa. The epithelium resembles intestinal mucosa. The clinical concern with Barrett's esophagus is its propensity to progress to dysplasia and then form adenocarcinoma (Figure 1.12). The incidence of adenocarcinoma is estimated to be one case per 441 patient years. However, in patients who show aneuploidy on flow cytometry, the 5-year cumulative incidence of cancer is 43%, compared to 5% in those with no aneuploidy.[1]

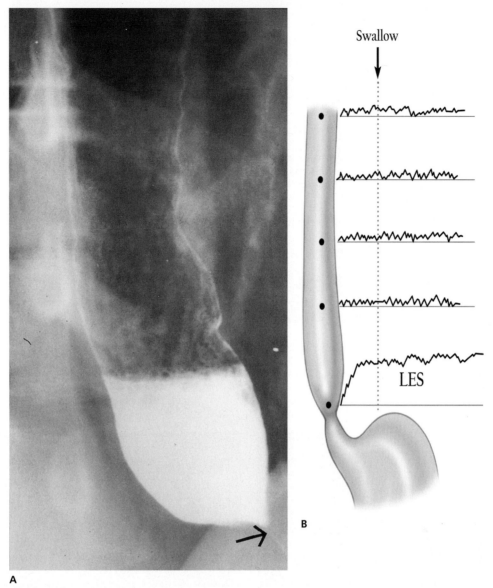

FIGURE 1.9. (A) In achalasia, the upper gastrointestinal (GI) series often demonstrates a dilated esophagus with retained food and fluids; the lower end of the column of barium has a "beak-like" appearance, with little barium entering the stomach (arrow). (B) In motility studies, the body of the esophagus exhibits feeble, uncoordinated contractions in response to swallowing, and the lower esophageal sphincter (LES), which may or may not be hypertensive, fails to relax. (Courtesy of Henry I. Goldberg, MD.)

Barrett's Ulcer

Uncommonly, a true peptic ulcer may develop within the Barrett's epithelium, causing a Barrett's ulcer. This is an infrequent cause of upper gastrointestinal hemorrhage.

Hypertensive LES

The isolated condition of hypertensive LES is rare. When it occurs, it causes retrosternal "squeezing" pain and dysphagia. The condition is sometimes referred to as "nut-

cracker esophagus." To diagnose this condition, it is necessary to confirm normal peristalsis of the esophageal body. Unlike achalasia, LES relaxation is normal.

Achalasia

Achalasia is characterized by abnormalities of both the esophageal body and the LES (see Figure 1.9). The abnormal motility of the esophageal body in achalasia is characterized by feeble, uncoordinated, aperistaltic contractions in response to swallowing. The cause is

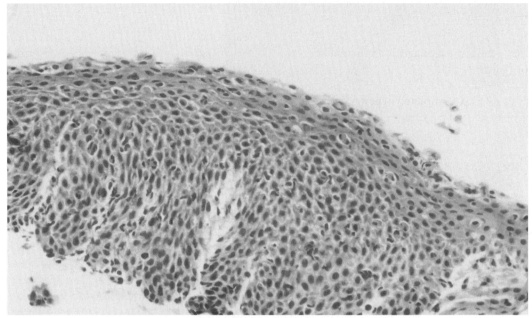

FIGURE 1.10. Esophagitis is caused by chronic reflux-associated damage to the mucosa. Low-grade esophagitis is characterized histologically by basal cell hyperplasia and lengthening of the papillae toward the surface. (Courtesy of Linda D. Ferrell, MD.)

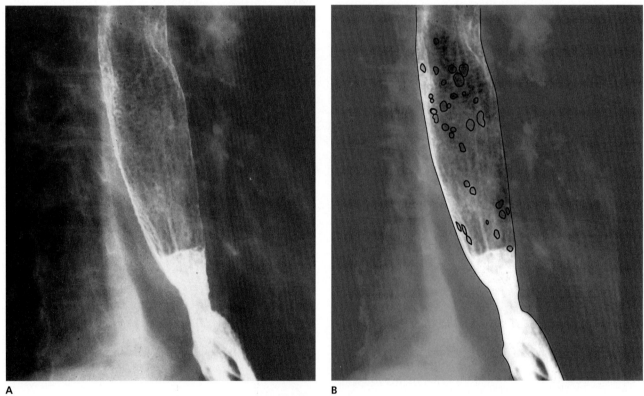

A   B

FIGURE 1.11. (A) Air-barium esophagram of an advanced case of esophagitis demonstrates roughened mucosal surface, small punctate ulcers, and distal esophageal stricture—all features of chronic esophagitis. (B) The diagram accentuates the ulcerated lesions. (Courtesy of Henry I. Goldberg, MD.)

unknown, but it is associated with degeneration of the myenteric plexus, perhaps as a result of autoimmune disease. Chagas' disease, caused by infection from *Trypanosoma cruzi*, causes esophageal abnormalities very similar to those of achalasia.

The most important abnormality of the LES in achalasia is its failure to relax completely when a patient swallows. This abnormality is not infrequently combined with increased LES pressure, hence the old name "cardiospasm." Occasionally in achalasia, the LES may demonstrate early relaxation but with premature contractions that prevent the swallowed bolus from entering the stomach. The most important symptom is dysphagia. Pain is a feature only in the rare condition referred to as vigorous achalasia, which is characterized by vigorous but aperistaltic esophageal contractions and a hypertensive LES.

CLINICAL DISORDERS

CARDINAL SYMPTOMS OF ESOPHAGEAL DISEASE

The cardinal symptoms of esophageal disease include dysphagia, pain, and heartburn. Each requires a different work-up and clinical approach to the patient to determine the proper course of management (Table 1.4).

Dysphagia

Difficulty in swallowing associated with the sensation that food sticks at some level of the esophagus is a most important symptom of esophageal disease. The patient will be able to indicate the level at which the food sticks, which is often the site of the pathology. In its early stages, dysphagia may be limited to solid foods and then progress to liquids. The patient may present with obstruction from ingested food as the first symptom of esophageal disease, in which case an underlying lesion must be ruled out after the food is removed.

Approach to the Patient with Dysphagia

In the patient with dysphagia, the most important point is to assume that carcinoma is present until proven otherwise. A chest x-ray and upper gastrointestinal (GI) series with barium are probably the best initial specific tests after a thorough history is recorded and physical examination is performed. Upper gastrointestinal flexible endoscopy with biopsy and brushings provide the most definitive information if the disease is mucosal. If the results of the barium swallow and esophagoscopy are negative, a motility disorder is a possibility, and esophageal manometry should be obtained. If the barium swallow study demonstrates the presence of an esophageal diverticulum, esophageal manometry studies must also be obtained, because the association of diverticula with motility disorder of the esophagus is high.

Chest Pain

Chest pain is an important symptom of esophageal disease. When chest pain is associated with swallowing (odynophagia), it is highly likely that the esophagus is the source of the pain. Otherwise, other causes of chest pain must be seriously considered. The pain may be mild or severe, steady or squeezing. The most common esophageal causes of chest pain are DES and reflux of gastric acid into the esophagus.

Approach to the Patient with Chest Pain

In evaluating the patient with chest pain, the first step is to rule out a cardiac cause by electrocardiogram (EKG), stress-EKG, or thallium scan. A chest x-ray is also necessary to rule out pulmonary or mediastinal lesions (e.g., dissecting thoracic aortic aneurysm), and abnormalities of the thoracic spine and ribs. If the above test results are normal, systematic investigation of the esophagus should be undertaken, using the following tests: barium swallow with cinefluorography, upper GI endoscopy with or without biopsy, and esophageal motility studies including 24-h pH monitoring. This latter investigation should facilitate the identification of either DES or reflux of acid as the cause of the chest pain. An acid infusion (Bernstein) test is useful if the 24-h pH-monitoring test is equivocal. Infusion through a nasoesophageal tube of 0.1 N HCl, but not saline, reproduces the chest pain if it is due to reflux of acid.

Heartburn

The classic symptom of gastroesophageal reflux is a burning, retrosternal sensation, often following ingestion of a meal, whether the patient is bending or supine. Heartburn may or may not be associated with a sensation of reflux that the patient is able to appreciate. Typically, the symptom rapidly responds to ingestion of antacids or milk. Mild initial symptoms do not require formal investigation and can be managed conservatively with such measures as antacids, the use of acid-reducing drugs, eating smaller meals, avoiding recumbence after eating, weight loss, and cessation of smoking.

Approach to the Patient with Heartburn

If symptoms persist, formal esophageal investigation is necessary, including barium swallow to determine the presence of hiatal hernia and gastroesophageal reflux. Upper GI endoscopy is also needed to assess the presence

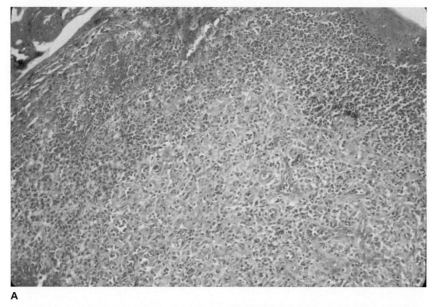

A

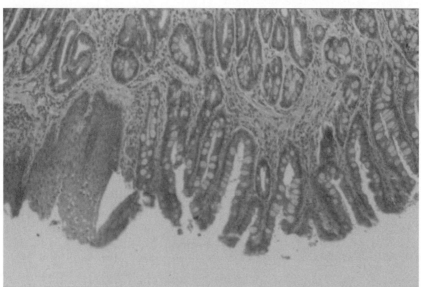

B

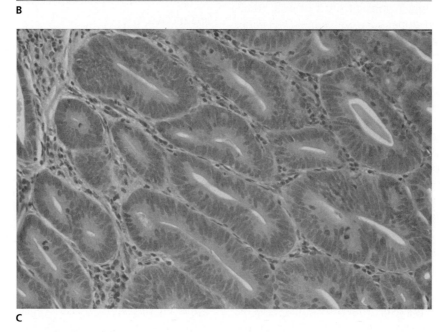

C

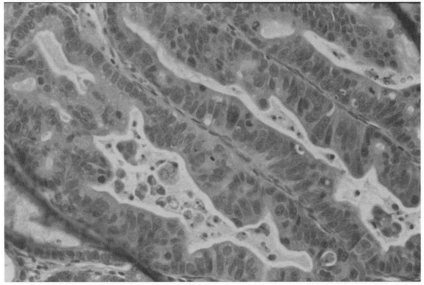

D

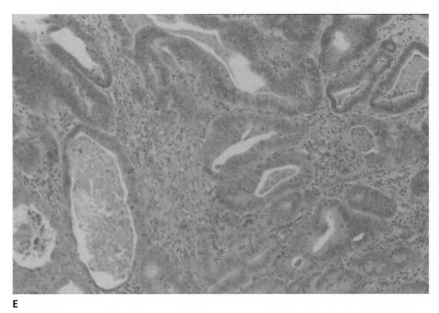

E

FIGURE 1.12. Progression of esophagitis to Barrett's esophagus to adenocarcinoma: (A) High-grade esophagitis is characterized by marked inflammation in the lamina propria and superficial mucosal ulceration. (B) Metaplasia of esophageal mucosa into Barrett's esophagus demonstrates formation of columnar, intestinal-type epithelium. (C) Low-grade dysplasia of Barrett's epithelium exhibits minor pseudostratification with elongated and crowded nuclei. (D) High-grade dysplasia shows more marked nuclear atypia, enlargement, and loss of polarity of cells. (E) Carcinoma in situ is characterized by glandular architectural changes and some necrosis. (Courtesy of Linda D. Ferrell, MD.)

and severity of esophagitis, the position of the gastro-esophageal junction, and whether or not metaplasia (also known as Barrett's epithelium) is present. Multiple biopsy samples are necessary to assess the severity of esophagitis microscopically, to confirm the presence of Barrett's epithelium, and to determine whether or not dysplasia is present. Esophageal manometry is usually necessary only if surgical correction of gastroesophageal reflux is being contemplated. It is prudent to establish preoperatively that esophageal motility and the "pump action" of the esophagus are normal before proceeding with antireflux procedures. Severe and disabling postoperative dysphagia can

result if a full Nissen procedure is performed in a patient with severe esophageal dysmotility.

MOTILITY DISORDERS OF THE ESOPHAGUS

Achalasia

Clinical Presentation

Patients with achalasia present with longstanding and progressive dysphagia. They may also complain of halitosis and regurgitation into the throat of sweet-tasting undigested food, in contrast to the sour taste associated with gastroesophageal reflux. Cases of acute esophageal obstruction are usually due to an ingested piece of meat. Over time, weight loss may occur. Pain is not a feature of classic achalasia. The occasional patient with so-called vigorous achalasia may experience substernal pain, but this condition is rare.

Diagnosis

The patient's medical history as described above is suggestive of achalasia. The physician's first goal is to exclude carcinoma. An upper GI series often shows a diffusely dilated esophagus with retained food and fluids. Typically, the lower end of the column of barium within the esophagus has a "beak-like" appearance, with little barium entering the stomach (see Figure 1.9). Upper GI endoscopy confirms esophageal dilatation and retention of food and fluid. Mucosal abnormality is absent. The lower end of the esophagus is contracted and provides a definite resistance to the passage of the endoscope. But suddenly, a characteristic "give" occurs and the endoscope enters the stomach. Even though no gross mucosal lesion might be visualized in the lower esophagus, it is prudent to take multiple biopsies to rule out carcinoma. Patients with achalasia have an incidence of esophageal cancer ten times higher than the general population.[2] The diagnosis of achalasia is most definitively established by esophageal manometry that demonstrates an aperistaltic esophageal body with feeble, uncoordinated contractions and failure of the LES to relax.

Treatment

Ordinary dilatation with bougies provides only transient benefit. Forceful dilatation with a balloon under fluoroscopy provides more prolonged relief, but it is associated with the complication of esophageal perforation in 1% to 10% of cases.[3] Injection of botulinum toxin into the LES provides only temporary relief. Botulinum toxin is believed to act by paralyzing the LES musculature by causing neurotoxicity.

Most patients eventually require modified Heller's myotomy, which is commonly performed either laparoscopically or thoracoscopically (Figure 1.13). It can also be performed by open surgery either via the thoracic or abdominal approach. Essential features of the operation include longitudinal division of the muscle over the distal 3 to 5 cm, pushing the muscle coat laterally for half the circumference of the esophagus, thus exposing the submucosal tube. Extension onto the stomach is limited to no more than a few millimeters, at which point the oblique sling fibers of the cardia are seen. Some surgeons routinely add an antireflux procedure, but this is rarely necessary unless a longer incision onto the stomach is made.

Diffuse Esophageal Spasm

Clinical Presentation

Dysphagia and chest pain are the usual presenting symptoms in patients with DES. The pain may or may not be associated with dysphagia, which usually develops over a long period of time. Any associated chest pain, which may be mild or severe with squeezing characteristics, must be distinguished from pain of cardiac origin. Regurgitation is not a typical symptom.

Diagnosis

Carcinoma (as the cause of dysphagia) and myocardial ischemia (as the cause of chest pain) must first be excluded with the appropriate tests—endoscopy, EKG, stress EKG, etc. Endoscopy is generally normal. Barium swallow, especially with cine-fluorography, might show tertiary waves, and in advanced cases, a "corkscrew esophagus" (see Figure 1.8). On occasion, an associated epiphrenic diverticulum may be demonstrated.

The diagnosis, however, is most definitively established by esophageal manometry, which shows that the distal esophagus contracts simultaneously without peristalsis. The contraction waves are usually strong and repetitive. The LES contracts normally during swallowing, although the LES pressure (LESP) may be higher than normal in many patients.

Treatment

Medical therapy with muscle relaxants may be attempted to relieve symptoms. Long-acting nitrate preparations

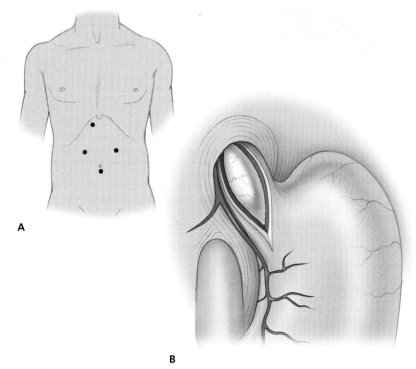

A

B

FIGURE 1.13. Heller's myotomy is performed to relieve achalasia. (A) The procedure is now commonly performed laparoscopically, using four ports in the abdomen and avoiding a large incision, although it can also be performed thorascopically. (B) The muscle layer in the contracted segment is divided longitudinally and separated to expose the submucosa for half the circumference of the esophagus.

(e.g., isosorbide dinitrate) and calcium-channel blockers (e.g., nifedipine) are said to produce symptomatic relief, but their efficacy has not been proven by prospective, controlled trials. Although bouginage is ineffective, pneumatic dilatation may be of temporary help in relieving dysphagia.

Selected patients with intractable severe symptoms may be candidates for surgical therapy. The procedure of choice is long esophageal myotomy, which is best performed thoracoscopically, thus avoiding thoracotomy. The length of the myotomy is determined based on the manometric findings, and it should extend above the level of muscular thickening. Myotomy should not include the LES. Esophagomyotomy is not always successful; in a larger clinical series, 80% to 90% of patients have benefited.[4]

Postoperative Complications

The most serious immediate postoperative complication is esophageal perforation, which nearly always requires immediate thoracotomy. Postoperative gastroesophageal reflux may be induced if the myotomy is carried into the LES. Symptoms recur or persist in 30% to 40% of patients.

ESOPHAGEAL DIVERTICULA

Two types of esophageal diverticuli are seen: traction and pulsion. Traction diverticuli are rarely, if ever, clinically

significant. Pulsion diverticuli, on the other hand, are often associated with motility disorders and are apt to cause clinical problems. Of these, two are important: Zenker's and epiphrenic diverticuli.

Zenker's Diverticulum

Clinical Presentation

Longstanding dysphagia in the upper esophagus is the primary symptom of Zenker's cricoesophageal diverticulum. The dysphagia may be progressive. Secondary symptoms include coughing or frank aspiration during swallowing and weight loss. An increased incidence of carcinoma is noted in patients with cricoesophageal diverticulum.

Diagnosis

An upper GI series demonstrates the presence of a Zenker's diverticulum with no or varying degrees of esophageal deviation (Figure 1.14). Endoscopy is best performed after barium studies to assess the degree of esophageal deviation. A flexible endoscope may be introduced into the esophagus past the mouth of the diverticulum. In some cases, however, intubation of the esophagus may be impossible. When manometry can be done successfully, the test findings demonstrate failure of the UES to relax in response to pharyngeal contraction. Often,

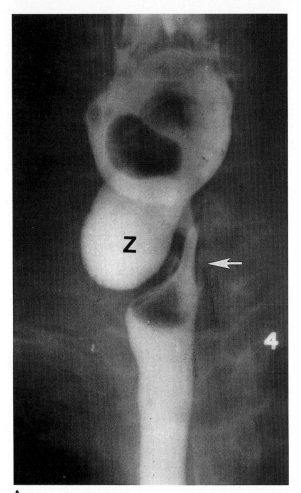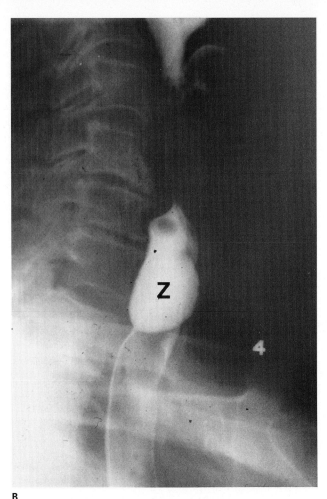

FIGURE 1.14. Zenker's diverticulum (Z), as demonstrated by upper an GI series, from both (A) anterior and (B) lateral views. The esophagus itself is slightly narrowed (arrow). The barium swallow test can further assess the degree of esophageal deviation and the feasibility of endoscopy. Endoscopic intubation of the esophagus may not be possible and, in fact, may be dangerous in some cases. (Courtesy of Henry I. Goldberg, MD.)

however, the manometric catheter cannot be passed into the UES and esophagus.

Treatment

Zenker's diverticula are treated surgically, using a left cervical approach. Because failure of the UES to relax is considered the underlying cause, an important goal of surgery is cricopharyngeal myotomy. If the diverticulum is small (<2 cm), resection may be unnecessary. Larger diverticula (2–4 cm) may be suspended upside-down through sutures to the retropharyngeal fascia after the myotomy. Diverticula larger than 4 cm are best excised using a stapler following myotomy.

Epiphrenic Diverticulum

Clinical Presentation

The most common presentation of epiphrenic diverticulum (Figure 1.15) is dysphagia in the lower esophagus.

Approximately 40% of patients have associated esophageal motility abnormality, most commonly DES. When DES is present, there may also be chest pain.

Diagnosis

The diverticulum is demonstrated by barium swallow studies. Endoscopy is necessary to rule out carcinoma. Esophageal manometry is essential when surgical resection is being considered to define any associated motility disorder. Performance of diverticulectomy without treating the associated DES may not only fail to relieve symptoms, but may also result in postoperative dehiscence of esophageal closure.

Treatment

Surgical treatment is reserved for patients with severe symptoms. The operation includes diverticulectomy and a procedure to treat the underlying motility disorder, either

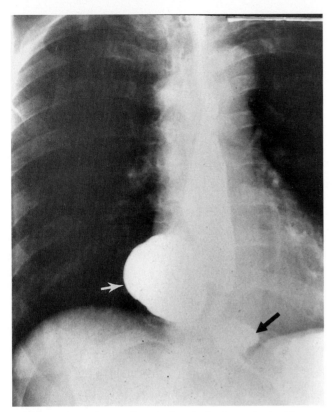

FIGURE 1.15. Epiphrenic diverticulum is demonstrated with barium swallow studies. The epiphrenic diverticulum in this patient (white arrow) projects to the right and is located just above a small hiatal hernia (black arrow). (Courtesy of Henry I. Goldberg, MD.)

long esophagomyotomy for DES or myotomy of the LES for achalasia. The operations may be done thoracoscopically or via thoracotomy.

HIATAL HERNIA

The two types of hiatal hernia are paraesophageal hernia and sliding hiatal hernia. Occasionally, the two types may coexist (Figure 1.16). Paraesophageal hernia is rare but, when present, causes mechanical problems of incarceration. Sliding hiatal hernia, on the other hand, is very common and becomes clinically significant only when associated with gastroesophageal reflux.

Paraesophageal Hernia

Anatomic Characteristics

In paraesophageal hernia, part or all of the stomach herniates into the chest through a defect in the hiatus, most commonly to the left of the gastroesophageal (GE) junction (Figure 1.17). Because a sac develops, this is a true hernia. The GE junction remains in its normal position in the abdomen, and its physiology is undisturbed. Hence, gastroesophageal reflux is not a common feature of classic

paraesophageal herniation. When the whole stomach herniates into the chest, the condition is sometimes referred to as an "upside-down stomach."

Pathophysiology

The symptoms of paraesophageal hernia are caused by the mechanical presence of the stomach in the chest. Severity of symptoms depends on whether or not the herniated stomach is obstructed. Intermittent mechanical obstruction of the neck of the herniated stomach may lead to venous congestion and chronic occult bleeding or even to moderate acute upper gastrointestinal bleeding. In extreme cases, arterial inflow is compromised, and the herniated segment may undergo necrosis and perforation with subsequent mediastinitis.

Clinical Features

Most patients present with symptoms after the fifth or sixth decade of life. Early symptoms include a sense of pressure in the lower chest and gaseous eructations. Chronic symptoms, such as chest pain and dysphagia, may intermittently become more acute as transient incarceration of the herniated segment occurs. As mentioned above, either chronic or acute bleeding may occur. The most serious complication is obstruction and strangulation, leading to acute emergency presentation. Strangulation may lead to perforation and severe sepsis.

Diagnosis

The diagnosis of paraesophageal hernia is established by barium study of the upper GI tract, which shows herniation of part or all of the stomach into the chest, while the GE junction remains in its normal abdominal location. Endoscopy shows a normal esophagus; the herniated pouch may be visible when the endoscope is retroflexed within the stomach. Rarely will paraesophageal and sliding hiatal hernia coexist, in which case gastroesophageal reflux may also be present.

Treatment

All symptomatic and most asymptomatic cases are best treated surgically to prevent complications. The operation can be done laparoscopically or through laparotomy. The hernia is reduced and the hiatal defect closed snugly around the esophagus. The herniated stomach is fixed in the abdomen by gastropexy. Some surgeons advocate the use of tube gastrostomy to further fix the stomach. This latter procedure may be more useful in the upside-down stomach, where the greater curvature has a tendency to roll back up into the chest. Other surgeons perform Nissen fundoplication in the belief that the procedure prevents reherniation.

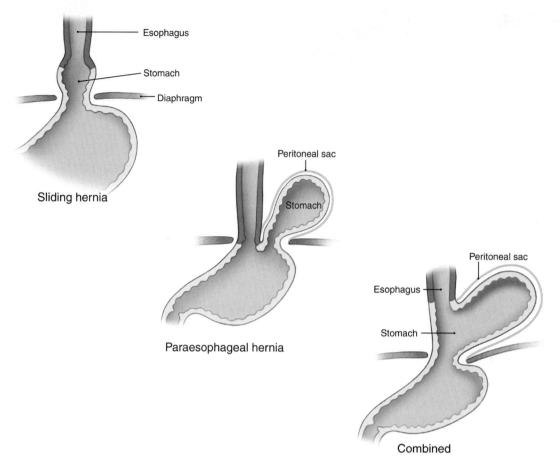

Esophagus

Stomach

Diaphragm

Sliding hernia

Peritoneal sac

Stomach

Paraesophageal hernia

Peritoneal sac

Esophagus

Stomach

Combined

FIGURE 1.16. Three types of hiatal hernia are seen, including sliding hernia, paraesophageal hernia, and a combination of the two.

Sliding Hiatal Hernia and Reflux Esophagitis

Clinical Presentation

The presence of a sliding hiatal hernia *per se* does not cause symptoms. Symptoms are caused when LES function is defective, and gastric contents reflux into the esophagus. Healthy individuals have "physiologic reflux" several times a day, but because the esophagus is able to clear the refluxate quickly, no symptoms develop. Prolonged irritation of esophageal mucosa from reflux of acid, pepsin, and bile acids in patients with defective LES causes symptoms of heartburn (i.e., retrosternal burning pain). Reflux is most prominent on recumbency and following the ingestion of large meals, particularly meals with a high-fat content. Many patients identify ingestion of onions as an inciting factor. Nighttime reflux can lead to aspiration, causing chronic cough, recurrent pneumonia, or asthma-like symptoms.

In advanced gastroesophageal reflux disease (GERD), dysphagia may develop as a symptom. Dysphagia is caused by inflammatory edema early on but often heralds benign stricture formation. Chronic acid reflux, as discussed earlier, may cause metaplasia of the esophageal squamous cell lining into columnar-type mucosa, which can subsequently undergo malignant degeneration. Thus, not all dysphagia in patients with known GERD is the result of benign stricture formation. Additionally, carcinoma must be ruled out (Table 1.5).

Diagnosis

Diagnostic strategies are aimed at assessing the degree of esophagitis, determining the presence or absence of Barrett's mucosa, and proving that the symptoms are due to gastroesophageal reflux. The methods for evaluating sliding hiatal hernia and reflux esophagitis are many, including barium swallow, upper GI endoscopy, esophageal manometry, 24-h pH monitoring, and scintigraphic assessment.

BARIUM SWALLOW The barium swallow test provides evidence of a sliding hiatal hernia and gastroesophageal reflux but is incapable of evaluating esophagitis until the late stages, as shown in Figure 1.11.

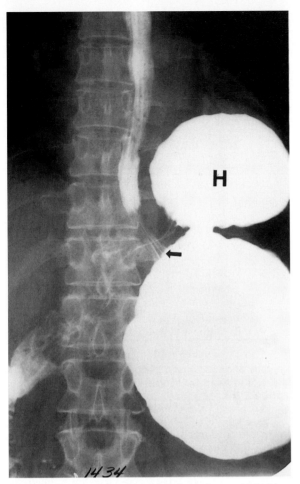

FIGURE 1.17. Paraesophageal hernia is best demonstrated by barium study of the upper GI tract, which shows herniation of all or part of the stomach into the chest through a defect in the hiatus. As in this patient, the herniation (H) is usually to the left of the gastroesophageal junction, which maintains its normal position below the diaphragm (arrow). (Courtesy of Henry I. Goldberg, MD.)

UPPER GI ENDOSCOPY Upper GI endoscopy is the best way to determine the presence of esophagitis and Barrett's mucosa and to evaluate the severity of the esophagitis. Multiple biopsy samples are required for adequate assessment.

ESOPHAGEAL MANOMETRY Manometry is a useful technique to detect hypotensive LES (i.e., <15 mm Hg); abnormal motility in the body of the esophagus; and abnormal UES function, which has been described in patients with respiratory complications of gastroesophageal reflux. Manometry is a vital preoperative investigation because it may identify coexisting motility disorders that rule out the use of unmodified Nissen fundoplication.

TWENTY-FOUR-HOUR pH MONITORING Twenty-four-hour pH monitoring is of paramount importance to determine the extent of acid reflux, to measure the ability of the esophagus to clear acid reflux, and most importantly, to correlate episodes of acid reflux with the patient's symptoms (Figure 1.18). This test records the percentage of time within a 24-h period when esophageal pH registers below 4 and correlates it with the extent of both reflux episodes and the presence of complications of esophagitis. In normal subjects, esophageal pH is below 4 about 2% of the time. This incidence increases to 8% in patients with uncomplicated GERD, to 12% in those with GERD and esophagitis, to 15% in those with GERD and stricture, and to almost 30% in those with GERD and Barrett's mucosa.[5]

SCINTIGRAPHIC ASSESSMENT Scintigraphic assessment of gastroesophageal reflux has the added value of assessing not only gastroesophageal reflux but also gastric emptying. It is useful only in selected patients.

Treatment

NONSURGICAL THERAPY Most patients with early symptoms of esophagitis can be managed effectively with medical therapy and other measures designed to minimize reflux, reduce production of gastric acid, neutralize acid in the esophagus, provide a mucosal barrier, or improve gastric emptying. Medical therapy must be well planned and is most effective if administered under the supervision of a gastroenterologist.

Minimizing Reflux Key strategies to minimize reflux include reduction of abdominal pressure by weight loss and avoidance of abdominal compression by articles of clothing. Other methods include elevating the head of the bed 6 in on blocks; avoiding large meals; taking evening meals at least 4 h before bedtime; avoiding fatty foods, which are potent releasers of CCK; and avoiding smoking because nicotine reduces LESP.

Reducing Acid Acid secretion can be effectively suppressed with histamine H_2-receptor antagonists or proton-pump inhibitors. Proton-pump inhibitors have

TABLE 1.5. Essentials: Consequences of Severe Gastrointestinal Reflux Disease (GERD)
Injurious refluxate
▪ Acid and pepsin
▪ Bile and pancreatic juice
▪ *Succus entericus*
Pathophysiologic responses
▪ Pain without inflammation
▪ Inflammation
Low-grade esophagitis
High-grade esophagitis
Stricture formation
▪ Metaplastic/dysplastic response
Columnar metaplasia (e.g., Barrett's mucosa)
Dysplasia
Adenocarcinoma in situ
Adenocarcinoma

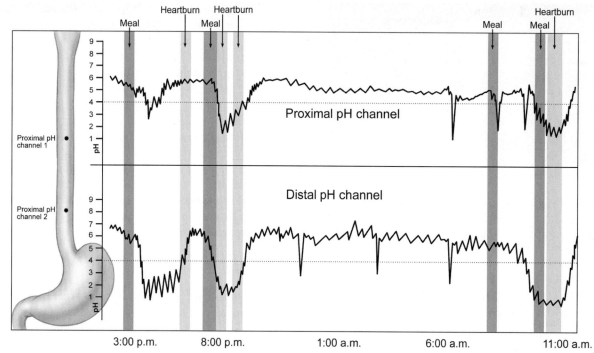

FIGURE 1.18. Monitoring esophageal pH measures the percentage of time during a 24-h period when the pH is outside the normal range and can be used to evaluate acid reflux incidents and correlate them with the patient's symptoms. (Courtesy of Marco G. Patti, MD.)

two advantages over H_2-receptor antagonists. First, they more effectively suppress acid secretion, often causing achlorhydria after several days of treatment. Second, theoretically, achlorhydria improves LES function by preventing gastric acidification, which reduces LESP; and by leading to hypergastrinemia, which enhances LESP. Omeprazole (20–40 mg/day) has become the drug of choice and can be administered for 6 to 8 weeks at a time.

Neutralizing Acid Neutralizing acid within the esophagus and stomach may be accomplished with antacids, which provide effective and cheap symptomatic therapy in most patients early in the disease. After an initial rigorous antacid therapy for some 12 weeks, patients can safely carry out self-medication with these drugs. Antacids containing calcium have the theoretical advantage of being potent releasers of gastrin, which increases LESP.

Providing Barrier Protection Sucralfate and alginic acid in combination with antacids are said to provide a barrier to the esophageal mucosa against the action of acid and other irritants in the refluxate.

Improving Gastric Emptying Metoclopramide, cisapride, and domperidone have been used because of their action to improve gastric emptying and LESP. The value of this therapy in severe disease is questionable.

INDICATIONS FOR SURGICAL THERAPY The essentials of surgical treatment of gastroesophageal reflux disease are given in Table 1.6.

Nonresponsiveness to Medical Therapy If a well-planned and administered program of medical therapy fails, usually after several months or years of therapy, both patient and physician may agree that more needs to be done. DeMeester et al. believe that a defective LES is the most important factor predicting failure of medical therapy.[6] They argue that antireflux surgery should be considered in the presence of a defective LES—irrespective of the presence or degree of esophagitis—providing that 24-h pH monitoring studies have proven that the symptoms are due to reflux. This recommendation is increasingly being put into practice as minimally invasive surgery has become the preferred surgical approach.

Severe Endoscopic Esophagitis A patient with severe endoscopic esophagitis, poorly controlled symptoms, and a structurally defective LES is a candidate for surgery.

Esophageal Stricture Esophageal strictures must be dilated by bougies. Malignancy in strictures must be excluded by endoscopy and biopsy. Although this condition can be successfully managed nonsurgically following stricture dilatation, the development of strictures often indicates severe disease that is best managed surgically. Strictures must be dilated adequately before antireflux surgery is done. Because of to the excellence of medical therapy, nondilatable strictures are now rare. When they do occur, strictures must be resected and an antireflux procedure or jejunal interposition performed.

Barrett's Esophagus The presence of Barrett's metaplasia, or Barrett's esophagus, indicates severe disease and

TABLE 1.6. Essentials: Surgical Treatment of Gastroesophageal Reflux Disease (GERD)

Indications
- Symptomatic failure of medical therapy
- Severe endoscopic esophagitis
- Esophageal stricture (following dilatation)
- Barrett's esophagus to arrest progression to cancer

Preoperative work-up
- Endoscopy and biopsy
- Motility studies to assess LESP and rule out associated motor disorder
- 24-h pH monitoring to ensure symptoms are caused by reflux

Principles of surgical treatment
- Reduce hernia into abdomen
- Restore LESP by fundoplication
- Narrow hiatus by crural approximation
- Anchor wrap to preaortic fascia (optional)

Surgical procedures
- Most now performed laparoscopically
- Nissen fundoplication most popular (complete wrap, 2–5 cm long)
- Toupet fundoplication (270° posterior wrap)
- Short esophagus: Collis-Nissen repair

Outcome
- Operative mortality 0.2%–0.3%
- Complication rate 3%–10%
- Long-term symptom relief in 90%–95%

Abbreviation: LESP, lower esophageal sphincter pressure.

TABLE 1.7. Objectives of Surgical Therapy for Hiatal Hernia and Gastroesophageal Reflux Disease (GERD)

- Restore gastroesophageal continence.
- Reduce the hiatal hernia and create a 5- to 6-cm length of abdominal esophagus.
- Improve LESP by wrapping the gastric fundus around the distal 2–3 cm of the esophagus, either totally or partially.
- Narrow the hiatus by approximating the crura.
- Anchor the wrap within the abdomen by suturing it to the preaortic fascia or crura, if this can be done expeditiously.
- Avoid damage to the vagus nerves, which not only regulate LES function but are critical for preservation of normal gastric emptying.

often tips the balance in favor of surgery. Antireflux surgery has not been shown to reverse Barrett's metaplasia, but it might arrest progression of the disease. Evidence is accumulating that the risk of progression to cancer may be reduced. Of course, if severe dysplasia or carcinoma in situ is present, esophageal resection is necessary.

SURGICAL PROCEDURES Some form of simple antireflux procedure is applicable to the patients just described, except the few with short esophagus and those with undilatable fixed stricture. The goals of surgery for patients with hiatal hernia and gastroesophageal reflux disease, also just described, are summarized in Table 1.7.

Nissen Fundoplication Nissen fundoplication (Figure 1.19), the most common antireflux procedure, can be

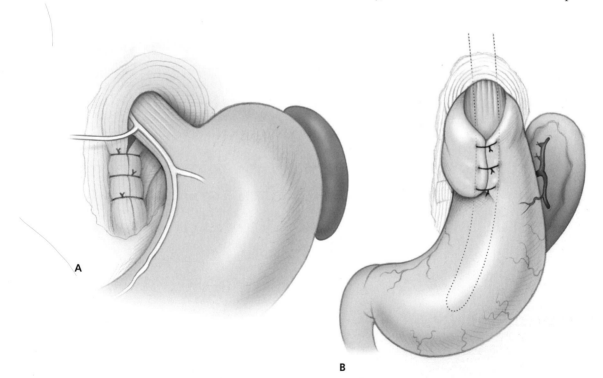

FIGURE 1.19. Nissen fundoplication is commonly performed to treat gastroesophageal reflux. (A) The esophagus is mobilized, the hiatal hernia reduced, and the crura approximated. (B) The gastric fundus is then mobilized and wrapped around the distal esophagus to augment the sphincteric function. The procedure is most commonly performed laparoscopically. The dotted line represents the bougie that has been introduced by mouth and passed into the stomach. It serves to prevent the wrap from being too tight.

performed laparoscopically or open by the abdominal or thoracic route. After esophageal mobilization with careful identification and preservation of the vagi, the hiatus is dissected and the crura identified. The surgeon then reduces the hiatal hernia and places, but leaves untied two to four large sutures to approximate the crura. The surgeon then mobilizes the gastric fundus by dividing several short gastric vessels between ligatures taking care not to injure the spleen. The surgeon next takes the fundus behind the esophagus to the right side and then wraps it around the distal 2 to 3 cm of the esophagus with sutures that incorporate the anterior fundus, part of the anterior esophageal wall, and the posterior fundus. Usually, two or three sutures are needed, placed 1 cm apart, with the distal-most suture

at the gastroesophageal junction. Before any sutures are tied, an assistant passes a 60 F bougie from the mouth into the stomach. The crural sutures are tied first, then the fundoplication sutures. The wrap should be loose and the hiatus not too tight.

The identical procedure can be done either open or laparoscopically. It has been previously thought that the wrap should be 3 to 5 cm. A current tendency is to limit the wrap to 1 to 2 cm, especially with laparoscopic fundoplication. Long-term outcome studies are needed to determine the optimal length of the wrap.

Nissen fundoplication can also be performed thoracically in special circumstances in which the abdominal approach is difficult or unsuitable.

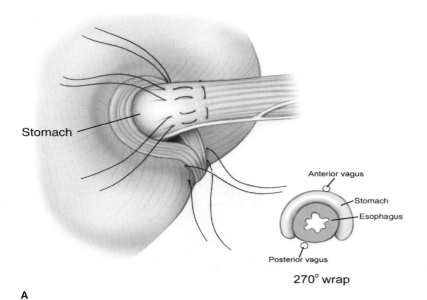

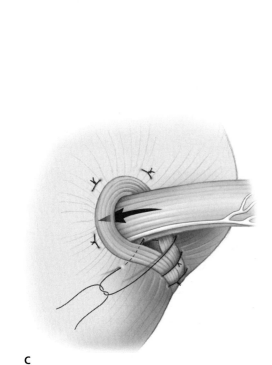

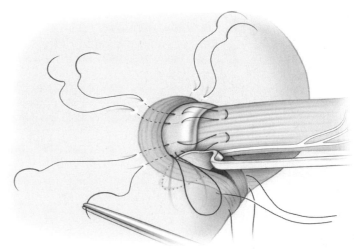

FIGURE 1.20. The Belsey Mark IV procedure, performed thoracically, accomplishes a 270° fundic wrap of the distal esophagus, (A) using "ink-welling" sutures, (B) reduction of the wrap below the diaphragm, and (C) narrowing of the hiatus. (Adapted from Jamieson GG, Debas HT, eds. Rob & Smith's Operative Surgery: Surgery of the Upper Gastrointestinal Tract. London: Chapman & Hall Medical; 1994.)

Belsey Mark IV   The Belsey Mark IV procedure is done thoracically (Figure 1.20) and involves a 270° wrap of the esophagus by the gastric fundus.

Hill Repair   An abdominal operation, the Hill repair (Figure 1.21) accomplishes a 90° anterior wrap of the esophagus by the stomach and anchors the wrap to the preaortic fascia.

Toupet Fundoplication   Also a partial fundoplication, Toupet fundoplication is usually performed laparoscopically, involving a 270° posterior wrap of the esophagus.

CHOICE OF SURGICAL PROCEDURE   The most popular operation and the one for which outcome data are most complete, the Nissen fundoplication, which accomplishes a 360° wrap of the esophagus, is contraindicated in patients in whom propulsive motility in the body of the esophagus is diminished or absent. Such patients may have an associated motility disorder such as achalasia or scleroderma. When the "pump action" of the body of the esophagus is lacking, Nissen fundoplication may result in obstruction that cannot be overcome by esophageal peristalsis. Significant postoperative dysphagia ensues. The major argument for performing preoperative esophageal manometry is to identify these patients. When identified, they are best treated by one of the procedures that accomplish a partial wrap (e.g., Belsey Mark IV, or Toupet).

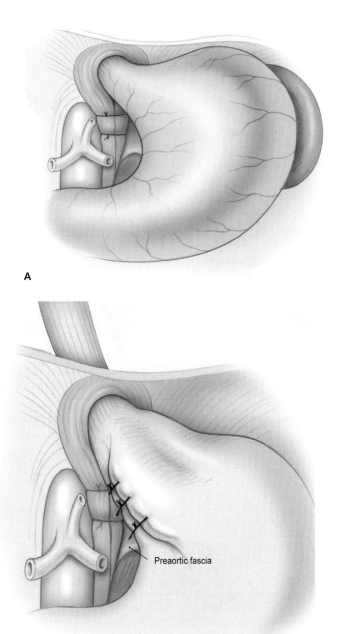

A

C

Preaortic fascia

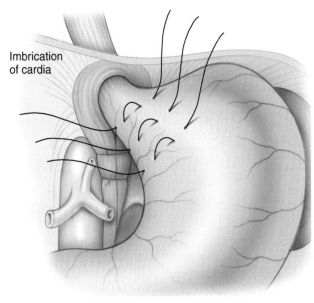

Imbrication of cardia

B

FIGURE 1.21. The Hill repair is performed abdominally and involves (A) approximation of the crura, (B) a 90° wrap of the esophagus at the anteromedial cardia, and (C) suturing the wrap to the preaortic fascia.

Long-Term Outcome of Surgical Therapy In most reported series, Nissen fundoplication results in a doubling of the resting LESP from about 10 mm Hg to more than 20 mm Hg. Similarly, symptomatic relief is accomplished in about 90% of patients. Persistent post-operative dysphagia occurs in 5% to 10% of patients. The incidence of postoperative dysphagia can be reduced by performing preoperative manometry and avoiding the Nissen procedure in patients with abnormal esophageal motility. The incidence of dysphagia is also reduced when the length of total wrap is less than 3 cm.

In patients with Barrett's esophagus, good-to-excellent symptomatic response is 80% to 90% following surgery, but postoperative regression of metaplasia is uncommon.

Increasing evidence, however, supports that progression to dysplasia and malignant degeneration is reduced after surgical correction of reflux. Nevertheless, all patients with Barrett's esophagus should undergo annual endoscopic surveillance.

Sliding Hiatal Hernia with Short Esophagus

Despite arguments to the contrary, the number of patients who have short esophagus because of GERD is low. In these patients, the surgical procedure of choice is the Collis-Nissen procedure (Figure 1.22). Performed thoracically, this operation lengthens the esophagus; a "neoesophagus" length of stomach is created by stapling

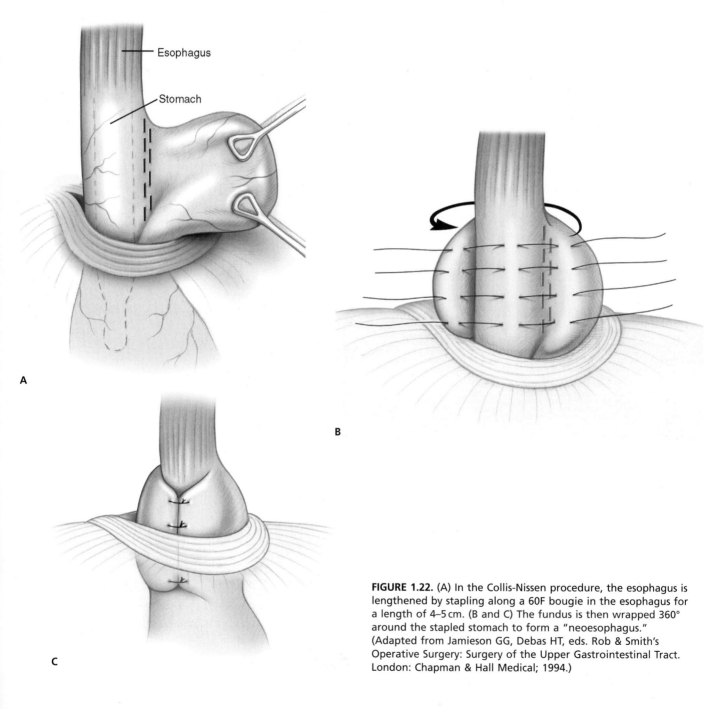

FIGURE 1.22. (A) In the Collis-Nissen procedure, the esophagus is lengthened by stapling along a 60F bougie in the esophagus for a length of 4–5 cm. (B and C) The fundus is then wrapped 360° around the stapled stomach to form a "neoesophagus." (Adapted from Jamieson GG, Debas HT, eds. Rob & Smith's Operative Surgery: Surgery of the Upper Gastrointestinal Tract. London: Chapman & Hall Medical; 1994.)

down (with or without cutting) 4 to 5 cm from the gastroesophageal junction distally, along a 60 F bougie within the lumen. The gastric fundus is then wrapped 360° around the "neoesophagus." Although the number of patients in individual reports is understandably small, the operation is reported to have an 80% success rate in relieving symptoms.

PERFORATED ESOPHAGUS

Early recognition and immediate operation are keys to the successful outcome in patients with esophageal perforation. Primary repair and drainage as well as provision of a route for early nutrition are important in early perforation. The nonoperative approach has a limited place in the management of this problem. Esophageal perforations seen late may be managed in a variety of ways from drainage alone, to closure with muscle flaps, to esophageal exclusion. In the few patients with underlying severe motility disorder or benign stricture, total esophagectomy with immediate esophagogastrostomy in the neck or delayed reconstruction may be necessary.

Clinical Presentation

Esophageal perforation can be caused iatrogenically, traumatically, and/or spontaneously by ingestion of a foreign body or by tumor (Table 1.8). It is associated with intense periesophageal inflammatory response and cytokine release.

The site of perforation determines the evolution of the clinical picture. For example, cervical perforation is associated with local pain, and the systemic response is slow to develop. Subcutaneous emphysema may be detectable clinically and/or radiologically. On the other hand, perforation of the thoracic esophagus is likely to present with

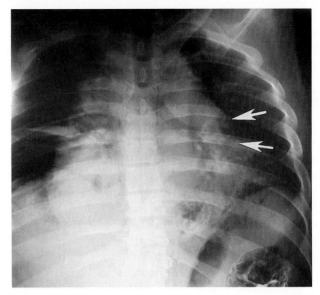

FIGURE 1.23. Esophageal perforation is best diagnosed radiologically. Chest x-ray often demonstrates a left pleural effusion; mediastinal widening (arrows); or free mediastinal air, which is manifest as dark vertical streaks overlying the left side of the heart. (Courtesy of Henry I. Goldberg, MD.)

more florid symptoms and signs. Chest pain, dysphagia, and fever develop early, and a most characteristic finding is tachycardia out of proportion to other systemic signs. Auscultation of the chest may reveal a crunching precordial sound (Hamman's sign), pathognomonic of free air in the mediastinum. The inflammatory response spreads rapidly from the site of perforation to cause spreading mediastinitis. Untreated, mediastinitis can lead to septic shock and associated multiorgan failure. By contrast, intraabdominal esophageal perforation causes generalized peritonitis akin to that following perforated peptic ulcer. Although presentation of esophageal perforation is sometimes obvious, diagnosis often necessitates a high index of suspicion.

Diagnosis

The diagnosis of perforated esophagus is best confirmed radiologically. Endoscopy plays only a secondary role when perforation is suspected but cannot be documented radiologically.

RADIOLOGICAL TESTING Chest radiography frequently shows a left pleural effusion, mediastinal widening, or free mediastinal air (Figure 1.23). The presence of perforation can be established by oral administration of Gastrografin. If a leak is not detected, the barium swallow test or endoscopy may be required. When perforation is suspected but no leak has been demonstrated radiologically, a follow-up computerized tomography (CT) scan may be helpful.

TABLE 1.8. Causes, Incidence, and Sites of Esophageal Perforation

Iatrogenic (54%)
- Instrumentation (44%)
- Intraoperative (8%)
- Radiation, sclerotherapy, and other therapies (2%)

Traumatic (19%)
- Penetrating
- Blunt
- Ingestion of caustic substance

Spontaneous, also known as Boerhaave syndrome (16%)

Ingestion of foreign body (7%)

Tumor (4%)

Site of perforation
- Thoracic (54%)
- Cervical (40%)
- Abdominal (6%)

ENDOSCOPY Endoscopic examination is used only when perforation is suspected and radiologic studies have failed to demonstrate it. Endoscopy must be performed carefully to avoid exacerbation of the perforation.

Management

PRINCIPLES OF MANAGEMENT The essential management principles of esophageal perforation are summarized in Table 1.9. Successful treatment depends on prompt diagnosis and immediate operation. Delays in diagnosis only increase the mortality. In all cases, broad-spectrum antibiotics should be administered immediately. The site of perforation can be identified by Gastrografin swallow, which facilitates selection of the proper incision: either thoracotomy (left or right), cervical incision, or laparotomy. Early perforations are closed in two layers after excising any devitalized tissue, and the closure is reinforced with adjacent tissue (i.e., pleural flap, omentum, or stomach). Adequate suction drainage is instituted. A decision must be made about the route for providing nutrition (i.e., either parenterally or enterally). Enteral nutrition is best provided via a feeding jejunostomy. When the jejunostomy is constructed, a gastrostomy tube should also be provided to obviate the need for nasogastric suction. The gastrostomy tube should be used for gastric decompression and not for feeding.

TABLE 1.9. Essentials: Management of Esophageal Perforation

Diagnosis
- Clinical: Chest pain, fever, tachycardia
- "Hamman's sign": Air in mediastinum

Radiologic
- Chest x-ray: (L) Pleural effusion, free mediastinal air, mediastinal widening
- Gastrografin swallow: Identifies leak
- Endoscopy: Only if suspected but not shown by Gastrografin or barium swallow

Principles of management

Early perforation
- Prompt diagnosis
- Institution of IV antibiotic therapy
- Early operation to close perforation with reinforcement (pleura, omentum, stomach) and establish adequate drainage
- Establish enteral or parenteral nutrition

Late perforation
- Individualized treatment
- Options: Simple drainage, transesophageal drainage, closure with muscle flap, esophageal exclusion

Nonsurgical management (rare)
- Small, contained perforation; drains well into esophagus; minimal symptoms; no sepsis

Role of esophageal resection
- Perforation in presence of severe, underlying motility disorder (e.g., achalasia)
- Proximity of perforation to severe benign stricture, or malignancy

---

NONSURGICAL MANAGEMENT Most esophageal perforations should be treated operatively; therefore, nonoperative management is only rarely employed. The conditions that must be present to undertake the nonoperative form of treatment include: (1) a perforation well contained within the mediastinum; (2) the cavity drains well back into the esophagus; (3) minimal symptomatology; and, (4) presence of no or minimal sepsis. Nonoperative treatment is appropriate only in tears caused by endoscopy or foreign bodies.

LATE ESOPHAGEAL PERFORATION There is little controversy about the approach to treatment of early perforation. Surgical management of late perforations, however, is complex and subject to considerable variation. Several options exist, including drainage only, transesophageal drainage by interventional radiology and irrigation, closure with muscle flap, and esophageal exclusion. Selecting the appropriate technique depends on the location of the perforation, the age and condition of the patient, the age of the perforation, and the degree of mediastinal sepsis and necrosis.

Drainage Only In patients who present several days after the perforation has occurred, closure is no longer an option. An immediate strategy is to perform pleural drainage through a chest tube, with adequate decompression of the stomach and nasoesophageal suction proximal to the perforation. This allows the patient to be transferred to a tertiary care center for further management. An early strategy for enteral or parenteral nutrition must be developed.

Transesophageal Drainage by Interventional Radiology On occasion, the periesophageal abscess may be drained by a tube placed into the abscess cavity through the mouth and esophagus. A chest tube may also be placed into the cavity. With time, an irrigation system can be established. A gastrostomy tube and a feeding jejunostomy can also be placed percutaneously.

Closure with Muscle Flap In patients with late perforation and established mediastinitis with or without tissue necrosis, extensive drainage and closure of the perforation may be accomplished with vascularized muscle flap. A rhomboid flap is used to close perforations in the upper third of the esophagus, while a serratus or latissimus dorsi flap is used in the mid- or lower third. Perforations in the distal esophagus may be closed by gastric fundus wrap, much as is done in the Nissen procedure.

Esophageal Exclusion In patients whose diagnosis was delayed or who are too sick for thoracotomy, esophageal exclusion is the treatment of choice. This procedure is also used for patients in whom a previous attempt at closure has failed or in whom sepsis is not controlled by drainage. The esophagus is divided in the neck, the proximal end is exte-

26 .... ESOPHAGUS

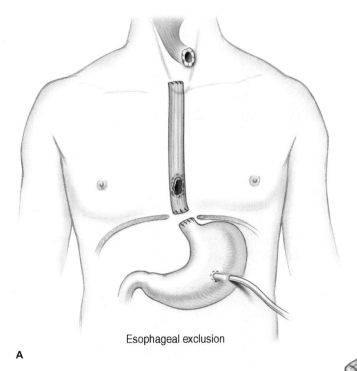

Esophageal exclusion

A

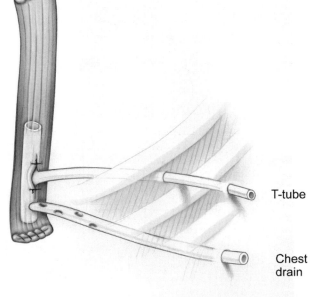

T-tube

Chest
drain

B

FIGURE 1.24. Esophageal exclusion is performed to isolate the perforated esophagus in selected patients. (A) Cervical esophagostomy and stapled division of the gastroesophageal junction are performed and a gastrostomy tube is inserted. (B) The perforation is approximated over a T-tube and the chest drained. (Adapted from Sabiston DC, ed. Textbook of Surgery: The Biological Basis of Modern Surgical Practice. Philadelphia: WB Saunders; 1997.)

riorized to create an esophagostomy, and the distal end is closed (Figure 1.24). A laparotomy or laparoscopy is then performed, and the gastroesophageal junction is stapled closed. A gastrostomy and feeding jejunostomy is also provided. Adequate tube drainage of the chest is accomplished. If the patient survives the procedure, esophageal reconstruction will be necessary many months later. This may require esophageal resection and esophagogastric reconstruction in the neck or colon interposition.

ROLE OF RESECTION Certain circumstances dictate that it is best to resect the perforated esophagus. Indications for resection include the presence of a severe underlying motility disorder such as achalasia or scleroderma, or proximity of the perforation to a severe benign stricture of the esophagus. Under these conditions, the preferred management strategy is to perform a total esophagectomy with either immediate esophagogastrostomy in the neck or delayed reconstruction.

Early perforation in the distal esophagus due to pneumatic dilatation can be safely managed by surgical closure and concomitant Heller's myotomy without resection.

CARCINOMA OF THE ESOPHAGUS

Incidence

The incidence of squamous cell carcinoma in the United States and Western Europe is about 20 per 100,000.[7] The incidence is higher among smokers, persons addicted to alcohol, and black men. The disease occurs with eight times this frequency in the Henan province of China and in the Transkei province of South Africa and is 20 to 30 times as high in some districts of Kazakhstan.[7] Nitrosamine compounds, fungal contamination of food, and deficiencies of zinc and molybdenum have been cited as possible explanations for the high frequency.

The incidence of adenocarcinoma of the esophagus in the West has increased steeply in recent years (Figure 1.25). In some areas, adenocarcinoma approaches or exceeds the incidence of squamous cell carcinoma. While the steep rise in the incidence of adenocarcinoma in the West has not been explained, GERD and its consequences and therapy may provide partial explanation.

Pathology

Premalignant conditions for squamous cell carcinoma (Figure 1.26) include achalasia, chronic iron deficiency, and congenital tylosis of the esophagus. The most important premalignant condition for adenocarcinoma is Barrett's epithelium, which is metaplastic columnar epithelium that results from chronic gastroesophageal reflux. About 10% of patients with GERD have Barrett's esophagus. Patients with Barrett's esophagus are 40 times more at risk to develop adenocarcinoma than those without Barrett's.

Preoperative staging of esophageal cancer has been made possible by endoscopic ultrasound, which can detect with 80% accuracy the presence of transmural invasion and periesophageal lymphadenopathy. Ultrasonographic evidence of wall penetration has been used to develop the WNM classification, which some prefer to the TNM classification. Five-year survival is well correlated to the stage of the disease (Table 1.10).[8]

Clinical Presentation

The level at which food seems to stick in the patient's esophagus usually indicates the location of the lesion. Weakness, weight loss, and iron deficiency anemia are frequently present. Late symptoms include regurgitation and aspiration, which indicate obstruction; chest pain, which indicates invasion of structures outside the esophagus; and coughing during swallowing, which might indicate the presence of a tracheoesophageal fistula.

Diagnosis

ENDOSCOPY AND BIOPSY Flexible endoscopy visualizes the lesion and facilitates evaluation of its luminal and circumferential extension as well as the degree of obstruction the lesion causes. The extent of transmural invasion, however, is poorly evaluated. The presence or absence of Barrett's esophagus should be assessed carefully. Multiple biopsies must be obtained from the lesion and adjacent or suspicious mucosa.

ENDOSCOPIC ULTRASOUND Endoscopic ultrasound is a useful guide to staging the lesion, as discussed earlier. It assesses the degree of extension of the tumor within the wall of the esophagus and to adjacent tissue outside. The presence or absence of lymphadenopathy is also indicated.

BARIUM SWALLOW Useful in indicating the extent of the lesion, the barium swallow test (Figure 1.27) can also provide the extent of any luminal narrowing and any angulation of the axis of the esophagus.

COMPUTERIZED TOMOGRAPHIC SCAN OF CHEST AND ABDOMEN CT scan of the chest and abdomen can be used to assess pulmonary metastases, extension of the tumor into adjacent structures, and presence or absence of any liver metastases. CT scan cannot accurately diagnose mediastinal and celiac lymphadenopathy.

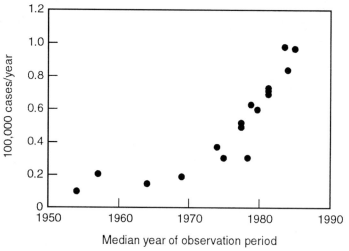

FIGURE 1.25. The increasing incidence of adenocarcinoma of the esophagus as determined by several studies of United States and European populations. The increase in the West is unexplained, but may be due to GERD, its consequences and its therapy. (Reprinted with permission from Pera M, Cameron AJ, Trastek VF, et al. Gastroenterology 1993;104:510–513.)

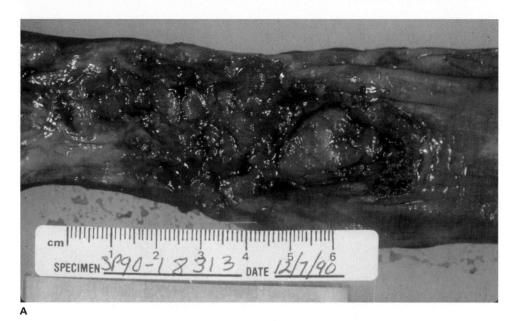

A

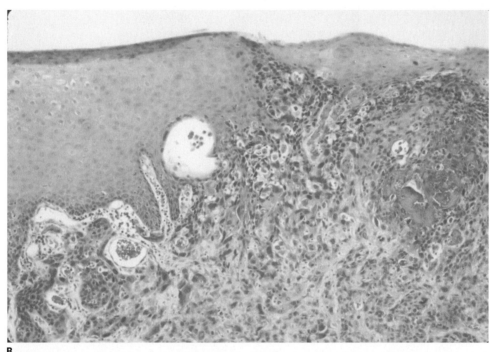

B

FIGURE 1.26. (A) Gross appearance of squamous cell carcinoma in the mid-esophagus, (B) manifest microscopically as poorly differentiated carcinoma invading the submucosa. (Courtesy of Linda D. Ferrell, MD.)

TABLE 1.10. Modified WNM Staging of Cancer of the Esophagus and Cardia and Survival

Stage	Classification	5-Year Survival Rate
0	$W_0N_0M_0$	88%
I	$W_0N_1M_0$	50%
II	$W_1N_1M_0$	22%
III	$W_2N_1M_0$	10%
IV	Any W, any N, M	0

Source: Reprinted with permission from Ellis FH Jr, Heatley GJ, Krasna MJ, et al. Esophagogastrectomy for carcinoma of the esophagus and cardia: a comparison of findings and results after standard resection in three consecutive eight-year intervals with improved staging criteria. J Thorac Cardiovasc Surg 1997;113:836–846.

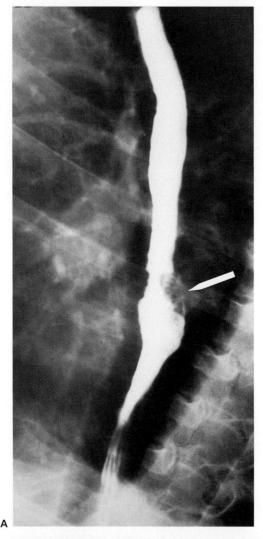

A

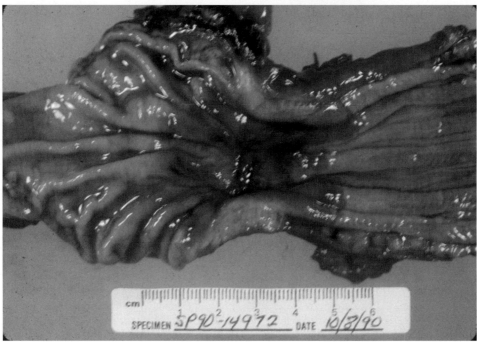

B

FIGURE 1.27. (A) In adenocarcinoma of the esophagus, the barium swallow test can be used to indicate the extent of the lesion, the extent of any luminal narrowing, and any angulation of the axis of the esophagus. The tumor in this patient is polypoid (arrow). (B) The surgical specimen is shown. (Courtesy of Linda D. Ferrell, MD, and Henry I. Goldberg, MD.)

BRONCHOSCOPY An important preoperative investigation in cancer of the upper and middle esophagus, bronchoscopy can determine whether or not the tracheopulmonary tree has been invaded.

Treatment

THERAPEUTIC OPTIONS Basic information regarding esophageal carcinoma is summarized in Table 1.11. The four therapeutic options for carcinoma of the esophagus are surgery, radiotherapy, chemotherapy, or a combination of methods. In patients who are good candidates for surgery and in whom no distant organ metastasis has been identified (stages I and II), surgical resection provides the best chance for cure and the best palliation when cure is not possible. Preoperative radiation is useful in stage III squamous cell carcinoma and may convert an unresectable lesion into a resectable one. Combined chemoradiotherapy has produced, in some studies, complete remission in 20% to 30% of patients.[9] Typically, fluorouracil, cisplatin, and mitomycin-C or vincristine are given in combination with 2500 to 3000 cGy external radiation directed at the lesion. This therapy may be given as the sole treatment or preoperatively. There is debate whether patients with complete endoscopic disappearance of the tumor after chemoradiotherapy should be subjected to resection. Adenocarcinoma is generally less responsive to radiotherapy, and surgical resection is the preferred method.

SURGICAL THERAPY Preoperative staging determines whether a patient is operable. Surgery is usually of little benefit in cases that involve distant organ metastasis (e.g., lung, liver), or invasion of the trachea or aorta. Esophagectomy can be accomplished with or without thoracotomy.

Ivor-Lewis Procedure A common procedure for resection of tumors in the distal half of the esophagus is the Ivor-Lewis operation (Figure 1.28). Through an abdominal approach, the stomach is completely mobilized, preserving the right gastric and right gastroepiploic vessels, and a pyloroplasty or pyloromyotomy is performed. The hiatus is opened and the distal esophagus mobilized within the mediastinum. A jejunostomy for eating is also performed. Right thoracotomy is then performed through the bed of the sixth rib, and the thoracic esophagus is mobilized. The stomach is then pulled up into the right chest for resection. At least 10 cm of proximal margin on the esophagus is needed. The resection line is distal to the gastroesophageal junction, and the portion of the stomach to be resected depends on tumor location within the esophagus. Gastroesophageal anastomosis is performed at or above the azygous vein.

The entire esophagus must be resected in the presence of more proximal thoracic lesions or extensive Barrett's metaplasia. In this case, the operation may be modified to

---

TABLE 1.11. Essentials: Carcinoma of the Esophagus

Incidence
- 20:100,000 population in North America and Europe
- 8 times more common in China

Type of cancer
- Squamous cell cancer: 95% worldwide
- Adenocarcinoma: >50% in North America

Risk factors
- Squamous: Tobacco, alcohol, tylosis, achalasia
- Adenocarcinoma: Barrett's esophagus and high-fat diet

Clinical presentation: Dysphagia, weight loss, weakness, anemia

Diagnosis: Endoscopy and biopsy

Staging
- Endoscopic ultrasound
- Barium swallow (axis)
- CT scan or MRI of chest and abdomen
- Bronchoscopy
- Thoracoscopy

Treatment
- Surgical: Stages I, II, following preoperative radiation of stage III
- Chemoradiotherapy: 5-FU, cisplatin and mitomycin-C in combination with 2500–3000 cGy external radiation

Choice of operation
- Distal one third: Transhiatal esophagectomy or Ivor Lewis procedure
- Middle one third: Ivor-Lewis procedure, transhiatal
- Upper one third: Total esophagectomy (three-cavity) with esophagogastrostomy in the neck

Outcome
- Stage I: 35% 5-year survival
- Stage II: 20% 5-year survival

Abbreviations: CT, computerized tomography; 5-FU, 5-fluorouracil; MRI, magnetic resonance imaging.

---

include a left cervical dissection of the esophagus with esophagogastric anastomosis in the neck.

Transhiatal Esophagectomy Alternatively, resection can be accomplished without thoracotomy. The procedure of choice is transhiatal esophagectomy, requiring abdominal and left cervical incisions. This procedure is best suited for carcinoma of the distal esophagus and is often the preferred procedure when associated Barrett's esophagus is extensive. The thoracic esophagus is mobilized with blunt transhiatal dissection. Esophagogastric anastomosis is performed in the neck (Figure 1.29) and has two advantages. First, thoracotomy and its attending disabilities are avoided. Second, the performance of the anastomosis in the neck is safer because anastomotic leak in the neck is less morbid and easily controlled.

Left Thoracic Esophagogastrectomy Esophagogastrectomy can also be accomplished through a left thoracic incision or a left thoraco-abdominal incision. The popularity of this approach has declined due to the difficulty of consistently achieving a proximal clear margin of resection.

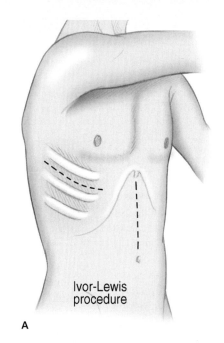

Ivor-Lewis
procedure

A

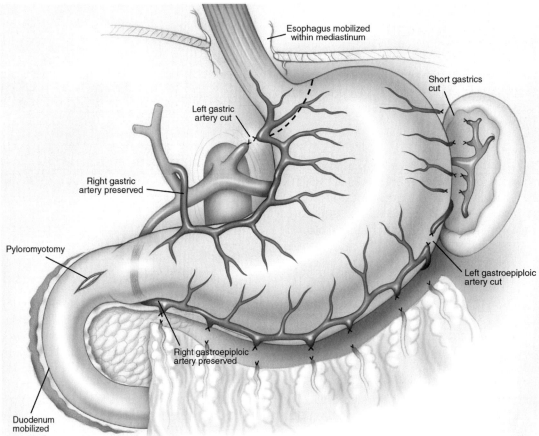

Esophagus mobilized
within mediastinum

Short gastrics
cut

Left gastric
artery cut

Right gastric
artery preserved

Left gastroepiploic
artery cut

Pyloromyotomy

Right gastroepiploic
artery preserved

Duodenum
mobilized

B

FIGURE 1.28. The Ivor-Lewis procedure is commonly performed for resection of tumors in the distal half of the esophagus. (A) Through a vertical upper abdominal incision, the stomach and duodenum are mobilized, all gastric vessels are divided (but sparing the right gastric and right gastroepiploic vessels), and (B) pyloromyotomy and feeding jejunostomy are performed. (C) Esophagogastric resection to the extent shown is accomplished in the chest through a right thoracotomy incision, and (D) esophagogastric anastomosis is performed at the level of the azygous vein. (Adapted from Jamieson GG, Debas HT, eds. Rob & Smith's Operative Surgery: Surgery of the Upper Gastrointestinal Tract. London: Chapman & Hall Medical, 1994; and Orringer MB, Sloan H. Substernal gastric bypass of the excluded thoracic esophagus for palliation of esophageal carcinoma. J Thorac Cardiovasc Surg 1975;70:836.)

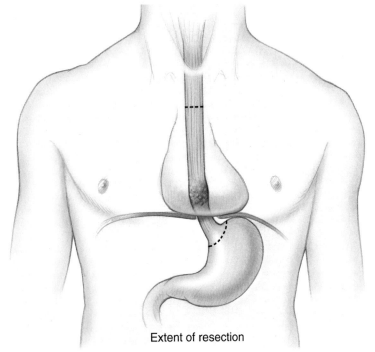

Extent of resection

C

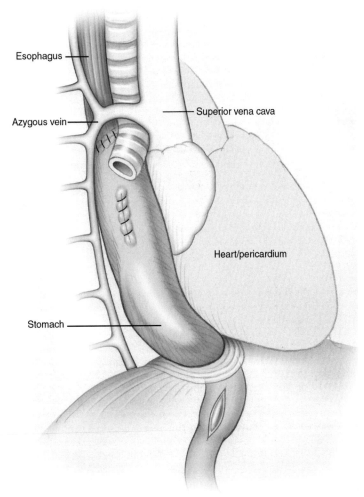

Esophagus

Azygous vein

Superior vena cava

Heart/pericardium

Stomach

D

FIGURE 1.28. *Continued*

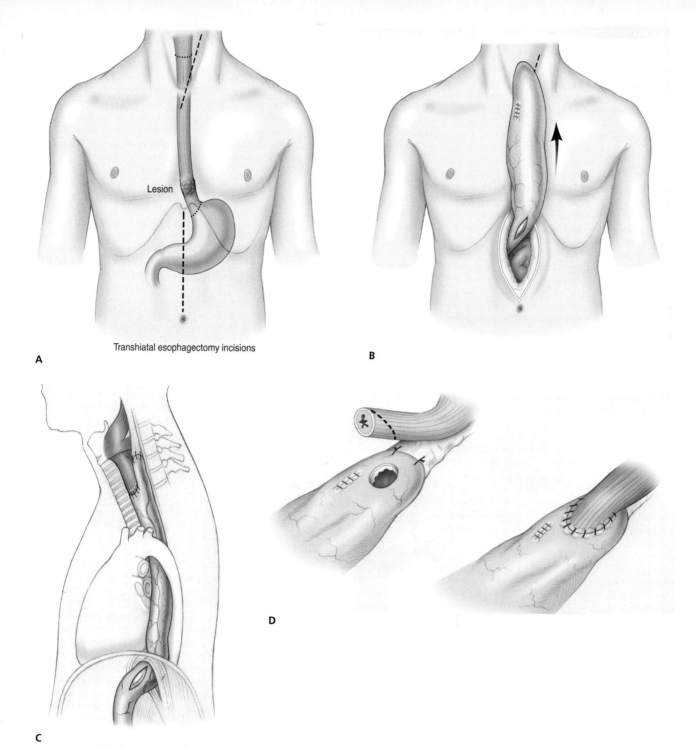

A

Lesion

Transhiatal esophagectomy incisions

B

C

D

FIGURE 1.29. Transhiatal esophagectomy is the procedure of choice in carcinoma of the distal esophagus. It is preferred in all cases when extensive Barrett's esophagus accompanies the cancer. (A) A vertical upper abdominal incision and a left cervical incision are employed. (The mobilization and vascular division of the stomach is the same as for the Ivor-Lewis procedure shown in Figure 1.28. (B) The stomach is divided 6–10 cm beyond the gastro-esophageal junction in such a way that the gastric remnant forms a tube that can reach the neck. (C) The gastric tube is passed to the neck through the posterior mediastinum and (D) esophagogastric anastomosis performed in the left neck. (Adapted from Jamieson GG, Debas HT, eds. Rob & Smith's Operative Surgery: Surgery of the Upper Gastrointestinal Tract. London: Chapman & Hall Medical, 1994; and Orringer MB, Sloan H. Esophagectomy without thoracotomy. J Thorac Cardiovasc Surg 1978;76:643.)

REFERENCES

1. Reid BJ, Levine DS, Longton G, et al. Predictors of progression to cancer in Barrett's esophagus: baseline histology and flow cytometry identify low- and high-risk patient subsets. *Am J Gastroenterol* 2000;95:1669–1676.
2. Wychulis AR, Woolam GL, Andersen HA, et al. Achalasia and carcinoma of the esophagus. *JAMA* 1971;215:1638–1641.
3. Vaezi MF, Richter JE. Current therapies for achalasia: comparison and efficacy. *J Clin Gastroenterol* 1998;27:21–35.
4. Vantrappen G, Hellemans J. Treatment of achalasia and related motor disorders. *Gastroenterology* 1980;79:144–154.
5. Younes Z, Johnson DA. Diagnostic evaluation in gastroesophageal reflux disease. *Gastroenterol Clin North Am* 1999;28:809–830.
6. DeMeester TR, Stein HJ, Fuchs KH. Physiologic diagnostic studies. In: Zuidema GD, ed. *Shackelford's Surgery of the Alimentary Tract.* 3rd ed, vol. 1. Philadelphia: WB Saunders; 1991:94–126.
7. Akiyama H. Surgery for carcinoma of the esophagus. *Curr Probl Surg* 1980;17:53–120.
8. Esophagus. In: Beahrs OH, Hansen DE, Hutter RVP et al., eds. *AJCC Cancer Staging Manual, American Joint Committee on Cancer.* 4th ed. Philadelphia: JB Lippincott, 1992:57.
9. Cooper JS, Guo MD, Herskovic A, et al. Chemoradiotherapy of locally advanced esophageal cancer: long-term follow-up of a prospective randomized trial (RTOG 85-01). Radiation Therapy Oncology Group. *JAMA* 1999;281:1623–1627.

SELECTED READINGS

Anatomy and Physiology

Castell DO, ed. *The Esophagus.* 1st ed. Boston: Little, Brown, 1992.

Castell DO, Richter JE, Dalton CB. *Esophageal Motility Testing.* New York: Elsevier, 1987.

DeMeester TR, Wang CI, Wernly JA, et al. Technique, indications, and clinical use of 24 hour esophageal pH monitoring. *J Thorac Cardiovasc Surg* 1980;79:656–670.

Duranceau A, Liebermann-Meffert C. Embryology, anatomy and physiology of the esophagus. In: Zuidema G, Yeo C, eds. *Shackelford's Surgery of the Alimentary Tract.* 3rd ed. Philadelphia: WB Saunders, 1991.

Emde C, Armstrong D, Castiglione F, et al. Reproducibility of long-term ambulatory esophageal combined pH/manometry. *Gastroenterology* 1991;100:1630–1637.

Gray SW, Rowe JS Jr, Skandalakis JE. Surgical anatomy of the gastroesophageal junction. *Am Surg* 1979;45:575–587.

Helm JF, Dodds WJ, Riedel DR, et al. Determinants of esophageal acid clearance in normal subjects. *Gastroenterology* 1983; 85:607–612.

Joelsson BE, DeMeester TR, Skinner DB, et al. The role of the esophageal body in the antireflux mechanism. *Surgery* 1982;92:417–424.

Kahrilas PJ, Dodds WJ, Hogan WJ. Effect of peristaltic dysfunction on esophageal volume clearance. *Gastroenterology* 1988;94: 73–80.

Siewert JR, Blum AL. The oesophagus. Part I: Surgery at the upper oesophageal sphincter, tubular oesophagus and lower oesophageal sphincter. *Clin Gastroenterol* 1979;8:271–291.

Stein HJ, DeMeester TR. Outpatient physiologic testing and surgical management of foregut motility disorders. *Curr Probl Surg* 1992;29:413–555.

Motility Disorders

Birgisson S, Richter JE. Achalasia: what's new in diagnosis and treatment? *Dig Dis* 1997;15(Suppl 1):1–27.

Bonavina L, Khan NA, DeMeester TR. Pharyngoesophageal dysfunctions. The role of cricopharyngeal myotomy. *Arch Surg* 1985;120:541–549.

Browning TH. Diagnosis of chest pain of esophageal origin. A guideline of the Patient Care Committee of the American Gastroenterological Association. *Dig Dis Sci* 1990;35:289–293.

Csendes A, Braghetto I, Henriquez A, et al. Late results of a prospective randomised study comparing forceful dilatation and oesophagomyotomy in patients with achalasia. *Gut* 1989;30:299–304.

Felix VN, Cecconello I, Zilberstein B, et al. Achalasia: a prospective study comparing the results of dilatation and myotomy. *Hepatogastroenterology* 1998;45:97–108.

Goldenberg SP, Burrell M, Fette GG, et al. Classic and vigorous achalasia: a comparison of manometric, radiographic, and clinical findings. *Gastroenterology* 1991;101:743–748.

Pellegrini CA, Leichter R, Patti M, et al. Thoracoscopic esophageal myotomy in the treatment of achalasia. *Ann Thorac Surg* 1993; 56:680–682.

Shimi SM, Nathanson LK, Cuschieri A. Thoracoscopic long oesophageal myotomy for nutcracker oesophagus: initial experience of a new surgical approach. *Br J Surg* 1992;79:533–536.

Waters PF, DeMeester TR. Foregut motor disorders and their surgical management. *Med Clin North Am* 1981;65:1235–1268.

Watson TJ, DeMeester TR, Kauer WK, et al. Esophageal replacement for end-stage benign esophageal disease. *J Thorac Cardiovasc Surg* 1998;115:1241–1249.

Esophageal Diverticula

Bonafede JP, Lavertu P, Wood BG, et al. Surgical outcome in 87 patients with Zenker's diverticulum. *Laryngoscope* 1997;107: 720–725.

Cook IJ, Gabb M, Panagopoulos V, et al. Pharyngeal (Zenker's) diverticulum is a disorder of upper esophageal sphincter opening. *Gastroenterology* 1992;103:1229–1235.

Debas HT, Payne WS, Cameron AJ, et al. Physiopathology of lower esophageal diverticulum and its implications for treatment. *Surg Gynecol Obstet* 1980;151:593–600.

Peracchia A, Bonavina L, Narne S, et al. Minimally invasive surgery for Zenker diverticulum: analysis of results in 95 consecutive patients. *Arch Surg* 1998;133:695–700.

Gastroesophageal Reflux Disease

Allison PR. Reflux esophagitis sliding hiatal hernia and the anatomy of repair. *Surg Gynecol Obstet* 1951;92:419.

Champault G. Gastroesophageal reflux. Treatment by laparoscopy. 940 cases—French experience. *Ann Chir* 1994;48:159–164.

Duranceau A, Ferraro P, Jamieson GG. The staging of severity in gastroesophageal reflux disease. *Chest Surg Clin N Am* 2001;11: 507–515.

Heitmiller RF, Redmond M, Hamilton SR. Barrett's esophagus with high-grade dysplasia. An indication for prophylactic esophagectomy. *Ann Surg* 1996;224:66–71.

Hill LD. An effective operation for hiatal hernia: an eight year appraisal. *Ann Surg* 1967;166:681–692.

Hinder RA, Filipi CJ, Wetscher G, et al. Laparoscopic Nissen fundoplication is an effective treatment for gastroesophageal reflux disease. *Ann Surg* 1994;220:472–483.

Kochhar R, Makharia GK. Usefulness of intralesional triamcinolone in treatment of benign esophageal strictures. *Gastrointest Endosc* 2002;56:829–834.

Lerut T, Coosemans W, Christiaens R, et al. The Belsey Mark IV antireflux procedure: indications and long-term results. *Acta Gastroenterol Belg* 1990;53:585–590.

Orlando RC. The pathogenesis of gastroesophageal reflux disease: the relationship between epithelial defense, dysmotility, and acid exposure. *Am J Gastroenterol* 1997;92(4 Suppl):3S–7S.

Peters JH. The surgical management of Barrett's esophagus. *Gastroenterol Clin North Am* 1997;26:647–668.

Pisegna JR. GERD and its complications. The pathogenic relationship between symptoms and disease progression. *Postgrad Med* 2001;19–23.

Sampliner RE. Updated guidelines for the diagnosis, surveillance, and therapy of Barrett's esophagus. *Am J Gastroenterol* 2002;97:1888–1895.

Carcinoma of the Esophagus

Akiyama H. Surgery for carcinoma of the esophagus. *Curr Probl Surg* 1980;17:53–120.

Akiyama H, Hiyama M, Miyazono H. Total esophageal reconstruction after extraction of the esophagus. *Ann Surg* 1975;182:547–552.

Bollschweiler E, Wolfgarten E, Gutschow C, et al. Demographic variations in the rising incidence of esophageal adenocarcinoma in white males. *Cancer* 2001;92:549–555.

DeMeester TR. Esophageal carcinoma: current controversies. *Semin Surg Oncol* 1997;13:217–233.

Dexter SP, Martin IG, McMahon MJ. Radical thoracoscopic esophagectomy for cancer. *Surg Endosc* 1996;10:147–151.

Krasna MJ. Advances in staging of esophageal carcinoma. *Chest* 1998;113(1 Suppl):107S–111S.

Law S, Wong J. New adjuvant therapies for esophageal cancer. *Adv Surg* 2001;35:271–295.

Lewis I. The surgical treatment of carcinoma of esophagus with special reference to new operation for growths of the middle third. *Br J Surg* 1946;34:18–31.

Orringer MB. Transhiatal esophagectomy without thoracotomy for carcinoma of the thoracic esophagus. *Ann Surg* 1984;200:282–288.

Stark SP, Romberg MS, Pierce GE, et al. Transhiatal versus transthoracic esophagectomy for adenocarcinoma of the distal esophagus and cardia. *Am J Surg* 1996;172:478–482.

Swisher SG, Wynn P, Putnam JB, et al. Salvage esophagectomy for recurrent tumors after definitive chemotherapy and radiotherapy. *J Thorac Cardiovasc Surg* 2002;123:175–183.

van Sandick JW, van Lanschot JJ, ten Kate FJ, et al. Indicators of prognosis after transhiatal esophageal resection without thoracotomy for cancer. *J Am Coll Surg* 2002;194:28–36.

Vigneswaran WT, Trastek VF, Pairolero PC, et al. Extended esophagectomy in the management of carcinoma of the upper thoracic esophagus. *J Thorac Cardiovasc Surg* 1994;107:901–907.

Walsh TN, Noonan N, Hollywood D, et al. A comparison of multimodal therapy and surgery for esophageal adenocarcinoma. *N Engl J Med* 1996;335:462–467.

Stomach and Duodenum

It is customary to consider the duodenum with the stomach because its most common affliction is peptic ulcer disease. This chapter first reviews the anatomy and physiology of the stomach. This information then forms the basis for discussion of the pathophysiology and management of secretory, motor, and neoplastic disorders of the stomach and duodenum.

ANATOMY

SURGICAL ANATOMY

Parts of the Stomach

Like the esophagus, the stomach is closed at each end with a sphincter, the LES proximally and the pyloric sphincter distally. Also like the esophagus, the musculature of the stomach consists of an inner circular muscle and an outer longitudinal smooth muscle. Unlike the esophagus, however, the stomach has a well-developed serosal layer. Just distal to the esophagogastric junction, the circular fibers are more robust and are arranged obliquely around the proximal stomach; they are often referred to as the "sling fibers." These oblique fibers may extend distally to form a third muscular layer. For ease of description, the stomach consists of four parts: the cardia, the fundus, the body, and the antrum (Figure 2.1).

Anatomic Relationships

The left lobe of the liver lies anterior to the proximal stomach. Thus, to obtain easy access to the proximal stomach and the hiatus, the left lobe of the liver is usually displaced to the right after division of the left triangular ligament (Figure 2.2). To the left, the stomach is closely related to the spleen, and several short gastric vessels attach the stomach to the splenic vessels at the splenic hilum. The rate of incidental splenectomy in gastric surgery can be high, particularly in reoperations if the adhesions and short gastric vessels are not carefully divided early in the operation. The inferior relationship of the stomach is to the transverse colon and the gastrocolic ligament. Due to proximity of the transverse colon and the potential of its being invaded by gastric malignancy, the prudent practice has evolved of preoperative bowel preparation when gastric resection for cancer is contemplated.

Behind the stomach is the lesser sac. Within it lies the pancreas, which extends transversely from the c-loop of the duodenum on the right to the hilum of the spleen on the left. Ligamentous bands of connective tissue attach the posterior of the stomach to the anterior of the pancreas. These bands, remnants of the mesogastrium in the embryo, must be divided to mobilize the stomach off the pancreas.

A key relationship is that of the pylorus to the distal common bile duct (CBD). In severe duodenal ulcer disease, in which the first portion of the duodenum is scarred and foreshortened, the antropyloric region is brought even closer to the CBD. Care must be taken not to injure the CBD during surgery for complex chronic duodenal ulcer disease and during suture control of bleeding duodenal ulcer.

Blood Supply

The blood supply of the stomach is pictured in Figure 2.3. The celiac axis provides the arterial supply in the following manner. The left gastric artery, a branch of the celiac itself, supplies the lesser curvature aspect of the body and cardia; the right gastric artery, a branch of the common hepatic, supplies the lesser curvature aspect of the antrum. The greater curvature of the stomach is supplied by the right gastroepiploic, a branch of the gastroduodenal, and the left gastroepiploic, a branch of the splenic artery.

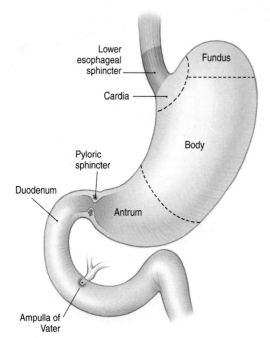

FIGURE 2.1. Anatomy of the stomach. The fundus and body of the stomach contain the parietal cell mass. The mucosa of the cardia is composed primarily of mucous and chief cells; the antral mucosa is the site of the gastrin-secreting cells and contains no parietal cells. A transitional zone exists between the body and antrum, where gastric ulcers tend to occur.

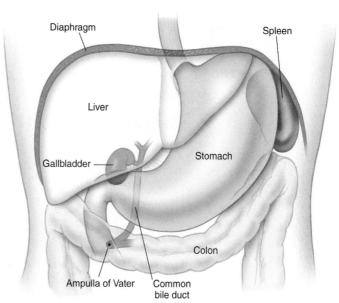

FIGURE 2.2. Anatomic relationships of the stomach. The esophagus emerges through the hiatus, where the abdominal esophagus and cardia are covered anteriorly by the left lobe of the liver. The spleen is intimately related to the gastric fundus through the short gastric vessels. The transverse colon is below the stomach and is draped with the greater omentum. The immediate space between the two organs is covered with the gastrocolic ligament, the division of which provides access to the lesser sac. Distally, near the junction of the stomach and duodenum, important relationships exist with the gall bladder and the common bile duct. Posterior to the stomach is the lesser sac, in which lies the pancreas with the splenic vessels.

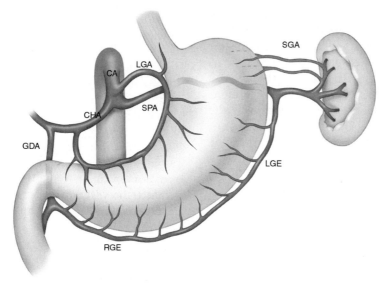

FIGURE 2.3. Arterial blood supply to the stomach. The stomach is supplied through branches of the celiac axis (CA). The left gastric artery (LGA) supplies the distal esophagus and the lesser curvature aspect of the cardia and body. The right gastric artery (RGA) and the gastroduodenal artery (GDA) are branches of the common hepatic artery (CHA). The right gastric artery supplies the lesser curvature aspect of the antrum and anastomoses with branches of the LGA. The GDA travels behind the pyloroduodenal area, where it is often eroded by a duodenal ulcer. Inferior to the pylorus, it leads to the right gastroepiploic (RGE) and the pancreaticoduodenal arteries. The RGE travels about 0.5 cm inferiorly to the greater curvature and supplies the greater curvature aspect of the antrum and body of the stomach. The left gastroepiploic artery (LGE), a branch of the splenic artery, courses 0.5 to 1.0 cm to the left of the stomach at the greater curvature and anastomoses with the RGE. Finally, the fundus of the stomach is supplied through several short gastric arteries (SGA), which originate from the splenic artery (SPA) as it branches in the splenic hilum.

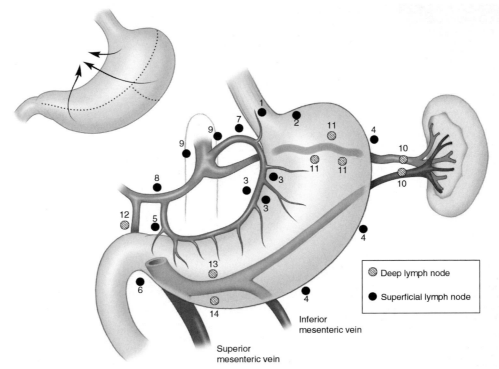

FIGURE 2.4. The lymphatic drainage of the stomach generally follows the blood supply, and the major groups of lymph nodes are named after the major vessels (e.g., celiac, left gastric, splenic, and so on). (Adapted from Barr H, Greenall MJ. Carcinoma of the stomach. In: Morris PJ, Wood WC, eds. Oxford Textbook of Surgery. 2nd ed. Oxford, UK: Oxford University Press; 2000:1313–1328.)

Venous drainage essentially follows the arterial supply, except on the lesser curvature aspect, where the venous drainage collects into the coronary vein before the latter drains into the portal vein.

Lymphatic Drainage

The lymphatic drainage of the stomach follows the blood supply (Figure 2.4), using the lymph node stations defined by the Japanese Research Society for Gastric Cancer, which were designed to accurately define metastatic spread to lymph nodes.[1] Unfortunately, however, because tumor spread is so unpredictable, the numerical designation is not as useful as might be expected.

The main lymphatic drainage of the stomach on the lesser curvature is to the left gastric nodes, then onward to the celiac nodes. The lesser curvature of the antrum drains to the suprapyloric nodes, then to the common hepatic nodes. Drainage of the gastric fundus is into the splenic and left gastroepiploic nodes. The posterior aspect of the stomach drains into nodes along the splenic artery, at the root of the mesentery and in the retropancreatic area.

The nodes can be primary (N_1) or secondary (N_2) drainage sites, depending on the location of the tumor. The primary and secondary lymphatic drainage of tumors in different regions of the stomach is shown in Table 2.1.

Nerve Supply

The nerve supply of the stomach consists of extrinsic, enteric (intrinsic), and sensory innervation.

Extrinsic Nervous System

Extrinsic innervation is supplied by vagal and sympathetic nerves; both systems playing a role in regulation of the secretory and motor functions of the stomach. The role of the vagus dominates.

VAGAL INNERVATION OF THE STOMACH Figure 2.5 shows the subdiaphragmatic distribution of the vagus nerve. The anterior and posterior vagal trunks are reconstituted over the distal esophagus. The left vagus nerve emerges at the hiatus, anterior to the esophagus, as either

TABLE 2.1. Lymphatic Drainage of the Stomach

Drainage site	N_1	N_2
Proximal third	1, 2, 3, 4	5, 6, 7, 8, 9, 10, 11
Middle third	3, 4, 5, 6, 12	1, 7, 8, 9, 10, 11
Distal third	3, 4, 5, 6	2, 7, 8, 11

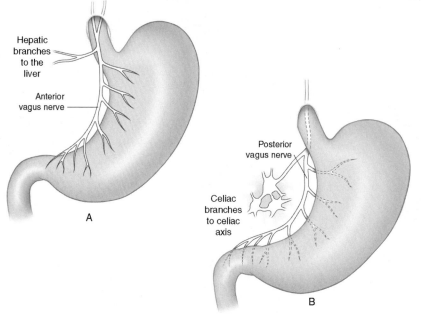

FIGURE 2.5. The subdiaphragmatic distribution of the vagus nerves. (A) The anterior vagus, which often emerges as more than one trunk from the hiatus, first gives the hepatic branches to the liver. It then continues distally 1.0 cm from the lesser curvature to end on the anterior surface of the antrum. The nerve of Latarjet provides the gastric branches from its left aspect to supply the anterior parietal cell mass. (B) The posterior vagus nerve nearly always emerges as a single trunk from the hiatus behind the esophagus and has divisions analogous to the anterior vagus but instead of the hepatic branches it sends the celiac branches to the celiac axis. (Adapted from Jamieson GG, Debas HT, eds. Rob & Smith's Operative Surgery: Surgery of the Upper Gastrointestinal Tract. London: Chapman & Hall Medical; 1994.)

a single trunk (70%) or multiple trunks (30%). The right vagus nerve lies behind the esophagus as it emerges from the hiatus and is nearly always a single trunk (94%). The first branches of the vagus in the abdomen are extragastric, including the hepatic branches (anterior vagus) and the celiac branches (posterior vagus). The vagus nerves then continue distally as the anterior and the posterior nerves of Latarjet, otherwise called the long nerves to the antrum. On reaching the antrum, the nerves of Latarjet become terminal branches that resemble a crow's foot. From the left side of the nerves of Latarjet, 12 to 20 gastric branches supply the acid-secreting part of the stomach.

SYMPATHETIC INNERVATION The sympathetic innervation of the stomach is derived from the celiac ganglion and is distributed on the adventitia of the arterial supply.

Enteric Nervous System

The enteric nervous system (ENS) is made up of the submucousal and myenteric ganglia, which contain the cell bodies of the nerves whose long axons then form a rich neuronal plexus. Preganglionic efferent vagal fibers terminate in these ganglia, from which emerge postganglionic fibers that are distributed to target cells (i.e., smooth muscle, epithelial), either directly or through interneurons. Neurotransmission at the ganglia is activated by the release of acetylcholine, which acts on the cell bodies of postganglionic neurons, which possess M3 receptors. It is now believed that the majority of postganglionic neurons are peptidergic, that is, they synthesize peptides in their cell bodies, transport the peptides along their axons, and release them in close proximity to the target cell. Part of Figure 2.6 illustrates the mechanism for smooth muscle relaxation and vagal release of gastrin. Postganglionic neurons that mediate smooth muscle relaxation are predominantly vasoactive intestinal polypeptidergic (VIP), while those responsible for gastrin release contain gastrin-releasing peptide (GRP). Immunohistochemical studies show that the ENS is rich in neurons containing a variety of peptides.

Sensory Nervous System

Unmyelinated sensory neurons, containing substance P (SP) and calcitonin gene-related peptide (CGRP) provide sensory innervation to the stomach. The cell bodies of these sensory neurons, which are located in paravertebral ganglia, also have axons that project into the posterior horn of the spinal chord. When these cell bodies are stimulated, SP and CGRP can be released simultaneously in the spinal cord and the stomach. As is discussed later, the sensory innervation of the stomach plays an important role in mucosal defense and blood flow.

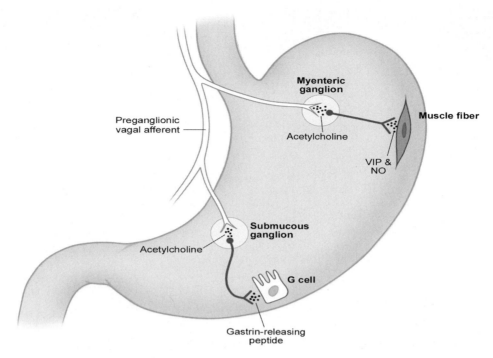

FIGURE 2.6. Vagal regulation of gastric function. Preganglionic vagal fibers terminate in the submucosal and myenteric ganglia of the stomach, where they are closely related to the postganglionic fibers, which supply the target cells (smooth muscle and epithelial). The neurotransmitter in the ganglia is acetylcholine. Relaxation of gastric smooth fibers is caused by the release of vasoactive intestinal polypeptide (VIP) and nitric oxide (NO) at the neuromuscular junction. Postganglionic vagal regulation of gastrin release is accomplished through postganglionic peptidergic fibers that release gastrin-releasing peptide at the basal lateral surface of the G cell.

MICROSCOPIC ANATOMY

The gastric mucosa is lined with mucous cells. Gastric pits in the mucosal surface provide openings for the gastric glands, which extend down to the muscularis mucosa (Figure 2.7). Five types of epithelial cells make up the gastric gland: surface mucous cells and mucous neck cells, both of which produce mucus and bicarbonate; parietal (oxyntic) cells, which secrete H^+ and intrinsic factor; chief cells, which produce pepsinogen; and endocrine cells, of which the most important are the enterochromaffin-like (ECL) cells. ECL cells make up 35% of the entire population of endocrine cells in the gastric gland, and they secrete histamine, a final common mediator of gastric acid secretion.

The stroma surrounding gastric glands make up the lamina propria. In gastritis, the lamina propria is invaded by inflammatory blood cells. The muscularis propria consists of three smooth muscle layers: the inner oblique, the middle circular, and the outer longitudinal layers. The stomach, unlike the esophagus, has a well-developed serosa.

PHYSIOLOGY

The essentials of the physiology of the stomach are summarized in Table 2.2.

EXOCRINE SECRETION

Regulation of Acid Secretion

Acid secretion is regulated by neural, endocrine, and paracrine mechanisms.

Neural Mechanisms

The vagus nerve plays a central role in both the stimulatory and inhibitory regulation of acid secretion.

VAGAL STIMULATION OF ACID SECRETION

Central Mechanisms The thought, sight, or smell of food stimulates medullary nuclei and then the dorsal motor nucleus (DMN) of the vagus nerve (Figure 2.8). The DMN

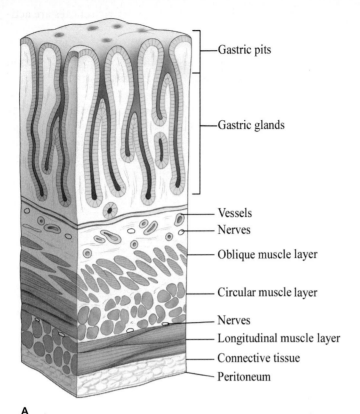

Gastric pits

Gastric glands

Vessels

Nerves

Oblique muscle layer

Circular muscle layer

Nerves

Longitudinal muscle layer

Connective tissue

Peritoneum

A

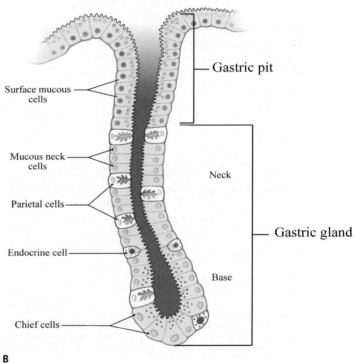

Surface mucous cells

Gastric pit

Mucous neck cells

Neck

Parietal cells

Gastric gland

Endocrine cell

Base

Chief cells

B

FIGURE 2.7. (A and B) Microscopic structure of the gastric wall. The gastric glands are the functional unit of the mucosa and communicate to the lumen by gastric pits. The luminal surface as well as the neck of the glands is covered with mucous cells. The gastric glands themselves contain both epithelial cells (e.g., parietal, chief) and endocrine cells (e.g., ECL cells). The muscular layer contains an outer longitudinal and an inner circular layer. Frequently, however, there are three layers, which include an innermost oblique muscle layer. (Adapted with permission from Ito S. Functional gastric morphology. In: Johnson LR, et al., eds. Physiology of the Gastrointestinal Tract. 2nd ed. Vol. 1. New York: Raven Press; 1987.)

TABLE 2.2. Essentials: Physiology of the Stomach

Motor function
  Myogenic mechanisms
  - Gastric pacemaker: Located in greater curvature
  - Basal electrical rhythm (BER): 1 per 20 s
  Neural mechanisms
  - Excitatory mechanisms: ACh, SP, 5-HT
  - Inhibitory neurotransmitters: VIP, NO (mediate receptive relaxation)
  Hormonal mechanisms
  - Stimulatory: Motilin
  - Inhibitory: CCK
  Gastric emptying control
  - Liquids: Mainly proximal stomach
  - Solids: Mainly distal stomach

Secretory function
  Exocrine
  H+
  - Secreted by parietal cells
  - Stimulated by histamine, gastrin, ACh
  - Inhibited by somatostatin, intestinal peptides (CCK, secretin, GIP)
  Pepsinogen
  - Secreted by chief cells
  - Stimulated primarily by ACh
  Mucus and bicarbonate
  - Secreted by mucous cells
  - Stimulated by prostaglandins, ACh, β-adrenergics
  - Inhibited by NSAIDs
  Intrinsic factor
  - Secreted by parietal cell
  - Stimulated by histamine, ACh, gastrin
  - Binds vitamin B_{12} for absorption in distal ileum
  Endocrine/paracrine/neurocrine (see Table 2.4)

Abbreviations: ACh, acetylcholine; SP, substance P; CCK, cholecystokinin; 5-HT, 5-hydroxy tryptamine; GIP, gastric inhibitory peptide; H^+, hydrogen ions; NO, nitric oxide; NSAIDs, nonsteroidal anti-inflammatory drugs; VIP, vasoactive intestinal polypeptide.

is activated by release of thyrotropin-releasing hormone (TRH) from neurons that project to the nucleus. DMN activation, in turn, stimulates the afferent vagal fibers.

Peripheral Mechanisms Vagal stimulation of acid secretion involves several peripheral mechanisms, as described below and in Figure 2.9:

1. Release of acetylcholine (ACh) at nerve endings triggers direct vagal stimulation of the parietal cell. ACh binds to M3 receptors on the parietal cell, resulting in a phospholipase C–activated rise in cytosolic calcium, elaboration of H^+/K^+–ATPase on the apical surface, and secretion of H^+.

2. Cholinergic stimulation of the ECL cell and release of histamine stimulate the parietal cell by binding to the histamine H_2 receptor.

3. Inhibition of somatostatin release from delta cells results in "disinhibition" of the parietal, ECL, and G cells.

4. Antral gastrin is released through stimulation of G cells by GRP from GRP-containing postganglionic neurons.

5. Vasovagal reflexes and short gastric reflexes are activated by gastric distension.

VAGAL INHIBITORY MECHANISMS Vagal stimulation results in the activation of several peptidergic inhibitory pathways, including VIP, neuropeptide Y, CGRP, SP, and galanin. The relative importance of these inhibitory peptidergic pathways has not been elucidated. Inhibitory vagal regulation is more apparent on the G cell than on the parietal cell. For example, basal and postprandial hypergastrinemia develops following all types of vagotomy. Postvagotomy hypergastrinemia is not fully explained by the reduction of acid and the rise of luminal pH postoperatively.

Humoral Mechanisms

STIMULATION OF ACID SECRETION The key humoral substances responsible for gastric acid secretion are histamine and gastrin.

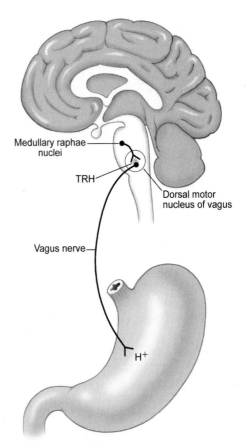

FIGURE 2.8. Central mechanisms of acid secretion control. Centrally located, the dorsal motor nucleus (DMN) of the vagus controls the stimulation of acid secretion. Neurons that project from the medullary raphae nuclei activate the DMN through release of thyrotropin-releasing hormone (TRH), which stimulates the preganglionic vagal fibers to release acetylcholine at the ganglia in the gastric wall. (Adapted with permission from Debas HT, Carvajal SH. Vagal regulation of acid secretion and gastrin release. Yale J Biol Med 1994;67:145–151.)

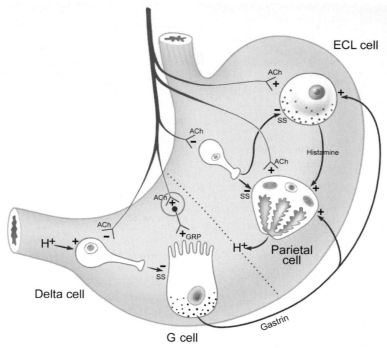

FIGURE 2.9. Peripheral mechanisms of acid secretion. The parietal cells secrete hydrogen ions (H⁺) when stimulated by histamine, gastrin, and acetylcholine (ACh). The main source of histamine, the enterochromaffin-like (ECL) cell, secretes histamine in response to stimulation by both the vagus nerve (ACh) and gastrin. Inhibitory regulation is accomplished chiefly by the release of somatostatin (SS) at the level of either the ECL cell or the parietal cell. In the antrum, gastrin release is stimulated by luminal food or by the vagus acting through the release of gastrin-releasing peptide (GRP). Inhibitory control of the G cell is through the release of somatostatin from delta cells. Antral acidification releases somatostatin from delta cells to shut off gastrin release. This constitutes the negative feedback regulation of gastrin release. (Adapted with permission from Debas HT, Carvajal SH. Vagal regulation of acid secretion and gastrin release. Yale J Biol Med 1994;67:145–151.)

Histamine Histamine has emerged as the common final pathway for both vagal- and gastrin-stimulated acid secretion, although both ACh and gastrin can act directly on the parietal cell through the M3 and cholecystokinin-B (CCK-B) receptors, respectively. Histamine is a paracrine agent. It is now believed that the physiologically relevant pool of histamine that lies within diffusion distance of the parietal cell is the histamine contained within ECL cells. The ECL cell contains receptors for ACh, gastrin, pituitary adenylate cyclase activating peptide (PACAP), and somatostatin. Histamine released from ECL cells diffuses to the parietal cell, binds to histamine H₂ receptors, and activates the adenylate cyclase system to stimulate acid secretion.

Gastrin Gastrin, produced by G cells in the antrum and proximal duodenum, is released by food and antral distension. It is responsible for most or all of the gastric phase of acid secretion and is synthesized in the cell as a preprohormone. Posttranslational processing results in production of several molecular sizes of the hormone; the 17-amino-acid C-terminal peptide (G-17) is the most important stimulant of acid secretion.

As mentioned earlier, gastrin acts through the CCK-B receptor, which is present on the parietal and ECL cells.

Although it can stimulate acid secretion *in vitro* from isolated parietal cells, its acid secretory action *in vivo* is probably mediated largely through histamine release from the ECL cell.

In addition to its acid secretory effect, gastrin stimulates growth of the acid-secreting portion of the gastric mucosa. The most important trophic action of gastrin is on the parietal cell (which explains parietal cell hyperplasia in Zollinger-Ellison syndrome) and the ECL cell (which explains ECL-cell hyperplasia and formation of carcinoid tumors in chronic hypergastrinemic states). Gastrin has no trophic effect on the antral mucosa.

The direct action of gastrin on the parietal cell through the CCK-B receptor is mediated through the cyclic guanosine monophosphate (GMP) pathway.

INHIBITION OF ACID SECRETION Processes and substances that regulate the release of gastrin and somatostatin are summarized in Table 2.3.

Inhibition of Gastrin Release Antral acidification, the most important mechanism for turning off gastrin secretion, releases somatostatin from antral D cells. Somatostatin acts on the G cell to inhibit gastrin release.

TABLE 2.3. Regulation of Gastrin and Somatostatin (SS) Release

	Stimulation	Inhibition
Gastrin	Proteins, amino acids GRP (vagus) Antral distension Antral alkalization	Somatostatin Antral acidification (SS) Galanin
Somatostatin	Antral acidification CCK PACAP VIP	Acetylcholine Vagal stimulation

Abbreviations: CCK, cholecystokinin; GRP, gastrin-releasing peptide; PACAP, pituitary adenylate cyclase-activating peptide; VIP, vasoactive intestinal polypeptide.

Secretion of Somatostatin in Oxyntic Mucosa Somatostatin released from D cells in the oxyntic mucosa inhibits acid secretion by directly acting on the parietal cell or indirectly by acting on the ECL cell to inhibit histamine release.

Intestinal Inhibitory Mechanisms (Enterogastrones) The introduction of fat or acid into the duodenum elicits the release of various inhibitory substances, some known and some unknown. Some of the known inhibitory peptides released from the intestine include CCK, secretin, VIP, somatostatin, and enteroglucagon. Infusion of glucose into the intestine also releases gastric inhibitory peptide (GIP).

Regulation of Pepsinogen Secretion

Pepsinogen is a proenzyme secreted mainly by the chief cells in the gastric mucosa. Seven types of pepsinogen have been classified into two groups. Pepsinogen I (PGI) contains PG1 through PG5 and is the dominant form in the oxyntic mucosa. PGI is not found in the cardia, antrum, or duodenum. PGII, containing PG6 and PG7, on the other hand, is found in all parts of the stomach and in the Brunner's glands of the duodenum. Both PGI and PGII are present in the serum but only PGI is excreted in the urine as "uropepsin."

Pepsinogen is converted by acid into the active enzyme pepsin. The pH optimum for PGI is 1.5 to 2.0 and for PGII 3.2. Once pepsin is generated, it autocatalyzes the conversion of pepsinogen into pepsin. The initial digestion of proteins is the primary function of pepsin. Pepsin hydrolyzes proteins to generate smaller protein fragments and some free amino acids. Protein digestion into amino acids is completed in the intestine mainly by pancreatic enzymes.

Primary regulation of pepsin secretion in vivo is under cholinergic control. Vagal stimulation and gastric distension release ACh, which activates chief cells by acting on M3 cholinergic receptors, utilizing calcium as the intracellular messenger. Histamine also leads to the release of pepsinogen into the gastric lumen. Whether this release represents true stimulation of the chief cell or a "wash-out phenomenon" has been debated for a long time. Gastrin and secretin also stimulate pepsinogen secretion, but stimulation of pepsinogen by hormones is not as important as that by cholinergic mechanisms.

Regulation of Mucus and Bicarbonate Secretion

Both mucus and bicarbonate are secreted by surface cells of the gastric mucosa. Mucus is secreted continuously by exocytosis mostly from mucous surface and mucous neck cells, and is stimulated by several agonists, including ACh, β-adrenergic agents, and prostaglandins. The mucus forms an aqueous gel on the surface of the epithelial cells.

Bicarbonate secretion is stimulated by prostaglandins. Compared with the amount of acid the gastric mucosa secretes, bicarbonate secretion is small, at most 10% of total acid output. Nevertheless, bicarbonate plays a critical protective role in the gastric mucosa because it is trapped beneath the "unstirred" mucous gel layer close to the surface of the mucosa. In this strategic location, the small amount of bicarbonate secreted plays a significant role in neutralizing acid at the luminal surface of gastric cells.

Nonsteroidal anti-inflammatory drugs (NSAIDs) eliminate the synthesis of prostaglandins, thereby inhibiting the production of both mucus and bicarbonate. Acidification of the duodenal bulb mucosa also results in increased synthesis and release of both mucus and bicarbonate—a mechanism believed to be important in preventing duodenal ulceration.

Regulation of Secretion of Intrinsic Factor

Intrinsic factor (IF) is secreted by the parietal cells of the stomach, stimulated by the same agents that stimulate acid secretion. It is then transported bound to R-protein of salivary origin. In the small intestine, IF is released from the binding protein by pancreatic proteases. Once released, IF binds vitamin B_{12}. The complex is carried into the ileal cell, and vitamin B_{12} is then released into plasma. In other words, IF is a necessary carrier glycoprotein for the absorption of vitamin B_{12} in the ileum. Failure of IF secretion leads to megaloblastic anemia. Conditions that contribute to such failure include atrophic gastritis, in which the parietal cell mass is critically small or nonexistent, and total gastrectomy and proximal gastrectomy, which remove the entire parietal cell mass. Following total and proximal gastrectomy, therefore, patients must receive parenteral vitamin B_{12} monthly.

ENDOCRINE/PARACRINE/ NEUROCRINE SECRETION

The discussion of the exocrine secretion of the stomach indicated that an integration of humoral and neural mechanisms regulate acid secretion. This section briefly discusses each of the important humoral agents. As a

TABLE 2.4. Major Humoral Products of the Stomach

Humoral agent	Cell of origin	Target (receptor)	Action
Endocrine			
Gastrin	G cell	ECL cell (CCK-B)	↑ histamine release
		Parietal cell (CCK-B)	↑ mucosal growth
Paracrine			
Histamine	ECL cell	Parietal cell (histamine, H-2)	↑ H^+ secretion
Somatostatin	D cell	ECL cell (SS-2)	↓ histamine release
		G cell (SS-2)	↓ gastrin release
Neurocrine			
Acetylcholine	Vagal efferents	ECL cell (M3)	↑ histamine release
		Parietal cell (M3)	↑ H^+ secretion
		Smooth muscle (M1)	Contraction
PACAP	ENS	ECL cell	↑ histamine release
VIP	ENS	Blood vessel	↑ blood flow
		Smooth muscle	Relaxation
GRP	ENS	G cell	↑ gastrin release
CGRP, SP	Vagal afferents	D cell	↑ somatostatin release
	ENS	Blood vessel	↑ blood flow
Galanin	ENS	G cell	↓ gastrin release
		ECL cell	↓ histamine release
Other local agents			
Prostaglandins	Endothelial cells	Mucous cell	↑ mucus, ↑ HCO_3
		Parietal cell	↓ H^+ secretion
Nitric oxide	ENS	Smooth muscle	Relaxation

Abbreviations: CCK-B, cholecystokinin-B; CGRP, calcitonin gene-related peptide; ECL, enterochromaffin-like; ENS, enteric nervous system; GRP, gastrin-releasing peptide; PACAP, pituitary adenylate cyclase-activating peptide; SS, somatostatin; VIP, vasoactive intestinal polypeptide.

preamble, notice that humoral agents may be released from endocrine cells or neurons. Endocrine cells may release their secretory products (e.g., peptides, amines) directly into the bloodstream or into the interstitial space. Humoral agents released into the bloodstream and carried by it to their target site are called *hormones*. Gastrin is a good example of a hormone. Substances secreted into the interstitial space diffuse through the interstitial fluid to reach their target are known as *paracrine agents*. Both histamine and somatostatin are examples of paracrine agents. *Neurocrine agents* are usually secreted at the nerve terminal and cross a short synaptic gap to reach their receptors on target cells. ACh and GRP are examples. The major humoral secretory products of the stomach are listed in Table 2.4.

Although somatostatin is classified here as a paracrine agent, it is also both a hormone and a neurocrine agent. Released into the bloodstream following antral acidification and intestinal perfusion with fat, somatostatin is also present in the enteric nervous system as shown by immunohistology. Whether its role as a hormone or neurocrine agent is important in gastric physiology is as yet unknown.

Most gastrointestinal peptides are neurocrine agents. In the stomach, CGRP and substance P are found in small-diameter sensory neurons and in the enteric nervous system. CGRP appears to play an important role in gastric mucosal defense and blood flow as well as in motility. Pituitary adenylate cyclase-activating peptide (PACAP) and VIP belong to the secretin family of peptides. Both are present in postganglionic neurons in the stomach, and both play a role in regulating the ECL and the D cells. Galanin, another peptide released from postganglionic nerve endings in the stomach, appears to be an inhibitor of the ECL cell and the G cell.

DEFENSE MECHANISMS OF THE GASTRODUODENAL MUCOSA

The gastric mucosa is continually exposed to acid, with luminal pH often approaching 1.0. Because this degree of acidity is one million times greater than that within the interstitial or intracellular spaces of the gastric mucosa, how does the gastric mucosa protect itself from peptic damage in this acidic environment? How does it prevent acidification of the gastric mucosa and submucosa? The development of peptic ulceration is explained as a disruption of the balance between the aggressive factors (acid and pepsin) and the defensive factors (to be described below), in which the equilibrium is tilted in favor of the former. Even after the discovery of *Helicobacter pylori* as an important cause of peptic ulcer, the imperative that gastric acid must be present to cause ulceration has not

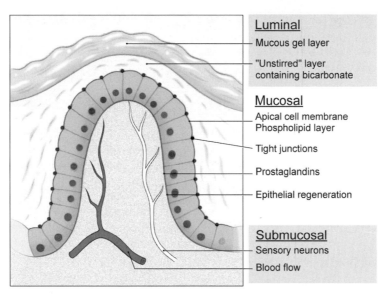

| Luminal |
| Mucous gel layer |
| "Unstirred" layer containing bicarbonate |

| Mucosal |
| Apical cell membrane Phospholipid layer |
| Tight junctions |
| Prostaglandins |
| Epithelial regeneration |

| Submucosal |
| Sensory neurons |
| Blood flow |

FIGURE 2.10. Defense mechanisms of the gastroduodenal mucosa. The luminal components include secretion of bicarbonate beneath the "unstirred" mucous gel layer applied to the apical surface. The mucosal components include the phospholipid bilayer of the apical membrane, the tight junctions, and the ability of the gastric mucosa to both secrete prostaglandins and undergo rapid epithelial regeneration. The submucosal components include the rich blood flow, which brings defense factors and disposes of noxious agents, as well as the sensory neurons, which are mainly responsible for cytoprotection of the mucosa.

changed. The old adage, "no acid, no ulcer," therefore, still holds. Not all patients who develop duodenal ulcer are acid hypersecretors. With *H. pylori*, inappropriate acid secretion occurs in the basal state because acid inhibitory mechanisms are deranged.

The term *defense mechanisms* is used here to describe all the elements that operate to prevent acid-peptic damage to the gastroduodenal mucosa. These mechanisms, described as gastric and duodenal, are depicted in Figure 2.10.

Defense Mechanisms of the Gastric Mucosa

Luminal Factors

The secretion of mucus from the mucous surface and neck cells and the formation of a continuous mucous gel layer that closely adheres to the mucosa has already been discussed. Between this gel layer and the apical surfaces of the mucosal cells is a small quantity of fluid that constitutes the "unstirred" layer, into which the surface mucous cells secrete bicarbonate. The mucous gel layer and the unstirred layer containing bicarbonate are important luminal defense factors.

Mucosal Factors

APICAL CELL MEMBRANE The gastric surface is coated by a phospholipid layer, similar to the surfactant found in the lung. The phospholipid bilayer lacks proteins capable of transporting protons and hence is acid resistant.

TIGHT JUNCTIONS In contrast to the leaky tight junctions of intestinal epithelium, the gastric epithelium contains "tight" tight junctions that are resistant to back diffusion of acid from the gastric lumen.

PROSTAGLANDINS The generation of prostaglandins by gastric mucosa is an important regulator of mucus and bicarbonate secretion. Small doses of exogenous 16,16-dimethyl prostaglandin E2 (PGE2) have been shown to protect the gastric mucosa against gross damage from subsequent application of injurious agents such as strong acid, strong alkali, alcohol, or heat. This phenomenon has been described as "cytoprotection." The means by which PGE2 confers cytoprotection is unknown, but it may involve as yet undescribed mechanisms beyond mucus and bicarbonate production.

Several types of prostaglandins are generated from arachidonic acid. Prostaglandins of the E type are potent inhibitors of acid secretion by acting on a G protein–coupled EP3 receptor. NSAID therapy abolishes the generation of prostaglandins from arachidonic acid by inhibiting Cox I. Recently, NSAID-type drugs that are selective Cox II inhibitors have been developed in the hope of preventing interference with the generation of prostaglandins by Cox I.

REGENERATIVE CAPACITY OF GASTRIC EPITHELIAL CELLS The entire gastric mucosa is renewed every 3 to 5 days by the twin processes of cell regeneration and cell desquamation. The rapid regenerative capacity of the mucosa is important in the process of healing erosions and ulcers. Inhibition of this cellular regenerative capacity of the gastroduodenal mucosa may explain, at least in part, why steroids aggravate peptic ulceration.

MUCOSAL RESTITUTION The gastric mucosa has a remarkable ability to establish epithelial integrity following mucosal damage. This process, known as *mucosal restitution*, is a rapid process of cell migration from the edges of the defect to cover it. The process is completed within minutes and cannot be explained by cell proliferation. The mechanisms underlying restitution are unknown but involve proteins of the basal lamina (e.g., laminin) and matrix receptors on epithelial cells.

Sensory Neurons and Calcitonin Gene-Related Peptide

The major sensory neurons in the stomach are small-diameter C-fibers containing CGRP and SP. Capsaicin, the sensory neurotoxin present in pepper, and other noxious agents are capable of releasing CGRP from sensory neurons in the stomach. CGRP, thus released, has been shown to protect against ulceration and to promote restitution. The mechanisms for the protective action of CGRP and CGRP-containing neurons may involve stimulation of blood flow, inhibition of acid secretion, release of somatostatin, and inhibition of motility.

Blood Flow

Not only does the gastric mucosa have rich blood flow, but the blood flow increases during stimulation of gastric acid secretion. The important role sensory neurons play in mucosal protection and the powerful vasodilatory effects of CGRP have been mentioned. Conditions that decrease gastric blood flow, such as hemorrhagic shock and sepsis, predispose to erosive gastritis and ulceration.

Postmucosal Factors

Circulating agents such as growth factors and antibodies probably also contribute to the protection of gastric mucosa from offending toxins and bacteria.

Duodenal Defense Mechanisms

The first few centimeters of the duodenal mucosa are frequently exposed to low pH levels and must be appropriately protected from acid and pepsin, particularly since the duodenal tight junctions are significantly leakier than those of the gastric mucosa. Three protective mechanisms appear to be important, as described below.

Mucosal Bicarbonate Secretion

The mucosa of the proximal duodenum secretes appreciable amounts of bicarbonate in response to luminal acidi-

fication. This response is diminished in patients with duodenal ulcer and in individuals with *H. pylori* infection.

Mucosal Dissipation of Acid

Unlike the stomach, the duodenum has a large capacity to dissipate acid across its mucosa. This probably is the result of paracellular pathways and the leaky tight junctions in the duodenal mucosa.

Pancreatic Bicarbonate Secretion

Acidification of the duodenal mucosa provokes rapid secretion of pancreatic bicarbonate. In this regard, the duodenum acts like a titrimeter, causing equivalent bicarbonate secretion from the pancreas to the acid load it receives. Duodenal acidification stimulates pancreatic secretion mainly through the release of secretin and CCK from the duodenum.

MOTOR FUNCTION OF THE STOMACH

Control of Gastric Motility

Myogenic, neural, and humoral mechanisms regulate gastric motility. The essential features of gastric motor function are listed in Table 2.5.

Myogenic Mechanisms

Myogenic mechanisms provide the most important control of stomach functions. The smooth muscle fibers of the stomach exhibit a basal electrical rhythm (BER) that oscillates every 20 seconds. The BER is controlled by a "pacemaker" located on the greater curvature aspect of the proximal stomach. It is believed that the pacemaker is made up of a concentration of interstitial cells of Cajal. The BER spreads from the pacemaker distally toward the

TABLE 2.5. Essentials: Gastric Motor Function
Regulation of gastric motility
Myogenic mechanisms
■ Gastric pacemaker: Greater curvature, proximal stomach
■ Basal electric rhythm (BER)
■ Action potential: Coordinated by BER
Neural mechanisms
■ Excitatory neurotransmitters: ACh, SP, neurokinin A
■ Inhibitory neurotransmitters: VIP, NO
Hormonal mechanism
■ Motilin: Accelerates gastric emptying
■ CCK: Inhibits gastric emptying
Gastric emptying
Liquids controlled by proximal stomach
Solids controlled by antropyloric segment
Abbreviations: ACh, acetylcholine; CCK, cholecystokinin; NO, nitric oxide; SP, substance P; VIP, vasoactive intestinal polypeptide.

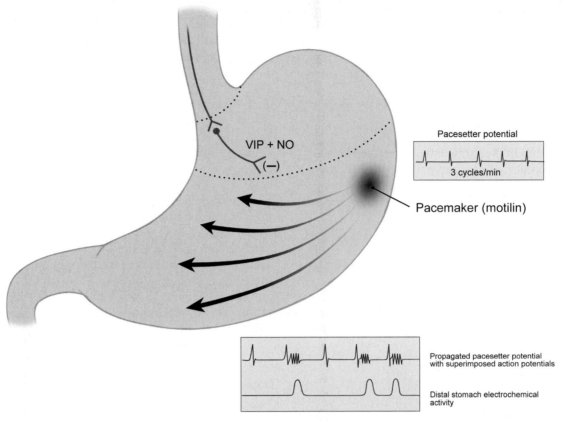

FIGURE 2.11. Gastric motility is controlled by a *pacemaker* located on the greater curvature aspect of the proximal stomach. The pacemaker generates the pacesetter potential (3 cycles per min), which sweeps down toward the antrum to organize and regulate the timing of the action potential, hence of muscular contraction. Receptive relaxation of the stomach is regulated by vagal reflexes with vasoactive intestinal polypeptide (VIP) and nitric oxide (NO) acting as the peripheral neurotransmitters. (Adapted from Freedlender AE, McCallum RW. The role of gastrointestinal hormones and neuropeptides in the physiological regulation of gastric emptying. Regul Pept Lett 1990;2.)

pylorus. The depolarization waves of the BER are sometimes referred to as "slow waves." The BER does not result in contractile muscle response. Muscle contraction is preceded by an action potential that occurs at specific points of the BER. Thus, the BER serves to organize and regulate the timing of the action potential, hence of muscular contraction. Figure 2.11 summarizes the regulation of gastric motor function.

Neural Mechanisms

Both extrinsic (vagal and sympathetic) and intrinsic (enteric nervous system) factors influence the motor function of the stomach through the release of excitatory and inhibitory neurotransmitters.

EXCITATORY NEUROTRANSMITTERS The main excitatory neurotransmitters include acetylcholine, neurokinins (substance P and neurokinin A), and 5-hydroxytryptamine (5-HT).

INHIBITORY NEUROTRANSMITTERS The most important inhibitory neurotransmitters are VIP and NO, with opioids, somatostatin, and adenosine triphosphate (ATP) playing a secondary role. Receptive relaxation of the proximal stomach in response to esophageal distension is mediated by VIP and NO and can be blocked experimentally by VIP antagonists and by NO synthase inhibitors.

Hormonal Mechanisms

Hormonal mechanisms are brought into play when they are released from the small intestine. The two most important hormones in regulating motility are motilin and cholecystokinin.

MOTILIN Motilin, a 22-amino-acid peptide released from the intestine in response to alkalinization, activates specific receptors on smooth muscle cells of the proximal stomach to cause contraction, hence accelerating the emptying of liquid from the stomach.

CHOLECYSTOKININ   One of the physiological actions of CCK is to delay gastric emptying. CCK is released from the duodenum in response to fat, amino acids, and acid. The mechanism of CCK inhibition of gastric emptying appears to be indirect, mediated through its effect on afferent sensory neurons (Figure 2.12).

Control of Gastric Emptying

Different regions of the stomach tend to be responsible for different functions. For example, the proximal stomach (fundus and body) primarily controls the emptying of liquids, while the distal stomach (antropyloric segment) handles the emptying of solids.

Emptying of Liquids

When a volume of liquid enters the stomach, it is "accommodated" in the proximal stomach, which relaxes to

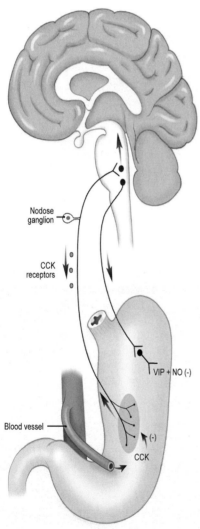

FIGURE 2.12. Cholecystokinin (CCK) is a major inhibitor of gastric emptying. This CCK action is mediated through its effect on long vagal reflexes. Abbreviations: NO, nitric oxide; VIP, vasoactive intestinal polypeptide.

receive it. As a result, the intragastric pressure is not elevated. To empty liquid from the stomach, contraction of the proximal stomach is necessary to create a pressure gradient between this region and the distal part of the stomach. This is accomplished through the release of excitatory neurotransmitters and motilin. Gastric emptying of liquids is accelerated following vagotomy and pyloroplasty because receptive relaxation of the proximal stomach is lost. The effect of proximal gastric vagotomy on the emptying of liquids is modest, indicating the importance of the pyloric sphincter. CCK is a potent inhibitor of the emptying of liquids.

Gastric emptying of liquid can be measured by instilling a liquid meal with a nonabsorbable marker through a nasogastric tube, then aspirating residual volume after fixed periods of time. Clinically, two other tests are more useful. Perhaps the best clinical test is a radioscintigraphic measurement using a gamma camera and a [133]In-labeled liquid meal (Figure 2.13A). Ultrasound is another useful technique but, unfortunately, this noninvasive test is difficult to standardize.

Emptying of Solids

The emptying of solids is primarily under the control of the antropyloric segment, which mixes, grinds, and propels food into the duodenum. Normally, the food has to be ground to particles of less than 1 mm before being emptied into the duodenum. The emptying of solids is also inhibited by CCK. A number of primary (e.g., idiopathic gastroparesis) and secondary (e.g., diabetic gastroparesis) motor disorders interfere with the normal emptying of solids.

Clinically, the rate of gastric emptying of solids can be estimated radiologically using solid food impregnated with barium. A more useful and quantitative technique is the use of the radioscintigraphic testing employing ^{99m}Tc-labeled solid meal (Figure 2.13B).

Pyloric Sphincter

The pyloric sphincter is interposed between the stomach and duodenum and lies at the level of T12, slightly to the right of the midline. It is made up of a condensation of circular muscle, which forms a palpable structure at the distal end of the stomach. As the antrum ends at the pyloric sphincter, the narrow pyloric channel is formed.

Pyloric contraction and relaxation are coordinated with gastric motility by the gastric pacemaker on the greater curvature of the stomach. In humans, the pyloric sphincter opens and closes every 20 seconds. Closure is accomplished by contraction of the sphincter, which is under sympathetic innervation with noradrenalin and, perhaps also, substance P as the neurotransmitters. Relaxation of the sphincter is under vagal control, with VIP and

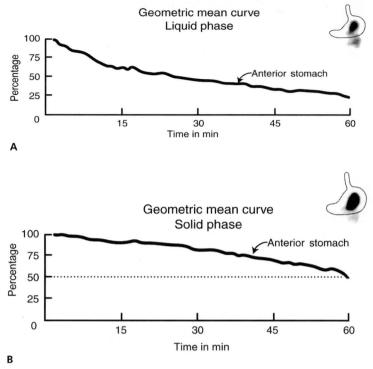

FIGURE 2.13. Measurement of gastric emptying of liquid. (A) One way the liquid can be measured is with a radioscintigraphic measurement using a gamma camera and a ^{133}In-labeled liquid meal. Fifty percent of the liquid meal had emptied from the stomach in approximately 23 minutes. (B) The rate of gastric emptying of solids can be measured using radioscintigraphic testing with a ^{99m}Tc-labeled solid meal. Fifty percent of the solid meal had emptied in 60 minutes. (Courtesy of Henry I. Goldberg, MD.)

NO acting as neurotransmitters. In addition, reflexes originating in the proximal part of the duodenum participate in both contraction and relaxation of the sphincter. Truncal vagotomy, which vagally denervates the entire stomach, including the antropyloric complex, causes closure of the sphincter due to unopposed action of sympathetic innervation. Unless vagotomy is accompanied by gastric drainage, accomplished by either destruction of the sphincter (pyloroplasty) or bypass (gastrojejunostomy), delayed gastric emptying and stasis result.

PATHOPHYSIOLOGY

Clinical abnormalities are associated with several disorders of secretion, motility, or cell growth.

SECRETORY DISORDERS

Abnormalities of Acid Secretion

Hypersecretion

Some 25% of duodenal ulcer patients are hypersecretors of acid; that is, they have a maximal acid output greater than 30 mEq/h following maximal stimulation with histamine or gastrin. Even so, it is not clear that hypersecretion of acid is the cause of these ulcers. Indeed, many of these patients may be infected with *H. pylori*, and the increased acid output in response to exogenous stimulants may represent an increased population of parietal cells secondary to *H. pylori*-induced chronic hypergastrinemia. Significant hypersecretion of acid occurs in Zollinger-Ellison syndrome and in the rare disease of systemic mastocytosis.

Altered Secretion

Infection with *H. pylori* (Figure 2.14) leads to a marked decrease in the number of somatostatin-secreting D cells. This, in turn, leads to hypergastrinemia because the negative feedback mechanism that depends on somatostatin release in response to acidification of antral D cells is diminished or lost. The resultant chronic basal hypergastrinemia has two consequences that may be important in

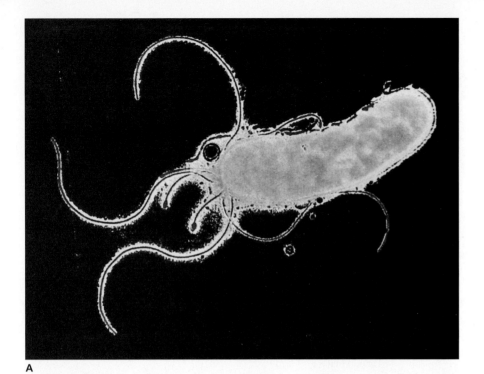

A

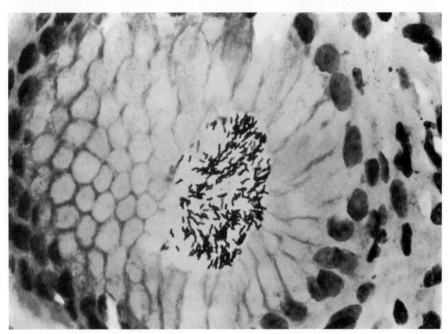

B

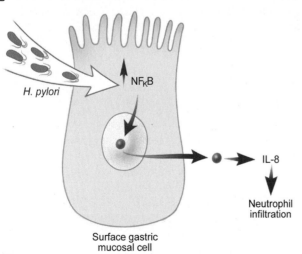

C

FIGURE 2.14. Identification and mechanism of *Helicobacter pylori*. (A) *H. pylori* is a gram-negative flagellate rod. (B) It can survive under the mucosal layer of the stomach and within gastric pits because of its ability to emit ammonium, which protects it from the acidic environment. The damage to surface gastric mucosal cells is mediated through the release of interleukin-8 (IL-8), elaborated through the action of NF$_K$B. (C) The same mechanism probably operates in the destruction of the delta cells in the antrum. (2.14B is reprinted with permission from Genta RM, Graham DY. Images in clinical medicine. Helicobacter pylori in a gastric pit. *N Engl J Med* 1996;335:250.)

Labels in figure C: H. pylori, NF$_K$B, IL-8, Neutrophil infiltration, Surface gastric mucosal cell causing peptic ulcer. First, an inappropriate level of acid secretion is present in the basal (fasting) state, when little or no acid should be secreted. Second, in response to the trophic action of chronic hypergastrinemia, parietal cell hyperplasia develops. Hence, the acid factor is important in peptic ulcer due to *H. pylori*.

Hyposecretion

Hyposecretion of acid is caused by atrophic gastritis, including that associated with pernicious anemia. More than two-thirds of patients with carcinoma of the stomach also have acid hyposecretion. The association of atrophic gastritis and pernicious anemia with carcinoma of the stomach is well known. Gastric acid hyposecretion is also seen in hypoparathyroidism and may develop following ulcer surgery (e.g., vagotomy, gastrectomy).

Abnormalities of Intrinsic Factor Secretion

Intrinsic factor (IF) is secreted by the parietal cells. Conditions in which the number of parietal cells is reduced, such as atrophic gastritis, are associated with pernicious anemia. IF is required as a cofactor for the absorption of vitamin B_{12} in the terminal ileum.

Acid-Peptic Disease

Erosions and Ulcers

As described above, the integrity of the gastroduodenal mucosa can be thought of as an equilibrium that must be maintained between the aggressive factors, principally acid and pepsin, and mucosal defense mechanisms. This equilibrium can be disturbed by either excessive or unregulated production of acid and pepsin secretion or by failure of one or more of the defense mechanisms. Erosions are defined as mucosal defects superficial to the muscularis mucosa, while ulcers are defects that reach deeper beyond the muscularis mucosa.

EROSIVE GASTRITIS The development of numerous mucosal erosions results in erosive gastritis. The most common cause of erosive gastritis is now the ingestion of NSAIDs. In the past, erosive gastritis was a frequent cause of massive upper gastrointestinal hemorrhage in certain clinical settings before the routine practice of prophylactic use of antacids, H_2-receptor antagonists, or proton-pump inhibitors in these clinical settings. Patients most susceptible to erosive gastritis and its complications include: (1) ICU patients with multiple organ system failure; (2) those with severe systemic sepsis; (3) those with major burns (e.g., Curling's ulcer); (4) those with widespread metastases; and (5) those with head injury or increased intracranial pressure (i.e., Cushing's ulcer).

Several different mechanisms probably underlie the pathogenesis of erosive gastritis. NSAIDs cause it by abolishing mucosal prostaglandin synthesis, which results in decreased production of bicarbonate and mucus and in disruption of the maintenance of the mucosal gel layer. The mechanisms by which systemic sepsis, major burn, and widespread metastases cause erosive gastritis are not well understood, but they probably include decreased mucosal defense due to reduced mucosal blood flow, interference with postmucosal defense mechanisms, and the effects of cytokines. Erosions and ulcers associated with head injury and increased intracranial pressure tend to be caused by increased vagal stimulation of acid and can be effectively prevented by the use of anticholinergics.

PEPTIC ULCERATION The discovery of *H. pylori* as a primary cause of peptic ulceration has revolutionized concepts of the pathophysiology of peptic ulcer. Overproduction of gastric acid is no longer thought to be the dominant factor in peptic ulceration. Acid and pepsin, however, are always required to cause ulceration. The old adage "no acid, no ulcer" is still valid today. Even in *H. pylori*—caused peptic ulcer, the production of acid in the fasting state is one important factor. Some 20%–25% of peptic ulcers are not caused by *H. pylori*. Next, the three important mechanisms in the etiology of peptic ulcer: *H. pylori*, NSAIDs, and acid hypersecretion are discussed.

Causes of Peptic Ulcer

The causes of peptic ulcer are summarized in Table 2.6.

HELICOBACTER PYLORI *H. pylori* is a spiral-shaped, gram-negative motile rod capable of penetrating the mucous gel layer lining the gastric mucosa to lie in the gastric pits (Figure 2.14). Its survival in this location is due to its potent urease activity, which splits ammonia from urea to create a neutral or alkali medium to surround and protect it from acid. The bacterium is found in 90% of patients with duodenal ulcer, 80% of those with gastric

---

TABLE 2.6. Causes of Peptic Ulcer

H. pylori
  Involved in 90% of duodenal ulcers, 80% of gastric ulcers
  Causes hypergastrinemia and increased basal acid secretion because of destruction of D cells that secrete somatostatin
  Also causes gastritis

Nonsteroidal anti-inflammatory drugs
  Increasingly important cause in elderly patients
  Damage mucosal defense mechanisms by inhibiting prostaglandin release, leading to decreased production of bicarbonate and mucus

Zollinger–Ellison syndrome
  Rare cause because of pancreatic or duodenal gastrinoma

Idiopathic acid hypersecretion

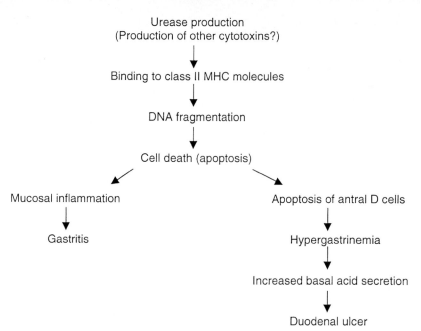

FIGURE 2.15. Mechanism of action of *Helicobacter pylori* as a cause of gastritis and duodenal ulcer. Abbreviation: MHC, major histocompatibility complex.

ulcer, and 100% of those with gastritis. Eradication of *H. pylori* effectively prevents ulcer recurrence after successful therapy with acid-reducing drugs.

Mechanisms of Action The mechanisms by which the bacterium causes gastritis and duodenal ulcer are likely to differ, because the infection in both cases is in the stomach only and not in both. The development of gastritis is thought to be related to urease activity, which binds to Class II major histocompatability complex (MHC) molecules to cause DNA fragmentation and apoptosis. Infection with *H. pylori* may also stimulate secretion of a variety of cytotoxins that damage mucosal membrane. The result is the development of inflammation. But how can we explain development of duodenal ulcer when the infection is in the antrum and not in the duodenum? A partial explanation can be given as follows: In the gastric antrum, D cells that release somatostatin are selectively destroyed, disrupting the inhibitory regulation somatostatin exerts on the G cells and abolishing the negative-feedback regulation of gastrin by antral acidification. The result is development of mild hypergastrinemia in the fasting state and postprandially. The fasting hypergastrinemia stimulates acid secretion continuously in the basal state. This altered secretion of acid is probably important in causing duodenal ulcer (Figure 2.15).

NONSTEROIDAL ANTI-INFLAMMATORY DRUGS NSAIDs have become an increasingly important cause of peptic ulcer and its complications of perforation and bleeding. Patterns of use of these drugs have given rise to an increased incidence of complicated peptic ulcer in the older population and in women.

Mechanisms of Action The mechanism by which NSAIDs cause ulceration is twofold: (1) prostaglandin generation within the gastric mucosa is abolished, and, as a result (2) the mucous gel layer is destroyed, with decreased production of mucus and bicarbonate. The incidence of bleeding from NSAIDs is twice as high as when the patient has concurrent infection with *H. pylori*.

ACID HYPERSECRETION Although some individuals are hypersecretors of acid for no known reason, the most common cause of hypersecretion is the Zollinger-Ellison syndrome. In addition, other rare causes of hypergastrinemia (Table 2.7) and systemic mastocytosis may cause hypersecretion of acid.

Abnormalities of Gastrin Secretion

Hypersecretion of Gastrin

Hypergastrinemia may be associated with acid hypersecretion or hyposecretion. From the surgeon's perspective, Zollinger–Ellison syndrome is the most important cause. In the days when gastrectomy was performed frequently, the "retained gastric antrum syndrome" used to be encountered. In this condition, now extremely rare, the terminal portion of the antrum is inadvertently left with the duodenum when Bilroth II gastrectomy is performed. The patient with the retained antrum, which is chronically bathed in alkaline pancreatic juice, develops G-cell hyperplasia that leads to hypergastrinemia. Hypergastrinemia can also be caused by gastric outlet obstruction and chronic renal failure. It may also develop after massive small bowel resection, perhaps because the site of produc-

TABLE 2.7. Essentials: Causes of Hypergastrinemia

Associated with gastric acid hypersecretion
  Zollinger–Ellison syndrome (gastrinoma)
  Retained gastric antrum syndrome
  Antral G cell hyperplasia/hyperfunction
  Gastric outlet obstruction
  H. pylori infection
  Chronic renal failure
  Post-massive small bowel resection

Associated with gastric acid hyposecretion
  Atrophic gastritis
  - Idiopathic pernicious anemia
  - Autoimmune pernicious anemia
  Iatrogenic
  - Antisecretory therapy
  - H^+K^+ATPase inhibitors
  - Histamine H_2-receptor antagonists
  - Postvagotomy

tion of inhibitory substances is removed and because the small bowel is an important site of gastrin degradation.

Two hypergastrinemic states associated with hyposecretion of acid are important for the surgeon to consider. First, the most common cause of hypergastrinemia in patients with gastroesophageal disease referred for surgical consultation is now chronic therapy with H^+K^+ATPase inhibitors. If the diagnosis of Zollinger–Ellison syndrome cannot be readily excluded, serum gastrin levels need to be measured again 2 to 3 weeks following discontinuation of H^+K^+ATPase inhibitor therapy. Alternatively, a secretin test may be performed. Intravenous administration of secretin causes an increase in plasma gastrin in Zollinger–Ellison syndrome but results in either no change or a decrease when the cause of hypergastrinemia is other than gastrinoma.

Hyposecretion of Gastrin

No known pathological condition is associated with hyposecretion of gastrin. Antrectomy lowers plasma gastrin level basally and in response to a meal. Even then, because gastrin is also formed in the duodenum, significant levels of plasma gastrin are maintained. However, the dominant molecular form of gastrin is now the larger form, and the levels of G-17 gastrin are significantly depressed. Release of gastrin is inhibited by an increase in levels of somatostatin brought about during therapy with the long-acting somatostatin analogue octreotide and in hypersomatostatinemia associated with somatostatinoma.

MOTOR DISORDERS OF THE STOMACH

Motor disorders of the stomach continue to be a major therapeutic challenge to the gastroenterologist as well as the surgeon. Both delayed and rapid gastric emptying can cause clinical problems. With the decline in ulcer surgery (vagotomy and drainage or gastrectomy), the incidence of pathologically rapid gastric emptying, known as "the dumping syndrome," has also declined. Problems related to poor gastric emptying, however, constitute a difficult and recalcitrant problem for clinicians.

Delayed Gastric Emptying

Delayed gastric emptying can be due to either primary or secondary motor disorders. The primary disorders include idiopathic gastroparesis, gastroparesis associated with pseudo-obstruction of the intestine, and gastroparesis due to functional dyspepsia. Few patients with this disorder are referred for surgical treatment. Of the secondary motor disorders, the surgeon is most familiar with postoperative and postradiation gastroparesis. Delayed gastric emptying can also be caused by a variety of clinical conditions, including diabetes mellitus (the diabetic gastroparesis syndrome), metabolic disorders (e.g., thyroid disease), and CNS diseases (e.g., psychogenic, intracranial lesions). Drugs, particularly opioids and tricyclics, can also delay gastric emptying. An uncommon form of gastroparesis occurs secondary to disturbed electrical rhythm of the stomach. These disturbances include tachygastria (BER frequency faster than 5 cycles/min); bradygastria (BER frequency slower than 2 cycles/min); or gastric arrhythmia, in which the rhythm is irregular and disorganized.

Rapid Gastric Emptying or "Dumping Syndrome"

The dumping syndrome is one of the undesirable sequelae of gastric surgery. The most common causes are truncal vagotomy and drainage, and gastrectomy with gastroduodenal (Bilroth I) or gastrojejunal reconstruction (Bilroth II). Vagotomy also leads to a loss of receptive relaxation (i.e., accommodation), so that ingestion of food, particularly liquids, raises the intragastric pressure and causes rapid emptying of chyme into the intestine. This is especially true when the pylorus has been destroyed or resected. The "dumping" of high osmolar chyme into the duodenum or jejunum causes two significant responses. First, fluid is drawn into the gut lumen from the circulation, causing hypovolemia, tachycardia, sweating, a sensation of epigastric bloating, and fatigue. Second, the rapid entry of hyperosmolar solution into the intestine causes the release of vasoactive amines and such peptides as VIP and neurotensin. Systemic vasodilation is induced, and this response causes further reduction of circulating volume. Another feature of the dumping syndrome is flushing, caused by increased levels of circulating vasoactive amines and peptides. The dumping syndrome may also cause urgent diarrhea.

It must be noted that proximal gastric (highly selective) vagotomy is not associated with increased incidence of rapid gastric emptying compared with preoperative prevalence.

ACID-PEPTIC DISORDERS

Erosive Gastritis

Prevention

The incidence of life-threatening bleeding in ICUs from erosive gastritis and stress ulceration has declined dramatically since the adoption of routine prophylactic acid-reducing therapy in all high-risk patients. The practice now is to keep the intragastric pH above 4.5 using antacids, H_2-receptor antagonists, or proton-pump inhibitors.

Clinical Presentation

The most important presenting problem is bleeding in the form of hematemesis. Many patients on NSAIDs may also complain of epigastric pain. The extent of bleeding may be minor or catastrophic. Occasionally, the bleeding may present as severe lower GI bleeding; therefore, as a precaution, a nasogastric tube is inserted in any patient with major lower GI bleeding. Invariably the surgeon is called upon when conventional attempts at controlling hemorrhage have failed.

Management

When bleeding is massive, the critically ill patient is treated with a well-known protocol of resuscitation techniques: protect the airway, assess the amount of blood loss, and correct blood volume before undertaking any serious investigation of the cause of bleeding. The ideal time to perform emergency upper GI endoscopy is when the patient is hemodynamically stable and when gastric lavage aspirates are pink. Endoscopy results usually show punctate erosions with or without bleeding (Figure 2.16). The lesions tend to cover the mucosa of the proximal stomach. At times, severe bleeding from one or more of the erosions may be visible.

Treatment is almost always nonsurgical and includes: (1) discontinuation of NSAIDs and treatment of underlying sepsis or multiple organ failure; (2) institution of acid-reducing measures to maintain gastric pH levels above 4.5; and (3) endoscopic control using vasoconstrictor injection therapy (adrenalin 1:1000), heater or laser coagulation therapy, and so on). Surgery is indicated only if all of the above measures fail and life-threatening bleeding continues. Surgical options include: (1) gastrotomy and suture control of major bleeding sites with or without addition of truncal vagotomy and pyloroplasty; and (2) total gastrectomy, which, although rarely used, may be the only life-saving procedure in certain cases.

Peptic Ulcer Disease

Gastric vs. Duodenal Ulcer

Many specialists consider gastric and duodenal ulceration to be two distinctly different diseases. Whether this is true or not, important clinical differences exist between a gastric and a duodenal ulcer. First, whenever faced with a patient who has gastric ulcer, the physician must rule out the diagnosis of carcinoma by endoscopic biopsy and brushing. The incidence of benign gastric ulcer turning malignant is extraordinarily small (<1.0%). Chances that a seemingly benign ulcerating gastric lesion may be malignant, however, are much higher.

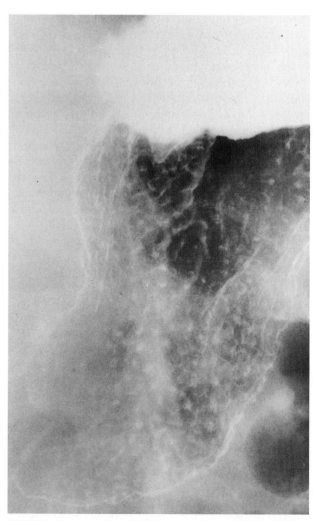

FIGURE 2.16. In erosive gastritis, upper GI endoscopy usually shows punctate erosions covering the mucosa of the proximal stomach. Bleeding from one or more of the erosions may be visible. Air-barium upper GI series also provides an overall map of the extent of gastric erosions (multiple punctate barium collections). (Courtesy of Henry I. Goldberg, MD.)

Other differences relate to complications caused by the two types of ulcer. Bleeding from a gastric ulcer may be more serious and less likely to stop spontaneously compared to a duodenal ulcer. Gastric outlet obstruction is more a feature of duodenal ulcer than of gastric ulcer. Perforation is more common with a duodenal ulcer and, at surgery, whenever possible, a gastric ulcer must be excised or removed with the gastrectomy specimen to be sure it is not malignant. In gastric ulcers located high in the body of the stomach, where resection of the ulcer is not feasible, four-quadrant biopsy is necessary.

Finally, the response to surgical therapy of the two types of ulceration is different. While proximal gastric vagotomy is a highly satisfactory operation for duodenal ulcer, it is less effective for treating gastric ulcer. In prepyloric ulcers, for example, proximal gastric vagotomy is associated with ulcer recurrence rates of 25% to 40%.[2] When surgery is indicated, the majority of gastric ulcers are most reliably treated by antrectomy and Bilroth I anastomosis, thus removing the ulcer completely.

Clinical Presentation

The characteristic ulcer symptom is a "burning" epigastric pain that usually develops when the stomach is empty, often waking the patient in the early morning hours. The pain is relieved by eating, drinking milk, or by taking antacids. Occasionally, pain is precipitated by eating food, but this is rare and is more likely to happen with a gastric ulcer. The pain may be aggravated by NSAIDs, spicy foods, and major life stresses. The pain is usually felt in the epigastrium over a limited area. When the pain radiates to the back (usually T12 to L1 region), it suggests the presence of a posterior penetrating ulcer. In peptic ulcer disease, physical findings are usually absent except for a mild epigastric tenderness and spasm of the right rectus. It is generally impossible to distinguish between gastric and duodenal ulceration on the basis of symptoms alone.

Occasionally, the first sign presented is the complication of either perforation or bleeding. Bleeding may be occult, with iron-deficiency anemia as the presenting problem. Physicians have often noticed that patients with acutely bleeding ulcer rarely complain of pain. The previous statements notwithstanding, most individuals with ulcer disease experience worsening of their pain preceding the development of perforation or bleeding. The development of gastric outlet obstruction is gradual over several months or even years. Patients first experience early satiety, particularly with meals containing meat. Vomiting is occasional in the early stages and typically occurs after the evening meal. With time, vomiting becomes progressive. Weight loss and fatigue follow. When vomiting is prolonged, dehydration and hypokalemic metabolic alkalosis develop.

Management of Uncomplicated Peptic Ulcer

Thanks to the pharmaceutical and microbiological advances of the past 15 to 20 years, nearly all patients with uncomplicated peptic ulcer are successfully treated with medications. Intractability of symptoms as an indication for surgery is now exceedingly rare. Ironically and somewhat historically significant is that the development of proximal gastric vagotomy, a physiologically-based elective ulcer operation without serious side effects, coincided with the advent of powerful and effective acid-reducing drugs—first the H_2-receptor antagonists and then the proton pump inhibitors.

UPPER GASTROINTESTINAL ENDOSCOPY Upper GI endoscopy, the most specific examination, can rule out esophageal diseases as well as gastritis, identify the ulcer, and obtain gastric mucosal biopsies for detection of *H. pylori*. If the ulcer is gastric, several biopsies and brushings of the ulcer need to be taken for cytological examination. The size of the pyloric channel can be assessed and the duodenum examined for presence of an ulcer.

BARIUM MEAL The use of the barium meal to diagnose peptic ulcer has declined with advances in fiberoptic endoscopy. A gastric ulcer usually shows as a niche along the lesser curvature, with the barium extending outward beyond the stomach. In contrast, the floor of an ulcer crater that is malignant does not extend outside the lesser curvature (Carlan's sign). Radiating mucosal folds from the ulcer may be apparent when seen *en face*. In duodenal ulcers, a barium-filled crater and deformity of the duodenal cap are typical signs. The presence of stenosis or gastric outlet obstruction can also be assessed.

DETECTION OF HELICOBACTER PYLORI Three tests are available to assess the presence of *H. pylori*: endoscopic biopsy, the breath test, and ELISA antibody testing.

Endoscopic Biopsy Mucosal biopsy specimens can be examined histologically for the presence of bacterium and gastritis. The best use of the biopsy specimen is to perform a urease test, in which the specimen is placed in a solution of urea containing a pH indicator. If urease is present, ammonia is generated from the urea, causing the solution to turn more alkali. The urease test is highly specific and sensitive. A biopsy specimen can also be cultured to grow the bacterium. While highly specific, culture has very low sensitivity.

Breath Test Urea labeled with either ^{14}C or ^{13}C is administered with a meal. If *H. pylori* infection is present, its urease will cleave the labeled urea, releasing labeled bicarbonate that is then converted into labeled expired CO_2. The great value of this test is that it can be used serially to assess the efficacy of *H. pylori* eradication therapy.

ELISA Antibody Test *H. pylori* infection leads to the development of antibodies that can be detected in the blood. The ELISA antibody test is not as useful as the breath test to monitor response to *H. pylori* eradication because antibody titers in the blood decrease slowly.

GASTRIC ACID SECRETORY STUDIES Gastric acid secretory studies were once used to determine the type of ulcer surgery to be performed. The premise has never been valid and the practice has been discontinued. At present, the most important use of gastric acid secretory studies is in determining whether hypergastrinemia detected by radioimmunoassay is associated with acid hypersecretion or with hypochlorhydria and achlorhydria. For example, patients with Zollinger–Ellison syndrome typically have high basal secretion of acid (20–30 mEq/h). The basal secretion is typically greater than 60% of the maximal acid output in response to histamine or pentagastrin (30–50 mEq/h). The only other clinical setting in which acid secretory studies may be useful is assessing the completeness of vagotomy in patients who have developed a recurrent ulcer after previous vagotomy. The best test in this regard is the "sham feeding test," in which patients are asked to chew but not to swallow food. This procedure activates the cephalic phase of acid secretion and, if intact vagal fibers are present, sham feeding stimulates acid secretion. Previously used tests that involved insulin-induced hypoglycemia to stimulate central vagal centers are rarely chosen because of the inherent danger of a hypoglycemic crisis.

ELECTIVE SURGERY FOR PEPTIC ULCER DISEASE As mentioned, elective surgery for duodenal ulcer is rare because of the efficacy of acid-reducing drugs and the eradication of *H. pylori*. Intractability is now rarely seen, but it has four prerequisites as determined by the patient and his or her doctor. These include: (1) the ulcer persists despite eradication of *H. pylori*; (2) pain persists despite well-planned medical management under the care of a gastroenterologist; (3) the patient is unable to work; and (4) the patient senses an inability to enjoy life and a serious loss of well being.

Intractability is easier to define in the case of a gastric ulcer because, in addition to the symptomatic criteria, the size of the ulcer and progress of healing can be followed endoscopically. If a gastric ulcer has diminished in size but has not healed completely after a course of 6 to 8 weeks of intense medical therapy with proton pump inhibitors, a second course of treatment for 6 to 8 weeks is indicated, provided that biopsy and brushings are negative for cancer. If, at the end of the second course of treatment, the ulcer has still not healed completely, the safest course of action is to perform resection because malignancy cannot be excluded. A list of the elective surgical options for peptic ulcer is shown in Table 2.8. In all nonhealing ulcers, fasting plasma gastrin levels should be measured.

TABLE 2.8. Types of Elective Peptic Ulcer Surgery

Type of ulcer	Operation	Operative mortality	Ulcer recurrence
Duodenal	PGV	<0.1%	10%–15%
	TV	<1.0%	8%–10%
	V & A	1.0%–2.0%	<0.5%
Gastric			
Type I	BI	1.0%	1.0%
Type II	BI	1.0%	Unknown
Type III	V & A	1.0%–2.0%	0.5%

Abbreviations: BI, Bilroth I gastrectomy; PGV, proximal gastric vagotomy; TV, truncal vagotomy; V & A, vagotomy and antrectomy.

ELECTIVE SURGICAL PROCEDURES FOR DUODENAL ULCER

Proximal Gastric Vagotomy It is generally agreed that proximal gastric vagotomy (PGV)—also known as highly selective vagotomy (HSV) or parietal cell vagotomy (PCV)—is the elective surgical treatment of choice for duodenal ulcer because it has the lowest operative mortality (<0.1%) and few, if any, side effects.[3] The long-term sequelae of vagotomy and gastrectomy (e.g., dumping syndrome, diarrhea, anemia, weight loss, and so on) are not seen with PGV. On the other hand, the operation must be performed meticulously by well-trained surgeons. PGV can be done via laparotomy or laparoscopically. The advantage of the laparoscopic approach is that visibility is improved by magnification, and both hospital stay and postoperative pain are significantly reduced. Again, it is important that only well-trained laparoscopic surgeons perform laparoscopic PGV. Whether the operation is done "open" or laparoscopically, the approach is identical (Figure 2.17).

Truncal Vagotomy and Drainage Truncal vagotomy and drainage should be used only for selected patients in the elective setting, usually if the operating surgeon's experience with PGV is limited. Before embarking on pyloroplasty, the surgeon should carefully inspect the first part of the duodenum. If there is an associated inflammatory mass or very severe distortion from strictures, the preferred drainage procedure is gastrojejunostomy rather than pyloroplasty. In this way, the surgeon avoids the problem of a difficult pyloroplasty or duodenal stump closure.

Selective Total Gastric Vagotomy Selective total gastric vagotomy divides the vagal trunks below the origin of the hepatic branches (anterior vagus) and celiac branches (posterior vagus). This procedure is now only of historic importance. Like truncal vagotomy, it requires a drainage procedure because the entire stomach is vagally denervated. Hence, it has the same potential to cause dumping syndrome. Unlike truncal vagotomy, however, it preserves the extragastric fibers that supply the liver, biliary tree, pancreas, and small intestine. Consequently, the incidence of postvagotomy diarrhea is significantly lower after selective total gastric vagotomy than after truncal vagotomy.

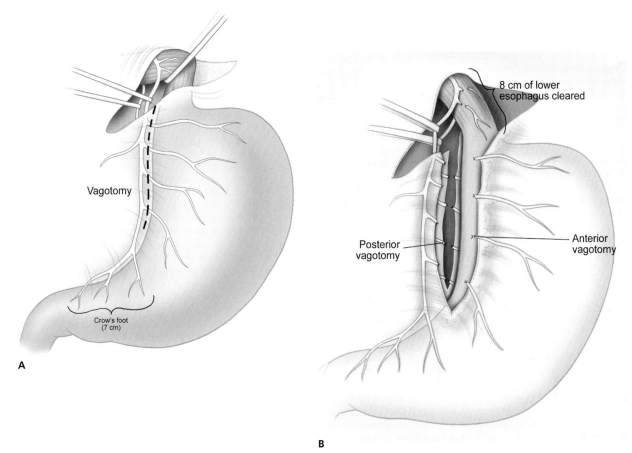

FIGURE 2.17. Proximal gastric vagotomy. (A and B) The key elements of proximal gastric vagotomy are to divide the gastric branches of the anterior and posterior vagi at the lesser curvature while preserving the nerve of Latarjet and the innervation of the antral pyloric mechanism. Another key feature of this operation is "skeletonization" of the distal 6–8 cm of the esophagus. (Adapted from Jamieson GG, Debas HT, eds. Rob & Smith's Operative Surgery: Surgery of the Upper Gastrointestinal Tract. London: Chapman & Hall Medical; 1994.)

Truncal Vagotomy and Antrectomy From the acid-reducing perspective and that of postoperative recurrence of ulcer, truncal vagotomy and antrectomy comprise the superior procedure for duodenal ulcer. It removes both the vagal (cholinergic) and gastrin drive of acid secretion. The ulcer recurrence rate is <0.5%.[4] The problem with the operation is that it creates the potential for the side effects of both vagotomy and gastrectomy. For this reason, it should be used rarely to treat uncomplicated duodenal ulcer.

Relative Merits of Operative Procedures Worldwide, PGV is the elective operation of choice for duodenal ulcer. It has the lowest operative mortality rate and is not associated with the undesirable side effects seen with other procedures (e.g., dumping syndrome, diarrhea). Unfortunately, patients treated with PGV have a higher recurrence rate (5% to 20%); now that elective surgery for duodenal ulcer is rare, few surgeons are appropriately trained to perform PGV.[5] Hence, truncal vagotomy and drainage

(TV), a simpler operation to do, has retained popularity, particularly in the United States. It has a low operative mortality, and the incidence of ulcer recurrence is 8% to 10%.[4] Looseness of bowel occurs in some 10% to 15% of patients after the operation, but 1% develop debilitating diarrhea postvagotomy.[4] The dumping syndrome is a problem in 5% to 10% of patients.[4] Selective total vagotomy is the most appropriate type of vagotomy to be combined with antrectomy because it preserves hepatic, biliary, pancreatic, and intestinal vagal innervation. It also reduces the incidence of postoperative diarrhea.

None of these operations are as effective as vagotomy and antrectomy (V & A) in preventing ulcer recurrence. Unfortunately, the low ulcer recurrence rate of <0.5% comes at the expense of long-term complications from both vagotomy and gastrectomy.

ELECTIVE SURGICAL PROCEDURES FOR GASTRIC ULCER
While vagotomy is the cornerstone of elective surgery for

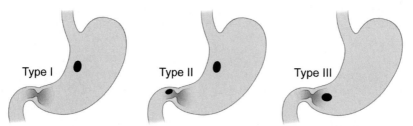

FIGURE 2.18. Types of gastric ulcer. Type I gastric ulcer, one of the most common varieties, occurs in the antrum of the stomach. In Type II gastric ulcer, the ulcer in the antrum is associated with an ulcer in the duodenum. Type III gastric ulcer is a prepyloric ulcer.

duodenal ulcer, gastric resection is often more appropriate to treat patients with gastric ulcer. Two reasons support this philosophy. First, unlike duodenal ulcer, where increased or inappropriate acid secretion is invariably a factor, gastric ulcer appears to be associated more with reduced mucosal defense. Second, although a duodenal ulcer is nearly always benign, a gastric ulcer can be malignant. Resection provides the best chance for the diagnosis and cure of gastric ulcer.

Types of Gastric Ulcer Three types of gastric ulcer have been described; they are designated as Type I, Type II, and Type III (Figure 2.18).

1. Type I, the most common type of gastric ulcer, occurs at the lesser curvature and is typically found in the transitional mucosa between the body of the stomach and the antrum.
2. Type II is a gastric ulcer that coexists with a duodenal ulcer.
3. Type III is a prepyloric or pyloric channel ulcer that seems to be associated with gastric acid hypersecretion.

Choice of Operation The operation of choice differs for these three types of gastric ulcer. The best surgical procedure for Type I ulcer is conservative distal gastrectomy, which can often be limited to antrectomy. A gastroduodenal anastomosis is associated with fewer long-term complications, and so is preferred over a gastrojejunal anastomosis.

Patients with Type II gastric ulcers are also best treated with conservative distal gastrectomy and gastroduodenal anastomosis. Some surgeons add truncal vagotomy to this procedure because gastric acid hypersecretion is frequently seen with this type of ulcer. Any benefits of truncal vagotomy may be outweighed by the long-term sequelae of postvagotomy diarrhea. A large clinical experience is now documented to indicate that PGV as the only operation is inappropriate in this setting because ulcer recurrence in patients approaches 40%.[4]

Patients with Type III gastric ulcers are more definitively treated with vagotomy and antrectomy. Ideally, a selective gastric vagotomy should be done to preserve extragastric vagal innervation and minimize the incidence of postvagotomy diarrhea.

Management of Complicated Peptic Ulcer

MANAGEMENT OF PERFORATED PEPTIC ULCER Perforation still occurs commonly and continues to be a lethal complication of peptic ulcer disease, particularly in elderly patients or when treatment is delayed. Its incidence in elderly patients is rising because of increased use of NSAIDs. Perforated duodenal ulcer is ten times more common than perforated gastric ulcer. The essentials of management are summarized in Table 2.9.

In all abdominal crises, as in multiple trauma, it is helpful to use a consistent approach that includes resuscitation, diagnosis, and treatment.

Resuscitation: Initial and Secondary Assessments The patient is in obvious pain and is anxious. Very quickly, the

TABLE 2.9. Essentials: Management of Perforated Peptic Ulcer
Trends
Overall incidence unchanged
Rising incidence in elderly patients
Mortality rate of 10%
Diagnosis
Usually presents with acute abdomen
If accompanied by hypotension, suspect other diagnoses (ruptured AAA, pancreatitis, mesenteric vascular accident)
If accompanied by blood in nasogastric aspirate, consider "kissing ulcer"
Only 75%–80% show pneumoperitoneum
Operative technique
Duodenal ulcer: Closure of perforation alone or with addition of PGV
Gastric ulcer: Distal gastrectomy to include ulcer or local excision of ulcer
Late perforation: Conservative management if
■ Ulcer is sealed
■ Peritonitis is absent

Abbreviations: AAA, abdominal aortic aneurysm; PGV, proximal gastric vagotomy.

airway and vital signs are assessed. The breathing is shallow and rapid as diaphragmatic movement is restricted, but airway is not usually a problem. A mild tachycardia is present, but during the early phases of perforation, hypotension should not be present. If hypotension is present, other diagnoses should be suspected. These include ruptured abdominal aortic aneurysm, severe acute pancreatitis, and mesenteric vascular accident. The initial survey also reveals the presence of an acute abdomen or peritonitis with board-like abdominal rigidity, tenderness and rebound tenderness, and hypoactive or absent bowel sounds. The patient lies perfectly still, often in the fetal position.

Once the initial examination is completed (it should take no more than 1 or 2 minutes), resuscitation is started with institution of intravenous fluid administration and insertion of a nasogastric tube to decompress the stomach and prevent aspiration.

Secondary assessment should include obtaining a full history and performing a thorough physical examination. A history of previously diagnosed peptic ulcer or peptic ulcer–type symptoms may or may not be present. Florid presentation of an acute abdomen may be absent in a number of patients with special circumstances. These include:

1. the very old or very young patient;
2. any patient who is receiving high-dose steroid therapy, which blunts the peritoneal response;

3. the paraplegic patient, in whom the only symptom may be tip of shoulder pain;
4. the comatose patient, in whom systemic manifestation of sepsis is often the first clue; and
5. the patient recovering from an abdominal operation, where the diagnosis is often delayed as signs and symptoms are assigned to causes related to the recent operation. Thus, the surgical ward may be the worst place for a patient to have a perforated ulcer.

Diagnosis A patient's diagnosis is often established with his or her medical history and the classic findings from the physical examination. The patient may have a slight leukocytosis with some shift to the left and a normal urinalysis, which often suffice in the typical case. Often, however, plain abdominal views (supine, upright, and right decubitus) and a chest x-ray are also obtained. Free gas in the peritoneal cavity is seen in about 75% of patients (Figure 2.19). When perforation is suspected but no free air is seen in the peritoneal cavity, a Gastrografin swallow may be useful. Endoscopy, however, should be avoided. When the presentation is not as clear-cut as described above, other conditions must be included in the differential diagnosis, particularly acute pancreatitis, acute cholecystitis, acute appendicitis, and even acute myocardial infarction. If the serum amylase level is elevated because of a perforated peptic ulcer, the elevation is usually lower than three times the normal level. Leukocytosis tends to be greater in acute pancreatitis. An abdominal ultrasound,

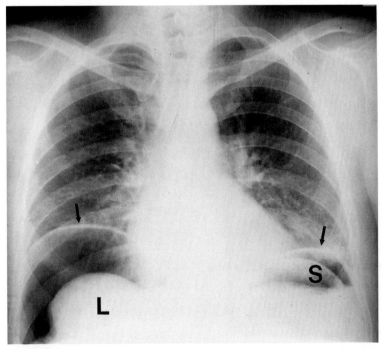

FIGURE 2.19. Perforated peptic ulcer. This condition may be evident from the history and demonstration of classic findings in physical examination. This patient's chest x-ray shows air between the right hemidiaphragm (arrow) and the liver (L) and between the left hemidiaphragm (arrow) and the stomach (S). (Courtesy of Henry I. Goldberg, MD.)

when indicated, is useful in ruling out acute cholecystitis. An electrocardiogram and serum enzymes may be necessary to exclude the diagnosis of acute myocardial infarction.

Once it is decided that an operation will be performed, analgesia and perioperative broad-spectrum antibiotics should be administered.

Surgical Management   Operative closure of the perforation is the definitive treatment. This operation can be done laparoscopically or through a limited epigastric incision, depending on the surgeon's experience. A classic approach to closing a perforated duodenal ulcer is the Graham patch technique (Figure 2.20). Alternatively, the ulcer can be closed primarily and an omental patch applied over the suture line.

A secondary approach is to perform an additional ulcer-reducing procedure. Several prospective randomized clinical trials[6] have documented that the addition of proximal gastric vagotomy (see Figure 2.17) to closure of perforation does not increase the mortality or morbidity of surgical therapy, but reduces postoperative ulcer recurrence from 40% to 50% to approximately 8%. The following conditions must be confirmed before PGV is added to the closure procedure.

1. The perforation must be less than 24 hours old;
2. The patient must be hemodynamically stable and free of any serious cardiac, pulmonary, or renal disease;
3. There must be evidence of ulcer chronicity in either the history or the operative findings of scarring and distortion of the duodenal bulb.

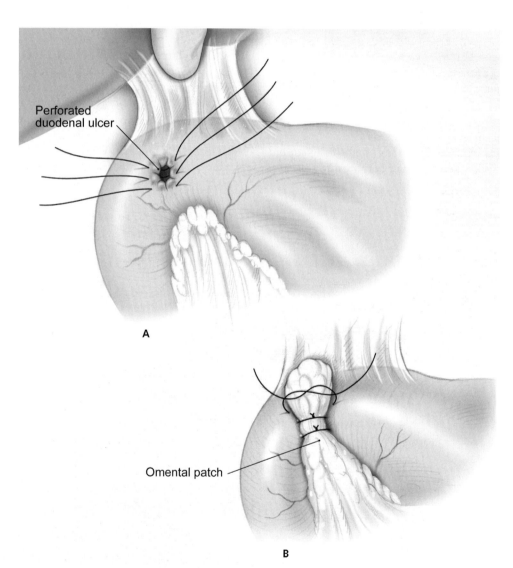

FIGURE 2.20. Graham patch technique. (A and B) This technique provides a safe and established method of closure of perforated duodenal ulcer. The ulcer is closed by sutures applied over a piece of omentum. (Adapted from Schwartz SI, Ellis H, Husser WC, eds. Maingot R. Maingot's Abdominal Operations. Stamford, CT: Appleton & Lange, 1989.)

It must be mentioned, however, that the studies demonstrating the usefulness of PGV were done before the recognition of *H. pylori* as a cause of ulcer and the development of effective eradication therapy to prevent recurrence. Prospective randomized studies are needed to determine whether PGV is necessary in the era of *H. pylori* eradication. The author's view is that performing truncal vagotomy and pyloroplasty when closing the perforation is not an optimal acid-reducing procedure because of the potential for troublesome long-term side effects.

Delayed Perforation A patient with a perforation of 48 hours duration or longer may be treated conservatively with nasogastric suction, intravenous antibiotics, and parenteral nutrition, as long as peritonitis is absent and Gastrografin swallow shows that the perforation is sealed. If a conservative management approach is decided upon, careful follow-up is necessary to detect early development of any abdominal abscess. If an abdominal abscess does develop, diagnosis and treatment by percutaneous catheter can be accomplished with the aid of an abdominal CT scan.

Nonsurgical Management of Perforation From time to time, published clinical studies claim that nonsurgical management is effective. When carefully scrutinized, however, these studies show flaws that make it difficult to accept their recommendations. For example, at the University of Southern California, the Gastrografin swallow test has been used to determine whether the perforation is sealed or not. If the perforation is sealed and peritonitis is not present, conservative management of these selected patients has been used successfully. While this approach may be necessary when operating room capacity is in short supply, it is not recommended for general use.

"Kissing Ulcer" Problem Infrequently, a patient who presents with a perforated duodenal ulcer is found to have blood in the stomach when nasogastric suction is performed. In these circumstances, the old adage applies: "Anterior ulcers perforate and posterior ones bleed." A patient with unequivocal findings of a perforated duodenal ulcer and concomitant bloody nasogastric aspirate must be suspected of having a "kissing ulcer," that is, a perforated anterior ulcer and a bleeding posterior ulcer. At the time of operation, the posterior wall of the first part of the duodenum must be examined by extending the hole from the perforation. In the presence of a bleeding duodenal ulcer, suture control of the bleeding must be accomplished. A definitive ulcer operation is also required. The choices are to close the perforation and duodenotomy with an omental patch and perform proximal gastric vagotomy; or to extend the duodenotomy incision across the pylorus into the stomach, close this with pyloroplasty, and perform truncal vagotomy.

Perforated Gastric Ulcer The above discussion on perforated duodenal ulcer applies equally well to perforated gastric ulcer with one difference.[7] Malignancy, which has an incidence of 15%, must always be ruled out in a perforated gastric ulcer. This can be accomplished by completely excising the ulcer or, alternatively, by four-quadrant biopsy if excision cannot be accomplished successfully. Conservative distal gastrectomy encompassing the ulcer is the initial therapy of choice. If the ulcer is malignant, a more radical type of gastrectomy will be needed.

HEMORRHAGE The most common cause of upper GI hemorrhage is peptic ulcer. Approximately 20% of patients with peptic ulcer will bleed. It is likely that, with *H. pylori* eradication and proton pump inhibitor therapy, the incidence of bleeding will decrease. To date, however, no convincing data support this contention.

Not all bleeding from ulcer is acute or massive. Indeed, some patients present with iron-deficiency anemia from occult blood loss. When acute hemorrhage occurs, patients present with hematemesis and/or melena. Infrequently, massive bleeding from a duodenal ulcer presents as lower gastrointestinal hemorrhage without hematemesis. If the bleeding is rapid, the blood issuing rectally may be red rather than black.

Some 90% of patients admitted with upper GI hemorrhage from an ulcer stop bleeding spontaneously within 8 hours of admission to a hospital. Of the remainder, about half are successfully treated endoscopically with injection therapy or with heater-probe or laser coagulation. The rare patient has such an exsanguinating hemorrhage that immediate operation and control of bleeding is necessary before volume resuscitation can be adequately accomplished. The management is summarized in Table 2.10.

TABLE 2.10. Essentials: Management of Peptic Ulcer Hemorrhage

General
  Bleeding duodenal ulcer: 10 times more common than bleeding gastric ulcer
  90% of patients stop bleeding within 8 h of admission

Endoscopic stigmata of possible further bleeding
  Arterial spurting
  Visible vessel
  Adherent fresh clot at ulcer base

Indications for surgery
  Exsanguinating hemorrhage
  Failure of control with endoscopically administered therapy
  Rebleeding after initial cessation

Choice of operations
  Duodenal ulcer
  ■ Suture control of bleeding and vagotomy and pyloroplasty, or
  ■ Duodenotomy, suture control, and proximal gastric vagotomy
  Gastric ulcer
  ■ Distal gastrectomy including the ulcer

Resuscitation Initial resuscitation should be accomplished quickly. If there is any question about the patient's level of consciousness, the airway must be protected with endotracheal intubation. In most circumstances, such drastic action is unnecessary. In the initial survey, the patient should also be carefully examined for any stigmata of chronic liver disease and oral mucosal hemangiomas.

Quickly, two large-bore intravenous catheters should be inserted, as well as a nasogastric tube and a Foley catheter. A blood sample is obtained for complete blood count (CBC), blood urea nitrogen (BUN), electrolyte levels, and for a crossmatch of 4 to 6 units. The speed and type of fluid resuscitation depends on the hemodynamic status of the patient. Most patients are moderately hypotensive, and the initial resuscitation can be successfully accomplished with crystalloids (saline or lactated Ringer's solution). When hypotension is extreme, however, immediate blood transfusion should be given, using either group specific, Rh-negative, or O-negative blood. Some severely hypotensive patients can be successfully resuscitated quickly with colloids (plasma, albumin, or Hespan) until fully crossmatched blood is available. When the patient is hemodynamically compromised, central venous pressure monitoring, or preferably, pulmonary artery pressure monitoring is necessary. The goal of resuscitation is to rapidly restore circulating volume and adequate urine output (>50 mL/h) and to establish monitoring of vital signs, urine output, and central venous or pulmonary arterial wedge pressure measurements.

Aspiration should be prevented by insertion of either a large nasogastric tube or an Ewald tube. The stomach is evacuated and lavaged with water or saline. When large amounts of blood are transfused, it is necessary to monitor coagulation factors (e.g., platelets, prothrombin time), and vitamin K administration may be necessary.

Diagnosis Early detection of the source of bleeding is a key step in management. The best way to identify the source is with upper GI endoscopy. The ideal time to perform this examination is (1) when the patient is hemodynamically stable, and (2) when the nasogastric aspirate following irrigation is pink. Endoscopy identifies the site of bleeding in about 90% of patients with upper GI bleeding. The esophagus is easily ruled out as the site of bleeding. Lesions in the stomach may be obscured by blood clot, but even then, with persistence and expertise, the entire stomach can be examined satisfactorily. Bleeding from duodenal ulcer may be evidenced by the presence of (1) active bleeding from a posterior ulcer crater; (2) a visible bleeding vessel; (3) a visible nonbleeding vessel with clot; or (4) an adherent fresh clot at ulcer base. In 2 and 3, the visible vessel is the gastroduodenal artery or one of its major branches (Figure 2.21).

Angiography has a role, but not a frequent one, in the early detection of the site of hemorrhage. Bleeding has to occur at the rate of 2 mL/min or more for the test to succeed. It is most useful when endoscopy has failed to

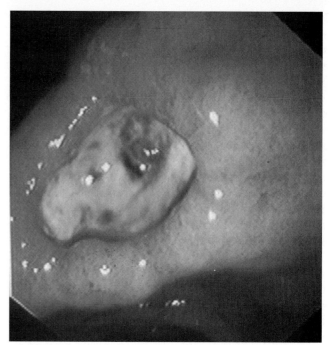

FIGURE 2.21. Endoscopic view of a visible vessel at the base of an active ulcer. (Courtesy of John P. Cello, MD.)

identify the cause of bleeding. On occasion, when bleeding is massive and a nonsurgical treatment approach is chosen, angiography can be useful not only in identifying the bleeding vessel but also in controlling bleeding by selective embolization.

Control of Bleeding As indicated earlier, 90% of patients stop bleeding spontaneously within 8 hours of admission to a hospital and can be managed conservatively. If bleeding persists, control with the aid of endoscopy can be achieved with coagulation (e.g., heater probe, laser), endoscopic sclerotherapy, or by endoscopic injection of alcohol or adrenaline.

Surgical Indications The following indications for surgery for the patient with a bleeding ulcer are generally accepted:

1. Exsanguinating hemorrhage when quick resuscitation is difficult.
2. Failure of control of hemorrhage with endoscopic-based methods.
3. Rebleeding that begins again while the patient is under treatment in a hospital after initial cessation. (This circumstance nearly always suggests bleeding from a gastroduodenal artery.) Even here, it is reasonable to attempt endoscopic control before surgery if the patient is stable and/or at high risk for surgery.
4. Loss of 6 units of blood or more where endoscopic therapy is unavailable or cannot be performed.

The principles of surgery in a bleeding peptic ulcer are to control bleeding and perform a definitive ulcer operation. Preferred options are available when the site of bleeding can be identified as either a duodenal or a gastric ulcer. When the site of bleeding is uncertain, a distal gastrotomy is first performed so that it can be extended into the duodenum if necessary.

Surgery for Bleeding Duodenal Ulcer If a duodenal ulcer is identified as the cause of bleeding, the two surgical options are (1) truncal vagotomy, pyloroplasty, and suture control of bleeding or (2) duodenotomy, suture control of bleeding, and PGV. In the elderly or unstable patient, the first option is more appropriate; the author prefers the second option in the young and stable patient.

The technique of controlling a bleeding duodenal ulcer with sutures is illustrated in Figure 2.22. Nonabsorbable 00 sutures on a stout needle are used. Interrupted sutures are placed at the proximal and distal parts of the ulcer and tied. This may control all or most of the bleeding. Then a U-stitch is used, as shown in the figure, to ligate branches of the gastroduodenal artery. Additional sutures, including figure-8 sutures, may be needed to arrest the bleeding completely. If these techniques fail to completely control the bleeding, the gastroduodenal artery must be dissected outside the duodenum as it branches off the hepatic artery and ligated in continuity using 0-silk suture.

In severe, chronic duodenal ulcer disease with advanced scarring and foreshortening of the first part of the duodenum, the application of sutures to control bleeding from the ulcer bed poses a potential risk to the common bile duct. If the risk is considered high, it is prudent to perform choledochotomy and leave a red rubber catheter in the CBD until after the hemostatic sutures are tied. At this point, the surgeon can ascertain whether the catheter is freely movable, indicating that no ligation of the duct has occurred. The choledochotomy is then closed over a T-tube.

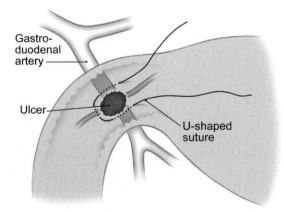

FIGURE 2.22. Suture control of bleeding ulcer requires the ligature of several branches of the gastroduodenal artery in the base of the ulcer. One technique uses the U-shaped suture as shown in the diagram.

Surgery for Bleeding Gastric Ulcer Although a bleeding gastric ulcer can be treated by underrunning the bleeding point and performing truncal vagotomy and pyloroplasty, the preferred surgical approach is to perform a distal gastrectomy that removes the ulcer. When the ulcer is higher up on the lesser curvature of the stomach, a sleeve resection of the lesser curvature may be performed, encompassing the ulcer. When the ulcer is very high and near the gastroesophageal junction, the Madlener procedure may be used. This procedure, which has been successfully utilized in the past, involves underrunning with sutures to control bleeding, a four-quadrant biopsy to rule out carcinoma, and a distal gastrectomy to treat the ulcer diathesis. If the surgeon can ascertain intraoperatively that the ulcer is *H. pylori*–associated, the gastrectomy may be avoided and eradication therapy administered postoperatively. At the present time, because no data are available to support this theoretical approach, it is not recommended.

MANAGEMENT OF GASTRIC OUTLET OBSTRUCTION
Gastric outlet obstruction results from fibrous scarring of chronic duodenal ulcer disease. Symptoms develop over a long period of time, occasionally more acutely due to edema caused by acute exacerbation of ulceration. But, even in the latter circumstance, preexisting scarring and stenosis are likely to be confirmed. Gastric outlet obstruction occurs less frequently than the complications of perforation and bleeding. It is likely that its incidence has decreased because of the advent of potent acid-reducing drugs and identification and eradication of *H. pylori*. Essentials of the management are listed in Table 2.11.

Clinical Presentation The symptoms of gastric outlet obstruction are usually insidious and accompanied by a chronic history of duodenal ulcer. The initial symptoms are early satiety, bloating, and halitosis. When vomiting eventually develops, it is usually after the last meal of the day. The vomitus may contain undigested food eaten 24 to 48 hours earlier. As the obstruction becomes more complete, vomiting may occur after any meal. Chronic weight loss, even emaciation, and chronic fatigue develop.

Physical examination may show the presence of "succussion splash" (i.e., a splashing sound in the epigastrium when the patient is shaken from side to side). Infrequently, particularly in the emaciated patient, gastric peristalsis may be visible in the epigastrium.

Investigation A barium meal confirms gastric outlet obstruction by showing a dilated stomach and a small amount of barium entering the duodenum (Figure 2.23). The use of upper GI endoscopy is necessary to exclude antral cancer as the cause. The endoscope cannot be passed into the duodenum, and no gastric pathology may be found. Antral biopsy for histology and *H. pylori* studies should be obtained.

The typical biochemical findings when prolonged vomiting is present are of hypochloremic, hypokalemic,

TABLE 2.11. Essentials: Management of Gastric Outlet Obstruction

Symptoms and signs
  Insidious clinical presentation
  Early satiety antedating vomiting
  Weight loss
  Fatigue

Biochemical goals of treatment
  Correction of hypovolemia and hypochloremic, hypokalemic, metabolic alkalosis

Diagnostic tests
  Barium meal
  Endoscopy

Conservative therapy (8–10 days)
  Continuous gastric decompression
  Suppression of acid secretion
  Nutritional support with parenteral or enteral nutrition (percutaneous feeding jejunostomy)
  Correction of anemia and vitamin K deficiency

Operative therapy
  Assess for "difficult" duodenum
  ■ If present, perform truncal vagotomy and gastrojejunostomy
  ■ If absent, perform truncal vagotomy and pyloroplasty
  Ancillary procedures
  ■ Feeding jejunostomy
  ■ Tube gastrostomy

and metabolic alkalosis. Vomiting results in loss of fluid, chlorides, and H^+. Severe dehydration develops, and the kidneys attempt to compensate by retaining Na^+. To accomplish this, potassium is initially exchanged, but as dehydration progresses and potassium stores become depleted, H^+ is exchanged for Na^+ in the renal tubules. Early in the evolution of biochemical derangements caused by gastric outlet obstruction, the urine is alkaline; however, paradoxic aciduria soon develops as H^+ is lost in the urine, even as systemic metabolic alkalosis is developing. An electrocardiogram may show the typical peaked T-waves of hypokalemia.

Starvation leads to hypoproteinemia and potential vitamin K deficiency. Therefore, nutritional status and coagulation factors need to be assessed.

Treatment The patient should be treated with nasogastric suction to prevent aspiration. Decompression of the stomach should also be started to restore gastric muscle tone. Acid secretion can be suppressed by parenteral administration of H_2-receptor antagonists or proton-pump blockers. This is an important step that helps to rapidly correct metabolic alkalosis.

The extracellular space volume is severely contracted and must be replenished by administration of normal saline (not lactated Ringer's, which contains fewer chloride ions). A Foley catheter and central venous pressure monitor may also be necessary.

Moderate electrolyte disturbances can be corrected through administration of saline and potassium chloride. When large amounts of potassium chloride must be administered rapidly, cardiac monitoring may be necessary. Very rarely, if the metabolic alkalosis is severe (blood pH > 7.6), either 0.01 N HCl or ammonium chloride solution may need to be given intravenously.

As blood volume is restored, significant hypoalbuminemia and even anemia may become evident. Early institution of parenteral or enteral nutrition is essential. The placement of an enteral catheter through the mouth is not likely to succeed. If enteral therapy is preferred, a feeding jejunostomy must be placed either percutaneously or laparoscopically. In addition, chronic obstruction is likely to be accompanied by vitamin K deficiency, which must be corrected.

Nonsurgical Management If a patient's gastric outlet obstruction is the result of edema from exacerbation of duodenal ulcer, conservative management as outlined above may relieve the obstruction in 8 to 10 days. During this time, it is necessary to maintain nasogastric suction and administer acid-reducing therapy and nutritional support. Any improvement in gastric emptying is assessed by the volume of gastric aspirate and by the use of the saline load test (Hunt's test). If obstruction does not resolve completely within 10 days, it is highly probable that surgical intervention will be necessary.

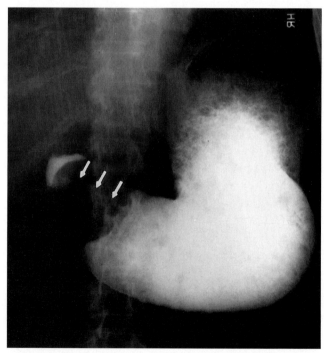

FIGURE 2.23. Gastric outlet obstruction. This condition can be confirmed by a barium meal, which demonstrates a dilated stomach, an abrupt narrowing of the gastric antrum (arrows), and scarce barium entering the duodenum. This is an example of late gastric cancer. (Courtesy of Henry I. Goldberg, MD.)

Operative Management   The following three considerations are paramount in the timing of surgery for gastric outlet obstruction:

1. Correction of fluid and electrolyte imbalance and anemia;

2. Improvement of nutritional status by hyperalimentation for 7 to 10 days monitored by measurement of serum albumin, ferritin, and so on;

3. Improvement of gastric tone by continuous nasogastric suction for 7 to 10 days in the totally atonic stomach. The clinical impression is that restoration of gastric tone preoperatively lessens the incidence of prolonged failure of gastric emptying following surgery.

The critical intraoperative step is to examine the duodenum for evidence of any inflammatory mass (often indicating localized perforation) or advanced scarring that would make closure of the duodenum unsafe. If inflammation or excessive scarring is present, the pyloroduode-

TABLE 2.13. Essentials: Recurrent Ulcer Following Surgical Therapy

Causes
  Incomplete vagotomy
  Inadequate gastric resection
  Gastrinoma
  Uncommon following distal gastrectomy for gastric ulcer
Diagnosis
  Best established by endoscopy
  Assess for *H. pylori* infection and initiate eradication therapy if present
  Evaluate for completeness of vagotomy
Surgical treatment
  Necessary if medical treatment fails
  Choice of procedure depends on type of initial operation:
  ▪ Antrectomy if PGV was initially performed
  ▪ Re-vagotomy with or without antrectomy if truncal vagotomy was initially performed
  ▪ Re-vagotomy with or without re-resection if V & A was initially performed

Abbreviations: PGV, proximal gastric vagotomy; V & A, vagotomy and antrectomy.

TABLE 2.12. Pathophysiologic Basis of Long-Term Complications of Ulcer Surgery

Complication	Pathophysiologic basis
Recurrent ulcer	Incomplete vagotomy Inadequate gastric resection Zollinger-Ellison syndrome Retained antrum syndrome
Postvagotomy diarrhea	Unknown
Dumping syndrome	Rapid gastric emptying Fluid shift into intestine, causing hypovolemia Release of vasoactive peptides and amines (VIP, neurotensin, bradykinin, 5-HT)
Reactive hypoglycemia	Excessive release of insulinotropic peptides from the gut (GLI, GIP) Secondary hyperinsulinemia
Gastroparesis	Unknown
Bile gastritis	Duodeno-jejuno-gastric bile reflux Bile-induced mucosal injury
Iron-deficiency anemia	Decreased absorption of dietary iron Chronic occult blood loss
Megaloblastic anemia	Decreased intrinsic factor secretion following radical subtotal or total gastrectomy
Malabsorption	Steatorrhea Rapid intestinal transit Blind-loop syndrome
Osteoporosis	Calcium malabsorption
Postgastrectomy carcinoma	Hypochlorhydria or achlorhydria

Abbreviations: 5-HT, 5-hydroxytryptamine; GIP, gastric inhibitory peptide; GLI, glucagon-like immunoactivity; VIP, vasoactive intestinal peptide.

num should be left undisturbed, and truncal vagotomy and gastrojejunostomy should be performed. If, on the other hand, pyloroplasty can be performed safely, then truncal vagotomy and pyloroplasty are the treatment of choice. In either case, a feeding jejunostomy and tube gastrostomy should be constructed in anticipation of a protracted recovery period to restore adequate gastric emptying. Some surgeons believe that vagotomy and antrectomy (V & A) is a superior option, but there are no good data to support the contention.

Long-Term Sequelae of Ulcer Surgery

With the exception of proximal gastric vagotomy (PGV), any ulcer surgery may be associated with undesirable long-term sequelae. These and their pathophysiologic bases are summarized in Table 2.12. The operation least likely to cause undesirable side effects, PGV, is associated with the highest incidence of ulcer recurrence. On the other hand, the operation most likely to cure the ulcer problem, V & A, can lead to long-term complications.

ULCER RECURRENCE   The causes of ulcer recurrence are incompleteness of vagotomy, inadequacy of gastric resection, or both. Occasionally, however, ulcer recurrence is due to an undiagnosed gastrinoma. Recurrence following distal gastrectomy for gastric ulcer is uncommon. The incidence of recurrent ulcer after surgery for duodenal ulcer is higher than other rates of recurrence and depends on the type of operative procedure used to treat the primary ulcer (Table 2.13). Following PGV and truncal vagotomy and pyloroplasty (V & P), the site of ulcer recurrence is usually the duodenum, although it may also be the stomach. Following truncal vagotomy and gastrojejunostomy (V & GJ), ulcer recurrence is nearly always in the jejunum, next to the stoma; hence, the names stomal and marginal ulcers.

The evaluation of ulcer recurrence includes endoscopy, measurement of plasma gastrin levels, assessment of completeness of vagotomy, and tests for presence of *H. pylori*.

Diagnosis with Upper Gastrointestinal Endoscopy Barium meal studies are usually not helpful in the diagnosis of recurrent ulcer. Upper GI endoscopy is the only reliable method of diagnosis.

Diagnosis with Plasma Gastrin Levels Following all types of vagotomy not associated with antral resection, both basal and postprandial hypergastrinemia develop. Thus, elevated plasma gastrin levels following vagotomy must be interpreted with caution. If there is concern that a gastrinoma may be present, a "secretin test" should be performed to detect a paradoxical rise in plasma gastrin level following intravenous injection of secretin. If hypergastrinemia is demonstrated in a patient who has had antrectomy, either a gastrinoma or retained antrum syndrome is present. The latter syndrome develops after Bilroth II gastrectomy, when antral tissue is left in continuity with the duodenum. Chronic exposure of this tissue to alkaline secretion leads to G-cell hyperplasia and hypergastrinemia. Again, the secretin test is needed to rule out the diagnosis of gastrinoma.

Assessment of Completeness of Vagotomy Although a high basal acid output (>5 mEq/h) is suggestive of an incomplete vagotomy, the sham feeding ("chew and spit") test is more definitive. It evaluates the cephalic phase of acid secretion.

Diagnosis with Helicobacter pylori *Testing* Evaluation for the presence of *H. pylori* may be accomplished with endoscopic biopsy, breath test, or serology. If *H. pylori* infection is present, eradication therapy is needed.

Treatment If infection with the bacterium *H. pylori* is diagnosed, eradication therapy should be started with the objective of effecting a permanent cure for the ulcer. Combination therapy with amoxicillin or with tetracycline, metronidazole and omeprazole is effective.

A histamine H_2-receptor antagonist or proton-pump inhibitor provides symptomatic relief but is unlikely to cure the recurrence of the ulcer.

The type of operation needed if medical therapy fails depends on the primary operation that was performed (see Table 2.13).

POSTVAGOTOMY DIARRHEA The incidence of incapacitating diarrhea following truncal vagotomy is 1% to 2%.[8] The cause is unknown. Symptomatic treatment includes avoidance of certain foods and the use of bulk-forming agents (Kaopectate), codeine, and Lomotil. Postvagotomy diarrhea has no satisfactory treatment and is best avoided by performing PGV rather than truncal vagotomy as the

primary procedure of choice. Surgical therapy for postvagotomy diarrhea is a last resort. If pyloroplasty was previously performed, pyloric sphincter reconstruction, which reverses the pyloroplasty, has had some success. If a gastrojejunostomy was performed, it can be taken down. The most controversial procedure is the interposition of a 6-inch segment of reversed jejunum between the stomach and duodenum or jejunum to slow intestinal transit. The reported results are not very encouraging and the procedure is rarely, if ever, recommended. Hence, the best form of treatment is prevention.

DUMPING SYNDROME Rapid entry of hyperosmolar chyme into the intestine as a result of destruction, resection, or bypass of the pyloric sphincter is the main cause of this side effect. Vagotomy, which interferes with gastric accommodation, contributes to rapid gastric emptying. Within 15 to 30 minutes of a meal, the patient experiences epigastric distress, sweating, flushing, and profound fatigue. Exaggerated bowel sounds (borborygmi) and sudden diarrhea may also be experienced. As described earlier, the underlying cause of the syndrome is the combination of fluid shift into the intestine, which causes hypovolemia, and the release of vasoactive substances from the intestine.

REACTIVE HYPOGLYCEMIA Patients may develop typical signs and symptoms of hypoglycemia 90 to 120 minutes after a meal. In extreme cases, hypoglycemic crisis may develop. This side effect used to be called the "late dumping syndrome." The pathophysiologic basis appears to be rapid absorption of glucose from the intestine, which leads to excessive secretion of insulin due to release of the insulinotropic peptide glucagon-like immunoactivity (GLI), which outlasts the hyperglycemic stimulus. Avoidance of carbohydrates in the diet is helpful. The long-acting somatostatin analogue octreotide is effective in controlling severe symptoms.

GASTROPARESIS A small percentage of patients may develop gastroparesis following vagotomy and/or gastric resection. The cause is unknown. Symptomatic therapy with prokinetic agents (e.g., dopamine antagonists, cisapride) may be helpful. Some patients require repeated gastric resections, eventually necessitating total gastrectomy with Roux-en-Y esophagojejunostomy. In some patients with disabling symptoms, total gastrectomy is the only definitive and successful treatment.

BILE GASTRITIS Regurgitation of bile into the stomach invariably occurs when the pylorus is destroyed, resected, or bypassed. Some patients develop epigastric pain and bilious vomiting presumably due to the resultant gastritis. Medical therapy includes bile salt antagonists and prokinetic agents. Bile reflux can be prevented or minimized by inserting a 60-cm Roux-en-Y jejunal limb between the stomach and upper jejunum. Unfortunately, the early encouraging results of this operation have not been sustained over time.

CHRONIC ANEMIA   Iron-deficiency anemia commonly occurs several years after gastrectomy, but it can also develop following truncal vagotomy. The causes may include chronic occult blood loss from gastritis and poor absorption of dietary iron. Megaloblastic anemia, due to vitamin B_{12} deficiency, may be seen after radical gastrectomy, indicating insufficient secretion of intrinsic factor. It can be successfully treated with monthly vitamin B_{12} administration parenterally.

MALABSORPTION   Postgastrectomy patients often undergo weight loss and sometimes show signs of malabsorption of fat, carbohydrates, vitamins, and metals. Mild steatorrhea tends to occur after Bilroth II gastrectomy. Vitamin deficiencies may be related to blind-loop syndrome. Lactose intolerance is unmasked in patients who have a mild preoperative lactase deficiency. A significant long-term complication of gastric surgery is calcium malabsorption, which over years may lead to osteoporosis, particularly in women.

POSTGASTRECTOMY CARCINOMA   A higher incidence of carcinoma of the stomach is seen in patients who had gastrectomy 20 years or more previously.[9] The cause is unknown but may be related to hypoacidity favoring bacterial overgrowth and a generation of carcinogenic nitrosamines from food.

NON-PEPTIC ULCER CAUSES OF UPPER GASTROINTESTINAL BLEEDING

Peptic ulcer and erosive gastritis are the most common causes of upper gastrointestinal hemorrhage, accounting for 85% of cases. But upper gastrointestinal bleeding may also be caused by lesions of the esophagus, stomach, and duodenum other than peptic ulcer or erosive gastritis.

Esophageal Causes

Esophageal Varices

Esophageal varices represent the most important cause of bleeding from the esophagus. Portal hypertension and esophageal varices are covered more fully in later chapters. Suffice it to say here that esophageal varices must be excluded whenever upper GI hemorrhage is encountered. A history of alcoholism, cirrhosis, or hepatitis is suggestive. The presence of jaundice and other stigmata of chronic liver disease (e.g., spider nevi, palmar erythema, gynecomastia, hepatosplenomegaly, dilated collateral veins around the umbilicus or caput medusae, ascites, testicular atrophy, and encephalopathy) make the diagnosis of variceal hemorrhage more likely, but do not prove it. Only

upper GI endoscopy can verify that esophageal varices are present and that they are the source of bleeding. As many as 30% to 40% of patients with proven esophageal varices may bleed from another source, most commonly a peptic ulcer or erosive gastritis. The management of variceal hemorrhage is discussed in Chapter 6.

Gastroesophageal Reflux Disease

Gastroesophageal reflux disease (GERD) can cause bleeding, either from erosive esophagitis or from development of Barrett's ulcer. Bleeding from erosive esophagitis can be significant but is rarely massive unless a coagulopathy coexists. Bleeding from a Barrett's ulcer, on the other hand, can be massive. The cause is development of a typical peptic ulcer in Barrett's epithelium in the esophagus. Both conditions are nearly always associated with a sliding hiatal hernia. The topic is covered in more detail in Chapter 1.

Paraesophageal Hernia

The cause of bleeding in paraesophageal hernia is almost always venous congestion of the mucosa caused by mechanical obstruction of venous outflow from the herniated segment of the esophagus. Bleeding tends to be slow but is occasionally severe enough to present as hematemesis and/or melena. The treatment is surgical correction of the hernia.

Miscellaneous Causes

Malignancy and aortoesophageal fistula are rare causes of bleeding. Bleeding from aortoesophageal fistula can be exsanguinating and must always be suspected in the patient who has had an aortofemoral graft.

Non-Peptic Causes of Gastric Bleeding

Mallory–Weiss Syndrome

A mucosal tear at the gastroesophageal junction can lead to arterial bleeding at the base of the tear. The cause is usually mechanical and precipitated by retching and vomiting. The patient usually indicates that he or she had retched repeatedly or vomited non-blood–containing fluid before vomiting blood. The diagnosis is made with endoscopy, and the bleeding can usually be controlled with endoscopic coagulation. If endoscopic control fails, the bleeding is readily controlled surgically using an abdominal approach. The gastroesophageal junction is mobilized and a gastrotomy is performed adjacent to the gastroesophageal junction. Brisk arterial bleeding is seen coming from the base of a mucosal tear that usually straddles the gastroesophageal junction. The bleeder is under-sewn using 00-silk sutures.

Dieulafoy Syndrome

Dieulafoy syndrome involves bleeding through apparently normal gastric mucosa from localized angiodysplasia in the submucosa. The bleeding is from a single vessel and is easily controlled by endoscopic injection of adrenaline around the site of bleeding.

Gastric Tumors

Benign or malignant tumors of the stomach occasionally cause upper GI bleeding. These include both mesenchymal tumors (leiomyoma and leiomyosarcoma) and epithelial tumors (adenocarcinoma and carcinoma).

Hemangioma

Gastric hemangiomas can be single or multiple and may occur as isolated gastric lesions or as hemangiomatosis syndromes that affect other parts of the gastrointestinal tract.

Gastric Varices

Gastric varices are most commonly associated with splenic vein thrombosis. Although nonsurgical techniques may control the bleeding temporarily, the definitive treatment is splenectomy. Acutely bleeding varices may require suture control via gastrotomy prior to splenectomy.

Duodenal Causes

Non-peptic ulcer bleeding from the duodenum is rare and is associated with pancreatic tumors that have eroded into the organ.

Liver and Pancreas Causes

Liver and pancreas are exceedingly rare causes of upper GI bleeding and are considered when all other causes are excluded. There may be bleeding into the bile ducts or pancreatic duct and then into the duodenum through the ampulla of Vater. When the liver is the source, hepatic trauma is the usual cause, and bleeding originates from branches of the hepatic artery. The bleeding site may be identified angiographically and controlled by angiographic embolization. Bleeding into the pancreatic duct is exceedingly rare and may result from either trauma or acute pancreatitis.

Small Intestinal Causes

Upper GI bleeding caused by lesions in the small intestine is discussed in Chapter 8. The three important causes are Meckel's diverticulum, tumors, and hemangioma. Bleeding distal to the ligament of Treitz does not present as hematemesis but as rectal bleeding or melena.

MOTOR DISORDERS OF THE STOMACH

Gastroparesis

Gastroparesis represents one of the most difficult management problems in gastroenterology. Patients are usually referred for surgical opinion when all forms of medical therapy have failed. Many of these patients have had previous ulcer surgery.

Nonsurgical Management

Medical treatment for motor disorders of the stomach includes the administration of dopamine antagonists, cholinergic agonists, or acetylcholine releasers to improve gastric emptying. Metoclopramide, domperidone, and cisapride may improve gastric emptying, but in true gastroparesis, and particularly in patients who have had previous ulcer surgery, the effectiveness of these drugs is neither impressive nor long-lived.

Surgical Management

Gastroparesis presents a special challenge, as the surgeon is being asked to perform a major operation with an uncertain outcome. On the other hand, extensive experience now exists to suggest that total gastrectomy with Roux-en-Y esophagojejunostomy is the best surgical option. When this operation is performed, a feeding jejunostomy should be provided because the patient may require a long adaptive phase to learn to eat without a stomach.

Dumping Syndrome

The syndrome has been described above. Fortunately, most cases are mild. When the syndrome is severe, however, no adequate treatment exists. Hence, prevention is important.

Prevention

The best way to prevent dumping syndrome is to avoid, whenever possible, performing operations that are likely to cause it, including gastrectomy and truncal vagotomy and drainage. Pharmacologic and bacteriologic advances have nearly eliminated the need for elective ulcer surgery. In an emergency situation, the surgeon must decide whether to perform the quickest and safest operation at that moment as opposed to a lengthier operation with less undesirable side effects. Whenever the condition of the patient allows, particularly in young patients and women, PGV is a better choice than truncal vagotomy and drainage. In the setting of hemorrhage, control of bleeding is accomplished through duodenotomy, leaving the pyloric sphincter intact. When perforation is the indication for emergent surgery, PGV is again preferred if an acid-reducing procedure is to be done.

Nonsurgical Management

Dietary measures often effectively control dumping syndrome. These include avoiding a high carbohydrate diet; eating small, frequent meals; not ingesting fluids with the meals; and lying down for about 60 minutes after eating. Patients with severe symptoms have been successfully treated with the long-acting somatostatin analogue octreotide. The problem with this form of treatment is cost and the long-term need for injection therapy.

Surgical Management

As always, surgical treatment for the dumping syndrome is a last resort. Some operative approaches are simple and have a chance to succeed. These include pyloric sphincter reconstruction when a pyloroplasty is present, or takedown of gastrojejunostomy when the stomach is otherwise intact. Other surgical options are more complex and should be undertaken only in extreme cases. These include conversion of Bilroth II gastrectomy to Bilroth I, and interposition of jejunum between the stomach and the duodenum. The latter procedures have had variable success.

GASTRIC MALIGNANCIES

Information regarding premalignant conditions and other factors of gastric malignancy is summarized in Table 2.14.

Premalignant Conditions

Helicobacter pylori

Patients with *H. pylori* infection have a six- to nine-fold increased risk of gastric cancer. The pathogenesis is thought to proceed from gastritis to dysplasia to cancer (Figure 2.24). The incidence of mucosa-associated lymphoid malignancy is higher than adenocarcinoma.

Atrophic Gastritis and Pernicious Anemia

The risk of developing adenocarcinoma is increased nearly six-fold in patients with atrophic gastritis and pernicious anemia. In a longitudinal prospective study, 1 in 80 patients with pernicious anemia developed cancer.[10] The achlorhydria that accompanies this condition favors bacterial proliferation, which generates carcinogenic nitrosamines from nitrates in food.

Gastric Polyps

Adenomatous polyps, which represent about 10% of all gastric polyps, pose significant risk for cancer. The cancer risk in small adenomatous polyps (<2 cm) is 2%, but the risk rises to 24% in polyps 2 cm or larger.

TABLE 2.14. Essentials: Gastric Malignancy

Premalignant conditions
  H. pylori infection
  Atrophic gastritis and pernicious anemia
  Gastric polyps
  Gastric ulcer
  Hypergastrinemia
  Blood group A
  Previous gastric resection
  Ménétrier's disease
Carcinoma of the stomach
  Falling incidence
  Gross appearance: Polypoid, ulcerative, colloid, or infiltrative
  Surgical treatment: Bilroth II or total gastrectomy
  Early gastric cancer
  ▪ No invasion of muscularis
  ▪ 10% of gastric cancers in U.S.
  ▪ 5-year survival of 70%–95%
  Advanced gastric cancer
  ▪ Invasion of muscularis and/or lymph node metastasis
  ▪ 80% of cases in U.S.
Gastric carcinoid tumors
  Classification
  ▪ Type I: Associated with atrophic gastritis
  ▪ Type II: Associated with MEN-I syndrome
  ▪ Type III: Sporadic; most are malignant and metastasize to liver
  Treatment
  ▪ Tumors <2 cm: Endoscopic excision
  ▪ Tumors >2 cm: Resection with 1-cm margin
Gastric lymphoma
  Non-Hodgkin's lymphoma of B-cell type
  Significant association with MALT and *H. pylori* infection
  40% present with bleeding, perforation or obstruction
  Cure rate of 65%–75% after curative resection and neoadjuvant therapy
  Treatment
  ▪ Responsive to chemotherapy and radiotherapy
  ▪ When confined to stomach: Curative resection followed by adjuvant chemo- or radiotherapy

Abbreviations: MALT, mucosa-associated lymphoid tissue; MEN-1, multiple endocrine neoplasia-1.

Gastric Ulcer

The incidence of malignant degeneration of a benign gastric ulcer is probably no higher than 1% to 2%. On the other hand, malignant lesions can masquerade as benign ulcers more frequently.

Hypergastrinemia

Hypergastrinemia can be caused by gastrinoma, by prolonged achlorhydria that occurs as a result of atrophic gastritis, and by long-term therapy with proton-pump inhibitors. Hypergastrinemia results in hyperplasia of the ECL cells and a tendency to cause carcinoid tumors. Gastric carcinoids occur more frequently in patients with atrophic gastritis and the Zollinger–Ellison syndrome. Long-term therapy with proton-pump inhibitor has caused carcinoid tumors in mice, but there has been no

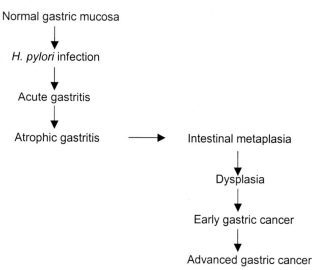

Normal gastric mucosa
↓
H. pylori infection
↓
Acute gastritis
↓
Atrophic gastritis ⟶ Intestinal metaplasia
↓
Dysplasia
↓
Early gastric cancer
↓
Advanced gastric cancer

FIGURE 2.24. *Helicobacter pylori* and genesis of gastric cancer.

reported incidence of carcinoid tumors in humans on long-term therapy. The clinical effects of long-term hypergastrinemia are listed in Table 2.15.

Blood Group A

A strong association exists between gastric cancer and individuals with blood Group A.

Previous Partial Gastrectomy

Patients who had partial gastrectomy 20 or more years ago have an increased risk of developing adenocarcinoma in the gastric stump.

Ménétrier's Disease

An undefined risk of gastric cancer exists in Ménétrier's disease.

Benign Neoplasms

Adenomatous Polyps

Adenomatous polyps, the most common benign neoplasms, are premalignant lesions. They may be single or multiple. They can cause bleeding or intussusception into the pylorus, causing gastric outlet obstruction. Lesions 2 cm or greater should be resected either endoscopically or

TABLE 2.15. Essentials: Clinical Effects of Long-Term Hypergastrinemia in Humans

Known effects
   Increased ECL cells
   Increased parietal cells
   Thickening of gastric mucosa

Probable risks
   Development of gastric carcinoids
   Accelerated growth of colonic neoplasms

Abbreviations: ECL, enterochromaffin-like.

surgically. A few patients with gastric polyposis (Figure 2.25) require total gastrectomy to prevent cancer.

Stromal Tumors

Leiomyomas are common stromal neoplasms of the gastric smooth muscle. Most are asymptomatic and found only at autopsy. Nearly 50% occur in the gastric corpus. They usually protrude into the lumen but can also grow outwardly. A central ulceration of the overlying mucosa may develop and may cause upper GI bleeding (Figure 2.26). Symptomatic lesions or those 3 cm or more in diameter should be surgically excised with a 2 to 3 cm margin of normal gastric wall.

Some 50% of unresectable malignant stromal tumors have been shown to respond to treatment with imatinib mesylate (Gleevec®), a selective tyrosine kinase inhibitor.[11] The tumors that respond express CD117, a marker for KIT-receptor tyrosine kinase, an enzyme critical in the pathogenesis of gastrointestinal stromal tumors including leiomyosarcoma.

Ménétrier's Disease (Hypertrophic Gastritis)

Ménétrier's disease is diffuse gastric mucosal hypertrophy that can lead to massive enlargement of rugal folds, usually sparing the antrum. No unanimity of opinion exists about the microscopic diagnostic criteria, but the disease involves expansion of the glandular stomach with elongated and branched gastric pits, often with focal cystic dilatation (Figure 2.27). The gastric hypertrophy can

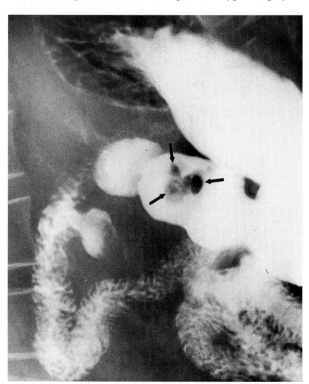

FIGURE 2.25. Gastric polyposis (arrows) is demonstrated with a barium upper GI series. If the polyposis is extensive, total gastrectomy may be required to prevent cancer. (Courtesy of Henry I. Goldberg, MD.)

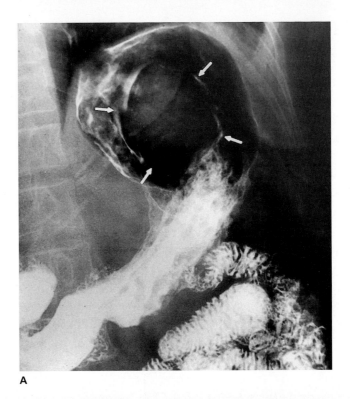

A

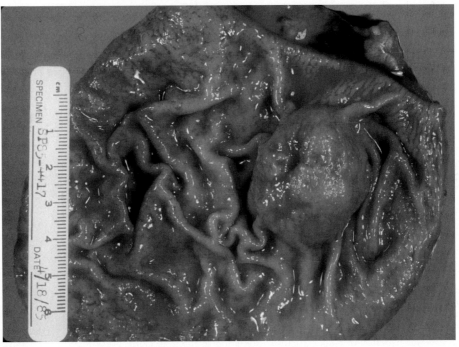

B

FIGURE 2.26. Gastric leiomyomas. These are common benign neoplasms of the gastric smooth muscle that are usually asymptomatic. (A) They may be detected by endoscopy and barium upper GI x-rays as a large round smooth mass (arrows), especially when they degenerate into leiomyosarcoma. (B) The partial gastrectomy surgical specimen shows a leiomyosarcoma that projects into the lumen as a polypoid mass. (Courtesy of Linda D. Ferrell, MD, and Henry I. Goldberg, MD.)

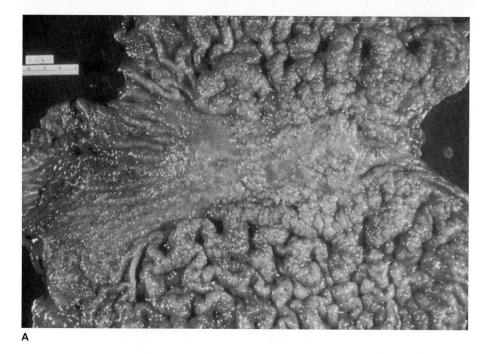

A

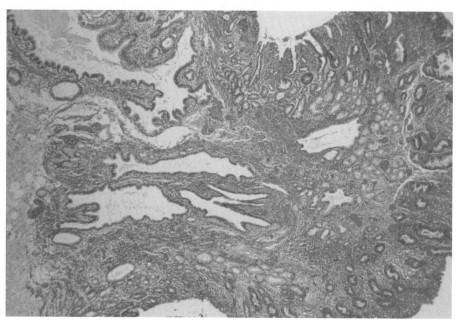

B

FIGURE 2.27. Ménétrier's disease. (A) Gross appearance of Ménétrier's disease shows hyperplastic, hypertrophic giant rugal folds involving mostly the body of the stomach. (B) Microscopic examination shows hypertrophic gastritis, with replacement of the normal mucosa by hyperplastic surface epithelial cells forming convoluted or cystic structures extending to the muscularis. (Reprinted with permission from Fenoglio-Preiser CM, Lantz P, Listrom M, et al., eds. Gastrointestinal Pathology Plus. 2nd ed. Philadelphia: Lippincott Williams & Wilkins, 1999.)

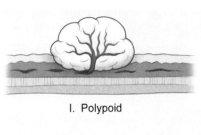

I. Polypoid

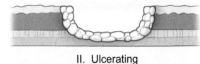

II. Ulcerating

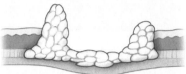

III. Ulcerating / infiltrating

IV. Infiltrating

FIGURE 2.28. Gross classification of gastric cancer. Gastric cancer can be polypoid, ulcerating, or infiltrating. Linitis plastica is the infiltrating type with the poorest survival outcome. (Adapted from Douglass HO, Nava HR. Gastric adenocarcinoma—management of the primary disease. *Semin Surg Oncol* 1985;12:32–45.)

mimic that seen in the Zollinger-Ellison syndrome, but there is no associated hypergastrinemia or acid hypersecretion. The hypertrophic mucosa may secrete proteins and lead to hypoalbuminemia. The primary clinical symptoms are abdominal pain, malnutrition, edema, and weight loss.

Antisecretory therapy (anticholinergics, H_2 blockers, proton-pump inhibitors) is used to decrease acid and fluid loss and thereby to limit protein loss. In rare circumstances, when symptoms are severe and uncontrollable, total gastrectomy with Roux-en-Y esophagojejunostomy is necessary.

Pseudolymphoma

In pseudolymphoma, lymphocytic infiltration of the gastric mucosa leads to diffuse thickening or enlargement of rugal folds. Microscopically, lymphoid follicles have clearly reactive germinal centers.

Carcinoma of the Stomach

Incidence

There is wide geographic variation in the incidence of gastric cancer. The number of cases per 100,000 population varies from 8 in the United States to 18 in England and Wales, 49 in Chile, over 50 in Japan and Russia, and 78 in Costa Rica.[12] In the United States, a remarkable decline in the incidence of gastric cancer has occurred over the past 70 years, from 40 per 100,000 men in the 1930s, to about 8 per 100,000 in the 1990s.[13] Gastric cancer accounted for 20% to 30% of all cancer deaths 50 years ago. Today, it accounts for only 3%.[14] This can be explained partly by the higher standard of living achieved, changing dietary habits, and perhaps the reduction in *H. pylori*

infections as a result of improved sanitation and food handling and increased use of antibiotics. Clearly, the incidence of gastric cancer is inversely related to the socioeconomic status of the populations it affects.

Pathology

Four macroscopic appearances (Figure 2.28) are seen in stomach cancer:

1. Malignant ulcer;
2. Polypoid tumor growing into the lumen;
3. Colloid tumor, which is gelatinous and capable of massive growth; and
4. Linitis plastica, a scirrhous cancer that infiltrates the submucosa to cause "leather-bottle stomach."

Microscopically, tumors are identified as adenocarcinoma with various degrees of differentiation. Linitis plastica is particularly anaplastic, manifesting clumps of bizarre-looking cells with surrounding fibrosis. Signet-ring cell carcinoma is particularly malignant in its behavior. Signet-ring cells result from intracellular mucus secretion (Figure 2.29).

Depth of Invasion

The depth of invasion has great prognostic significance in gastric cancer and is the basis for classifying gastric cancer as "early" or "advanced."

EARLY GASTRIC CANCER Cancer detected in patients early involves only the mucosa and submucosa and does not penetrate the muscularis propria (Figure 2.27). Even the presence of lymph node metastasis does not severely

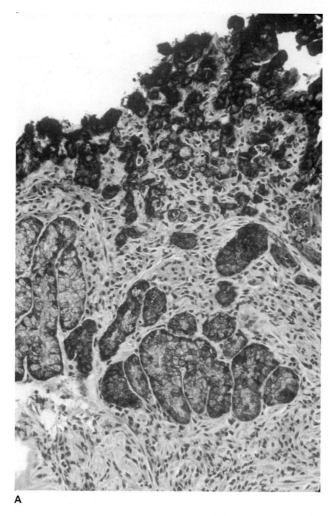

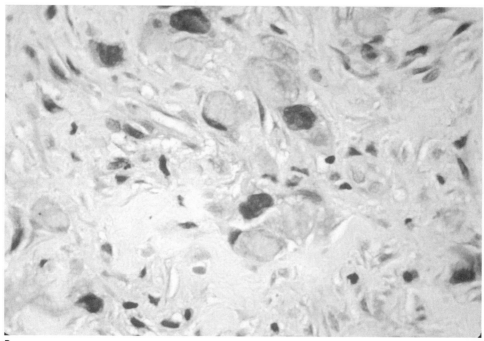

FIGURE 2.29. Gastric adenocarcinoma. Microscopic appearance of two types of gastric adenocarcinoma: (A) Superficial carcinoma with keratin stain demonstrates a tumor that has not invaded the muscularis mucosa and has an excellent prognosis. (B) By contrast, linitis plastica with signet-ring cells has a very poor prognosis but, fortunately, accounts for only 10% of gastric cancer. (Courtesy of Linda D. Ferrell, MD.)

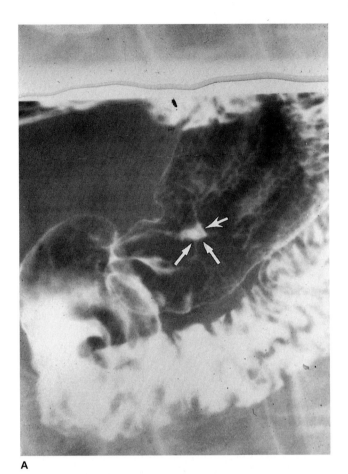

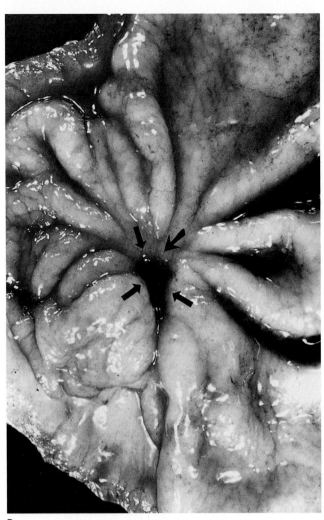

FIGURE 2.30. Late gastric cancer. (A and B) Once the muscularis propria is involved, the prognosis is considerably worsened. Even an apparently superficial malignant ulcer, seen on a double-contrast upper GI series (arrows in A), may be found to penetrate the muscularis propria when surgical resection is performed (arrows in B). (Courtesy of Henry I. Goldberg, MD.)

A

B

affect the good prognosis of early gastric cancer. The 5-year survival rate is 70% to 95%, depending on whether or not lymph nodes are involved.[15] Unfortunately, only 10% to 15% of all gastric carcinomas are early cancers at diagnosis. Endoscopic screening to diagnose gastric cancer at this early stage is too expensive and has a low yield, even in countries like Japan, where the disease is endemic.

ADVANCED GASTRIC CANCER Once the invasion penetrates the muscularis propria, prognosis declines (Figure 2.30). Unfortunately, more than 80% of all gastric cancers encountered in the United States are advanced at the time of diagnosis.

Clinical Presentation

Symptoms are insidious. Abdominal pain and weight loss are seen in 50% and 60% of patients, respectively. Other symptoms include anorexia and early satiety. The relative incidence of proximal gastric cancers has been increasing, and some 25% of these patients present with dysphagia. Approximately 10% of the patients present with disseminated disease as evidenced by an enlarged left supraclavicular node (Virchow's node), rectal shelf (Bloomer's shelf), hepatomegaly, jaundice, or ascites.

Investigations

A double-contrast barium meal test is the most economical preliminary examination in patients with nonspecific symptoms (Figure 2.31). About 15% of those so examined require endoscopy. Endoscopy with multiple biopsies and brushing is the most specific way to establish the diagnosis. Endoscopic ultrasonography indicates the depth of wall invasion with 80% to 90% accuracy, but its ability to detect involved lymph nodes is less than 70%.

Computed tomography is a useful examination. It may not only show the gastric lesion and thickening of the

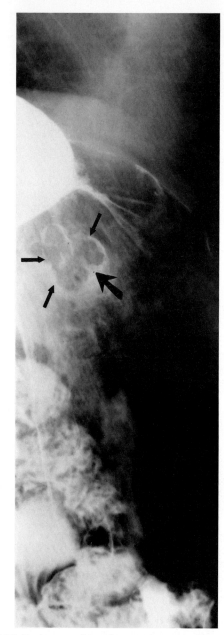

FIGURE 2.31. Barium meal test for gastric cancer. Nonspecific symptoms that may be indicative of gastric cancer are best and most economically evaluated at the outset with a double-contrast barium meal test. This double-contrast upper GI radiography demonstrates a Type I, slightly raised, lobulated early gastric cancer (arrows) in the body of the stomach. (Courtesy of Henry I. Goldberg, MD.)

stomach wall but indicates the presence of extragastric extension. Its most important role, however, is to detect the presence of metastases in the liver and in other abdominal organs.

Staging

Accurate staging is possible only after surgery. The use of laparoscopy to stage the disease is promising but its role is yet undefined. The most widely used staging method is the

TABLE 2.16. TNM Classification of Carcinoma of the Stomach	
Primary tumor (T)	
TX	Primary tumor cannot be assessed
T0	No evidence of primary tumor
Tis	Carcinoma in situ: intraepithial tumor without invasion of the lamina propria
T1	Tumor invades lamina propria or submucosa
T2	Tumor invades muscularis propria or subserosa
T2a	Tumor invades mucularis propria
T2b	Tumor invades subserosa
T3	Tumor penetrates serosa (visceral peritoneum) without invasion of adjacent structures
T4	Tumor invades adjacent structures
Regional lymph nodes (N)	
NX	Regional lymph node(s) cannot be assessed
N0	No regional lymph node metastasis
N1	Metastasis in 1 to 6 regional lymph nodes
N2	Metastasis in 7 to 15 regional lymph nodes
N3	Metastasis in more than 15 regional lymph nodes
Distant metastasis (M)	
MX	Distant metastasis cannot be assessed
M0	No distant metastasis
M1	Distant metastasis

Source: Reprinted with permission from the American Joint Committee on Cancer (AJCC), Chicago, Illinois. The original source for this material is the *AJCC Cancer Staging Manual*, Sixth Edition (2002) published by Springer-Verlag New York, www.springer-ny.com.

TNM classification and clinical staging (Tables 2.16 and 2.17).

Surgical Treatment

Surgical resection provides the only hope for curing gastric cancer. Even then, some patients show criteria of inoperability at the time of presentation. These include the presence of Virchow's node, obvious liver metastasis, rectal shelf, and ascites.

The type of gastric resection needed depends on location of the tumor (Figure 2.32). In all cases, proximal and distal surgical margins should be clear of tumor for at least

TABLE 2.17. Relating TNM Classification to Clinical Staging of Gastric Cancer			
Stage		*TNM classification*	
0	T1S	N0	M0
IA	T1	N0	M0
IB	T1	N1	M0
	T2	N0	M0
II	T1	N2	M0
	T2	N1	M0
	T3	N0	M0
IIIA	T2	N2	M0
	T3	N1	M0
	T4	N0	M0
IIIB	T3	N2	M0
	T4	N1	M0
IV	T4	N2	M0
	Any T	Any N	M1

STOMACH AND DUODENUM

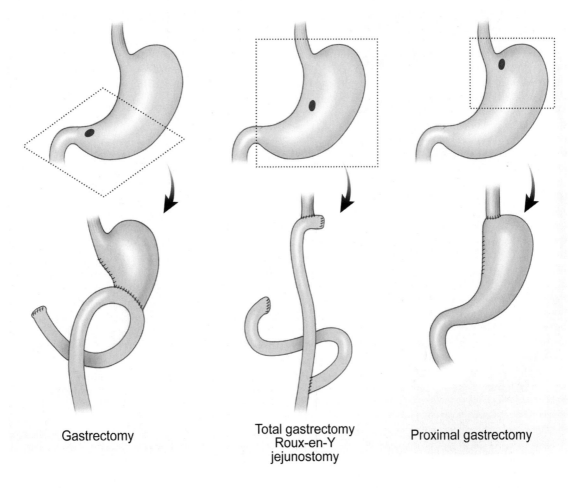

Gastrectomy

Total gastrectomy
Roux-en-Y
jejunostomy

Proximal gastrectomy

FIGURE 2.32. Surgical resection for stomach cancer. Most antral cancers can be resected by subtotal gastrectomy with Bilroth II anastomosis. Key aspects of the operation are removal of adequate proximal and distal margins, division of the left and right gastric arteries at their origin, and resection of the greater omentum. When the lesion is in the mid-body of the stomach or involves extensively the body of the stomach, total gastrectomy with Roux-en-Y jejunostomy is required. Some lesions of the cardia or fundus of the stomach may be amenable to proximal gastrectomy performed through a left thoraco-abdominal incision.

4 to 6 cm. When the resection required is distal gastrectomy, the following surgical strategies should also be employed:

1. Resection of the duodenal bulb and Bilroth II reconstruction.
2. Division of left and right gastric arteries at their origin, and
3. Removal of the greater omentum. It is always useful to do preoperative bowel preparation in the event that the transverse colon has to be resected *en bloc.*

The main controversy relates to the extent of lymph node dissection. Types of resective surgery have been classified based on this criterion as follows:

1. R1: complete removal of perigastric lymph nodes;
2. R2: resection of perigastric nodes and those along the left gastric, splenic, and right hepatic arteries;
3. R3: R2 with dissection of celiac axis nodes;
4. R4: R3 with dissection of paraaortic nodes.

Survival Rates

There is dispute about the usefulness of R4 gastrectomy. The importance of resection of all regional nodes (i.e., R2), however, has been demonstrated by the 5-year survival rate of patients treated surgically at Memorial Sloan-Kettering Cancer Center (see Table 2.18).[16]

TABLE 2.18. Five-Year Survival Rate of Patients with Stomach Cancer

Tumor stage	% Survival	
	R1 Tumors	R2 Tumors
IA	88	91
IB	56	85
II	39	58
IIIA	7	30
IIIB	0	12

Source: Reprinted with permission from Smith JW, Brennan MF. Surgical treatment of gastric cancer. Proximal, mid and distal stomach. Surg Clin North Am 1992;72:381–399.

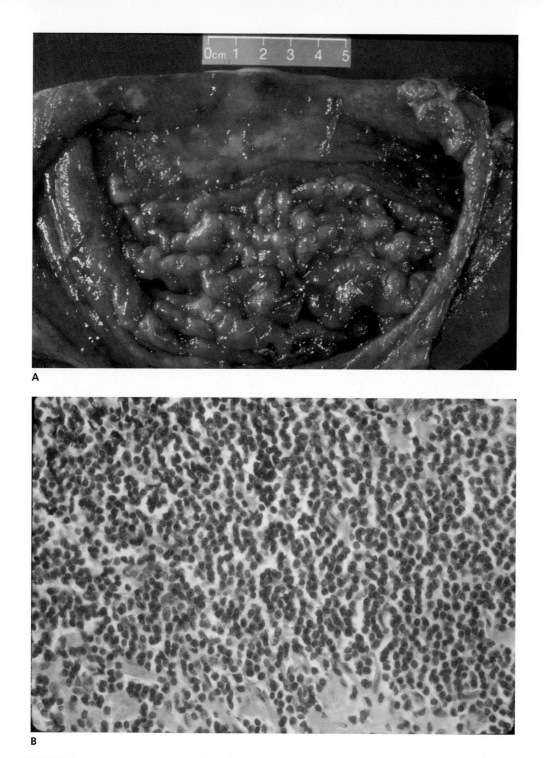

FIGURE 2.33. Gastric lymphoma. (A) The surgical specimen of extensive gastric lymphoma resembles hypertrophic rugal folds. (B) The microscopic appearance demonstrates that the lymphoma is a B-cell type. (Courtesy of Linda D. Ferrell, MD.)

Adjuvant Therapy

Carcinoma of the stomach is poorly responsive to chemotherapy or radiotherapy. Many randomized clinical trials have evaluated chemotherapy alone (5-fluorouracil, doxorubicin hydrochloride, mitomycin) or a combination of chemotherapy and radiotherapy. Although treatment advantages have been seen in some clinical trials, the picture is generally pessimistic for cure.

Palliative Treatment

Occasionally, palliative gastrectomy is required to treat bleeding or obstruction, even though tumor may be left behind. At other times, gastroenterostomy is performed to bypass an obstructing distal gastric cancer. Obstructing tumors at the cardia may be palliated by endolaser therapy.

Gastric Carcinoid Tumors

Gastric carcinoid tumors represent about 10% of all GI carcinoid syndromes. Three types are recognized:

1. Type I: associated with chronic atrophic gastritis and hypergastrinemia;
2. Type II: associated with multiple endocrine neoplasia syndrome (MEN-I); and
3. Type III: sporadic. Type III carcinoid tumors, the sporadic type, are the most malignant and have frequently metastasized to the liver by the time they are diagnosed.

Diagnosis

Diagnosis is often made incidentally during endoscopic examination. Most of these tumors are located in the body and fundus and may be single or multiple. They are often submucosal. Biopsy and histologic examination establish the diagnosis. When symptoms are present, they are often nonspecific, although some patients may present with bleeding. Nearly 20% of gastric carcinoids have metastasized at the time of diagnosis.

Treatment

Small tumors can be removed endoscopically. Those larger than 2 cm should be surgically resected with a 1-cm margin of normal tissue. If metastases are present, they should be resected whenever possible. Patients with unresectable lesions may be treated with doxorubicin. Streptozocin is not effective.

Gastric Lymphoma

Gastric lymphoma arises from mucosa-associated lymphoid tissue (MALT) and is usually a non-Hodgkin's lymphoma of the B-cell type. A significant association exists between MALT tumors and *H. pylori*–induced gastritis. Symptoms, similar to those of carcinoma, include abdominal pain, anorexia, and weight loss. Patients with diffuse disease may have the additional symptoms of night sweats and fevers. Approximately 40% present with the complications of bleeding, perforation, or obstruction. The appearance of gastric lymphoma (Figure 2.33) is characterized by hypertrophic rugal folds.

Unlike adenocarcinoma, gastric lymphoma is responsive to chemotherapy (with cyclophosphamide, vincristine, nitrogen mustard, procarbazine, and prednisone) and to radiotherapy. Nevertheless, when the disease is confined to the stomach and regional lymph nodes (stages I and II), curative resection followed by adjuvant chemo- and/or radiotherapy appears to provide the best results. The role of surgery in stages III and IV is to treat complications. Following chemo-radiotherapy, gastric perforation may occur, requiring gastrectomy. Resection may also be indicated when there is residual resectable disease following chemo-radiotherapy of stage III and IV tumors.

Five-year survival rates for stage I and II disease following resection alone are 30% to 45%, but improve to 65% to 75% if adjuvant therapy is added.[17]

REFERENCES

1. Barr H, Greenall MJ. Carcinoma of the stomach. In: Morris PJ, Wood WC, eds. *Oxford Textbook of Surgery*. 2nd ed. Oxford, UK: Oxford University Press; 2000:1313–1328.
2. Jordan PH Jr. Surgery for peptic ulcer disease. *Curr Probl Surg* 1991;28:265–330.
3. Stabile BE. Current surgical management of duodenal ulcers. *Surg Clin North Am* 1992;72:335–356.
4. Mulholland MW, Debas HT. Chronic duodenal and gastric ulcer. *Surg Clin North Am* 1987;67:489–507.
5. Hoffmann J, Olesen A, Jensen HE. Prospective 14- to 18-year follow-up study after parietal cell vagotomy. *Br J Surg* 1987;74: 1056–1059.
6. Boey J, Lee NW, Koo J, et al. Immediate definitive surgery for perforated duodenal ulcers: a prospective controlled trial. *Ann Surg* 1982;196:338–344.
7. Donovan AJ, Vinson TL, Maulsby GO, et al. Selective treatment of duodenal ulcer with perforation. *Ann Surg* 1979;189:627–636.
8. Gray JL, Debas HT, Mulvihill SJ. Control of dumping symptoms by somatostatin analogue in patients after gastric surgery. *Arch Surg* 1991;126:1231–1236.
9. Hansson LE. Risk of stomach cancer in patients with peptic ulcer disease. *World J Surg* 2000;24:315–320.
10. Kato I, Tominaga S, Ito Y, et al. A prospective study of atrophic gastritis and stomach cancer risk. *Jpn J Cancer Res* 1992;83: 1137–1142.
11. Demetri GD, von Mehren M, Blanke CD, et al. Efficacy and safety of imatinib mesylate in advanced gastrointestinal stromal tumors. *N Engl J Med* 2002;347:472–480.
12. Pisani P, Parkin DM, Bray F, et al. Estimates of the worldwide mortality from 25 cancers in 1990. *Int J Cancer* 1999;83:18–29.

13. Parker SL, Tong T, Bolden S, et al. Cancer statistics, 1997. *CA Cancer J Clin* 1997;47:5–27.
14. SEER cancer statistics review 1973–1996. U.S. Department of Health and Human Services. Bethesda, MD: Public Health Institute, National Institutes of Health, National Cancer Institute, 1999.
15. Hundahl SA, Phillips JL, Menck HR. The National Cancer Data Base Report on poor survival of U.S. gastric carcinoma patients treated with gastrectomy: Fifth Edition American Joint Committee on Cancer Staging, proximal disease, and the "different disease" hypothesis. *Cancer* 2000;88:921–932.
16. Smith JW, Brennan MF. Surgical treatment of gastric cancer. Proximal, mid, and distal stomach. *Surg Clin North Am* 1992; 72:381–399.
17. Frazee RC, Roberts J. Gastric lymphoma treatment. Medical versus surgical. *Surg Clin North Am* 1992;72:423–431.

SELECTED READINGS

Anatomy

Griffith CA. Anatomy. In: Harkins HN, Nyhus LM, eds. *Surgery of the Stomach and Duodenum.* 2nd ed. Boston: Little, Brown, 1969.

Helander HF. Parietal cell structure during inhibition of acid secretion. *Scand J Gastroenterol Suppl* 1984;101:21–26.

Ito S. Functional gastric morphology. In: Johnson LR, ed. *Physiology of the Gastrointestinal Tract.* Vol 1. New York: Raven Press, 1981:517–550.

Michels NA. Blood supply of the stomach and the esophagus. In: *Blood Supply And Anatomy Of Upper Abdominal Organs.* Philadelphia: Lippincott; 1955.

Physiology

Allen A, Flemstrom G, Garner A, et al. Gastroduodenal mucosal protection. *Physiol Rev* 1993;73:823–857.

Chuang CN, Chen MC, Soll AH. Gastrin-histamine interactions: direct and paracrine elements. *Scand J Gastroenterol Suppl* 1991; 180:95–103.

Code CF. Reflections on histamine, gastric secretion and the H2 receptor. *N Engl J Med* 1977;296:1459–1462.

Debas HT, Carvajal SH. Vagal regulation of acid secretion and gastrin release. *Yale J Biol Med* 1994;67:145–151.

Dragstedt LR. The physiology of the gastric antrum. *Arch Surg* 1957; 75:552.

Edkins JS. The chemical mechanism of gastric secretion. *J Physiol* 1906;34:183.

Feldman M, Richardson CT. Role of thought, sight, smell, and taste of food in the cephalic phase of gastric acid secretion in humans. *Gastroenterology* 1986;90:428–433.

Fordtran JS, Walsh JH. Gastric acid secretion rate and buffer content of the stomach after eating. Results in normal subjects and in patients with duodenal ulcer. *J Clin Invest* 1973;52:645–657.

Forte JG, Machen TE, Obrink KJ. Mechanisms of gastric H+ and Cl– transport. *Annu Rev Physiol* 1980;42:111–126.

Kirkwood KS, Debas HT. Physiology of gastric secretion and emptying. In: Miller TA, ed. *Modern Surgical Care: Physiologic Foundations and Clinical Applications.* 2nd ed. St. Louis: Quality Medical Publishing, Inc; 1998:362–377.

Lloyd KCK, Debas HT. Peripheral regulation of gastric acid secretion. In: Johnson LR, ed. *Physiology of the Gastrointestinal Tract.* 3rd ed. New York: Raven Press; 1994:1185–1226.

Miller TA, Jacobson ED. Gastrointestinal cytoprotection by prostaglandins. *Gut* 1979;20:75–87.

Silen W, Ito S. Mechanisms for rapid re-epithelialization of the gastric mucosal surface. *Annu Rev Physiol* 1985;47:217–229.

Taché Y. Central nervous system regulation of gastric acid secretion. In: Johnson LR, ed. *Physiology of the Gastrointestinal Tract.* 2nd ed. New York: Raven Press, 1987.

Thompson JC. Humoral control of gut function. *Am J Surg* 1991; 161:6–18.

Wolfe MM, Soll AH. The physiology of gastric acid secretion. *N Engl J Med* 1988;319:1707–1715.

Peptic Ulcer Disease

Allison MC, Howatson AG, Torrance CJ, Lee FD, Russell RI. Gastrointestinal damage associated with the use of nonsteroidal antiinflammatory drugs. *N Engl J Med* 1992;327:749–754.

Casas AT, Gadacz TR. Laparoscopic management of peptic ulcer disease. *Surg Clin North Am* 1996;76:515–522.

Covacci A, Telford JL, Del Giudice G, et al. *Helicobacter pylori* virulence and genetic geography. *Science* 1999;284:1328–1333.

Emas S, Grupcev G, Eriksson B. Six-year results of a prospective, randomized trial of selective proximal vagotomy with and without pyloroplasty in the treatment of duodenal, pyloric, and prepyloric ulcers. *Ann Surg* 1993;217:6–14.

Graham DY. NSAIDs, Helicobacter pylori, and Pandora's Box. *N Engl J Med* 2002;347:2162–2164.

Grossman MI, ed. *Peptic Ulcer: A Guide for the Practicing Physician.* Chicago: Year Book Medical Publishers, 1981.

Grossman MI, Kurata JH, Rotter JI, et al. Peptic ulcer: new therapies, new diseases. *Ann Intern Med* 1981;95:609–627.

Isenberg JI, Selling JA, Hogan DL, et al. Impaired proximal duodenal mucosal bicarbonate secretion in patients with duodenal ulcer. *N Engl J Med* 1987;316:374–379.

Jensen DM. Management of severe ulcer rebleeding. *N Engl J Med* 1999;340:799–801.

Jordan PH Jr, Thornby J. Twenty years after parietal cell vagotomy or selective vagotomy antrectomy for treatment of duodenal ulcer. Final report. *Ann Surg* 1994;220:283–296.

Lau JY, Sung JJ, Lam YH, et al. Endoscopic retreatment compared with surgery in patients with recurrent bleeding after initial endoscopic control of bleeding ulcers. *N Engl J Med* 1999; 340:751–756.

Malfertheiner P, Megraud F, O'Morain C, et al. Current concepts in the management of Helicobacter pylori infection—the Maastricht 2-2000 Consensus Report. *Aliment Pharmacol Ther* 2002;16:167–180.

Mertz HR, Walsh JH. Peptic ulcer pathophysiology. *Med Clin North Am* 1991;75:799–814.

Parsonnet J. *Helicobacter pylori. Infect Dis Clin North Am* 1998; 12:185–197.

Suerbaum S, Michetti P. Helicobacter pylori infection. *N Engl J Med* 2002;347:1175–1186.

Valen B, Dregelid E, Tonder B, et al. Proximal gastric vagotomy for peptic ulcer disease: follow-up of 483 patients for 3 to 14 years. *Surgery* 1991;110:824–831.

Walsh JH, Peterson WL. The treatment of *Helicobacter pylori* infection in the management of peptic ulcer disease. *N Engl J Med* 1995;333:984–991.

Gastric Carcinoma

Cuschieri A, Weeden S, Fielding J, et al. Patient survival after D1 and D2 resections for gastric cancer: long-term results of the MRC randomized surgical trial. Surgical Co-operative Group. *Br J Cancer* 1999;79:1522–1530.

Eid R, Moss SF. Helicobacter pylori infection and the development of gastric cancer. *N Engl J Med* 2002;346:65–67.

Farley DR, Donohue JH, Nagorney DM, et al. Early gastric cancer. *Br J Surg* 1992;79:539–542.

Fendrick AM, Chernew ME, Hirth RA, et al. Clinical and economic effects of population-based *Helicobacter pylori* screening to prevent gastric cancer. *Arch Intern Med* 1999;159:142–148.

Fiocca R, Luinetti O, Villani L, et al. Molecular mechanisms involved in the pathogenesis of gastric carcinoma: interactions between genetic alterations, cellular phenotype and cancer histotype. *Hepatogastroenterology* 2001;48:1523–1530.

Fuchs CS, Mayer RJ. Gastric carcinoma. *N Engl J Med* 1995;333:32–41.

Hermann RE. Newer concepts in the treatment of cancer of the stomach. *Surgery* 1993;113:361–364.

Kim JP. Current status of surgical treatment of gastric cancer. *J Surg Oncol* 2002;79:79–80.

Moreaux J, Msika S. Carcinoma of the gastric cardia: surgical management and long-term survival. *World J Surg* 1988;12:229–235.

Nakamura K, Ueyama T, Yao T, et al. Pathology and prognosis of gastric carcinoma. Findings in 10,000 patients who underwent primary gastrectomy. *Cancer* 1992;70:1030–1037.

Pacelli F, Sgadari A, Doglietto GB. Surgery for gastric cancer. *N Engl J Med* 1999;341:538–539.

Parsonnet J, Friedman GD, Vandersteen DP, et al. *Helicobacter pylori* infection and the risk of gastric carcinoma. *N Engl J Med* 1991;325:1127–1131.

Siewert JR, Fink U, Sendler A, et al. Gastric cancer. *Curr Probl Surg* 1997;34:835–939.

Wanebo HJ, Kennedy BJ, Chmiel J, et al. Cancer of the stomach. A patient care study by the American College of Surgeons. *Ann Surg* 1993;218:583–592.

Gastric Lymphoma

Coiffier B, Lepage E, Briere J, et al. CHOP chemotherapy plus rituximab compared with CHOP alone in elderly patients with diffuse large-B-cell lymphoma. *N Engl J Med* 2002;346:235–242.

Kodera Y, Yamamura Y, Nakamura S, et al. The role of radical gastrectomy with systematic lymphadenectomy for the diagnosis and treatment of primary gastric lymphoma. *Ann Surg* 1998;227:45–50.

Kodera Y, Yamamura Y, Shimizu Y, et al. The number of metastatic lymph nodes: a promising prognostic determinant for gastric carcinoma in the latest edition of the TNM classification. *J Am Coll Surg* 1998;187:597–603.

Shutze WP, Halpern NB. Gastric lymphoma. *Surg Gynecol Obstet* 1991;172:33–38.

Surgery for Morbid Obesity

Approximately 100 million Americans are overweight. Obesity is a major public health problem that is responsible for increased risk of cardiac disease and type II diabetes. The annual cost of treating obesity in the United States exceeds $30 billion.[1] Ideal body weights, based on actuarial studies from the Metropolitan Life Insurance Company,[2] define obesity as body mass index (BMI) greater than 30 kg per m^2 and morbid obesity as BMI greater than 40 kg per m^2. Approximately 1.5 million Americans are morbidly obese.

The cause of obesity is unknown, but genetic, endocrine, and psychogenic factors are probably important. The role of genetics is indicated from studies of monozygotic twins and from observations that overweight mothers have children who become overweight. Experimental studies have shown that hereditary obesity in mice is due to mutated ob gene, which encodes leptin. A glycoprotein secreted from fat cells, leptin is a primary regulator of satiety. It is believed to act by suppressing neuropeptide Y (NPY) release from the hypothalamus. NPY is a satiety factor, and its suppression results in overeating. Leptin also mediates peripheral insulin resistance and altered hypothalamic-pituitary-adrenal equilibrium, leading to obesity. The human obesity gene and the leptin-receptor gene have been cloned. The pharmaceutical industry is making a major effort to develop anti-obesity drugs based on leptin and its receptors.

MORBIDITY OF SEVERE OBESITY

Severe obesity is associated with several morbid conditions (Table 3.1). Obesity is a major risk factor for coronary artery disease. The Framingham Heart Study of the National Heart, Lung, and Blood Institute has shown that a 10% weight reduction lowers the risk of coronary artery disease by 20%.[3] In addition, hypertension is commonly associated with obesity and may be related to increased renin secretion, caused by decreased cardiac output, a direct consequence of elevated intra-abdominal and intrathoracic pressures. The incidence of adult-onset (type II) diabetes is also significantly increased by obesity. The main feature appears to be resistance to insulin as a result of down-regulation of peripheral receptors for insulin. Further, the incidence of obstructive sleep apnea is increased 20-fold or greater in obese individuals. The upper airway is narrowed by deposits of adipose tissue in the oropharynx. Hypoventilation and hypoxic episodes in obese individuals contribute significantly to cardiac dysfunction. Obesity aggravates and perhaps also precipitates gastroesophageal reflux. It increases the incidence of cholelithiasis and a variety of cancers, particularly those of the colon, breast and uterus, and accelerates development of degenerative arthritis. Obesity increases operative risk in gastrointestinal surgery, not only because of the attendant comorbid conditions, but also because the procedures become technically more difficult, leading to operative complications.

TABLE 3.1. Morbid Conditions Associated with Severe Obesity

Cardiovascular Conditions
- Coronary artery disease
- Hypertension
- Thromboembolism

Other Conditions
- Type II diabetes
- Obstructive sleep apnea
- Gastroesophageal reflux
- Cholelithiasis
- Cancer (colon, breast, uterine)
- Osteoarthritis
- Increased operative risk

TABLE 3.2. Essentials: Bariatric Surgery

Indications
- Morbid obesity: BMI >35 kg/m²
- Severe obesity with comorbid conditions

Procedures
- Vertical-banded gastroplasty (VBGP)
- Horizontal gastroplasty (HG)
- Roux-en-Y gastric bypass (RYGB)
- Biliopancreatic bypass
- Biliopancreatic bypass with duodenal switch
- Jejunoileal bypass

Outcomes
- RYGB and VBGP most popular
- RYGB more effective but has more complications
- Both reduce weight (>40% excess weight) and reverse diabetes and hypertension
- HG not as effective
- Jejunoileal bypass abandoned because of serious hepatic injury

Abbreviation: BMI, body mass index.

The primary treatment for obesity is nonsurgical, with surgical treatment indicated only in morbidly obese patients or very obese patients with comorbid conditions.

MEDICAL TREATMENT

Medical treatment of obesity is based on caloric restriction, exercise, and lifestyle and long-term behavior modifications. Several drugs have been used to curb appetite, sometimes with disastrous side effects. The search for the ideal drug continues and, with improved understanding of the mechanisms of satiety signals, success is likely. A variety of diets (e.g., liquid diets, protein diets) are in vogue with mixed results. The major problem is recidivism.

SURGICAL TREATMENT

Recommendation for surgical treatment of morbid obesity is not taken lightly. Most bariatric surgeons team up with psychiatrists, psychologists, and social workers for optimal patient selection and postoperative follow-up. Candidates for surgery are those with a BMI of 35 to 40 kg/m² and those with comorbid conditions.

Several procedures have been used. The two most popular operations in the United States are vertical banded gastroplasty (VBGP) and Roux-en-Y gastric bypass (RYGB). Gastric bypass is more successful as a weight-reducing operation but is associated with a higher incidence of complications. Both operations can be performed by the open method and, increasingly, laparoscopically. Jejunoileal bypass is no longer used as a primary operation for obesity because of serious long-term hepatic complications. The essentials of bariatric surgery are summarized in Table 3.2.

Jejunoileal Bypass

One of the first popular operations for treating obesity, the jujunoileal bypass procedure bypasses most of the absorptive surface of the small intestine by end-to-side anastomosis of a short segment of jejunum (8–14 inches) to the distal ileum, 4 to 12 inches proximal to the ileocecal valve (Figure 3.1). Early complications, such as intussusception of the bypassed small intestine, were handled by anastomosing the proximal end of the bypassed small intestine to the colon. Although satisfactory levels of weight loss were achieved, the operation was associated with severe late complications such as cirrhosis, rheumatoid-like arthritis, cholelithiasis, hypocalcemia, vitamin B_{12} deficiency, kidney stones, nephritis, and bacterial overgrowth in the bypassed segment. The most serious complication has been cirrhosis, which in some patients has caused liver failure. The procedure has now been abandoned, and most patients who have previously undergone jejunoileal bypass are advised to have the bypass reversed and replaced, if necessary, by VBGP or RYGP.

Vertical-Banded Gastroplasty

The goal of vertical-banded gastroplasty is to create, using staples, a small gastric pouch of 15 to 30 ml volume, 5 cm from the gastroesophageal junction (Figure 3.2). A stapled stoma is created to connect the pouch with the distal stomach, and a 1.5 cm × 5 cm collar of polypropylene mesh is wrapped around the stoma on the lesser curve to prevent widening of the stoma with time. This procedure is currently one of the two most popular in the United States for treating obesity. Postoperative complications of VBGP

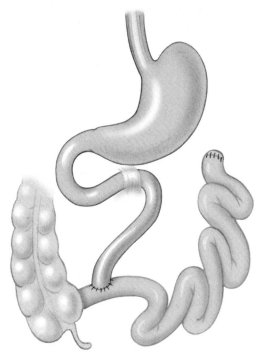

FIGURE 3.1. Jejunoileal bypass. (Adapted from Greenfield LJ, ed. Surgery: Scientific Principles and Practice, 2nd ed. Philadelphia: Lippincott-Raven; 1997.)

include staple-line dehiscence (2–7%), leak (0.5%), band erosion (2%), and outlet obstruction wound infection (1–2%). The operation's 30-day mortality rate is less than 1%.[4]

Loss of more than 50% of excess weight is seen in only 30% to 40% of patients following VBGP. Several reasons have been proposed for the failure to maintain weight loss, including enlargement of the gastric pouch with time, dehiscence of the staple line, and the ability of patients to consume excessive quantities of sweet liquids, thereby

overcoming the restrictions of the small gastric reservoir. On the other hand, because no part of the gastrointestinal tract is bypassed, long-term complications are few.

Horizontal Gastroplasty

The concept of horizontal gastroplasty (HG) is the same as for VBGP, except that the restricted pouch is created by a double application of staples horizontally across the proximal stomach; then either a central or lateral prolene-reinforced stoma is constructed (Figure 3.3). Other variations of this type of HG exist. Failure rates (loss of less than 40% excess weight) have been reported in 42% to 71% of patients. Controlled trials have shown that HG is not as effective as VBGP in achieving weight loss, but the procedure is associated with less vomiting as a side effect.

Roux-en-Y Gastric Bypass

In RYGB, the stomach is partitioned using a linear four-row non-cutting stapler applied from a point 2.5 to 3 cm below the gastroesophageal junction on the lesser curve to the angle of His on the greater curve (Figure 3.4). The vagi are identified and protected. The goal is to create a 15- to 30-ml proximal gastric pouch, which is anastomosed side-to-side with a 60-cm Roux-en-Y jejunal limb brought up retrocolically. Some surgeons prefer to completely divide the proximal pouch from the distal stomach.

Pories and colleagues,[5] in a study of 608 patients with 97% follow-up over 14 years, have shown a mean weight loss of nearly 50% of excess weight. The diabetic state was reversed in 91% of 298 of their patients. Similarly, blood

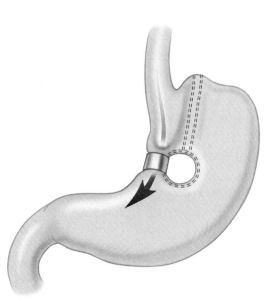

FIGURE 3.2. Vertical-banded gastroplasty.

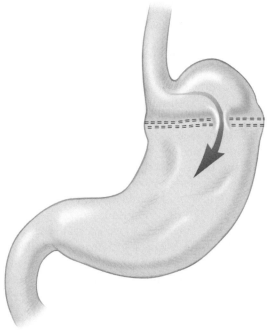

FIGURE 3.3. Horizontal gastroplasty.

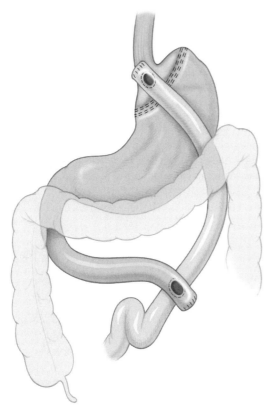

FIGURE 3.4. Roux-en-Y gastric bypass. (Adapted from Greenfield LJ, ed. Surgery: Scientific Principles and Practice, 2nd ed. Philadelphia: Lippincott-Raven, 1997; and Sabiston DC, Jr, ed. Textbook of Surgery: The Biological Basis of Modern Surgical Practice, 15th ed. Philadelphia: WB Saunders, 1997.)

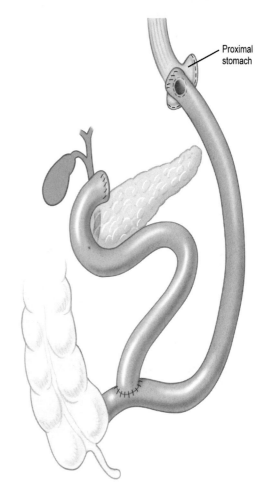

FIGURE 3.5. Biliopancreatic bypass.

pressure returned to normal levels in 86% of 353 hypertensive patients. Other studies have shown similar success rates. Complications include injury to the spleen (2%), anastomotic leak (1%–3%), and thromboembolism (0.6%–2%). Late complications include stenosis or obstruction of the gastrojejunostomy (3%–15%), small bowel obstruction (4%–5%), marginal ulceration (0.2%–13%), and gallbladder disease (10%). Vitamin deficiencies (B_{12}, A, D, E) occur unless appropriate supplementation is taken.

In the United States, gastric bypass is the most popular operation. It is superior to VBGP in its effectiveness to treat obesity but is associated with a higher complication rate.

Biliopancreatic Bypass

Biliopancreatic bypass involves performing a distal gastrectomy, leaving a proximal stomach that has a capacity of 200 to 500 ml. The stomach is then anastomosed with a Roux-en-Y retrocolic limb of distal ileum 250 cm proximal to the ileocolic valve. The proximal ileum is then anastomosed end to side with the distal ileum 50 cm proximal to the ileocolic junction (Figure 3.5). The largest experience reported was by Scopinaro et al in Italy.[6] Long-term success in loss of body weight in 1356 patients was 78% at 14 years. The procedure is not popular in the United States.

REFERENCES

1. Health implications of obesity. National Institutes of Health Consensus Development Conference Statement. *Ann Intern Med* 1985;103:1073–1077.
2. Measurement of overweight. *Stat Bull Metrop Insur Co* 1984; 65:20–23.
3. Eckel RH, Krauss RM. American Heart Association call to action: obesity as a major risk factor for coronary heart disease. AHA Nutrition Committee. *Circulation* 1998;97:2099–2100.
4. Mason EE. Vertical banded gastroplasty for obesity. *Arch Surg* 1982;117:701–706.
5. Pories WJ, Swanson MS, MacDonald KG, et al. Who would have thought it? An operation proves to be the most effective therapy for adult-onset diabetes mellitus. *Ann Surg* 1995;222:339–352.
6. Scopinaro N, Adami GF, Marinari GM, et al. Biliopancreatic diversion. *World J Surg* 1998;22:936–946.

SELECTED READINGS

Alvarez-Cordero R. Treatment of clinically severe obesity, a public health problem: introduction. *World J Surg* 1998;22:905–906.

Andersen T, Backer OG, Stokholm KH, et al. Randomized trial of diet and gastroplasty compared with diet alone in morbid obesity. *N Engl J Med* 1984;310:352–356.

Andersen T, Pedersen BH, Dissing I, et al. A randomized comparison of horizontal and vertical banded gastroplasty: what determines weight loss? *Scand J Gastroenterol* 1989;24:186–192.

Buchwald H. A bariatric surgery algorithm. *Obes Surg* 2002;12: 733–750.

Fisher BL, Schauer P. Medical and surgical options in the treatment of severe obesity. *Am J Surg* 2002;184:9S–16S.

Hall JC, Watts JM, O'Brien PE, et al. Gastric surgery for morbid obesity. The Adelaide Study. *Ann Surg* 1990;211:419–427.

Kellum JM, DeMaria EJ, Sugerman HJ. The surgical treatment of morbid obesity. *Curr Probl Surg* 1998;35:791–858.

MacLean LD, Rhode BM, Sampalis J, et al. Results of the surgical treatment of obesity. *Am J Surg* 1993;165:155–162.

Sugerman HJ, Londrey GL, Kellum JM, et al. Weight loss with vertical banded gastroplasty and Roux-Y gastric bypass for morbid obesity with selective versus random assignment. *Am J Surg* 1989;157:93–102.

Wittgrove AC, Clark GW, Schubert KR. Laparoscopic gastric bypass, roux-en-Y: technique and results in 75 patients with 3–30 months follow-up. *Obes Surg* 1996;6:500–504.

4

Pancreas

The pancreas, sometimes referred to as the queen organ, plays a major role in digestion and metabolism. Two separate components accomplish these functions: the exocrine pancreas, which secretes powerful enzymes that break down carbohydrates, fat, and proteins; and the endocrine pancreas, made up of the islets of Langerhans, which elaborate insulin and glucagon, hormones that regulate the level of blood glucose.

Lying in its retroperitoneal position, with a temperament that is unpredictable, the pancreas continues to present major challenges to the surgeon. The pathophysiology of its inflammatory conditions is incompletely understood and their therapy inconclusive. Although pancreaticoduodenectomy and total pancreatectomy are now performed with a low mortality rate, the ability of these major operations to cure pancreatic cancer is disappointingly low.

ANATOMY

DEVELOPMENT OF THE PANCREAS

The pancreas develops as a dorsal and ventral bud from the foregut during fourth week of fetal life (Figure 4.1). The duct of the ventral pancreas joins the distal common bile duct. During gestation, the duodenum rotates clockwise in its long axis, and the ventral pancreas and common duct come to lie to the left of the duodenum and fuse with the dorsal pancreas. In the process of rotation, the ventral pancreas, which forms most of the head of the pancreas, encloses the superior mesenteric vessels, which come to lie between the uncinate process posteriorly and the pancreatic head anteriorly. Most of the duct that drains the dorsal pancreas joins the duct of the ventral pancreas to form the main pancreatic duct called the duct of Wirsung. The most medial portion of the duct of the dorsal pancreas becomes the accessory pancreatic duct—the duct of Santorini—and enters the duodenum about 1 in proximal to the entrance of the duct of Wirsung into the duodenum.

There was once a theory that the endocrine pancreas was derived from the neural crest of the embryo and that endocrine cells migrated to the abdomen along with the sympathetic chain and with the cells that comprise the adrenal medulla. There is now conclusive evidence derived from studies in molecular genetics that the endocrine cells derive from endoderm cells of the primitive embryonic foregut. The genes for insulin, glucagon, and somatostatin are expressed in the foregut at the site where the future diverticulum forms. The same is true for exocrine cells, although the genes for exocrine enzymes are expressed a little later. Furthermore, the mesenchyma surrounding the primitive endoderm cells, from which the pancreas form, exerts significant influence on differentiation of the pancreas. In the absence of mesenchyme—which is required for differentiation into exocrine cells—the endoderm cells differentiate only into endocrine cells.

SURGICAL ANATOMY

The pancreas is a retroperitoneal organ consisting of two distinct functional units, exocrine and endocrine pancreas. The exocrine pancreas is comprised of acini and ducts, while the endocrine pancreas comprises approximately 1 million islets of Langerhans interspersed among the exocrine glands and ducts throughout the pancreas. The endocrine pancreas constitutes approximately 1% of the total organ. The surgical anatomy is shown in Figure 4.2.

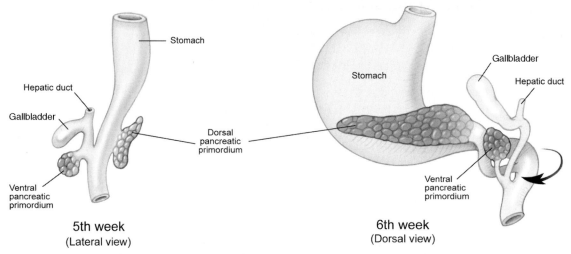

FIGURE 4.1. Development of the pancreas from the dorsal and ventral bud of the foregut. Lateral view at week 5 shows development of the ventral pancreas and biliary tree from the ventral bud. The dorsal view at week 6 shows how, with rotation of the duodenum clockwise, the ventral pancreas and common duct come to lie posteriorly and fuse with the dorsal pancreas.

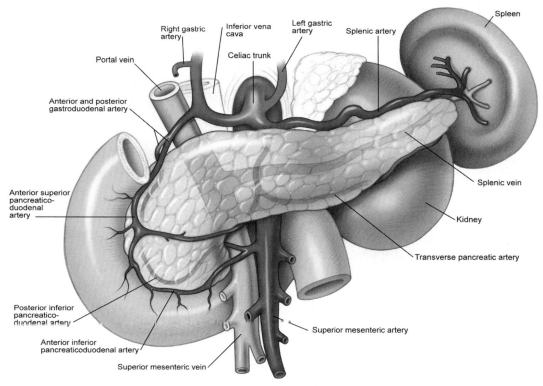

FIGURE 4.2. Surgical anatomy of the pancreas. The head of the pancreas lies in the concavity of the C-loop of the duodenum, from which the body and tail extend to the left upper quadrant. Blood supply to the head of the pancreas is from branches of the gastroduodenal artery, while that to the body and tail is primarily from branches of the splenic vessels. Behind the neck of the pancreas lies the junction of the superior mesenteric and splenic veins, forming the portal vein. Other important posterior relations of the pancreas include the left kidney, left renal vessels, and the left adrenal gland. (Adapted from Warren KW, Jenkins RL, Steele GD. Atlas of Surgery of the Liver, Pancreas, and Biliary Tract. Norwalk, CT: Appleton & Lange; 1991.)

Anatomic Relationships of the Pancreas

The pancreas lies transversely in the retroperitoneum across the upper abdomen, extending from the pancreatic head in the C-loop of the duodenum medially to the tail, which is closely related to the hilum of the spleen. Its anatomic relationships are as follows:

1. Anteriorly, the lesser sac and the stomach.
2. Medially, the C-loop of the duodenum.
3. Laterally, the splenic hilum.
4. Posteriorly, from right to left: The inferior vena cava (IVC) lies deep slightly to the right of the second portion of the duodenum and, more medially, the aorta. The left renal vein enters the IVC after running immediately behind the body, neck, and head of the pancreas from the left kidney. The superior mesenteric artery (SMA) and vein (SMV) run behind the head of the pancreas but anterior to the uncinate process. The SMV joins the splenic vein, which runs along the superior edge of the pancreas to form the portal vein (PV); the PV runs superiorly behind the head to the porta hepatis. The inferior mesenteric vein joins the splenic vein to the left and behind the neck of the pancreas. On the extreme left and more deeply lie the kidney with its hilar structures and the left adrenal gland.

Anatomic Points of Surgical Importance

Three salient points of pancreatic anatomy and its relationships are particularly important for the surgeon:

1. The tail of the pancreas is closely related to the hilum of the spleen. Care must be taken not to injure the pancreas when hilar vessels are divided in splenectomy.
2. No veins enter the anterior surface of the SMV and PV. Thus, an avascular window can be dissected behind the head of the pancreas and anterior to the PV and SMV. The dissection of this window, sometimes referred to as the portal tunnel, is a critical step in determining resectability during pancreaticoduodenectomy.
3. A substituted hepatic artery arises from the SMA rather than from the celiac axis in approximately 5%–10% of the population. To avoid inadvertent injury, the presence or absence of a substituted hepatic artery should be determined early in the dissection during pancreaticoduodenectomy.

Blood Supply

The arterial supply of the pancreas is derived from branches of the celiac axis and the superior mesenteric artery (SMA). The head of the pancreas shares its blood supply with the duodenum. The major blood supply to the head comes from the anterior and posterior pancreaticoduodenal arteries, which form arcades of vessels just inside the C-loop of the duodenum. These arteries originate from the gastroduodenal artery (a branch of the hepatic artery) and from the SMA, respectively. The body and tail of the pancreas are supplied by the superior and inferior pancreatic arteries, branches of the SMA, and branches of the splenic and left gastroepiploic arteries. Venous drainage corresponds to the arterial supply and eventually flows into the portal vein. The blood supply is shown in Figure 4.2.

Lymphatic Drainage

The head of the pancreas drains into nodes in the pancreaticoduodenal groove and then into subpyloric, portal, mesocolic, mesenteric, and aortocaval nodes. The body and tail of the pancreas drain into retroperitoneal and splenic hilar nodes, and to the celiac, mesenteric, and para-aortic nodes.

Innervation

The vagus and sympathetic nerves provide the principal extrinsic innervation. The preganglionic fibers of both the parasympathetic (celiac branches of the vagus) and sympathetic (the greater and lesser splanchnics) systems terminate in the celiac ganglia. Postganglionic vagal fibers are peptidergic as well as cholinergic and include neurons containing CCK, somatostatin, CGRP, neuropeptide Y, and gastrin-releasing peptide. Sensory innervation is via unmyelinated C-fibers containing substance P and CGRP.

MICROSCOPIC ANATOMY

Exocrine Pancreas

The exocrine pancreas is made up of grape-like glands called acini. These acini drain into ductules that join each other to make progressively larger ductules and ducts, which eventually drain into the main or accessory pancreatic ducts (Figure 4.3). The acinus is made up of polyhedral cells sitting on a basement membrane. The apical surfaces of these cells have microvilli and face the lumen of the acinar gland. The nuclei of acinar cells are located basally, and their cytoplasm contains several types of organelles. The rough endoplasmic reticulum (RER) and Golgi bodies are particularly prominent. Other structures in the cytoplasm include mitochondria, condensing vacuoles, numerous secretory granules, and lysosomes. The secretory granules are contained within cytoplasmic membranes and are transported to the apical membrane. The cytoplasmic membrane of the granules fuses with the apical membrane to initiate the process of exocytosis, by which the secretory proteins (proenzymes) are delivered to the acinar lumen. This intracellular transport or trafficking system of proteins is shown in Figure 4.4.

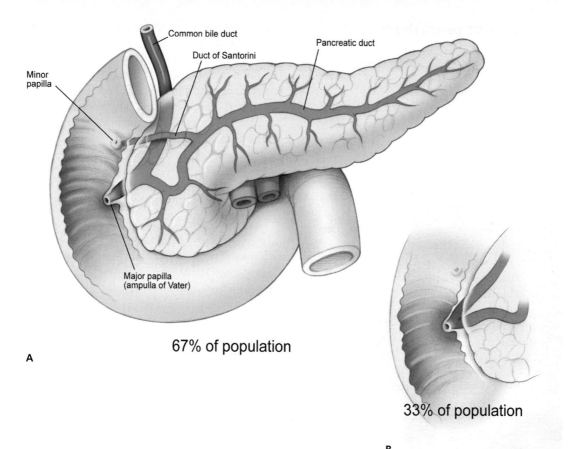

Common bile duct

Duct of Santorini

Pancreatic duct

Minor papilla

Major papilla (ampulla of Vater)

67% of population

A

33% of population

B

FIGURE 4.3. Pancreatic ductal system. The main pancreatic duct (the duct of Wirsung) joins the distal common bile duct to form a common channel (0.5–1.0 cm in length) before emptying into the duodenum at the major papilla (ampulla of Vater). The duct of Santorini drains separately into the duodenum at the minor papilla 1.0–1.5 cm proximal to the ampulla of Vater. (A) This common channel pattern is seen in 67% of the population. (B) In the remaining third of the population, no common channel exists and the two ducts drain into the ampulla separately.

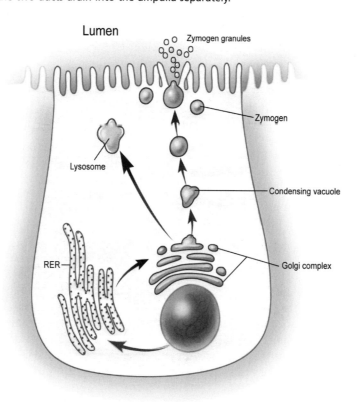

Lumen

Zymogen granules

Zymogen

Lysosome

Condensing vacuole

RER

Golgi complex

FIGURE 4.4. Intracellular trafficking of proteins.

Structure of Islets of Langerhans

The islet of Langerhans is made up of four types of cells: (1) glucagon-secreting alpha cells, (2) insulin-secreting beta cells, (3) somatostatin-secreting delta cells, and (4) pancreatic polypeptide (PP)-secreting cells. The beta cells comprise 80% of the islet cells. The islet architecture is designed to facilitate islet portal circulation (Figure 4.5). The beta cells comprise a central core; the three other cell types are arranged as a mantle surrounding the central core of beta cells. Arterial blood is delivered to the beta-cell core, from which venules carry the blood to the peripheral alpha, delta, and PP cells. This portal circulation allows for local paracrine influences between the cells. The islets are innervated with intrinsic neurons, which are cholinergic and peptidergic, and extrinsic neurons, which are cholinergic, peptidergic, and adrenergic.

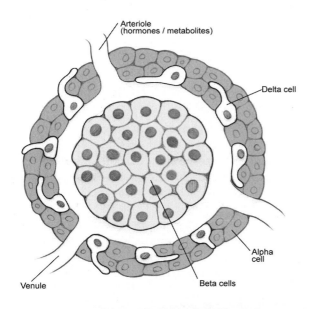

FIGURE 4.5. Structure of the islet of Langerhans. The islet of Langerhans consists of an inner core of insulin-secreting beta cells surrounded by a mantle of glucagon-secreting alpha cells interspersed with somatostatin-secreting delta cells and pancreatic polypeptide (PP)-secreting cells. The PP-secreting cells are few in number, located primarily in the outer layer, and some are located within nerves. Arterioles enter the core of the islet, from which venules carry the blood to the peripheral alpha, delta, and PP cells, thus establishing a portal circulation.

PHYSIOLOGY

EXOCRINE PANCREAS

Composition of Pancreatic Juice

The exocrine secretion of the pancreas consists of water, bicarbonate, and enzymes. Pancreatic juice is alkaline due to its bicarbonate content and typically has a pH of 8.2. Bicarbonate secretion is mainly derived from ductal cells, while enzyme secretion comes from acinar cells. Table 4.1 lists the major secretory products of the exocrine (and endocrine) pancreas and their normal function. The proteolytic enzymes are secreted as proenzymes or zymogens and remain in this inactive form until they reach the duodenum, where, by the action of the mucosal enzyme enterokinase, they are converted into active enzymes.

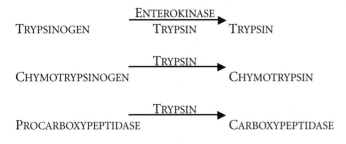

To ensure that these potent active enzymes are not generated within the pancreatic duct, pancreatic juice contains trypsin inhibitors.

Secretory Process

Bicarbonate Secretion

Bicarbonate is secreted primarily by ductal cells through catalytic conversion of carbon dioxide and water by carboxypeptidase.

$$CO_2 + H_2O \xrightarrow{\text{CARBOXYPEPTIDASE}} H_2CO_3 \longrightarrow HCO_3 + H^+$$

The bicarbonate so generated is then secreted into pancreatic ductules, while the H^+ crosses the basolateral membrane to enter the circulation.

Pancreatic Protein (Enzyme) Synthesis and Secretion

Pancreatic proenzymes are synthesized by ribosomes on the rough endoplasmic reticulum. The careful process of packaging and intracellular trafficking described above (Figure 4.4) then ensues to deliver these proteins to the apical membrane. Here, by the process of exocytosis, they

TABLE 4.1. Essentials: Exocrine and Endocrine Pancreas

Exocrine pancreas
  Constitutes 99% of pancreas
  Functional unit: Acinus
  Secretory products
    H_2O + bicarbonate: pH >8
      ▪ Main stimulant: Secretin

  Proenzymes
    Converted to active enzymes by enterokinase and pepsin
      ▪ Trypsinogen
      ▪ Chymotrypsinogen
      ▪ Procarboxypeptidase
Main stimulants: Vagus, CCK

Endocrine pancreas
  Constitutes 1% of pancreas
  Functional unit: Islet of Langerhans
  Cell composition: A, B, D, and PP cells
  Secretory products
    ▪ Insulin: Released from B cells in response to hyperglycemia and insulinotropic gut peptides (GLP, GIP, CCK, secretin)
    ▪ Glucagon: Released from A cells in response to hypoglycemia, sympathomimetics, enteral amino acids, CCK, GIP, glucocorticoids
    ▪ Somatostatin: Released from D cells; exerts inhibitory control on A and B cells
    ▪ Pancreatic polypeptide: Released from PP cells under cholinergic neurocrine regulation

Abbreviations: A, alpha cells; B, beta cells; CCK, cholecystokinin; D, delta cells; GLP, glucagon-like peptide; GIP, gastric inhibitory peptide; PP, pancreatic polypeptide cells.

---

are secreted into the acinar lumen to be carried down ductules to the pancreatic duct and then into the duodenum. Lysosomal hydrolases are also synthesized by ribosomes on the rough endoplasmic reticulum. These powerful activating enzymes are immediately packaged separately and transported to the lysosomes in the cytoplasm of the acinar cell. In this way, they are segregated from the proenzymes to ensure that activation of the latter does not occur within the acinar cell.

Synthesis of pancreatic proenzymes is stimulated by a number of gastrointestinal peptides and by acetylcholine secreted at cholinergic nerve terminals. The major stimulant of the synthesis and release of pancreatic proenzymes is CCK, although a number of other peptides also have similar effects. The latter peptides include neurotensin, PACAP, secretin, and VIP.

Summary of Mechanisms that Protect the Pancreas from Autodigestion

The pancreas is normally protected from autodigestion by the powerful enzymes it secretes in three ways:

1. The proteolytic enzymes are secreted as inactive proenzymes (zymogens) and must reach the duodenum before they are activated by enterokinase. Once trypsin is generated, it also promotes activation of proezymes.
2. The proenzymes are packaged into membrane-bound organelles and transported within the acinar cell to the apical membrane segregated from lysosomal enzymes, which are similarly packaged into lysosomes.
3. Trypsin inhibitors are synthesized and secreted with the proenzymes to ensure that premature activation of proenzymes within the pancreas does not occur.

Regulation of Pancreatic Exocrine Secretions

Complex interaction between nerves and humoral agents regulates pancreatic secretion. Separate mechanisms regulate basal secretion, stimulation, and inhibition of pancreatic secretion. The mechanisms that regulate pancreatic secretion are summarized in Figure 4.6.

Basal Pancreatic Secretion

The pancreas secretes small amounts of proteins (proenzymes) and bicarbonate under basal (fasting) conditions. The amount of basal secretion tends to increase with the migrating motor complex (MMC). Somatostatin exerts inhibitory tone on the action of intrapancreatic CCK-ergic neurons to regulate low levels of basal secretion. The mechanism is depicted in Figure 4.7. Administration of monoclonal somatostatin antibodies to fasting rats causes a significant increase in basal pancreatic secretion. This enhanced basal secretion is blocked by specific CCK-A receptor antagonist, suggesting a key role for intrapancreatic CCK in basal secretion.

Stimulation of Bicarbonate Secretion

The most powerful stimulant of pancreatic bicarbonate secretion is the hormone secretin. Secretin is released from the duodenum mainly by means of acid entering the duodenum. The amount of secretin released and the amount of bicarbonate secreted is directly proportionate to the amount of acid load in the duodenum. Another stimulant of secretin release from the duodenum is luminal fat.

The action of secretin on pancreatic cells is direct, via the secretin receptor. Binding of secretin to its receptor activates adenylate cyclase, resulting in the generation of cyclic adenosine monophosphate (cAMP), which acts as the intracellular messenger.

The action of secretin on water and bicarbonate secretion is amplified by CCK. This synergistic interaction is likely to be important physiologically, since the main releaser of secretin, that is, acid, also releases CCK.

Stimulation of Pancreatic Enzyme Secretion

Pancreatic enzyme secretion is stimulated both by neural and humoral mechanisms.

NEURAL MECHANISMS Direct vagal as well as regional reflexes stimulate pancreatic enzyme secretion.

Vagal Stimulation The vagus-mediated cephalic phase of pancreatic secretion in humans and experimental

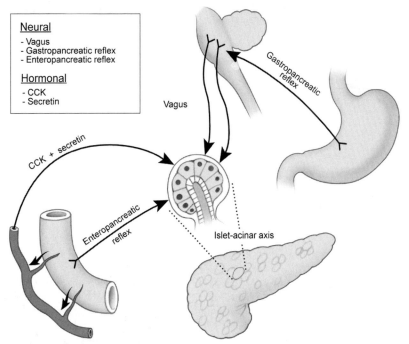

FIGURE 4.6. Regulation of pancreatic exocrine secretion. Neural regulation of exocrine pancreatic secretion involves direct vagal pathways as well as reflex pathways from both the stomach (gastropancreatic reflex) and duodenum (enteropancreatic reflex). Hormonal control is by the pancreatic peptides CCK and secretin. Enzyme secretion is stimulated largely by vagal mechanisms and CCK, while water and bicarbonate secretion is primarily under the control of the hormone secretin.

animals results in low-volume pancreatic secretion that is high in enzyme content. The final event of vagal stimulation at the level of the acinar cells is activation of cholinergic, muscarinic receptors (M3) with resultant generation of intracellular cyclic guanosine monophosphase (cGMP) and calcium. However, vagal stimulation of the acinar cell is not as simple as once thought. It is blocked not only by cholinergic nicotinic and muscarinic receptor antagonists, but also by specific CCK-A receptor antagonist. The action of CCK-A receptor antagonist appears to be on intrapancreatic CCK-ergic neurons, because the inhibition is seen in the isolated, vascularly perfused preparation of rat

pancreas where duodenal CCK is excluded. A proposed mechanism is shown in Figure 4.8.

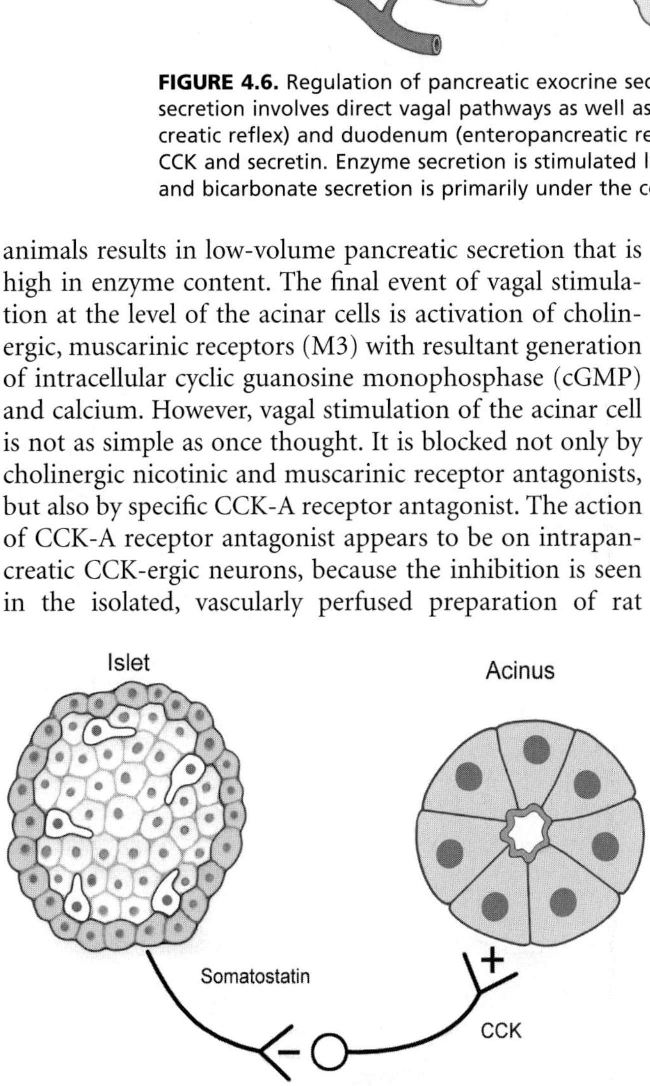

Reflex Pathways Antral distention elicits pancreatic enzyme secretion by activation of an *antropancreatic reflex*, that is, a long vagovagal reflex. The antropancreatic reflex is an important component of the gastric phase of pancreatic secretion. Food entering the duodenum stimulates not only the release of agonist peptides but also another reflex mechanism, the *enteropancreatic reflex.*

HUMORAL MECHANISMS A number of peptides stimulate pancreatic enzyme secretion. These peptides may be hormones (e.g., CCK, secretin, neurotensin) or neurocrine agents (e.g., GRP, PACAP).

Cholecystokinin CCK is released from I cells of the duodenum primarily by protein digest, fat, and acid. (For a more complete discussion of CCK, see Chapter 5). CCK is the most important mediator of the intestinal phase of pancreatic secretion. Its action on pancreatic secretion is mediated via the CCK-A receptor, which is present on acinar cells, intrapancreatic neurons, and cholinergic afferent neurons. At low physiological levels, CCK stimulates pancreatic enzyme secretion by acting on afferent cholinergic pathways originating from the gastroduodenal mucosa. At higher doses, CCK may act directly on acinar cells or on intrapancreatic neurons to stimulate enzyme secretion. In humans, pancreatic enzyme secretion in response to CCK stimulation, particularly to low doses, is inhibited by atropine. Similarly, pancreatic enzyme secre-

FIGURE 4.7. Regulation of basal pancreatic secretion. Basal pancreatic secretion is regulated by the interaction of stimulatory CCK-ergic and inhibitory somatostatin-ergic intrapancreatic neurons, indicating an important islet-acinar axis.

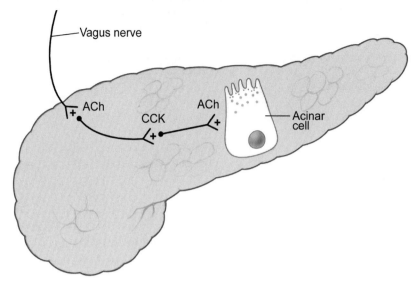

FIGURE 4.8. Vagal stimulation of pancreatic secretion. The mechanism by which the vagus stimulates pancreatic secretion involves preganglionic cholinergic neurons acting on CCK-ergic intrapancreatic interneurons, which, in turn, act on muscarinic cholinergic neurons. Thus, vagal stimulation of pancreatic secretion can be inhibited both by anticholinergic drugs and by CCK-A antagonists.

tion in response to food can be blocked completely by atropine. These observations suggest that CCK action on the pancreas is dependent on cholinergic mechanisms.

Other Humoral Stimulants of Enzyme Secretion A number of other peptides—including PACAP, GRP, and neurotensin—stimulate pancreatic enzyme secretion in vitro and in vivo. To what extent these peptides are important in physiologic control of pancreatic enzymes in humans is unknown. The action of GRP, the mammalian analogue of bombesin, is partly or wholly mediated through the release of CCK.

Inhibition of Pancreatic Secretion

A number of peptides are known to inhibit exocrine pancreatic secretion. These include somatostatin (SS), pancreatic polypeptide (PP), peptide YY (PYY), neuropeptide Y (NPY), pancreastatin, and glucagon. The action of these peptides is indirect through the activation of inhibitory intrapancreatic neurons. None of these peptides exert inhibitory action in vitro in the isolated acinar preparation. The tonic inhibitory role that somatostatin plays in basal pancreatic secretion was discussed earlier. It is likely that the main source of somatostatin in the pancreas is the delta cells of the islets of Langerhans, from which the peptide would diffuse out in a paracrine manner to inhibit acinar cells. Because somatostatin is also found in intrapancreatic neurons, the importance of a neural source of somatostatin cannot be excluded.

ENDOCRINE PANCREAS

The interplay between insulin and glucagon is responsible for maintaining blood sugar levels under normal and adverse circumstances. Thus, the control of secretion of these two peptides is critical.

Insulin Release

Insulin release is regulated by: (1) islet innervation, (2) circulating insulinotropic gut hormones, and (3) local paracrine and neurocrine mechanisms.

Islet Innervation

Splanchnic nerve stimulation causes glucagon release and inhibits insulin release, a response necessary for hypoglycemic crisis situations.

Circulating Insulinotropic Gut Hormones

These include glucagon-like peptide (GLP), gastric inhibitory peptide (GIP), cholecystokinin (CCK), and secretin. These peptides are released by nutrients (fat, proteins) in the gut. They amplify insulin release from the islets and are responsible for the observation that insulin response to an ingested meal is greater than the response to intravenously administered nutrients, known as the incretin effect.

Local Paracrine and Neurocrine Mechanisms

Somatostatin secretion from the delta cells of the islets exerts inhibitory control on insulin release. Under all conditions, the major stimulant of insulin secretion is glucose. The amino acids leucine and arginine are also stimulants. Inhibitory regulation of insulin is accomplished not only by somatostatin but also by the alpha-adrenergic effect of catecholamines.

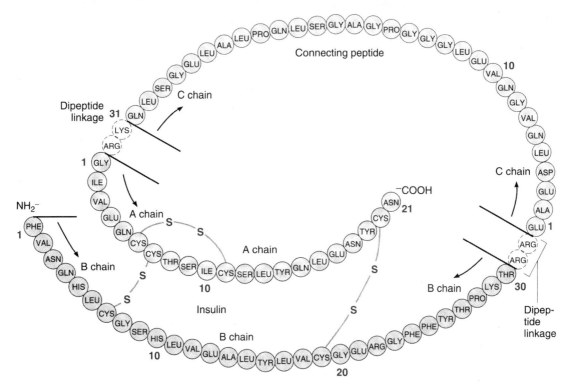

FIGURE 4.9. Structure of human insulin C-peptides and insulin molecules connected at two sites by disulfide links. (Reprinted with permission from Greenspan FS, ed. Basic and Clinical Endocrinology. 6th ed. Los Altos, CA: Lange Medical Publications; McGraw-Hill Companies 2001.)

Glucagon Release

Glucagon secretion is increased by both sympathetic and parasympathetic stimulation. Hypoglycemia is a potent releaser of glucagon, as are several amino acids (e.g., arginine, alanine). The gastrointestinal peptides CCK and GIP, as well as glucocorticoids, also release glucagon. Glucose exerts inhibitory regulation over glucagon. Somatostatin and gamma-aminobutyric acid (GABA) also inhibit glucagon secretion.

BIOCHEMICAL STRUCTURES

Insulin

Insulin is a 51-amino acid peptide consisting of A- and B-chains connected by two disulfide bonds (Figure 4.9). It is the result of posttranslational processing of pre-proinsulin

into proinsulin and then into insulin. Proinsulin is converted into insulin by splitting off the C-peptide and, hence, every molecule of endogenously secreted insulin is accompanied by the release of a molecule of C-peptide. The presence of elevated levels of proinsulin or C-peptide in the blood, therefore, indicates an overproduction of endogenous insulin, a useful indicator in distinguishing the presence of insulinoma from that of factitious hyperinsulinism.

Glucagon

Glucagon, a single-chain peptide of 29 amino acids, also is derived from the processing of a large precursor molecule secreted by alpha cells. Besides glucagon, this proglucagon molecule contains glycentin-related peptide, glucagon-like peptide 1 (GLP-1), and GLP-2.

PATHOPHYSIOLOGY

ACUTE PANCREATITIS

It is generally agreed that, no matter what the primary etiology in acute pancreatitis might be, the final common event is activation of pancreatic proenzymes into nascent

enzymes within the pancreas itself. Once pancreatic parenchymal damage occurs as a result of autodigestion, acute inflammatory cell infiltration begins and is accompanied by the release of cytokines, which further aggravates the inflammatory reaction.

Theories Regarding Initiation of Pancreatitis

What is not generally agreed upon is the mechanism by which pancreatic enzymes are activated within the pancreas. Several of the proposed explanations can be grouped into three theories: (1) secretory block resulting in intracellular activation of enzyme; (2) either bile or duodenal secretion refluxes into the pancreatic duct, causing activation first within the pancreatic ductal system; and (3) damage of pancreatic tissue by toxic or ischemic mechanisms.

Secretory Block Theory

The chapter described above how the intracellular transport of proenzymes in zymogen granules from the Golgi apparatus to the apical membrane is carefully segregated from lysosomal enzymes in lysosomes. An attractive theory popularized by Steer and colleagues that acute pancreatitis arises from a secretory block preventing exocytosis and leading to protein accumulation within the cytoplasm of acinar cells.[1] This leads to fusion of zymogen granules with lysosomes, leading in turn to activation of proenzymes. Also, zymogen granules take an abnormal path to the basolateral membrane and become discharged into the intercellular space. The presence of activated enzymes in the interstitial tissue causes tissue damage and inflammation, resulting in infiltration with activated neutrophils and macrophages and generation of cytokines. These cytokines include TNF-alpha, interleukin-1 beta (IL-1 beta), IL-6, IL-8, and intercellular adhesion molecule-1 (ICAM-1). The stage is then set not only for local inflammation but also for distant damage to organs such as the lung. Intracellular activation has been demonstrated in experimental pancreatitis caused by cerulein or by a choline-deficient diet. It has yet to be demonstrated in human pancreatitis.

Reflux Theory

Experimental pancreatitis can be caused by injection of bile (particularly infected bile) or bile salts into the pancreatic duct. Because approximately 67% of individuals have a common channel pattern, it is possible that a stone obstructing the ampulla of Vater could lead to reflux of bile into the pancreatic duct. Conversely, passage of a stone into the duodenum may temporarily leave the ampulla patulous, allowing duodenal fluid to reflux into the pancreatic duct. Duodenal fluid, of course, contains enterokinase, which could activate the proenzymes within the pancreas.

Pancreatitis occurs as a complication of endoscopic retrograde cholangiopancreatography (ERCP), with an approximate 1% incidence. The mechanism for this type of pancreatitis is not known, although excessive pressure of injection rather than postprocedure reflux of bile or duodenal juice is the probable cause.

Direct Damage of Pancreas

Toxic or ischemic damage of the pancreas may cause acute pancreatitis. One of the mechanisms proposed for alcohol-induced pancreatitis is acetaldehyde toxicity. Alcohol is metabolized into acetaldehyde, which has been shown experimentally to damage the pancreas by leading to increased permeability of ductal epithelium, which allows pancreatic enzymes to escape into the interstitial tissue. Acetaldehyde can also serve as a substrate for generation of toxic-free oxygen radicals. Other possible but less likely mechanisms for alcohol-induced pancreatitis include direct toxic damage of acinar cells and stimulation of pancreatic secretion at a time when spasm of the sphincter of Oddi has been caused by the presence of alcohol in the duodenal lumen. Hypertriglyceridemias are also thought to cause pancreatitis by leading to generation of toxic metabolites.

Ischemia causes tissue damage and capillary permeability. Ischemic insult capable of causing pancreatitis is seen in shock, hypothermia, during cardiopulmonary bypass surgery or in diseases causing small-vessel abnormalities (e.g., lupus, other collagen diseases). Conditions that cause ischemia, particularly those with systemic effects, lead to massive catecholamine response releasing alpha-adrenergic constrictors, which accentuate ischemia and initiate necrosis.

Etiologic Factors in Acute Pancreatitis

Several known etiologic factors in acute pancreatitis probably share more than one of the pathogenetic mechanisms for in situ enzyme activation described above. Alcohol and gallstones account for over 90% of cases of acute pancreatitis in the United States.[2]

Gallstones

The most common cause of pancreatitis, gallstones account for 60% of all cases of acute pancreatitis seen. Approximately 5% of individuals with gallstones develop acute pancreatitis. The likelihood is increased in those with small stones, those with a long common channel, and those with choledocholithiasis. Intraoperative cholangiogram associated with reflux into the pancreatic duct increases the likelihood of acute pancreatitis.

The great majority of patients who develop gallstone pancreatitis are not found to have a stone impacted at the lower end of the CBD. The question then is, how do stones cause pancreatitis? The two possible mechanisms are: (1) bile reflux into the pancreatic duct while the stone is going through the sphincter; or (2) reflux of enterokinase-containing duodenal fluid through the sphincter, left patulous after passage of the stone.

Three types of biliary (gallstone) pancreatitis may be recognized, based on severity of clinical presentation:

1. Type A. Biochemical pancreatitis or hyperamylasemia is found without associated abdominal findings. The hyperamylasemia is transient, lasting no more than 24 to 48 h.
2. Type B. Hyperamylasemia with moderate pancreatitis is associated with abdominal signs, often lasting 4 to 7 days and not associated with respiratory or other organ failure.
3. Type C. Type C disease indicates severe pancreatitis with multiple organ failure.

It is now clear that biliary pancreatitis can be cured with cholecystectomy and, if present, removal of CBD stones, with an extremely low risk of future recurrence or development of chronic pancreatitis.

Alcohol

Alcohol is the second most common cause of acute pancreatitis overall, but the most common in the population of patients seen in county and city hospitals. An acute attack often follows an episode of binge drinking. Alcoholic pancreatitis varies in its severity, but alcohol is the cause of some of the most severe cases of pancreatitis. Following an initial acute attack, alcoholic pancreatitis has a greater propensity than biliary pancreatitis to cause recurrent attacks and lead to chronic pancreatitis.

Postoperative and Post-ERCP Pancreatitis

Operations on and around the pancreas are associated with a small but significant incidence of postoperative or postprocedure acute pancreatitis. Gastric and hepatobiliary operations are associated with the highest incidence following operations on the pancreas itself. Postoperative pancreatitis can be severe and is associated with significant mortality.

The overall incidence of post-ERCP pancreatitis is 1%, but the incidence is higher when extensive instrumentation or manipulation of the papilla is required. Endoscopic sphincterotomy is associated with acute pancreatitis in 3% to 4% of cases.[3]

Hyperlipidemia

A higher incidence of acute pancreatitis has been recognized in several types of hyperlipidemias, especially Types I, IV and V. Some patients have milky serum during an attack of acute pancreatitis, due to massive elevation of triglycerides. This phenomenon can be seen in individuals without familial hyperlipidemia, presumably secondary to severe acute pancreatitis. Hence, when familial hyperlipidemia is suspected, full investigation should await total resolution of the pancreatitis. Patients with familial hyperlipidemia show high serum triglyceride levels but normal cholesterol. Hyperlipidemia may be associated with some of the severest attacks of necrotizing pancreatitis.

Hypercalcemia

Both primary and secondary hyperparathyroidism may be associated with acute pancreatitis. Although the mechanism is unknown, calcium is not only a potent releaser of the peptides that stimulate the pancreas, but it is also the intracellular secondary messenger leading to synthesis and secretion of pancreatic enzymes.

Drugs

Several drugs are associated with acute pancreatitis. The most common are thiazide diuretics, corticosteroids, estrogens, azathioprine, angiotensin-converting enzyme (ACE), sulfonamides, and tetracycline.

Carcinoma of the Pancreas

Occasionally, carcinoma of the pancreas presents with an attack of acute pancreatitis, presumably because of pancreatic duct obstruction by the tumor.

Idiopathic Pancreatitis

No demonstrable cause is seen in a significant number of patients with acute pancreatitis.

Other Causes

Acute pancreatitis may follow trauma, organ transplantation, or infection with viruses such as mumps, Epstein-Barr, or coxsackie virus. Bacterial infection with *Campylobacter* and infestation with ascariasis and *Clonorchis sinensis* have also been associated with acute pancreatitis. The association of pancreas divisum with acute pancreatitis has not been supported by incidence studies in large groups of patients.

Evolution of the Clinical Picture

The evolution of the full clinical picture in severe acute pancreatitis is described below and in Table 4.2. Not all attacks are severe and mild attacks will not have the discernible phases described here.

Hypovolemic Phase

The first 24 h or more of an acute attack are characterized by variable degrees of hypovolemia, with hypovolemic shock developing in severe cases. Several causes of hypovolemia may be identified:

1. Sequestration of fluid. Fluid may be sequestered in and around the pancreas, in the retroperitoneal space, in the peritoneal cavity, and within intestinal lumen due to paralytic ileus.
2. Systemic vasodilatation. Vasodilatation may occur as a result of release into the circulation of vasoactive sub-

TABLE 4.2. Essentials: Clinical Course of Acute Pancreatitis

Hypovolemic phase
  First 24 h, characterized by:
  - Sequestration of fluid (hypovolemia)
  - Systemic vasodilatation
  - Abdominal pain, vomiting, fever
  - Release of myocardial depressing factor
  - Hypotension

Respiratory phase
  Within 48–72 h, characterized by:
  - Tachypnea
  - Hypoxemia
  - Acute respiratory distress syndrome (in severe cases)

Septic phase
  Usually during second or third week
  Septic complications may include:
  - Infected necrosis
  - Pancreatic abscess
  - Infected pseudocyst
  - Acute cholangitis

stances such as bradykinin. This leads to reduction in circulating volume.

3. Abdominal pain, vomiting, and fever.

4. Myocardial depressing factor. Hypovolemia may be aggravated by decreased cardiac output secondary to release of myocardial depressing factor (MDF) from the injured pancreas. In addition to its systemic effects, hypovolemia contributes to pancreatic necrosis. Hemorrhagic pancreatitis is not seen as frequently now as it was 20 to 30 years ago, possibly because of the preventive effect of aggressive volume resuscitation now practiced in the early stages of the disease.

Respiratory Phase

Acute respiratory distress syndrome (ARDS), as evidenced by tachypnea and hypoxemia, is a common feature of severe acute pancreatitis, usually seen within 48 to 72 hours of onset. The more severe the attack, the earlier the signs and symptoms of respiratory distress develop, and the sooner the patient requires assisted ventilation. Two factors are important in the development of respiratory failure:

1. Lung injury. Lung injury is believed to be caused by cytokines released from activated neutrophils and macrophages. The important cytokines that have been implicated include TNF-alpha, IL-1, IL-6, IL-8, and IL-10, and the intercellular adhesion molecule (ICAM-1). Phospholipase A_2 (PLA_2) released from the injured pancreas is one of the factors that activates macrophages and neutrophils. Other toxic substances released by the injured pancreas, such as free fatty acids, may also contribute.

2. Decreased diaphragmatic movement. Abdominal pain limits diaphragmatic excursion, and the mechanics of breathing become intercostal.

Respiratory failure is a bad prognostic sign but, thanks to excellent treatment in intensive care units, most patients with this complication now survive. Occasionally, respiratory failure may develop later in the course of the disease or recur after initial improvement. This type of clinical setback in the course of the disease is invariably associated with infected pancreatic necrosis.

Septic Phase

Not all patients with acute pancreatitis develop sepsis, even in the presence of pancreatic necrosis. The overwhelming number of patients who develop septic complication, however, have pancreatic necrosis. The septic phase usually occurs in the second or third week, although it may occur even in the first week. Four types of septic complications are seen:

1. Infected necrosis. Infection of the necrotic pancreas or peripancreatic fat is the most serious complication. It is more serious and occurs earlier (within the first 2 weeks) than other types of septic complications. Infected necrosis is often associated with respiratory and other organ failure and may carry a mortality as high as 30%.[4] The source of bacterial infection is the gut, as evidenced experimentally by significant reduction in infection when either the gut is sterilized or the pancreas is mechanically shielded from the colon.

2. Pancreatic abscess. Abscess, a walled-off collection of pus in or around the pancreas, usually occurs after the second week. In a large study from Bittner and colleagues,[5] the average time to surgery from onset of pancreatitis was 2 weeks for infected necrosis and 5 weeks for pancreatic abscess.

3. Infected pseudocyst. This complication tends to occur late and represents infection of preexisting pseudocyst. The clinical course is neither as severe nor as fatal as infected necrosis or pancreatic abscess.

4. Acute cholangitis. This complication, which occurs when the CBD is obstructed, is seen almost exclusively in patients with biliary pancreatitis. The clinical picture is characterized by fever, chills, jaundice, increased pain, and mental obtundation.

Development of Other Complications

Several other complications are possible.

Pseudocysts

The wide utilization of CT scan has demonstrated that pseudocysts form in over 50% of patients with severe acute pancreatitis. Most of these cases resolve spontaneously.

Pseudocysts represent a collection of fluid associated with loss of integrity of a pancreatic duct.

Pseudocysts that do not resolve spontaneously proceed to form mature wall and become clinically significant when they persist beyond 4 to 6 weeks or achieve a size of 5 cm or more. Pseudocysts also become clinically significant if they: (1) perforate, causing peritonitis or pancreatic ascites; (2) erode into a blood vessel, causing a pseudoaneurysm that might rupture freely into the peritoneal cavity or into an adjacent viscus; or (3) compress an adjacent organ, either the CBD or duodenum, to cause obstruction.

Hemorrhage

Life-threatening hemorrhage occurs in 1% to 2% of patients with severe acute pancreatitis.[2] This complication may be associated with acute pseudocyst as described above, or it may occur in the absence of a pseudocyst.

Metabolic Complications

1. Hypocalcemia. A sign of severe pancreatitis, hypocalcemia may be caused by removal of calcium from circulation as calcium soaps, parathyroid hormone dysfunction, and increased deposition in bone due to increased calcitonin activity.

2. Hyperglycemia. A transient picture of hyperglycemia and glycosuria may be seen. An attack of acute pancreatitis is unlikely to lead to diabetes unless major necrosectomy has to be done. In patients with greater than 50% necrosectomy, more than 50% develop diabetes.

Hepatobiliary Complications

A mild picture of hepatocellular dysfunction or obstructive jaundice may occur. Acalculous cholecystitis occurs infrequently, usually at the time oral feeding is started. Although extremely rare, portal vein or hepatic artery thrombosis may occur, causing severe hepatobiliary and systemic dysfunction.

Gastrointestinal Complications

1. Upper GI bleeding. Bleeding may complicate the development of erosions or peptic ulcer or represent rupture of a pseudoaneurysm due to pseudocysts into the upper GI tract. It may also indicate bleeding from gastric varices due to splenic vein thrombosis, although this is rare in acute pancreatitis.

2. Bowel necrosis. Bowel necrosis leading to perforation, fistula formation, or stricture is a well-known complication. The transverse colon is at most risk.

3. Bowel obstruction. Bowel obstruction may occur due to compression from pseudocysts, adhesion formation, or development of stricture.

Vascular Complications

Several vascular complications may develop in acute pancreatitis:

1. Massive hemorrhage during acute attack. This uncommon complication represents necrosis and vascular wall digestion by nascent pancreatic enzymes during the early course of severe acute pancreatitis. Bleeding has occurred from the gastroduodenal, pancreaticoduodenal, or other pancreatic vessels. Still other vessels that may be involved include the hepatic, gastric, or even the splenic arteries.

2. Pseudoaneurysm formation. This complication can develop either as a result of partial damage to the wall of an artery or secondary to the erosion of a pseudocyst into an adjacent vessel. The latter is more serious because hemorrhage invariably follows.

When a pseudocyst erodes into a vessel, it suddenly enlarges, becomes pulsatile, and causes increased pain. This erosion, in essence the formation of a thin-walled pseudoaneurysm, causes bleeding in one of three ways: (1) free bleeding into the abdominal cavity; (2) erosion into adjacent viscus, leading to gastrointestinal hemorrhage; or, rarely, (3) bleeding back into the pancreatic duct in the presence of significant communication between the pseudocyst and the main pancreatic duct. In the latter case, bleeding occurs into the duodenum through the ampulla of Vater, a condition known as hemosuccus pancreaticus.

3. Left-sided portal hypertension and gastric varices. Splenic vein thrombosis sometimes complicates the course of acute pancreatitis. This condition leads to venous hypertension in the area drained by the splenic vein and, therefore, results in splenomegaly and gastric varices. Gastric varices may bleed, leading to upper gastrointestinal hemorrhage.

4. Portal vein thrombosis. An uncommon complication, portal vein thrombosis may contribute to ascites, sometimes present in acute pancreatitis.

CHRONIC PANCREATITIS

Although chronic pancreatitis can follow acute pancreatitis, two epidemiologic observations suggest that the two diseases are different. First, patients with chronic pancreatitis are, on average, 10 years younger than patients with acute pancreatitis. Second, alcohol is the cause of chronic pancreatitis in 70% to 80% of cases.[6] Other causes of acute pancreatitis (e.g., gallstones, hyperlipidemia, drugs) are infrequently associated with chronic pancreatitis.

Pathogenesis

The common final physical event in the pathogenesis of chronic pancreatitis appears to be the development of

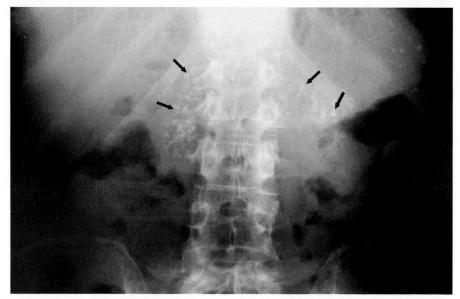

FIGURE 4.10. The common final physical event in the pathogenesis of chronic pancreatitis is the development of viscous pancreatic juice, leading to formation of protein plugs and secondary calcification (arrows), visible on x-ray. (Courtesy of Henry I. Goldberg, MD.)

viscous pancreatic juice, which subsequently leads to formation of protein plugs and secondary calcification (Figure 4.10). Two theories have been advanced:

1. Direct action of alcohol on the exocrine pancreas. This theory proposes that alcohol causes an increase in secretion of pancreatic proteins (enzymes) and a decrease in secretion of water, bicarbonate, and trypsin inhibitors.

2. Decreased secretion of pancreatic stone protein (lithostatin). The proposal is that chronic pancreatitis is associated with a lowered concentration of pancreatic stone protein. In patients with chronic pancreatitis, the concentration of pancreatic stone protein has been reported to be lowered, thus allowing calcium crystals and proteins to precipitate. Pancreatic stone protein (14,000-Da protein) is normally secreted in pancreatic juice and functions to prevent precipitation of calcium to form stones.

The essential features of this pathophysiology are summarized in Figure 4.11. Progression of disease includes:

1. Progressive inflammation and ductal injury, leading to progressive fibrosis, ductal obstruction, and stricture formation.
2. Calcification of proteinaceous plugs.
3. Progressive destruction of functional exocrine and endocrine pancreas, leading to pancreatic exocrine insufficiency (steatorrhea) and diabetes.
4. Development of pain, which gradually becomes intractable.

Etiologic Factors in Chronic Pancreatitis

Alcohol

The leading cause of chronic pancreatitis, alcohol accounts for 70% to 80% of all cases. National statistics in England and Wales have shown a close and direct correlation between the per capita consumption of alcohol and the incidence of hospital discharges for chronic pancreatitis. Between 1960 and 1988, both alcohol consumption and the incidence of chronic pancreatitis doubled in England and Wales.[7]

Familial Pancreatitis

Familial pancreatitis, a rare familial condition with Mendelian dominant inheritance, may lead to cancer in up to 25% of family members.

Tropical Pancreatitis

Seen in young people in the tropics, this form of chronic pancreatitis is thought to be caused by the combination of malnutrition and the presence of toxins in the diet (cassava and sorghum).

Hyperparathyroidism

Hyperparathyroidism is a rare cause of chronic pancreatitis.

Biliary Tract Disease

Although there is no clear evidence that chronic pancreatitis is caused by biliary tract disease, chronic

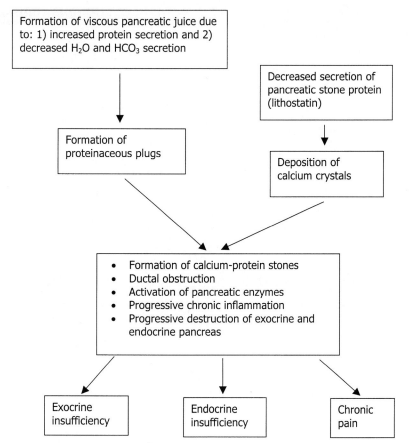

FIGURE 4.11. Essential features in the pathophysiology of chronic pancreatitis include formation of viscous pancreatic juice and decreased secretion of lithostatin, leading to exocrine and endocrine insufficiency and pain.

pancreatitis itself can lead to biliary disease due to stasis and stone formation in the common bile duct.

Obstructive Causes

Chronic pancreatic ductal obstruction from any cause may lead to chronic pancreatitis. Obstruction can be caused by post-traumatic or post-acute pancreatitis stricture, neoplasia, and perhaps also pancreas division, in which the entrance of the main pancreatic duct is strictured.

Cystic Fibrosis

Tenacious pancreatic juice is associated with defective chloride and water secretion in this congenital disease.

Idiopathic Causes

No cause is known in as many as 20% of patients with chronic pancreatitis.

Morphological Changes

A variety of morphological changes occur in the pancreas (Figure 4.12A), from minimal to end-stage fibrosis and destruction of the exocrine pancreas. Chronic inflamma-

tion is superimposed with acute necrosis. Single or multiple strictures of the pancreatic ducts may develop, and ducts may be obstructed with proteinaceous plugs or calculi. In the investigation of patients with chronic pancreatitis using ERCP or CT or MRI scans, two forms of chronic pancreatitis are recognizable depending on the size of the main pancreatic duct:

1. Small duct disease, in which no significant dilatation of the pancreatic duct occurs (Figure 4.12B); and
2. Large duct disease, in which the pancreatic duct is dilated (>6mm) uniformly or in parts, with intervening fibrosis giving the impression of a chain of lakes (Figure 4.12C).

As discussed later, these two morphological types have a significant impact both on the choice and outcome of surgical treatment.

Functional Disturbances in Chronic Pancreatitis

Pain

Pain from chronic pancreatitis, the most important symptom, is present in more than 90% of patients.

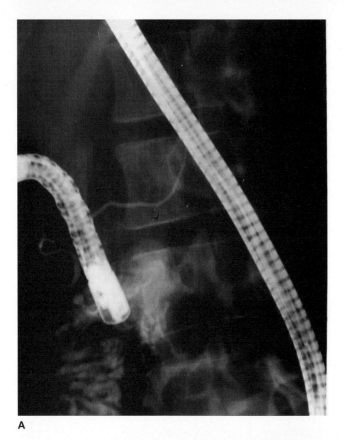

A

B

FIGURE 4.12. (A) In comparison with a normal pancreatic duct, (B) endoscopic appearance of small duct chronic pancreatitis demonstrates minimal dilatation (diameter <6 mm), tortuosity, and irregular contour of the main pancreatic duct and side branches. (C) Endoscopic appearance of large duct disease is characterized by pancreatic duct dilatation of >6 mm with intervening fibrosis and chain of lakes appearance. (Courtesy of Henry I. Goldberg, MD.)

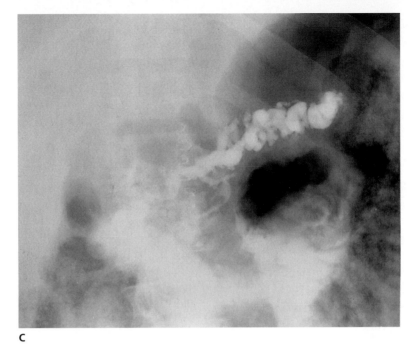

C

FIGURE 4.12. *Continued*

Immunohistochemical studies of pancreata with chronic pancreatitis have demonstrated the presence of large amounts of calcitonin gene-related peptide and serotonin. CGRP-containing neurons are the sensory neurons, and the increased accumulation of CGRP is believed to be related to increased pain sensation. Other mechanisms may also operate.

Exocrine Pancreatic Insufficiency

Most patients have decreased secretion of pancreatic enzyme. Some develop overt steatorrhea, which results when pancreatic enzyme secretion is inadequate to provide complete digestion of fat and protein. Large quantities of fat are secreted in the stool, which becomes greasy and foul-smelling. Stools typically float in the toilet bowl, and may be difficult to flush. With the failure in fat digestion, variable deficiencies of the fat-soluble vitamins (A, D, E, K) may develop. Weight loss may be significant.

Endocrine Insufficiency

Diabetes develops in most patients with severe chronic pancreatitis lasting more than 10 to 15 years. The incidence of diabetes is dramatically increased by resective surgery. Patients with total pancreatectomy, in particular, are likely to have "brittle" diabetes and are susceptible to sudden death. Hence, it is important to consider concomitant islet cell transplantation when total pancreatectomy is the treatment of choice. Recent advances in islet cell transplantation, both in islet harvesting techniques and specific immunosuppression, are very promising.

Other Complications of Chronic Pancreatitis

Chronic Pseudocyst

More than two-thirds of pseudocysts requiring surgical management are associated with chronic pancreatitis. Pseudocysts are a feature of the clinical picture of chronic pancreatitis in 25%–30% of cases. They may be single or multiple, and a communication to the main pancreatic duct is identified by ERCP in at least 50% of pseudocysts larger than 5 cm in diameter. Important complications of pseudocyst include: (1) free rupture, which occurs when the pseudocyst communicates with the pancreatic duct, and results in pancreatic ascites; (2) erosion into adjacent vessel, which leads to formation of pseudoaneurysm and hemorrhage; (3) distal common duct obstruction; and (4) duodenal obstruction.

Portal Hypertension

Splenic vein thrombosis may cause left-sided portal hypertension and gastric varices. This complication can lead to upper GI hemorrhage.

Biliary Obstruction

CBD obstruction, due to fibrosis and stricture of the intrapancreatic portion of the CBD, leads to obstructive jaundice.

Intestinal Obstruction

The duodenum and transverse colon are susceptible to obstruction. The latter may mimic carcinoma.

Carcinoma of the Pancreas

There is no convincing evidence that chronic pancreatitis causes pancreatic cancer. The two conditions, however, may coexist. It is estimated that 4% of patients with chronic pancreatitis develop pancreatic cancer within 20 years of the onset of the pancreatitis.[8]

CLINICAL MANAGEMENT

ACUTE PANCREATITIS

Although no major breakthrough has occurred in our understanding of the etiology and pathogenesis of acute pancreatitis, significant advances in management of the disease have improved survival. Clinical management (Table 4.3) is guided by answering the following four critical questions: (1) Is this acute pancreatitis and what is the cause (i.e., diagnosis)? (2) How severe is the attack (i.e., severity assessment)? (3) Is pancreatic necrosis present? (4) Is pancreatic sepsis present?

Diagnosis

Clinical Features

Upper abdominal pain radiating to the back in the region of L1 is a predominant feature of acute pancreatitis. The pain often develops 2 to 3 h after ingestion of a large fatty meal or alcohol. Nausea and vomiting are frequent. Abdominal pain tends to get worse in the supine position and improves when the patient sits up and leans forward. When the attack is severe, the clinical picture is that of the acute abdomen. Because of the retroperitoneal location of the pancreas, however, abdominal rigidity is not as marked as in the case of a ruptured viscus. Severe cases may be associated with hypovolemic shock, anuria, and respiratory failure. In the rare occurrence of retroperitoneal hemorrhage, blood may track along fascial planes and produce discoloration of the flank (Cullen's sign) or around the umbilicus (Grey-Turner's sign). Low-grade fever is common. The differential diagnosis includes perforated peptic ulcer, acute cholecystitis, appendicitis, mesenteric infarction, ruptured ectopic pregnancy, and myocardial infarction.

Laboratory Investigation

A complete blood count should be obtained. The white blood count is elevated, sometimes above 20,000 cells/hpf. Elevated serum amylase, present in more than 90% of patients on admission, is the most helpful finding. The amylase levels are highest in the first 8 to 24 hours and tend to be higher in biliary pancreatitis. Serum amylase may not be elevated in very severe disease or in patients with preexisting chronic pancreatitis. The elevation in acute pancreatitis starts to fall within 24 h and may return to normal within 48 to 96 h.

TABLE 4.3. Essentials: Management of Acute Pancreatitis

Diagnosis
  Clinical features: Abdominal pain, peritoneal signs, nausea and vomiting, fever, hypovolemia, hypotension, anuria, respiratory failure, Cullen's sign, Grey-Turner's sign (if hemorrhagic)
  Laboratory: Leukocytosis, hyperamylasemia, hypocalcemia
  Imaging studies:
   - Abdominal ultrasound: Assesses biliary tree, may show pancreatic enlargement or fluid collection
   - Abdominal CT scan: Best method to assess pancreatic inflammation, necrosis

Assessment of severity
  Clinical criteria: Ranson, Imrie (Glasgow), or APACHE II (see Table 4.4)
  CT criteria: Grades A to E

Initial therapy
  Volume and electrolyte (calcium) resuscitation
  Prevention of aspiration (nasogastric suction)
  Respiratory support: Endotracheal intubation, assisted ventilation
  Pain control

Subsequent management
  Intravenous antibiotics in severe disease
  Nutritional support
  Monitoring for pancreatic necrosis (CE-CT)
  If necrosis exists, rule out pancreatic infection (FNA: Gram stain, culture, and sensitivity)
  If biliary pancreatitis exists, perform early endoscopic sphincterotomy, followed later by cholecystectomy

Management of complications
  Infected necrosis: Surgical debridement and drainage
  Pancreatic abscess: Surgical debridement and drainage
  Infected pseudocyst: Percutaneous catheter drainage
  Pancreatic hemorrhage: Attempt angiographic control; if unsuccessful, operative control
  Cholangitis: Endoscopic drainage, followed by definitive biliary tract disease treatment, if present

Abbreviations: CE, contrast-enhanced; CT, computerized tomography; FNA, fine-needle aspiration cytology.

Hyperamylasemia may be seen in several nonpancreatic conditions; important among these are perforated peptic ulcer, mesenteric infarction, and ruptured ectopic pregnancy. It is rare for serum amylase levels to be elevated more than three times the normal level in these nonpancreatic causes of hyperamylasemia. Measuring urinary amylase is important because its level tends to stay elevated longer and rules out renal failure as a cause of hyperamylasemia. When low urinary amylase level is associated with high serum amylase level but serum creatinine is normal, the condition of macroamylasemia should be suspected. The serum lipase level is more specific than serum amylase and tends to stay elevated longer. It has a sensitivity and specificity of 90% and is the best test when uncertainty exists. Other tests necessary for severity assessment include blood glucose, liver function tests, blood urea nitrogen, serum albumin, and arterial oxygen saturation.

Imaging Studies

Abdominal ultrasound is an important early examination in acute pancreatitis to assess for gallstones, the presence of which is highly suggestive of biliary pancreatitis. Its ability to assess the severity of pancreatitis is severely limited by gas in the intestine. Nevertheless, ultrasound identifies most significant fluid collections in and around the pancreas.

Plain films of the abdomen (supine, upright, and decubitus) are useful to rule out perforated viscus. Specific findings that support the presence of pancreatitis are a dilated, fluid-filled stomach, duodenum, and ileus; and a dilated, air-filled transverse colon—sometimes a cut-off sign when gas is seen in the ascending and descending but not in the transverse colon. Occasionally, a sentinel loop of jejunum is seen, which represents localized ileus in a loop of bowel adjacent to the inflamed pancreas.

CT scan of the abdomen, the best imaging study both to diagnose and to estimate the severity of acute pancreatitis, should be delayed until circulating volume is restored to avoid renal failure. CT scan is most useful when enhanced by intravenous injection of a bolus of contrast agent. If the diagnosis of acute pancreatitis is evident, contrast-enhanced CT (CE-CT) is usually delayed 48 to 72h, at which time severity of disease can be properly evaluated.

Severity of Pancreatitis

Determining the severity of pancreatitis is a key step in management. It is best done by a combination of clinical and CT criteria. A useful practice is to obtain a clinical score within 48h of admission and a CT scan within 72h if the pancreatitis is severe. Routine use of these methods has facilitated comparison of various treatments in various centers.

Clinical Criteria

Three clinical criteria are in use: Ranson, Imrie (Glasgow), and the APACHE II scores (Table 4.4). Any of these three

TABLE 4.4. Clinical Scoring to Assess Severity of Acute Pancreatitis

Ranson criteria
0–2 = mild, 3–5 = moderately severe, >5 = very severe
On admission
- Age >55 years
- WBC ≥16,000
- Blood glucose >200 mg/dL
- LDH >300 IU/L
- SGOT >250 μm/dL

During initial 48 hours
- Hematocrit fall >10%
- Arterial oxygen saturation (P_aO_2) <60 mm Hg
- BUN rise >5 mg/dL
- Serum Ca^{++} <8 mg/dL
- Fluid sequestration >6000 mL

Imrie (Glasgow) criteria
On Admission
- Age >55 years
- WBC >15,000
- Blood glucose >10 nmol/L
- Serum urea >16 mmol/L (no response to IV fluids)
- Arterial oxygen saturation (P_aO_2) <60 mm Hg

During initial 48 h
- Serum calcium <2 mmol/L
- Serum albumin <32 g/L
- LDH >600 μL
- Aspartate aminotransferase/alanine aminotransferase >100 μm/L

APACHE II scoring
Acute physiology score = total points (0–4) for each of 12 variables:

Temperature:	0 = 36.0°–38.4°; 4 = <30.0° or >40.9°
Mean arterial pressure:	0 = 70–109; 4 = <50 or >159
Heart rate:	0 = 70–109; 4 = <40 or >179
Respiratory rate:	0 = 12–24; 4 = <6 or >49
FiO_2:	0 = >70; 4 = <55
Arterial pH:	0 = 7.33–7.49; 4 = <7.15 or >7.69
Serum sodium:	0 = 130–149; 4 = <111 or >179
Serum potassium:	0 = 3.5–5.4; 4 = <2.5 or >6.9
Serum creatinine:	0 = 53–129; 4 = ARF >305
Hemoglobin (g/L):	0 = 100–153; 4 = <67 or >200
WBC (per mm³):	0 = 3.0–14.9; 4 = <1.0 or >39.9
Glasgow coma score (GCS):	Actual points

Abbreviations: APACHE II, acute physiology and chronic health evaluation; BUN, blood urea nitrogen; Ca^{++}, ionized calcium; FiO_2, fraction of inspired oxygen; IV, intravenous; LDH, lactate dehydrogenase; SGOT, serum glutamic-oxaloacetic transaminase; WBC, white blood cell.

may be used, the important point being that the same criteria must be used over time.

When the Ranson criteria are used, a score of 2 or lower indicates mild pancreatitis, 3 to 5 moderately severe pancreatitis, and above 5 very severe pancreatitis. The mortality rate rises with the severity score.

CT Criteria

The severity of pancreatitis on CT scan has been graded as follows:

1. Grade A (score = 0): normal pancreas (Figure 4.13A).
2. Grade B (score = 1): pancreatic enlargement (Figure 4.13B).
3. Grade C (score = 2): grade B plus inflammation in the peripancreatic tissue (Figure 4.13C).
4. Grade D (score = 3): phlegmon and one fluid collection (Figure 4.13D).
5. Grade E (score = 4): phlegmon and two or more fluid collections (Figure 4.13E).

CE-CT scan is the best way to follow the course of severe pancreatitis that does not resolve, while ultrasonography is reserved to follow the course of any fluid collection.

Diagnosis of Pancreatic Necrosis

Pancreatic and peripancreatic necroses are the most important predisposing factors for pancreatic sepsis. Necrosis is associated with mortality rates of 5% to 20%, but virtually all patients with pancreatitis who do not have necrosis survive.[4] If patient does not improve in the first 2 weeks of the disease, it is critical that he or she be evaluated for pancreatic necrosis to determine whether any necrotic tissue is infected.

Numerous methods have been used in the attempt to confirm an early diagnosis of pancreatic necrosis. Most tests are based on serum concentrations of various indicators, including elevations in poly-[C]-specific ribonuclease (RNA-ase), alterations of alpha-1-protease inhibitor and alpha-2 macroglobulin, and decreases in complement factor C_3 and C_4. Unfortunately, none of these serum markers provide accurate diagnosis. Imaging with ultrasound and ^{111}In white-cell scan are likewise unsatisfactory.

The best available method at present is CE-CT, which correctly identifies the presence of necrosis in 90% of patients with severe pancreatitis. When a bolus of contrast is rapidly injected during CT scanning of the pancreas, vascularized pancreatic tissue is enhanced while areas of necrosis show as perfusion defects (Figure 4.14). The presence of pancreatic necrosis should lead to the next important question: Is the necrosis infected? Infected necrosis is more common than abscess formation.

Diagnosis of Sepsis in Acute Pancreatitis

1. Infected necrosis. The most serious complication of necrosis is infection. Mortality rates double when necrosis becomes infected. Once necrosis occurs, the likelihood of infection is as high as 50% to 70%.[4] Infection tends to occur within 1–2 weeks of onset of acute pancreatitis.

A clinical picture of deteriorating symptoms such as spiking fever, tachycardia, high leukocytosis with a shift to the left, and diminishing oxygen saturation should indicate the presence of infected necrosis. Unless diagnosis is made rapidly and treatment instituted, the patient becomes progressively confused and mentally obtunded. Septic shock with multiple organ failure and death may ensue. This type of end-stage deterioration can be prevented by regular follow-up of the sick patient with CE-CT and, when necrosis is diagnosed, fine-needle aspiration (FNA) for bacteriological studies.

CE-CT may demonstrate air bubbles associated with areas of poor or no perfusion, which is a late finding. Once CE-CT demonstrates necrosis, a CT-guided FNA is indicated to obtain aspirate for culture and sensitivity and for an examination with a Gram stain slide. CT- or ultrasound-guided FNA has proven to be safe and nearly always diagnostic. The finding of bacteria on Gram stain or culture indicates the need for surgical debridement.

2. Pancreatic abscess and infected pseudocyst. A pancreatic abscess probably results from infection of localized necrosis that undergoes liquefaction (Figure 4.15). It typically develops later than infected necrosis, often from 3 to 5 weeks after the acute attack. Pancreatic abscess develops in 1% to 4% of all patients with acute pancreatitis. The systemic manifestations of sepsis tend to be milder than those of infected necrosis. Another cause of pancreatic abscess is secondary infection of a preexisting pseudocyst. Diagnosis is established by CT or ultrasound scan with FNA to identify the infecting agent.

3. Acute cholangitis. Acute cholangitis accompanying acute pancreatitis is nearly always caused by CBD obstruction due to a gallstone. It is theoretically possible that obstruction of the distal CBD may be caused by edema in the head of the pancreas or an acute pseudocyst, leading to ascending cholangitis. Symptoms are fever with chills, abdominal pain, jaundice, and changes in the level of consciousness.

Ultrasonography usually shows stones within the gallbladder, rarely within the CBD, and modest dilatation of the extrahepatic biliary tree. Emergent ERCP may be required for diagnostic and therapeutic purposes.

General Treatment

Initial Therapy

Therapy in the first 24 to 48 h—the so-called hypovolemic phase of acute pancreatitis—is directed at volume resuscitation, prevention of aspiration, treatment of established or impending respiratory failure, and alleviation of pain.

1. Volume and electrolyte resuscitation. Patients with a severe attack of acute pancreatitis require major volume resuscitation that may need to be monitored by central venous pressure or pulmonary artery catheterization and urine output using a Foley catheter. The goal of therapy is to restore an adequate circulating volume and urine output (>50 mL/h) as quickly as possible. Such an aggressive approach to volume resuscitation is likely to prevent

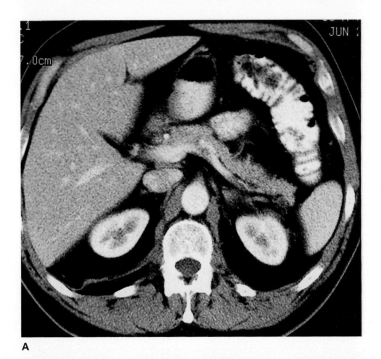

A

B

FIGURE 4.13. CT criteria for grading the severity of pancreatitis (A) compared with the normal pancreas. (B) Pancreatic enlargement with no fluid accumulation demonstrates grade B acute pancreatitis. (C) Grade C severity in acute pancreatitis includes enlargement of the pancreas and inflammation (arrows) in the peripancreatic tissue. (D) Pancreatic phlegmon with one fluid collection (arrows) demonstrates grade D disease and, (E) with two or more fluid collections (letter F), grade E disease. The pancreatic head is also enlarged (letter P). (Courtesy of Henry I. Goldberg, MD.)

(Continued)

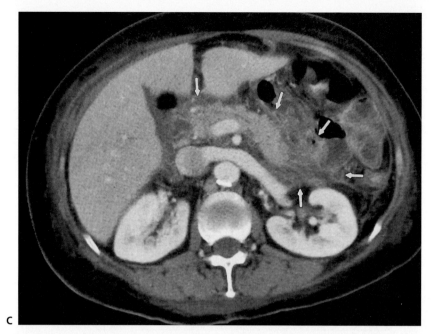

C

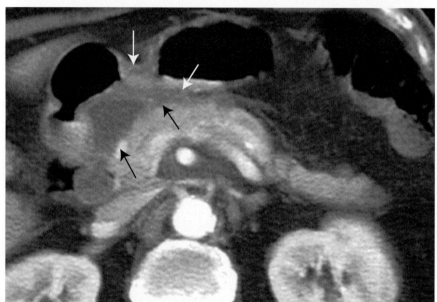

D

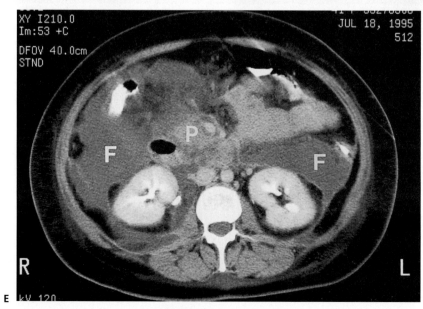

FIGURE 4.13. *Continued*

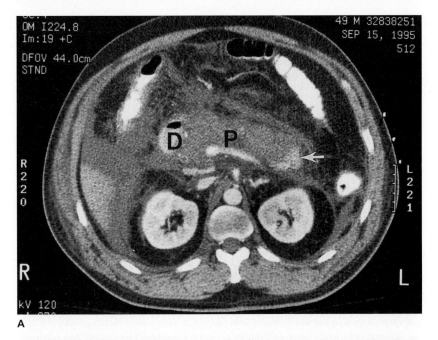

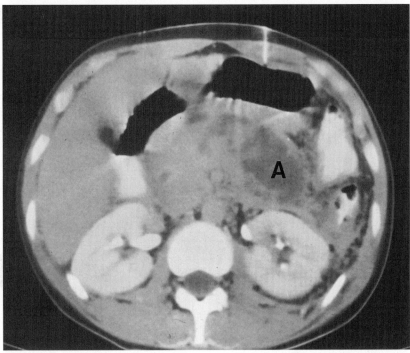

FIGURE 4.14. CE-CT scan demonstrates the presence of necrosis in severe pancreatitis. (A) A bolus of contrast is rapidly injected during CT scanning of the pancreas, enhancing vascularized pancreatic tissue (arrow) while areas of necrosis show as darker perfusion defects (letter P). The duodenum (letter D) marks the border with the necrotic head of the pancreas. (B) Even more extensive pancreatic necrosis is shown, with a large confluence of poorly perfused areas suggesting the presence of pancreatic abscess (letter A). (Courtesy of Henry I. Goldberg, MD.)

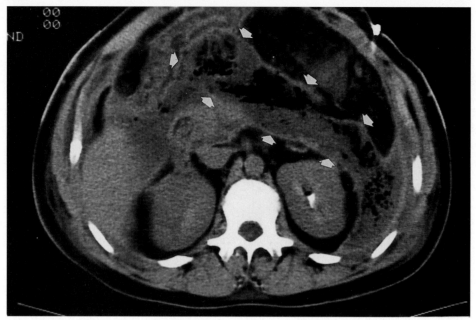

FIGURE 4.15. Pancreatic abscess with air fluid level and air bubbles (arrows) as demonstrated by CT scan may be a result of infection of localized necrosis that undergoes liquefaction in acute pancreatitis. (Courtesy of Henry I. Goldberg, MD.)

pancreatic ischemia and subsequent hemorrhage. Most patients can be adequately resuscitated with crystalloids, although colloids may be necessary in cases of hypovolemic shock. Transfusion of blood is used only if the hematocrit is low (<25%).

Serum calcium and magnesium levels should be measured and, if low, both should be corrected with the administration of calcium gluconate and magnesium sulfate, respectively. Occasionally, persistent hyperglycemia may develop. Hyperglycemia need not be treated unless ketosis develops.

2. Prevention of aspiration. Aspiration is an important complicating factor in severe acute pancreatitis. A nasogastric tube should be inserted in the patient to decompress the stomach. Gastric decompression is the more important reason for the use of nasogastric suction, but it also reduces pancreatic secretion by limiting duodenal acidification. Early intubation of the patient with respiratory failure and/or mental obtundation is another important strategy to prevent aspiration.

3. Respiratory support. Most patients can be supported with the administration of oxygen without intubation. Endotracheal intubation is necessary if arterial oxygen tension cannot be maintained above 60 mm Hg or if the patient has to work too hard to breathe and demonstrates a high respiratory rate (>30/min) for several hours or days.

4. Pain control. Rapid control of pain is best achieved with the intravenous administration of morphine or meperidine HCl (Demerol®). Theoretically, opiates should be avoided because they produce spasm of the sphincter of Oddi. Nevertheless, these drugs are the most effective in controlling the pain of acute pancreatitis.

Subsequent Therapy

If the patient's condition fails to improve within 72 to 96 h, not only must the initial treatment described above be continued, but additional therapeutic interventions must be considered, including prevention of sepsis, nutritional support, and peritoneal lavage.

1. Antibiotics. Prophylactic use of antibiotics was once considered ill-advised because it might possibly promote infection with resistant organisms and fungi. Recently, however, the use of prophylactic antibiotics in patients with severe pancreatitis has been condoned for two reasons. First, liberal use of CE-CT and FNA studies has shown that pancreatic necrosis is subsequently frequently infected with enteric organisms, suggesting that a preventive strategy may be valid. Second, recent experimental and clinical studies have shown that infection in acute pancreatitis can be prevented with antibiotics. In a recent controlled trial reported from the Netherlands by Luiten et al, selective gut decontamination with norfloxacin, colistin, and amphotericin B significantly reduced mortality rates (from 35%–22%) and the need for laparotomy in severe acute pancreatitis.[9] Other studies have shown that broad-

spectrum antibiotics given intravenously can significantly reduce infectious complications and mortality rates in severe acute pancreatitis. These studies suggest that antibiotics with good penetration into pancreatic juice are a better choice.[10,11] While no conclusive prospective trials are available, antibiotics such as clindamycin and ofloxacin are likely to be useful. Prophylactic antibiotics should be used judiciously and only in severe acute pancreatitis. Their use increases the incidence of systemic fungal infection.

2. Nutritional support. Parenteral hyperalimentation should be started if the patient is unable to take oral nutrition within 3 to 5 days and a protracted clinical course appears likely.

3. Therapeutic peritoneal lavage. Although pancreatic lavage is very effective in controlling pain, its therapeutic efficacy is still in doubt. Earlier studies showed that patients improved faster but developed sepsis with greater frequency after the initial improvement following peritoneal lavage. At present, therefore, therapeutic peritoneal lavage is rarely used.

4. Pharmacologic suppression of pancreatic inflammation. Several agents have been tried because of the obvious theoretical usefulness they appeared to have. Glucagon inhibits pancreatic and gastric secretion and increases pancreatic blood flow. Trasylol prevents activation of trypsin. Somatostatin suppresses pancreatic secretion directly and indirectly through inhibition of stimulant hormones. Unfortunately, prospective clinical trials with each of these three agents have failed to show therapeutic advantage. Indeed, once pancreatitis develops, no pharmacologic intervention to limit inflammation appears to work.

Specific Surgical Treatment

Treatment of Necrotizing Pancreatitis

INDICATIONS FOR SURGERY Surgical intervention is indicated in severe necrotizing pancreatitis in two circumstances: (1) when infected necrosis is diagnosed, usually based on CE-CT and FNA; and (2) when the patient's condition deteriorates, despite the inability to establish the presence of infection.

GOALS OF SURGERY The goals of surgery are threefold: (1) to remove all dead and liquefied pancreas, peripancreatic fat, and retroperitoneal tissue; (2) to establish adequate drainage of the lesser sac with or without continuous irrigation; and (3) to create a tube gastrostomy and feeding jejunostomy.

PROCEDURE A large vertical midline or bilateral subcostal incision is usually needed. The lesser sac is opened and all dead tissue removed by blunt dissection with the finger or laparotomy sponges. Formal pancreatic resection is to be avoided because it has an unacceptably high mor-

tality rate. When the extent of necrosis is too massive to manage in one procedure, subsequent second look operations are scheduled. As many as four or five operations may be needed, in which case the surgeon must decide whether to pack the abdomen open or close it. Some have used a zipper to allow easy reentry.

Once debridement is satisfactorily accomplished, the lesser sac should be drained with two or three large, soft sump tubes to establish closed-suction drainage. An alternative method is to strategically place two sump drains in the lesser sac (Figure 4.16) and use continuous irrigation postoperatively.

Provision of a tube gastrostomy avoids the need for prolonged use of a nasogastric tube. Construction of a feeding jejunostomy is advisable in the event of protracted duodenal ileus.

OUTCOME The mortality rate is high, especially when more than one operation is needed and when complications such as hemorrhage or small- or large-bowel fistula supervene. In a 1991 review of surgical treatment and the mortality rate in pancreatic necrosis and sepsis, D'Egidio and Schein reported the following outcomes: The mortality rate of patients treated with necrosectomy and lavage in 216 patients was 23%. However, when resection, necrosectomy, and drainage were performed in 516 patients, the mortality rate was 38%.[12] Necrosectomy without formal pancreatic resection and with continuous postoperative irrigation of the lesser sac appeared to provide the best outcome.

Treatment of Pancreatic Abscess

A pancreatic abscess that develops in the course of severe pancreatitis differs from a pseudocyst that becomes secondarily infected. In the latter, percutaneous tube drainage may prove satisfactory. True pancreatic abscess is not adequately managed with percutaneous catheters because it usually contains infected debris and dead tissue that cannot be drained with tube suctioning. Abdominal exploration with formal debridement and drainage is necessary.

Therapeutic Strategies in Biliary Pancreatitis

The simple classification of biliary pancreatitis given earlier provides useful guidelines for the therapeutic approach (Table 4.5). Type A patients have hyperamylasemia but no abdominal signs or any detectable inflammation of the pancreas. These patients are best treated with laparoscopic cholecystectomy and operative cholangiogram done on an urgent basis, usually when the hyperamylasemia subsides, which generally happens within 24 to 48 h.

Patients with Type B biliary pancreatitis have significant abdominal findings. On conservative treatment, the

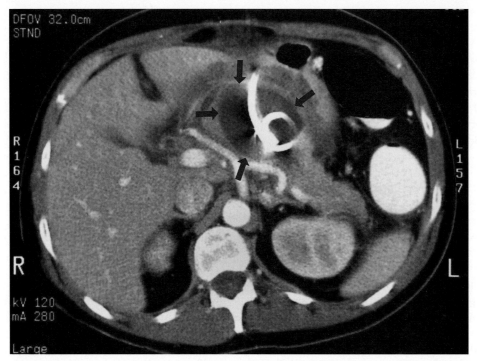

FIGURE 4.16. Necrotizing pancreatitis may be treated with surgical debridement and drainage, followed by strategic placement of two sump drains in the lesser sac to provide continuous irrigation postoperatively. The CT scan illustrates a large necrotic cavity (arrows) containing two drains (bright tubular structures). (Courtesy of Henry I. Goldberg, MD.)

abdominal findings usually resolve within 5 to 7 days. In the past, such patients were discharged home for readmission 6 to 8 weeks later for cholecystectomy. Unfortunately, acute pancreatitis, sometimes with fatal consequences, recurred too often during the waiting period. It is now generally accepted that patients with Type B biliary pancreatitis should have cholecystectomy and operative cholangiogram as soon as abdominal signs subside but during the same admission.

Patients with Type C biliary pancreatitis present more of a challenge because of the significant mortality. It was once advocated that these patients should be operated upon within 48 hours. This approach was associated with high morbidity and mortality. Treatment of this type of pancreatitis has been revolutionized by the advent of endoscopic sphincterotomy, which, in severe cases, if performed within 72 h, reduces morbidity and mortality. Rapid resolution of pancreatitis often follows, at which time definitive surgery can be performed.

Treatment of Acute Pseudocyst

Not all acute pseudocysts require specific treatment. As mentioned above, most cysts that develop in the course of acute pancreatitis resolve spontaneously. The indications for intervention and the nature of intervention are described below:

1. Rapid enlargement. When acute pseudocysts enlarge rapidly to 6 cm or more, especially when the enlargement is associated with increased pain, ultrasound- or CT-guided catheter drainage may be prudent to prevent spontaneous rupture.

2. Persistence of pseudocyst. Any pseudocyst 6 cm or more in size that persists for 8 weeks or longer after formation, especially if associated with symptoms, is an indi-

TABLE 4.5. Biliary Pancreatitis: Management Strategies

Classification	Features	Treatment
A	• Hyperamylasemia only • No peritoneal signs	Urgent cholecystectomy and operative cholangiogram
B	• Hyperamylasemia • Mild/moderate peritoneal signs • Ranson score <3	• Allow peritoneal signs to subside • Cholecystectomy during same admission
C	Severe pancreatitis ± multiple organ failure	• Endoscopic sphincterotomy within 3–5 days • Definitive operation when condition is optimal

cation for internal drainage (cyst-gastric or cyst-enteric). A well-formed mature cyst wall is needed to create the anastomosis.

3. Infected pseudocyst. An infected pseudocyst must first be distinguished from pancreatic abscess. The infected pseudocyst may be treated by percutaneous catheter drainage and, if that fails, by operative external drainage. Pancreatic abscess, however, nearly always requires debridement and external drainage, accompanied by institution of appropriate antibiotic therapy.

4. Pseudocyst hemorrhage. Pseudocyst hemorrhage is usually due to erosion of an adjacent vessel and the formation of a pseudoaneurysm or cyst-aneurysm. This development usually causes acute worsening of pain. The cyst-aneurysm may rupture into the free peritoneal cavity, causing an acute abdomen and hypovolemic shock, or into an adjacent viscus, causing upper or lower gastrointestinal hemorrhage. Angiography is immediately indicated after resuscitative measures are instituted. Angiographic control of bleeding with metal coils (Gianturco) or embolization is the most expedient and often successful mode of therapy (Figure 4.17). When angiographic control is unsuccessful, abdominal exploration is necessary to accomplish either transcystic ligation of the bleeder and/or ligation of the feeding vessel.

5. Obstruction. Infrequently, a pseudocyst may obstruct an adjacent organ, usually the duodenum or common bile duct. Obstruction may be successfully resolved by cyst-duodenal or cyst-jejunal drainage. Rarely will a bypass procedure be necessary.

CHRONIC PANCREATITIS

Clinical Presentation

Abdominal pain is the main presenting symptom of chronic pancreatitis. The pain, often in the epigastrium or the left subcostal region, typically radiates to the back in the T12–L1 region. The pain waxes and wanes and, with time, may become persistent and lead to narcotic addiction. Weight loss can be severe. Steatorrhea occurs in advanced disease and may lead to malabsorption of fat-soluble vitamins (A, D, E, K). Sometimes, this chronic disease is punctuated with intermittent acute attacks requiring hospitalization.

Patients are referred for surgical treatment, either because of the severity and unresponsiveness of pain, or because a complication has developed. Obstructive jaundice occurs in 5% to 10% of patients. Pseudocysts may present as an abdominal mass or are discovered by imaging techniques in the investigation of worsening pain. Other less frequent complications include development of pancreatic ascites or bleeding gastric varices. The essentials of managing chronic pancreatitis are summarized in Table 4.6.

Investigation

The objectives of investigation are to establish the diagnosis, to evaluate the degree of pancreatic dysfunction, to assess the severity of pancreatic damage, to detect complications, and to assess the status of the pancreatic duct. Studies include biochemical analysis, pancreatic function tests, x-ray, and other imaging studies.

Biochemical

Serum amylase levels are usually normal unless the pancreatitis becomes acutely exacerbated or a pseudocyst develops. Liver function tests are assessed to rule out common bile duct obstruction. Prothrombin time should be assessed, particularly in the presence of steatorrhea, which can lead to vitamin K malabsorption.

Pancreatic Function

1. Endocrine pancreas. The status of pancreatic endocrine function should be assessed by performing fasting and 2-h postcibal blood glucose levels. A glucose tolerance test is rarely needed.

2. Exocrine pancreas. Exocrine pancreatic function studies are limited in establishing diagnosis and are usually useful only when the diagnosis is suspected and imaging studies are negative. The two more popular tests measure duodenal bicarbonate and enzyme secretion: one in response to a meal (the Lundh test), the other in response to intravenous secretin with or without cholecystokinin. These tests are cumbersome to perform and difficult to standardize. Pancreatic enzymes (trypsin and chymotrypsin) can also be measured in the blood or feces. Pancreatic enzyme action can also be measured indirectly by the N-benzoyl-tryosyl-p-aminobenzoic acid (NBT-PABA; bentiromide) breath test.

Plain Abdominal X-Ray

Speckled pancreatic calcification or calcium stones within the pancreas provide strong confirmatory evidence of chronic pancreatitis (see Figure 4.10).

Imaging Studies

1. Ultrasonography. This study can assess the size and texture of the pancreas and presence or absence of pancreatic duct dilatation and pseudocysts. Its major value, however, may be assessment of the biliary tract for associated pathology.

2. Computed tomography. CT is the most sensitive and specific imaging study for diagnosing chronic pancreatitis. CT examination evaluates the presence of calcifications,

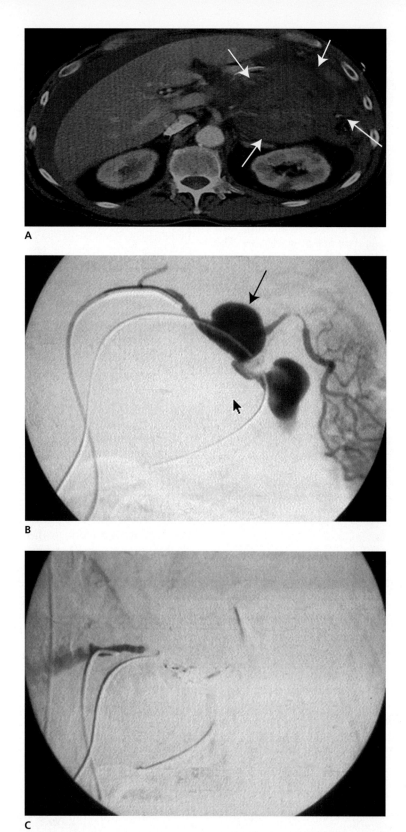

FIGURE 4.17. Pseudocyst hemorrhage can be treated with angiography. (A) The CT scan shows a large area of hemorrhage (arrows) in the region of the lesser sac. With metal coils (Gianturco), the bleeding pseudoaneurysm of the splenic artery (B, arrow) was embolized to control bleeding (C). (Courtesy of Henry I. Goldberg, MD.)

TABLE 4.6. Essentials: Management of Chronic Pancreatitis

Diagnosis
  Clinical
    - Chronic abdominal pain
    - Recurrent back pain (T12–L1)
    - History of alcoholism
    - Diarrhea, weight loss
  Laboratory
    - Serum amylase may be intermittently elevated
    - Pancreatic function tests
  Imaging
    - Plain abdominal films (calcification)
    - Ultrasound (PD: Dilatation, pseudocysts, gallstones)
    - CT scan (PD: Dilatation, pseudocysts, calcification)
    - ERCP: Most reliable and diagnostic study (pancreatic ductal anomalies, dilatation, chain of lakes, stones, pseudocysts)

Treatment
  Conservative
    - Abstinence from alcohol
    - Pain control
    - Patient education, counseling
    - Pancreatic enzyme therapy if steatorrhea present
    - Dietary restriction of fat and large meals
    - Vitamin E supplementation
    - Control of diabetes if present
  Endoscopic
    - Sphincterotomy and stone extraction
    - Dilatation of stenotic proximal duct
    - Stenting
  Surgical indications
    - Intractable pain
    - Pancreatic pseudocysts
    - Biliary obstruction
  Procedures (see Table 4.8)

Abbreviations: CT, computerized tomography; ERCP, endoscopic retrograde cholangiopancreatography; PD, pancreatic duct.

dilated pancreatic duct, and pseudocysts (Figure 4.18). It is also the best way to rule out the presence of pancreatic cancer. Helical CT provides even better images than traditional CT scans.

3. Endoscopic retrograde cholangiopancreatography. ERCP is not only the most reliable way to diagnose chronic pancreatitis, but it is also the best way to visualize pancreatic ductal anatomy, providing key information in surgical decision making. Pancreatic ductal abnormality may be mild and involve only peripheral ductules (Figure 4.12B). Or it may involve the main pancreatic duct, which may be dilated, sometimes with chain-of-lakes deformity when the duct is intermittently dilated between sites of stricture or impacted stones (Figure 4.12C). ERCP also assesses the presence or absence of common bile duct obstruction or other biliary tract pathology.

4. Angiography. Angiography is used only when there is either bleeding or suspicion of portal vein and splenic vein thrombosis. The latter information can be obtained more easily with the use of CE-CT scan or Doppler ultrasonography.

Management

Conservative Management

Most patients undergo medical management for years before they are eventually referred to surgery. Several aspects of conservative management are important.

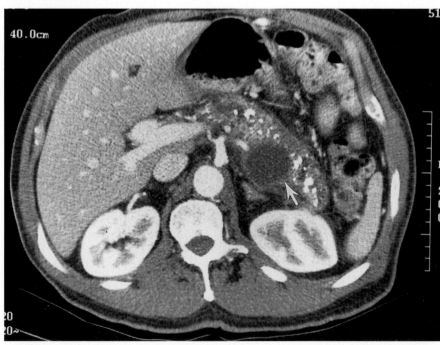

FIGURE 4.18. Chronic pancreatitis is best diagnosed with CT scan, which reveals the presence of calcifications, dilatated pancreatic duct, and pseudocysts (arrow). (Courtesy of Henry I. Goldberg, MD.)

1. Abstinence from alcohol. This important aspect of management is also the most difficult to institute. Patient education, counseling, group support, and psychiatry are all helpful.

2. Pain control. The cause of pain in chronic pancreatitis is unknown. Opioid drugs are invariably required and, with chronic use, addiction becomes a problem. Percutaneous celiac axis blockade with alcohol or phenol has proved disappointing. Three plausible causes for the pain have been described:

a. Ductal hypertension. Intraoperative measurements of pressure in dilated ducts have been shown to be elevated. The rationale for pancreatic drainage to ameliorate pain is based on reduction of ductal pressure. Unfortunately, many patients with pain do not have dilated ducts.

b. Perineural inflammation. In many specimens examined, perineural inflammation is striking. Recent studies with immunohistochemistry also show an increase in CGRP- and substance P-containing sensory neurons.

c. Peripancreatic inflammation. Chronic inflammation extending to the retroperitoneum is probably an important cause of back pain.

3. Pancreatic enzyme therapy. The finding that duodenal trypsin inhibits the release of CCK-releasing peptide and, thereby, secretion of CCK has led to the use of oral pancreatic enzyme supplements in chronic pancreatitis. The theory is that pancreatic stimulation is reduced, leading to pain relief. Unfortunately, the therapeutic effect on pain relief is sporadic. Pancreatic enzyme therapy, however, does play an important role in the treatment of steatorrhea.

4. Diet. Restriction of fat and large meals is useful in reducing pain. Vitamin supplements, especially fat-soluble vitamins, are also useful.

5. Control of diabetes. Appropriate measures are needed to control diabetes, when present, with either insulin or oral hypoglycemics.

Endoscopic Management

Advances in interventional endoscopy have provided a new alternative to surgical therapy. In addition to sphincterotomy, endoscopic procedures include sphincterotomy extraction of stones from the pancreatic duct, dilatation, and stenting of strictures. Good judgment and superior technical expertise are required. So far, anecdotal reports suggest that, under the right circumstances, these procedures result not only in relief of pain but also in some recovery of pancreatic endocrine function.[13]

Surgical Management

This section discusses the surgical options for treatment of chronic pancreatitis and its complications. Complications of surgery are listed in Table 4.7.

TABLE 4.7. Surgical Complications in Chronic Pancreatitis
Exocrine pancreatic insufficiency and steatorrhea
Diabetes mellitus
Pseudocyst formation
Pancreatic ascites
Hemorrhage due to vascular erosion, usually due to pseudocyst
Splenic vein thrombosis and gastric varices
CBD obstruction and obstructive jaundice
Duodenal obstruction
Carcinoma?

Abbreviation: CBD, common bile duct.

Intractable pain is the most common indication for surgery. Pancreatic pseudocysts and their complications are a second important indication. Biliary obstruction occurs in a significant percentage of patients but is severe or complete in only 5% to 10%.[6] Other complications that may require surgical intervention include bleeding gastric varices from splenic vein thrombosis, duodenal or colonic obstruction, pancreatic ascites, and sometimes, suspicion of pancreatic cancer.

PRINCIPLES OF SURGICAL THERAPY

1. The goals of surgery must be clearly explained to the patient. They include alleviating pain and bypassing or removing complications. Reversal of loss of pancreatic exocrine or endocrine function cannot be promised.

2. Pancreatic drainage procedures are based on the premise that ductal obstruction leads to distension and pain; therefore, the presence of dilated pancreatic duct is necessary to embark on a pancreatic drainage procedure.

3. Resecting procedures are indicated when disease is largely confined to one region and the pancreatic duct is not dilated. Any amount of pancreatic resection increases the incidence of postoperative diabetes.

4. A well-planned procedure should be executed only by an expert pancreatic surgeon after a thorough investigation that includes proper imaging studies and ERCP to provide information on the pancreatic duct and biliary tree.

5. The operative procedure with the greatest chance of success must be selected.

6. Continued use of alcohol or addicting drugs by the patient is a relative contraindication for elective surgery.

SURGICAL OPTIONS FOR TREATMENT OF CHRONIC PANCREATITIS
The two surgical options are pancreatic drainage and resection, various procedures for which are summarized in Table 4.8. In general, pancreatic drainage is reserved for cases in which the pancreatic duct is larger than 7 mm in diameter.

TABLE 4.8. Surgical Options in Treatment of Chronic Pancreatitis

Type of procedure	Comments
Pancreatic drainage procedures (require PD >7 mm)	
Longitudinal pancreaticojejunostomy (Peustow)	Relieves pain in 70%
End-to-side pancreaticojejunostomy (DuVal)	Relieves pain in 40%
Pancreaticogastrostomy	Infrequently performed
Sphincteroplasty	Low success rate
Pancreatic resection procedures	
Distal pancreatectomy	Rarely indicated
Near-total pancreatectomy (Child's)	Suboptimal
Pylorus-preserving pancreaticoduodenectomy	When disease is confined to the pancreatic head
Duodenum-preserving pancreatectomy	
■ Beger procedure	■ Excision of head and end-to-end pancreaticojejunostomy
■ Frey procedure	■ Excision of head and longitudinal pancreaticojejunostomy

Abbreviation: PD, pancreatic duct.

Pancreatic Drainage Procedures

1. Longitudinal pancreaticojejunostomy (the Peustow procedure). The lesser sac is opened through the gastrocolic ligament, and the pancreas is visualized from the head, at the duodenal C-loop, to the tail at the splenic hilum. The pancreatic duct can often be readily palpated; if not, intraoperative ultrasound helps in its identification. The duct is opened (filleted) along its entire length from tail to head, going as far as possible to the right of the superior mesenteric and portal veins and into the uncinate process. Any stones and sludge in the pancreatic duct are removed. A 40-cm retrocolic Roux-en-Y limb of jejunum is then fashioned and a side-to-side pancreaticojejunal anastomosis constructed along the entire length of the filleted pancreatic duct (Figure 4.19). Nonabsorbable sutures are used to construct the anastomosis between the opened Roux-en-Y jejunal limb and the pancreas, whose fibrosed capsule provides the necessary tissue of substance for the anastomosis.

Longitudinal pancreaticojejunostomy is a safe procedure with negligible mortality and morbidity rates. Long-term relief of pain has been reported in up to 70% of patients by several groups.[14]

2. End-to-side pancreaticojejunostomy (the DuVal procedure). Retrograde drainage of the pancreas into a Roux-en-Y limb of the jejunum is accomplished, following amputation of the tail of the pancreas and splenectomy (Figure 4.20). This procedure has not been as successful as longitudinal pancreaticojejunostomy, perhaps because multiple strictures and stones, often present in the duct in the head and body of the pancreas, prevent adequate drainage. Reported success in pain relief has been about 40%, and the procedure is not frequently used.[15]

3. Pancreaticogastrostomy. This procedure is used rarely and when the pancreatic duct has a single site of obstruction.

4. Sphincteroplasty. Transduodenal sphincteroplasty is useful only when the obstruction is in the area divided by sphincterotomy. When the operation was popular, temporary pain relief was achieved in 25% to 30%.

Pancreatic Resection

1. Distal pancreatectomy. This is a useful operation when disease involves only the body and tail. These circumstances rarely exist.

2. Near-total distal pancreatectomy (Child's procedure). This operation, which saves only a rim of pancreatic tissue along the duodenum, is only of historical importance. It does not have a high rate of success and can lead to postoperative diabetes.

3. Pylorus-preserving pancreaticoduodenectomy. When the main locus of disease is in the head of the pancreas and the major pancreatic duct is not dilated, pylorus-preserving pancreaticoduodenectomy is the operation of choice. The procedure also treats common bile duct obstruction if present. Pain relief has been accomplished in some 82% of reported cases.[16]

4. Duodenum-preserving resection of the head (the Beger procedure). The pancreas is divided over the superior mesenteric vein and the head of the pancreas cored out. The body of the pancreas is drained with a Roux-en-Y limb of jejunum to create an end-to-end anastomosis (Figure 4.21).

5. Frey procedure. This is another variant of duodenum-preserving resection of the pancreatic head, combined with longitudinal pancreaticojejunostomy (Figure 4.22). The Frey procedure addresses the difficulty of draining adequately with longitudinal pancreaticojejunostomy along the head of the pancreas when it is enlarged and the locus of major disease.

6. Total pancreatectomy. Total pancreatectomy inevitably creates total exocrine and endocrine insufficiency and is, therefore, used as a last procedure when

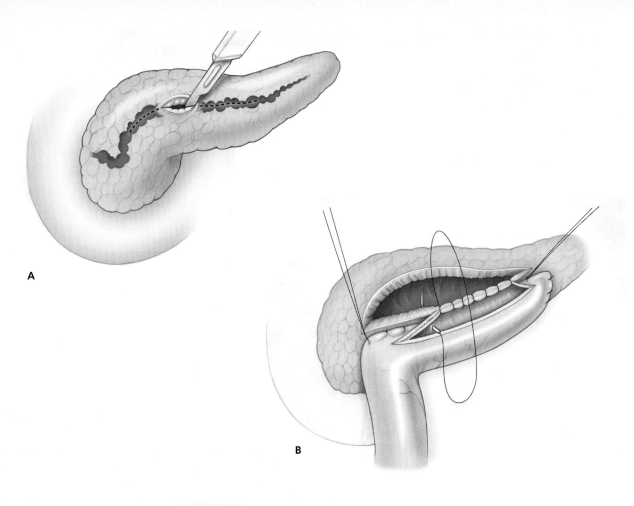

A

B

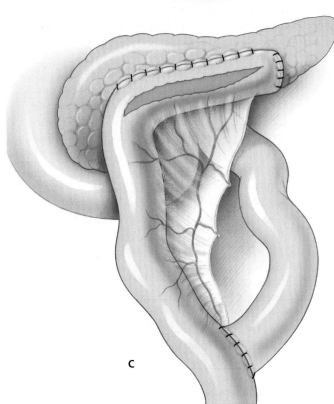

C

FIGURE 4.19. Longitudinal pancreaticojejunostomy (Peustow) procedure. (A) The dilated pancreatic duct is opened along its entire length. (B) A 40-cm Roux-en-Y limb of jejunum is fashioned and anastomosed side-to-side to the entire length of the filleted pancreatic duct. (C) The completed procedure is shown. (Adapted from Warren KW, Jenkins RL, Steele GD. Atlas of Surgery of the Liver, Pancreas, and Biliary Tract. Norwalk, CT: Appleton & Lange; 1991.)

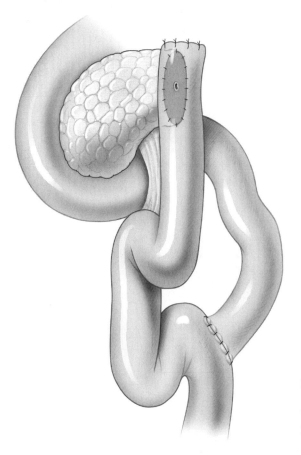

FIGURE 4.20. End-to-side pancreaticojejunostomy (DuVal) procedure. Following distal pancreatectomy, the cut edge of the pancreas is anastomosed end-to-side with a Roux-en-Y limb of jejunum. (Adapted from Warren KW, Jenkins RL, Steele GD. Atlas of Surgery of the Liver, Pancreas, and Biliary Tract. Norwalk, CT: Appleton & Lange; 1991.)

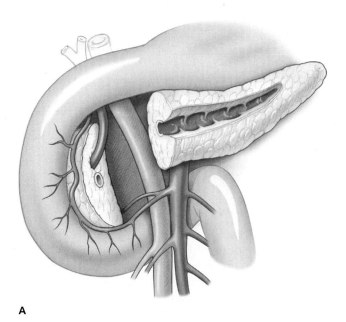

A

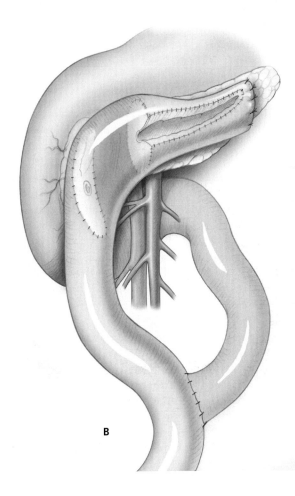

B

FIGURE 4.21. Duodenum-preserving resection of the head of the pancreas (Beger procedure). (A) The pancreas is divided over the superior mesenteric vein and the head of the pancreas excised. The pancreatic duct is opened longitudinally along the body and tail. (B) A Roux-en-Y limb of jejunum is then anastomosed to the cut end of the residual head and the body and tail of the pancreas.

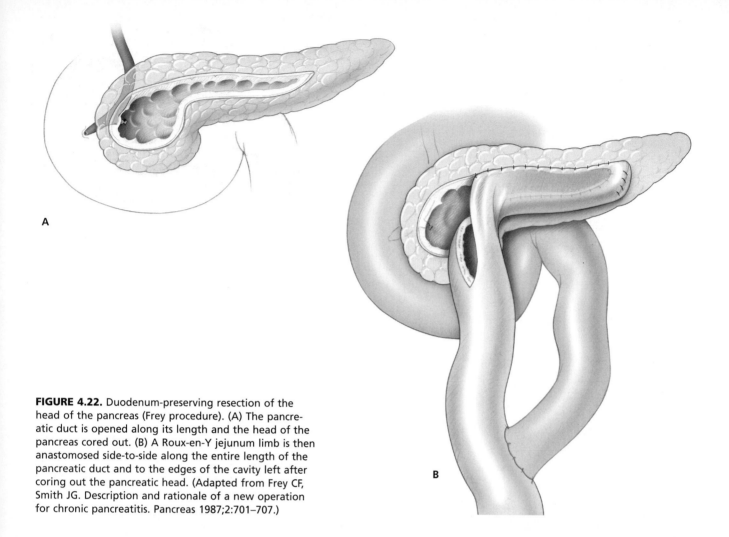

FIGURE 4.22. Duodenum-preserving resection of the head of the pancreas (Frey procedure). (A) The pancreatic duct is opened along its length and the head of the pancreas cored out. (B) A Roux-en-Y jejunum limb is then anastomosed side-to-side along the entire length of the pancreatic duct and to the edges of the cavity left after coring out the pancreatic head. (Adapted from Frey CF, Smith JG. Description and rationale of a new operation for chronic pancreatitis. Pancreas 1987;2:701–707.)

pancreaticoduodenectomy and distal resection fail. Even with total pancreatectomy, complete pain relief is achieved in only 65% to 80% of patients.[1]

CHOICE OF PROCEDURE IN CHRONIC PANCREATITIS
Different procedures are indicated depending on the location of major disease and whether or not the pancreatic duct is dilated.

1. Uniformly dilated pancreatic duct. When the pancreatic duct is uniformly dilated, the procedure of choice is longitudinal pancreaticojejunostomy. When the major locus of disease is the head of the pancreas, causing it to be bulky and thickened, and the duct within the head cannot be adequately drained, the Frey procedure may be more suitable.

2. Small pancreatic duct. The choice of procedure in this situation depends on the main locus of disease. For disease located mainly in the body and tail, distal pancreatectomy is indicated. For disease located mainly in the head, either pylorus-preserving pancreaticoduodenectomy or the Beger procedure may be selected. If the CBD is obstructed, the former procedure is indicated.

When subtotal resection fails, total pancreatectomy is considered as a last resort. This operation may be associated with brittle diabetes and longterm sudden death. Transplantation of the patient's own islet cells into the liver may offer a solution to this vexing problem.

Outcome in Chronic Pancreatitis

It is estimated that about 50% of patients with chronic pancreatitis die of their disease or of problems associated with alcoholism, diabetes, infection, or suicide within 20 to 25 years. Surgical treatment results in significant pain relief in about 75% of patients. Long-term results depend more on the patient's habits of drinking alcohol and using drugs than on the type of surgery performed.

PANCREATIC NEOPLASMS

Classification

Pancreatic neoplasms may be benign or malignant and may be derived from ductal cells, acinar cells, islet cells, or

TABLE 4.9. Classification of Pancreatic Neoplasms

Cell of origin	Benign	Malignant
Ductal cell	Adenoma Cystadenoma	Adenocarcinoma Cystadenocarcinoma
Acinar cell	Acinar cell adenoma Acinar cystadenoma	Acinar cell carcinoma Acinar cystadenocarcinoma
Mesenchymal cell	Fibroma Leiomyoma	Fibrosarcoma Leiomyosarcoma
Islet cell	Insulinoma Glucagonoma Gastrinoma Somatostatinoma VIPoma Islet adenoma	Insulinoma Glucagonoma Gastrinoma Somatostatinoma VIPoma Nonfunctioning islet cell carcinoma

mesenchymal cells. A working classification is given in Table 4.9.

Adenocarcinoma of the Pancreas

Adenocarcinoma accounts for 90% of pancreatic malignancy. The tumor is located in the head of the pancreas in two-thirds of cases. Unlike gastric cancer, the incidence of pancreatic cancer has been rising and now accounts for about 1 patient per 10,000 of the American population.[8] It is twice as common in men as in women. Dietary and occupational factors are believed to be associated with the higher incidence and include smoking; obesity, high-fat and high-protein diet; and exposure to benzidine, beta-naphthalene, and ethylene chloride. Mutation of K-ras genes is found in more than 85% of cases. Mutations of the p16[INK4] gene on chromosome 9p21 is also seen in pancreatic cancer. Surgical resection is the only hope for cure, but even then only 5% to 10% of patients survive for 5 years.[17] The essentials of management are summarized in Table 4.10 and pathological staging of pancreatic cancer is given in Table 4.11.

TABLE 4.10. Essentials: Cancer of the Pancreas

Clinical
  Pancreatic malignancies are 90% adenocarcinoma
  Clinical picture depends on tumor location
    Head
      ▪ Painless jaundice (>90%)
      ▪ Weight loss and pain (>66%)
      ▪ Hepatomegaly, sometimes Courvoisier's sign
    Body and tail
      ▪ Pain, weight loss
      ▪ Migratory thrombophlebitis (5%–10%)

Diagnosis
  Ultrasound
    ▪ Dilated biliary tree
    ▪ Hypoechoic pancreatic mass in some cases
  CT scan
    ▪ Visible mass if >2 cm
    ▪ Dilatation of extrahepatic biliary tree
    ▪ Liver and lymph node metastasis if present
    ▪ Arterial phase may show hepatic artery invasion
    ▪ CT-guided needle biopsy not recommended
  ERCP
    ▪ May show biliary dilatation and pancreatic duct obstruction or encasement
    ▪ Needle biopsy, brush cytology, pancreatogram possible
    ▪ Biliary drainage with stent possible

Management: See algorithm, Figure 4.26

Long-term outcome
  Five-year survival after pancreaticoduodenectomy: 12%
    ▪ Diploid tumors: 40%
    ▪ Aneuploid tumors: <10%
    ▪ Periampullary: 21%–56%

Abbreviations: CT, computerized tomography; ERCP, endoscopic retrograde cholangiopancreatography.

TABLE 4.11. TMN Staging of Exocrine Pancreatic Cancer

Primary tumor (T)
TX	Primary tumor cannot be assessed
T0	No evidence of primary tumor
Tis	Carcinoma in situ
T1	Tumor limited to the pancreas, 2 cm or less in greatest dimension
T2	Tumor limited to the pancreas, more than 2 cm in greatest dimension
T3	Tumor extends beyond the pancreas but without involvement of the celiac axis or the superior mesenteric artery
T4	Tumor involves the celiac axis or the superior mesenteric artery (unresectable primary tumor)

Regional lymph nodes (N)
NX	Regional lymph nodes cannot be assessed
N0	No regional lymph node metastasis
N1	Regional lymph node metastasis

Distant metastasis (M)
MX	Distant metastasis cannot be assessed
M0	No distant metastasis
M1	Distant metastasis

Source: Reprinted with permission from the American Joint Committee on Cancer (AJCC), Chicago, Illinois. The original source for this material is the *AJCC Cancer Staging Manual*, Sixth Edition (2002) published by Springer-Verlag New York, www.springer-ny.com.

Clinical Presentation

The classical presentation depends on the location of the tumor. Tumors in the head of the pancreas tend to present earlier and are often associated with painless obstructive jaundice. Adenocarcinoma of the body and tail presents late, often with pain and weight loss but without jaundice. Migratory thrombophlebitis (Trousseau's sign) is seen in 5% to 10%, more commonly with adenocarcinoma of the body and tail.

In adenocarcinoma of the head of the pancreas, jaundice is present in more than 90% of patients; weight loss and abdominal pain are seen in more than two-thirds. Typically, abdominal pain radiates to the back in the region of T12–L1. Hepatomegaly is detectable in some 80% of patients, and the gallbladder may be palpable (Courvoisier's sign). Anorexia, nausea, and vomiting are also common.

Diagnosis

Abdominal ultrasonography is usually the first diagnostic test to be obtained. It shows extrahepatic obstruction with dilated common bile duct and gallbladder in more than 75% of patients. A hypoechoic pancreatic mass may or may not be seen. Abdominal CT is then obtained, and a mass is usually visible if the tumor is larger than 2 cm in diameter (Figure 4.23). Dilatation of the extrahepatic biliary tree is also seen. CT may show the presence of hepatic metastasis and regional lymphadenopathy. The arterial phase of dynamic CT scan is shown in Figure 4.24.

In the past, a direct diagnostic approach with CT-guided fine-needle aspiration biopsy was advocated. This procedure, however, is now known to cause peritoneal and abdominal wall tumor spread and is recommended only in patients in whom abdominal exploration is not contemplated. Magnetic resonance imaging (MRI) provides no advantage over CT, but endoscopic ultrasound may detect lesions less than 2 cm in diameter more reliably than CT.

ERCP is often performed and is indispensable in patients with obstructive jaundice in whom neither tumor nor stone is visualized. It facilitates the performance of needle aspiration biopsy, brush cytology, and pancreatogram when the findings are equivocal. Visualization of the pancreatic duct is possible in over two-thirds of patients (Figure 4.25). ERCP also allows the placement of a drainage stent to provide relief of obstructive jaundice.

Use of these imaging techniques has increased resectability rates from less than 25% to over 75%.[18]

Treatment

An algorithm showing how treatment should be managed for carcinoma of the head of the pancreas is given in Figure 4.26. The options depend on several factors, including resectability, the presence of metastasis, and whether or not the tumor can be visualized.

INOPERABLE TUMOR Pancreatic cancer is inoperable if it is associated with clinical evidence of ascites or distant metastasis. Inoperability may also be indicated with imaging studies that demonstrate the presence of liver or abdominal metastasis and invasion of the portal vein. In these latter circumstances, metastasis and portal vein involvement should be confirmed by laparoscopy.

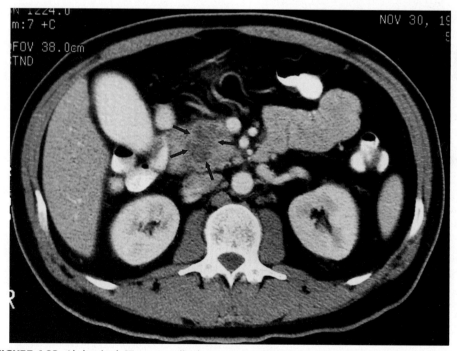

FIGURE 4.23. Abdominal CT can usually demonstrate pancreatic cancer if the mass is larger than 2 cm in diameter (arrows). (Courtesy of Henry I. Goldberg, MD.)

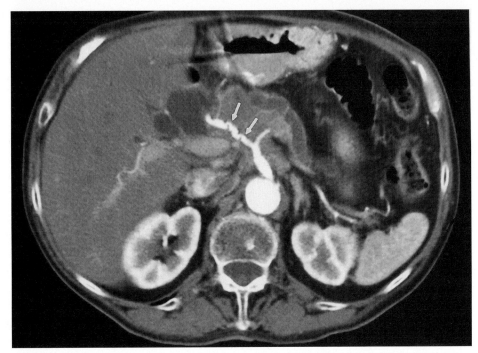

FIGURE 4.24. The arterial phase of dynamic CT scan may provide information about hepatic artery invasion (arrows) as well as portal vein involvement. (Courtesy of Henry I. Goldberg, MD.)

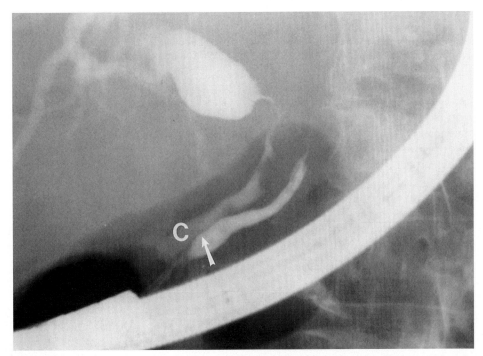

FIGURE 4.25. ERCP is useful in investigating pancreatic disease. The pancreatic duct can be visualized in more than two-thirds of patients. The usual findings are pancreatic duct obstruction or encasement (arrow). In this case, the common bile duct (C) is also obstructed. (Courtesy of Henry I. Goldberg, MD.)

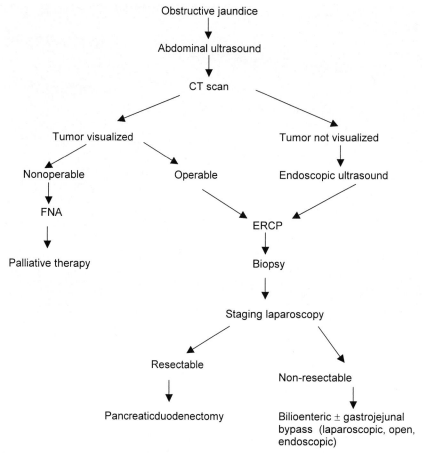

Obstructive jaundice

↓

Abdominal ultrasound

↓

CT scan

Tumor visualized   Tumor not visualized

Nonoperable   Operable   Endoscopic ultrasound

FNA   ERCP

Palliative therapy   Biopsy

Staging laparoscopy

Resectable   Non-resectable

Pancreaticduodenectomy   Bilioenteric ± gastrojejunal
                            bypass (laparoscopic, open,
                            endoscopic)

FIGURE 4.26. Algorithm for management of carcinoma of the head of the pancreas. *Abbreviations*: CT, computed tomography; FNA, fine needle aspiration; ERCP, endoscopic retrograde cholangiopancreatography.

If a patient's tumor is deemed nonresectable, palliation may be obtained with endoscopic or transhepatic biliary drainage using expandable stents or with operative biliary and gastric bypass performed either laparoscopically or with open abdominal operation. Although endoscopic and surgical bypass are equally effective in the short term, surgical bypass is associated with a lower incidence of recurrent jaundice and cholangitis. Following biliary bypass alone, 15% to 20% of patients develop duodenal obstruction.[19] Another advantage of surgical palliation is that gastric bypass can be done in addition to biliary bypass. Radiation and chemotherapy are relatively ineffective in providing palliation and, in any individual patient, the benefits must be compared with the side effects.

RESECTABLE TUMOR Patients with no demonstrable hepatic metastasis or other evidence of spread are candidates for pancreaticoduodenectomy. Resectability is determined during surgical exploration when the following are demonstrated:

1. The portal and superior veins are not invaded by tumor, and a tunnel can be developed anterior to these vessels and behind the head of the pancreas.
2. The tumor is not fixed to surrounding organs.

3. The transverse mesocolon is free of invasion.
4. No hepatic metastasis is demonstrated by palpation and intraoperative ultrasound.
5. There is no tumor deposit in lymph nodes that cannot be encompassed in en bloc excision.

SURGICAL PROCEDURES Three types of resection are possible: the classic Whipple pancreaticoduodenectomy (Figure 4.27), pylorus-preserving pancreaticoduodenectomy, and total pancreatectomy. Regional pancreatectomy, in which the portal vein is resected and replaced with a vein graft, has not improved survival.

Although there is concern about the adequacy of resection when pylorus-preserving pancreaticoduodenectomy is performed, this operation is associated with better nutritional status than the classic Whipple procedure. Postoperative delayed gastric emptying, however, is more common. The macrolide antibiotic erythromycin is useful in improving gastric emptying after pancreaticoduodenectomy.

Total pancreatectomy has no survival advantage and is associated with a higher mortality rate and a higher incidence of brittle diabetes than the Whipple procedure. Its use may be indicated, however, in the following clinical situations:

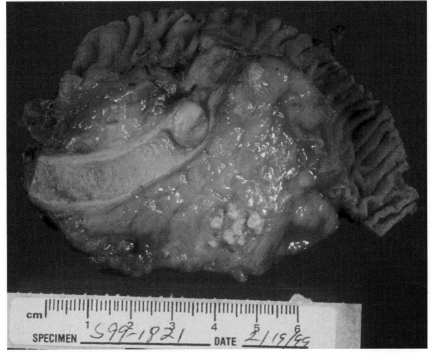

FIGURE 4.27. A Whipple resection specimen of ampullary carcinoma shows a polypoid lesion in the ampullary region obstructing the common bile duct. (Courtesy of Linda D. Ferrell, MD.)

1. The pancreas is so friable that it is unsuitable for anastomosis.
2. Frozen section reveals the presence of tumor at the resection line.
3. Diffuse involvement of the entire pancreas is present.
4. The patient already has insulin-dependent diabetes.

The operative mortality rate for pancreaticoduodectomy is now below 5% and in some centers below 2%, but this low mortality rate appears to be achieved only in hospitals where significant numbers of these procedures are performed.

Long-Term Outcome

The 5-year actuarial survival rate after pancreaticoduodenectomy is 12%.[17] The prognosis is better in small, well-differentiated and node-negative tumors, and the DNA content of the tumor cells has a significant implication. The 5-year survival rate of patients whose tumor cells are diploid is nearly 40% but less than 10% in those with aneuploid cells.

The 5-year survival rate is higher in periampullary tumors (21%–56%) than in tumors of the head of the pancreas.[8] Among periampullary tumors, duodenal tumor has the best prognosis.

The overall prognosis of pancreatic cancer is dismal; only 10% of patients are alive 12 months after the diagnosis is made.[17]

Cystic Neoplasms of the Pancreas

Cystic neoplasms of the pancreas account for 1% of all pancreatic cancers and for 10% of all cystic lesions of the pancreas (Figure 4.28). They may be mucinous (50%), cystadenoma (30%), and neuroendocrine (20%). A resected specimen of mucinous cystadenoma is shown in Figure 4.29. They can develop without eliciting many symptoms, and the only symptom they do produce is usually vague upper abdominal pain. They frequently grow to large sizes and can reach 25 cm in diameter.

The important clinical challenge is distinguishing the cystic neoplasms from benign pseudocysts (Figure 4.30). A history of pancreatitis, increased serum amylase levels, and CT findings of pancreatitis are helpful in suggesting the diagnosis of benign pseudocyst. When presumed pseudocysts recur after cyst-gastric or cyst-enteric drainage, a cystic neoplasm must be excluded. The best strategy is to routinely obtain biopsy samples of the wall of a pseudocyst when a drainage procedure is being performed.

All cystic tumors of the pancreas are potentially malignant and should be resected.

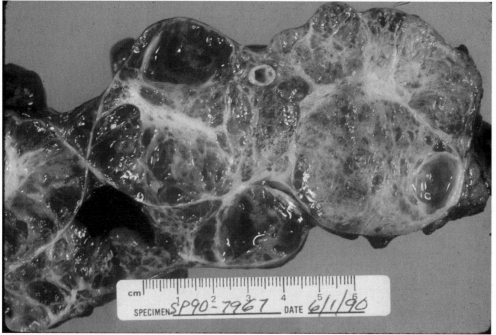

A

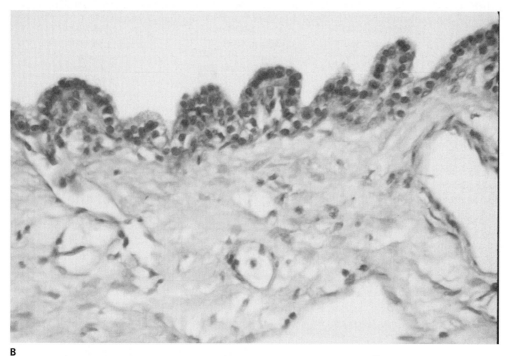

B

FIGURE 4.28. (A) Gross appearance of serous cystadenoma, also known as microcystic adenoma. (B) The typical microscopic feature is glycogen-containing cuboidal epithelial cells lining the wall of the cysts. The tumor tends to occur in the tail of the pancreas and is often benign. (Courtesy of Linda D. Ferrell, MD.)

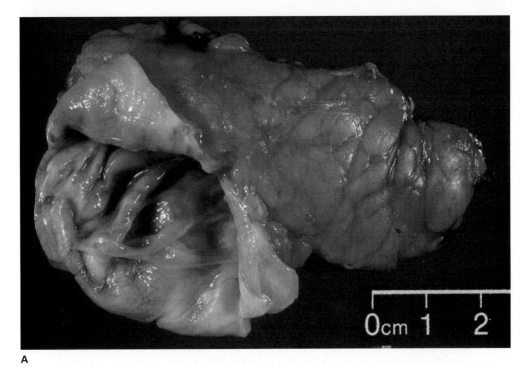

A

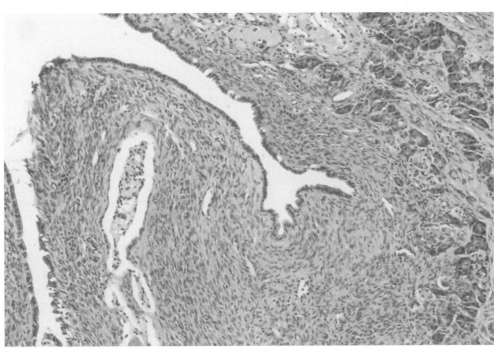

B

FIGURE 4.29. (A) Pancreas resection specimen from a large mucinous cystadenoma was opened to show the trabeculated cyst lumen. (B) Microscopically, the cyst wall shows ovarian-type stroma. This rare tumor tends to occur more commonly in women. (Courtesy of Linda D. Ferrell, MD.)

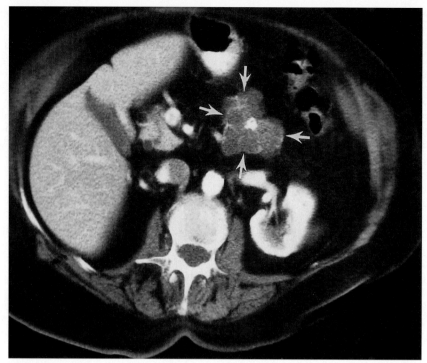

FIGURE 4.30. Cystic neoplasm. In patients with a history of pancreatitis, increased serum amylase levels, and CT findings characteristic of pancreatitis, such lesions are suggestive of benign pseudocyst. Neoplasm can be ruled out definitively with biopsy. These cystic neoplasms have septa and some have central calcification (arrows). (Courtesy of Henry I. Goldberg, MD.)

REFERENCES

1. Steer ML, Waxman I, Freedman S. Chronic pancreatitis. *N Engl J Med* 1995;332:1482–1490.
2. Baron TH, Morgan DE. Acute necrotizing pancreatitis. *N Engl J Med* 1999;340:1412–1417.
3. Sherman S, Lehman GA. ERCP- and endoscopic sphinctero-tomy-induced pancreatitis. *Pancreas* 1991;6:350–367.
4. Beger HG, Buchler M, Bittner R, et al. Necrosectomy and post-operative local lavage in patients with necrotizing pancreatitis: results of a prospective clinical trial. *World J Surg* 1988; 12:255–262.
5. Bittner R, Block S, Buchler M, et al. Pancreatic abscess and infected pancreatic necrosis. Different local septic complications in acute pancreatitis. *Dig Dis Sci* 1987;32:1082–1087.
6. Sarles H, Bernard JP, Johnson C. Pathogenesis and epidemiology of chronic pancreatitis. *Annu Rev Med* 1989;40:453–468.
7. Johnson CD, Hosking S. National statistics for diet, alcohol consumption, and chronic pancreatitis in England and Wales, 1960–88. *Gut* 1991;32:1401–1405.
8. Yeo CJ, Cameron JL. Pancreatic cancer. *Curr Probl Surg* 1999 Feb;36:59–152.
9. Luiten EJ, Hop WC, Lange JF, et al. Controlled clinical trial of selective decontamination for the treatment of severe acute pancreatitis. *Ann Surg* 1995;222:57–65.
10. Pederzoli P, Bassi C, Vesentini S, et al. A randomized multicenter clinical trial of antibiotic prophylaxis of septic complications in acute necrotizing pancreatitis with imipenem. *Surg Gynecol Obstet* 1993;176:480–483.
11. Sainio V, Kemppainen E, Puolakkainen P, et al. Early antibiotic treatment in acute necrotising pancreatitis. *Lancet* 1995; 346:663–667.
12. D'Egidio A, Schein M. Percutaneous drainage of pancreatic pseudocysts: a prospective study. *World J Surg* 1992;16:141–146.
13. Smits ME, Badiga SM, Rauws EA, et al. Long-term results of pancreatic stents in chronic pancreatitis. *Gastrointest Endosc* 1995;42:461–467.
14. Greenlee HB, Prinz RA, Aranha GV. Long-term results of side-to-side pancreaticojejunostomy. *World J Surg* 1990;14:70–76.
15. Ihse I, Borch K, Larsson J. Chronic pancreatitis: results of operations for relief of pain. *World J Surg* 1990;14:53–58.
16. Buchler MW, Friess H, Muller MW, et al. Randomized trial of duodenum-preserving pancreatic head resection versus pylorus-preserving Whipple in chronic pancreatitis. *Am J Surg* 1995;169:65–70.
17. Cameron JL. Long-term survival following pancreaticoduodenectomy for adenocarcinoma of the head of the pancreas. *Surg Clin North Am* 1995;75:939–951.
18. Yeo CJ, Cameron JL, Lillemoe KD, et al. Pancreaticoduodenectomy for cancer of the head of the pancreas. 201 patients. *Ann Surg* 1995;221:721–733.
19. Lillemoe KD, Barnes SA. Surgical palliation of unresectable pancreatic carcinoma. *Surg Clin North Am* 1995;75:953–968.

SELECTED READINGS

Acute Pancreatitis

Ashley SW, Perez A, Pierce EA, et al. Necrotizing pancreatitis: contemporary analysis of 99 consecutive cases. *Ann Surg* 2001;234: 527–580.
Bassi C, Falconi M, Talamini G, et al. Controlled clinical trial of pefloxacin versus imipenem in severe acute pancreatitis. *Gastroenterology* 1998;115:1513–1517.

Bradley EL 3rd, Allen K. A prospective longitudinal study of observation versus surgical intervention in the management of necrotizing pancreatitis. *Am J Surg* 1991;161:19–25.

Brown A, Baillargeon JD, Hughes MD, et al. Can fluid resuscitation prevent pancreatic necrosis in severe acute pancreatitis? *Pancreatology* 2002;2:104–107.

Buchler MW, Gloor B, Muller CA, et al. Acute necrotizing pancreatitis: treatment strategy according to the status of infection. *Ann Surg* 2000;232:619–626.

Folsch UR, Nitsche R, Ludtke R, et al. Early ERCP and papillotomy compared with conservative treatment for acute biliary pancreatitis. The German Study Group on Acute Biliary Pancreatitis. *N Engl J Med* 1997;336:237–242.

Gerzof SG, Banks PA, Robbins AH, et al. Early diagnosis of pancreatic infection by computed tomography-guided aspiration. *Gastroenterology* 1987;93:1315–1320.

Lee SP, Nicholls JF, Park HZ. Biliary sludge as a cause of acute pancreatitis. *N Engl J Med* 1992;326:589–593.

London NJ, Leese T, Lavelle JM, et al. Rapid-bolus contrast-enhanced dynamic computed tomography in acute pancreatitis: a prospective study. *Br J Surg* 1991;78:1452–1456.

McKay CJ, Imrie CW. Staging of acute pancreatitis. Is it important? *Surg Clin North Am* 1999;79:733–743.

Ranson JH, Rifkind KM, Roses DF, et al. Prognostic signs and the role of operative management in acute pancreatitis. *Surg Gynecol Obstet* 1974;139:69–81.

Steinberg W, Tenner S. Acute pancreatitis. *N Engl J Med* 1994; 330:1198–1210.

Chronic Pancreatitis

Ammann RW, Heitz PU, Kloppel G. Course of alcoholic chronic pancreatitis: a prospective clinicomorphological long-term study. *Gastroenterology* 1996;111:224–231.

Leung JW, Bowen-Wright M, Aveling W, et al. Coeliac plexus block for pain in pancreatic cancer and chronic pancreatitis. *Br J Surg* 1983;70:730–732.

Nealon WH, Townsend CM Jr, Thompson JC. Preoperative endoscopic retrograde cholangiopancreatography (ERCP) in patients with pancreatic pseudocyst associated with resolving acute and chronic pancreatitis. *Ann Surg* 1989;209:532–540.

Reinhold C. Magnetic resonance imaging of the pancreas in 2001. *J Gastrointest Surg* 2002;6:133–135.

Sakorafas GH, Tsiotou AG. Proximal pancreatectomy in the surgical management of chronic pancreatitis. *J Clin Gastroenterol* 2002; 34:72–76.

Sarles H, Adler G, Dani R, et al. The pancreatitis classification of Marseilles-Rome 1988. *Scand J Gastroenterol* 1989;24:641–642.

Sharer N, Schwarz M, Malone G, et al. Mutations of the cystic fibrosis gene in patients with chronic pancreatitis. *N Engl J Med* 1998;339:645–652.

Witt H, Becker M. Genetics of chronic pancrestitis. *J Pediatr Gastroenterol Nutr* 2002;34:125–136.

Witzigmann H, Mark D, Uhlmarn D, et al. Quality of life in ohronic pancreatitis: a prospective trial comparing classical Whipple procedure and duodenum-preserving pancreatic head resection. *J Gastrointest Surg* 2002;6:173–180.

Pseudocysts

Adler J, Barkin JS. Management of pseudocysts, inflammatory masses, and pancreatic ascites. *Gastroenterol Clin North Am* 1990;19:863–871.

Frantzides CT, Ludwig KA, Redlich PN. Laparoscopic management of a pancreatic pseudocyst. *J Laparoendosc Surg* 1994;4:55–59.

Spivak H, Galloway JR, Amerson JR, et al. Management of pancreatic pseudocysts. *J Am Coll Surg* 1998;186:507–511.

Vitas GJ, Sarr MG. Selected management of pancreatic pseudocysts: operative versus expectant management. *Surgery* 1992;111: 123–130.

Yeo CJ, Bastidas JA, Lynch-Nyhan A, et al. The natural history of pancreatic pseudocysts documented by computed tomography. *Surg Gynecol Obstet* 1990;170:411–417.

Pancreatic Tumors

Birk D, Beger HG. Neoadjuvant, adjuvant, and palliative treatment of pancreatic cancer. *Curr Gastroenterol Rep* 2001;3:129–135.

Brennan MF, Moccia RD, Klimstra D. Management of adenocarcinoma of the body and tail of the pancreas. *Ann Surg* 1996; 223:506–512.

Ghaneh P, Kawesha A, Howes N, et al. Adjuvant therapy for pancreatic cancer. *World J Surg* 1999;23:937–945.

Glimelius B. Chemotherapy in the treatment of cancer of the pancreas. J Hepatobiliary Pancreat Surg 1998;5:235–241.

Hilgers W, Kern SE. Molecular genetic basis of pancreatic adenocarcinoma. *Genes Chrom Cancer* 1999;26:1–12.

Lichtenstein DR, Carr-Locke DL. Endoscopic palliation for unresectable pancreatic carcinoma. *Surg Clin North Am* 1995;75:969–988.

Lillemoe KD. Current management of pancreatic carcinoma. *Ann Surg* 1995;221:133–148.

Lillemoe KD, Kaushal S, Cameron JL, et al. Distal pancreatectomy: indications and outcomes in 235 patients. *Ann Surg* 1999;229:693–700.

Loftus EV Jr, Olivares-Pakzad BA, Batts KP, et al. Intraductal papillary-mucinous tumors of the pancreas: clinicopathologic features, outcome, and nomenclature. Members of the Pancreas Clinic, and Pancreatic Surgeons of Mayo Clinic. *Gastroenterology* 1996;110:1909–1918.

Mannell A, van Heerden JA, Weiland LH, et al. Factors influencing survival after resection or ductal adenocarcinoma of the pancreas. *Ann Surg* 1986;203:403–407.

Martin I, Hammond P, Scott J, et al. Cystic tumours of the pancreas. *Br J Surg* 1998;85:1484–1486.

Neoptolemos JP, Kerr DJ. Adjuvant therapy for pancreatic cancer. *Br J Surg* 1995;82:1012–1014.

Pfau PR, Chak A. Endoscopic ultrasonography. *Endoscopy* 2002;34: 21–28.

Pitt HA. Curative treatment for pancreatic neoplasms. Standard resection. *Surg Clin North Am* 1995;75:891–904.

Sarr MG, Cameron JL. Surgical management of unresectable carcinoma of the pancreas. *Surgery* 1982;91:123–133.

Traverso LW, Longmire WP Jr. Preservation of the pylorus in pancreaticoduodenectomy. *Surg Gynecol Obstet* 1978;146:959–962.

Warshaw AL, Fernandez-del Castillo C. Pancreatic carcinoma. *N Engl J Med* 1992;326:455–465.

Zerbi A, Balzano G, Patuzzo R, et al. Comparison between pylorus-preserving and Whipple pancreatoduodenectomy. *Br J Surg* 1995;82:975–979.

Gastrointestinal Peptides and Peptide-Secreting Tumors (Apudomas)

Complex neurohumoral interactions regulate the functions of the gastrointestinal tract. These functions include secretion, motility, absorption, sensation, mucosal proliferation, mucosal defense, immune regulation, and inflammatory response (Table 5.1). They are mediated by peptides secreted from endocrine cells and nerves in the gastrointestinal tract (Figure 5.1).

Gastrointestinal peptides become clinically significant in several pathological states, most importantly when they are oversecreted by tumors arising from the cells that produce them. Growing evidence also indicates that abnormalities in the secretion and distribution of gastrointestinal peptides underlie several motility disorders. As described later, these peptides are important in clinical practice because they are used in the diagnosis as well as in the therapy of disease states.

NEUROENDOCRINE DESIGN OF THE GASTROINTESTINAL TRACT

Three components comprise the neuroendocrine system: the endocrine cells; the enteric nervous system (ENS); and the extrinsic nervous system, including the peptidergic components of the parasympathetic and sympathetic nervous systems.

ENDOCRINE CELLS

Endocrine cells are scattered throughout the mucosal lining of the gut and are found in clusters only in the islet cells of Langerhans in the pancreas. Some—like the gastrin-secreting G cell of the antrum (Figure 5.2)—are of the *open* type, having apical microvilli that reach the lumen. Most are of the *closed* type, meaning they have no microvilli and do not reach the lumen. They synthesize the peptides in the rough endoplasmic reticulum, package them in granules, and transport them to the cell membrane for exocytotic release into the interstitial fluid. From there, the peptides diffuse either directly to their target site (paracrine) or enter capillaries to be carried by the blood to their target organ (endocrine). Endocrine cells are stimulated to synthesize and/or release their secretory peptides, usually by activation of receptor-mediated, G-protein-coupled signaling mechanisms. The

exocytosis process has been studied extensively in the beta cell of the pancreas. When the beta cell is stimulated (e.g., by glucose), its membrane depolarizes due to the closing of ATP-sensitive potassium-ion (K^+) channels. This, in turn, leads to the opening of voltage-dependent calcium channels, resulting in increased concentration of cytosolic Ca^{++} and insulin release. The same or similar mechanism likely operates in the secretory process of all endocrine cells.

ENTERIC NERVOUS SYSTEM

The enteric nervous system (ENS) is vast, comprising as many nerve cells as the spinal cord. The term ENS is used to describe the intrinsic innervation not only of the intestine but also of the esophagus, stomach, and pancreas. It is made up of cell bodies, usually located in ganglia, and of neural processes or axons that form the plexus. Within the hollow gastrointestinal tract, the ganglia are arranged in two groups: the submucosal ganglia and the myenteric ganglia between the circular and longitudinal muscle layers (Figure 5.3). The nerve processes of these two systems of ganglia produce the submucosal and myenteric plexus, respectively.

TABLE 5.1. Examples of Gastrointestinal Peptide Regulation of Function

Function	Action	Peptide(s)
Exocrine secretion		
Gastric	Stimulation	Gastrin, GRP, PACAP
	Inhibition	Somatostatin
Pancreatic	Stimulation	CCK, secretin, VIP
	Inhibition	Somatostatin
Intestinal	Stimulation	VIP
	Inhibition	Somatostatin
Endocrine secretion	Stimulation	GRP (bombesin)
	Inhibition	Somatostatin
Motility	Stimulation	CCK, gastrin, motilin, neurotensin
	Inhibition	Somatostatin, VIP, PYY
Absorption	Stimulation	—
	Inhibition	Somatostatin, GIP
Sensation	Stimulation	Substance P, CGRP
	Inhibition	Somatostatin
Mucosal proliferation	Stimulation	Gastrin, CCK, enteroglucagon
	Inhibition	Somatostatin
Mucosal defense	Stimulation	CGRP, EGF, TGF-β, IFN-γ
	Inhibition	—
Immune/inflammatory regulation	Stimulation	Substance P, cytokines (TNF, IL-1, IL-6, IL-8)
	Inhibition	?
Inflammatory response	Stimulation	CGRP, substance P, cytokines
	Inhibition	Somatostatin
Food intake	Stimulation	—
	Inhibition	CCK, NPY

Abbreviations: CCK, cholecystokinin; CGRP, calcitonin gene-related peptide; EGF, epidermal growth factor; GIP, gastric inhibitory peptide; GRP, gastrin-releasing peptide; IFN-γ, interferon-gamma; IL-1, interleukin-1; IL-6, interleukin-6; IL-8, interleukin-8; NPY, neuropeptide Y; PACAP, pituitary adenylate cyclase-activating polypeptide; PYY, peptide YY; TGF-β, transforming growth factor-beta; TNF, tumor necrosis factor; VIP, vasoactive intestinal polypeptide.

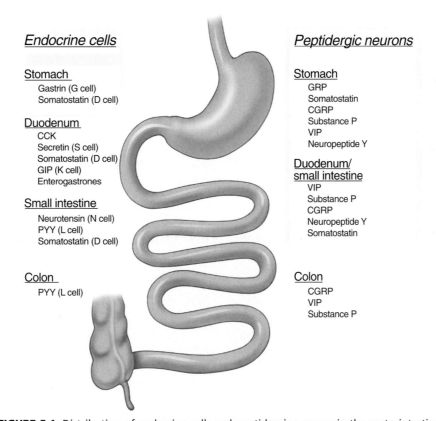

FIGURE 5.1. Distribution of endocrine cells and peptidergic neurons in the gastrointestinal tract. *Abbreviations*: CCK, cholecystokinin; CGRP, calcitonin gene-related peptide; GIP, gastric inhibitory polypeptide; GRP, gastrin-releasing peptide; PYY, peptide YY; VIP, vasoactive intestinal polypeptide.

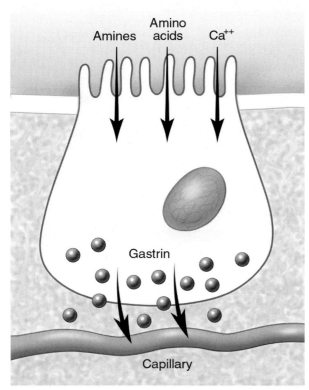

FIGURE 5.2. The gastrin-secreting G cell of the antrum is an open-type endocrine cell with luminal microvilli. Gastrin is secreted through the basal lateral membrane into capillaries.

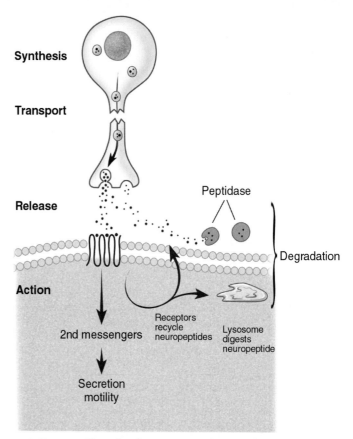

FIGURE 5.4. Life cycle of a neuropeptide. Peptidergic neurons synthesize neuropeptides in their cell bodies and transport them down the axons to be released at nerve terminals in close proximity to receptors on muscle, neural, and epithelial cells. Binding of the neuropeptide to its receptor stimulates the production of intracellular signals that eventuate in secretion or motility. Neuropeptidases at the external membrane of cells are strategically placed to degrade neuropeptides. This degrading mechanism, combined with internalization of the peptide receptor complex, terminates the action of the neuropeptide.

Most of the ENS neurons are peptidergic, that is, they synthesize peptides in their cell bodies, transport them along their axons, and release them at the nerve terminals, whence the peptides diffuse to bind to receptors on the target cells to effect a response. Figure 5.4 depicts an enteric neuron to demonstrate the life cycle of a neuropeptide, a peptide released by a neuron. Immunohistochemical techniques have facilitated the identification and mapping of the enteric neurons.

The neuropeptides of the ENS serve as important chemical messengers to regulate gastrointestinal function.

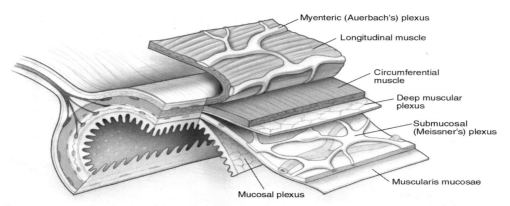

FIGURE 5.3. The enteric nervous system is composed of submucosal and myenteric ganglia connected by a network of neurons. (Adapted from Debas HT, Mulvihill SJ. Neuroendocrine design of the gut. Am J Surg 1991;161:244.)

A partial summary of the nonpeptide and peptide chemical messengers in the gastrointestinal tract is given in Table 5.2.

EXTRINSIC NERVOUS SYSTEM

The extrinsic innervation of the gastrointestinal tract derives mostly from the sympathetic and parasympathetic nervous systems. The sympathetic nervous system is distributed via the paravertebral ganglia and the greater and lesser splanchnic ganglia. Sympathetic innervation reaches target organs along the adventitia of arteries and arterioles. The parasympathetic system consists of the vagus, which supplies all the organs derived from the foregut and midgut and the lumbosacral outflow, which supplies the structures derived from the hindgut.

These details have been well understood for a long time. In recent years, however—thanks to immunohistochemical and anterograde and retrograde tracing techniques—it has been established that the sympathetic and parasympathetic systems are not only adrenergic and cholinergic, respectively, but also peptidergic, that is, they contain neuropeptides. In addition, it has been demonstrated that the sensory innervation of the gastrointestinal

TABLE 5.2. Neurotransmitters of the Gastric Inhibitory Tract
Nonpeptides
Acetylcholine (ACh)
γ-aminobutyric acid (GABA)
Nitric oxide (NO)
Noradrenaline
Serotonin
Peptides
Calcitonin gene-related peptide (CGRP)
Cholecystokinin (CCK)
Dynorphin
Enkephalin
Galanin
Gene-releasing peptide (GRP)
Neuropeptide Y (NPY)
Somatostatin (SS)
Tachykinins
Vasoactive intestinal polypeptide (VIP)

tract is mediated through unmyelinated C-fibers that predominantly contain substance P and CGRP.

The functional integration of peptidergic innervation is diagrammed in Figure 5.5. The role of sensory innervation in reflex control of the gut is shown in Figure 5.6.

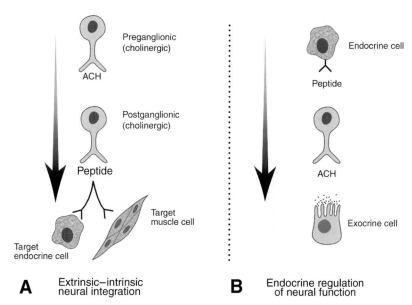

A   Extrinsic–intrinsic neural integration

B   Endocrine regulation of neural function

FIGURE 5.5. Functional integration of peptidergic innervation. Preganglionic neurons from the vagus or spinal cord activate enteric ganglia through the release of acetylcholine. (A) The postganglionic neurons then act on target cells (e.g., endocrine or muscle cells), again through cholinergic neurotransmission. A different type of integration involves the release of a peptide from an endocrine cell. (B) The peptide then acts on intrinsic muscurinic neurons to activate exocrine secretion (e.g., pancreatic secretion). (C) The third type of integration involves preganglionic cholinergic neurons acting on postganglionic peptidergic neurons to release peptides, which then act on target cells (e.g., release of gastrin by gastrin-releasing peptide). (D) The final type of integration is exemplified by the release of histamine in stimulation of acid secretion. The peptide gastrin or cholinergic neurons act on ECL cells to release histamine.

(Continued)

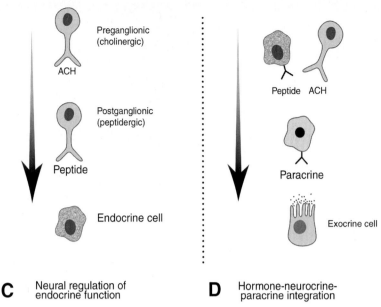

C Neural regulation of endocrine function

D Hormone-neurocrine-paracrine integration

FIGURE 5.5. *Continued*

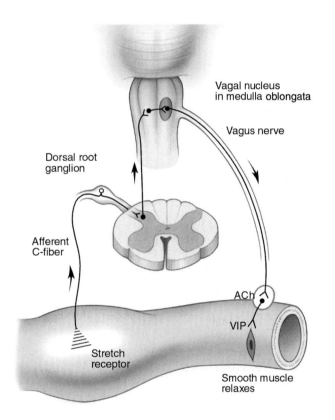

FIGURE 5.6. Role of sensory innervation in reflex control of the gut. Stretch receptors in the gut wall are stimulated by distention. The response is transmitted through afferent C-fibers to the dorsal root ganglia and then to the posterior horn. Spinal neurons then carry the message to the vagal nucleus in the medulla oblongata. Efferent vagal neurons carry the response to the intestinal wall, which, through cholinergic transmission, activates the release of vasoactive intestinal polypeptide (VIP) from intrinsic peptidergic neurons. The VIP then acts to relax the enteric smooth muscle. *Abbreviation*: ACh, acetylcholine.

CLASSIFICATION OF GASTROINTESTINAL PEPTIDES

Gastrointestinal peptides may be classified either by chemical structure or by mode of action. Structurally, they have been classified into several families, which share structural similarities (e.g., the CCK/gastrin family; the secretin family [secretin, VIP, PHI]; and the PP family [PP, NPY, PYY]). A classification of gastrointestinal peptides based on their mode of action is given in Table 5.3.

Endocrine peptides are secreted into the circulation and transported in the bloodstream to reach their target organ or cell. Paracrine agents are secreted into the inter-

TABLE 5.3. Classification of Gastrointestinal Peptides

Endocrine
  Cholecystokinin (CCK)
  Gastric inhibitory peptide (GIP)
  Gastrin
  Motilin
  Neurotensin
  Pancreatic polypeptide
  Peptide YY
  Secretin
  Somatostatin

Paracrine
  Somatostatin
  Vasoactive intestinal polypeptide (VIP)

Neurocrine
  Calcitonin gene-related peptide (CGRP)
  Cholecystokinin (CCK)
  Galanin
  Gastrin-releasing peptide (GRP)
  Neuropeptide Y
  Opioid peptides
  Somatostatin
  Substance P
  Vasoactive intestinal polypeptide (VIP)

stitial fluid and reach their target site by diffusion over distances that can be measured in nanometers or millimeters. Neurocrine agents are released at nerve endings and usually have to cross only a short synaptic gap to reach the target cell. This classification is imperfect because several peptides have more than one mode of action. For example, CCK acts as both a hormone and a neuropeptide, while somatostatin acts in all three capacities as an endocrine, paracrine, and neurocrine agent. Only gastrin and secretin appear to act solely as endocrine peptides within the gastrointestinal tract.

GASTRIN

The existence of gastrin was hypothesized by Edkins in 1905, when he demonstrated that antral extract stimulated acid secretion in the cat.[1] Many attributed the observation to contaminant histamine until 1938, when Komorov prepared histamine-free extract that retained acid-stimulatory effect.[2] In 1964, Gregory and Tracy purified porcine gastrin and characterized its amino acid sequence.[3]

Distribution

Gastrin is produced by G cells, which are located primarily in the mid-layer of the antral mucosa. These cells are also present in the duodenum, particularly in the first portion. Gastrin, present in the pancreas of the fetus, is not in the adult pancreas. Gastrin-like immunoreactivity is also found in the brain.

Structure and Synthesis

The gene that encodes gastrin has been isolated and characterized from porcine antrum and from a human genomic DNA library, as well as from a human antral cDNA library. A single gene produces a single progastrin sequence from which all molecular forms of gastrin are derived by post-translational processing. The human gene, located on chromosome 17, is about 4100 base pairs long. Gastrin cDNA contains 620 nucleotides, including an open reading frame of 312 nucleotides that encode preprogastrin. Gastrin gene expression in the antrum is regulated by luminal contents and pH in parallel with gastrin release. Post-translational processing of gastrin produces the various molecular forms and involves several cleavage steps and C-terminal amidation (Figure 5.7). Human preprogastrin consists of 101 amino acids. From this, an 80-amino acid progastrin is cleaved (preprogastrin 22–101). Progastrin is processed further in the Golgi complex and secretory granules into mature gastrin, G-17 and G-34. These peptides are amidated at the C-terminus. The final step in producing biologically active gastrin is deamidation of the C-terminal phenylalanine residue. About half of the gastrins isolated from the human antrum and duodenum are sulfated.

HUMAN PRE-PRO-GASTRIN

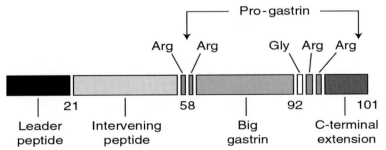

FIGURE 5.7. Post-translational processing of gastrin (preprogastrin). A number of molecular forms of gastrin are processed from the human preprogastrin. These molecular forms (e.g., big gastrin, G17) have C-terminal amide extension, which is removed by the action of amidase to release the active peptide.

The most abundant form of gastrin in the blood is G-34, comprising two-thirds of circulating gastrin in the fasting state and half in the postprandial state. The remainder is primarily G-17, with small amounts of G-14 and component I. Circulating G-34 and G-17 have similar potency for stimulating acid secretion. The C-terminal tetrapeptide retains acid-stimulating property but is 25 times less potent than G-17.

Release of Gastrin

Gastrin is released by peptides, amino acids, and calcium in the antral lumen. It is also released by gastric distension, which activates vasovagal nervous reflexes. Other releasers of gastrin include catecholamines and gastrin-releasing peptide (bombesin). Inhibition of gastrin is caused by antral acidification, which acts by releasing somatostatin from delta cells in close proximity to G cells. While sham feeding does release gastrin, the more dominant action of the vagus on gastrin release is inhibitory. Thus, following all types of vagotomy, hypergastrinemia develops.

Receptors and Postreceptor Signaling

The gastrin receptor has been cloned from canine parietal cells. It is also known as the CCK-B receptor because of its close structural relationship to CCK-A receptor, with which it shares 50% amino acid identity. CCK-B receptors, like the CCK-A receptors, have a seven membrane-spanning region and belong to the class of G protein-coupled receptors. When the receptor is activated by gastrin binding, phospholipase C is stimulated, resulting in the production of diacylglycerol and inositol 1,4,5

triphosphate in the cytoplasm of the target cell. This, in turn, leads to increased intracellular calcium concentration and activation of protein kinase C. The gastrin CCK-B receptor does not distinguish between gastrin and CCK, or between sulfated or unsulfated gastrin and CCK. In contrast, gastrin does not bind or binds little to the CCK-A receptor. The receptor and postreceptor mechanisms are diagrammed in Figure 5.8.

Gastrin CCK-B receptors are found on parietal cells, ECL cells, gastric oxyntic mucosal proliferative cells (stem cells), the lower esophageal sphincter muscle, gastric antral smooth muscle, and a subpopulation of pancreatic acinar cells. The gastrin CCK-B receptor is also found throughout the brain.

Biological Actions of Gastrin

The major biological actions of gastrin include the following items:

1. Acid secretion. Gastrin mediates most of the acid response to a meal during the gastric phase of acid secretion. In the dog, acid response to a meal can be prevented by pretreatment with monoclonal antibody to gastrin. Gastrin acts on CCK-B receptors on the ECL cell to release histamine, which then stimulates the parietal cell by acting on the histamine H_2-receptor. Gastrin also acts directly on the parietal cell, but the dominant mechanism for its acid secretory function is through activation of the ECL cell in the gastric oxyntic mucosa.

2. Trophic action. Gastrin is the primary growth regulator of the oxyntic gland mucosa. Hypergastrinemic states cause growth of the oxyntic mucosa and parietal cell hyperplasia. Gastrin also acts on the crypt cells in the duo-

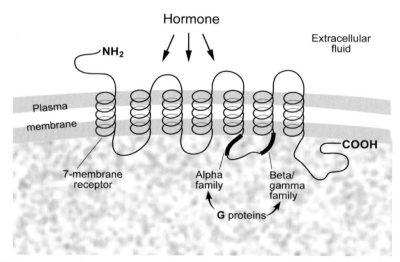

FIGURE 5.8. Receptors and postreceptor processes of gastrin. The gastrin receptor is a typical seven-membrane spanning, G-protein–coupled receptor.

denum to promote growth of the duodenal mucosa. The trophic action of gastrin is independent of its secretory effect. Gastrin is also trophic to the colonic mucosa, and the colonic cancer cells may elaborate gastrin that may act on them in autocrine fashion.

3. Motor effects. Gastrin causes contraction of the lower esophageal sphincter, but higher doses are required than those that stimulate its secretory action. It also stimulates antral motility. In vitro, gastrin stimulates smooth muscle contraction. In pharmacologic doses, as seen in Zollinger-Ellison syndrome (ZES), gastrin stimulates small intestinal peristalsis and shortens intestinal transit time.

4. Stimulation of pancreatic enzyme secretion. Gastrin stimulates the secretion of pancreatic enzyme, an action that is far less marked in humans than in dogs.

5. Stimulation of somatostatin release. Gastrin stimulates release of somatostatin from fundic endocrine cells but is less potent in this action than CCK.

CHOLECYSTOKININ

One of the longest known gastrointestinal peptides, cholecystokinin (CCK) was first described in 1928 by Ivy and Oldberg, who demonstrated that perfusion of fat into the intestine stimulated contraction of the gallbladder.[4] In 1943, Harper and Raper showed that intestinal perfusion of proteins and injection of small intestinal mucosal extracts into rats stimulated pancreatic enzyme secretion; they called the active substance *pancreozymin*.[5] In 1966, Mutt and Jorpes purified CCK from intestinal extracts and demonstrated that it is identical to pancreozymin.[6] For historical reasons, the name *CCK* has been adopted.

Distribution

CCK is released by I cells, which are endocrine cells located mostly in the mucosa of the duodenum and upper jejunum. CCK is present in high concentrations in the cerebral cortex, especially in layers II and III. It is colocalized with dopamine. In the peripheral nervous system, CCK is found in pancreatic neurons and in the nerves of the colon and ileum. CCK is also abundant in the celiac plexus and in the vagus. Human CCK has also been found in some pituitary and adrenal medullary cells.

Structure and Synthesis

CCK exists in multiple molecular forms (CCK58, CCK39, CCK33, CCK25, CCK22, CCK18, CCK8, CCK7, and CCK5). The major biological form of large CCK is CCK58. Cleavage at mono and dibasic residues of CCK58 releases smaller forms. In the brain, CCK exists primarily as CCK8 and CCK58. In humans, the gene for CCK is located on chromosome 3 (Figure 5.9). The third exon on chromosome 3 encodes the biologically active region of the peptide, including CCK58. CCK mRNA is about 750 bases, of which 345 encode protein. All the smaller forms of CCK are subsequently derived from CCK58. All molecular forms of CCK must be sulfated at the seventh amino acid from the carboxyl terminal in order to have biological function.

Release of CCK

CCK is released from the I cells of the duodenum and jejunum in response to luminal fat, peptides, amino acids and acid. Proteins must undergo partial digestion, and triglycerides must be hydrolyzed to become effective releasers of CCK. CCK is also released by GRP (bombesin). Monitor peptide, a CCK-releasing peptide, has been isolated from rat pancreatic juice and can release CCK in vitro from duodenal mucosal cells. Its role in vivo is uncertain. Trypsin in the duodenum inhibits CCK release, presumably by inactivating a CCK-releasing peptide

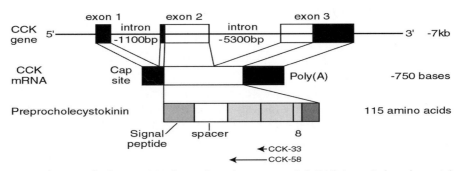

FIGURE 5.9. The gene for human CCK, located on chromosome 3, is 7 kilobases in length, containing three exons and two introns.

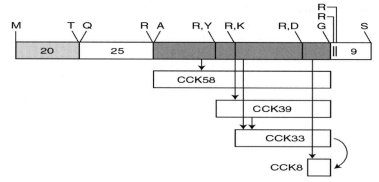

FIGURE 5.10. Intracellular processing of CCK. Post-translational processing releases multiple molecular forms of CCK (CCK58, CCK39, CCK33, and CCK8).

in the duodenal mucosa. Trypsin inhibitors release CCK by preventing inactivation of CCK-releasing peptide. Recent evidence in rats suggests that vagal electrical stimulation releases CCK from intrapancreatic neurons and that the so-released CCK acts as a neurotransmitter in vagal stimulation of enzyme secretion.

Receptors and Postreceptor Signaling

The action of CCK is mediated by two types of receptors, the CCK-A and CCK-B receptors, both from the 7-transmembrane, G-protein-linked receptor family. CCK-A receptor has a high affinity for sulfated CCK analogues and is the principal receptor that mediates pancreatic enzyme secretion and gallbladder contraction. CCK-B receptor has high affinity for both gastrin and CCK. Both receptors are coupled to phospholipase C, and activation produces diacylglycerol (DAG) and inositol triphosphate (IP$_3$). The subsequent intracellular processes are similar to those described for gastrin (Figure 5.10). Receptors for CCK are present on acinar cells; on gallbladder, ileum, and colon muscle; on lower esophageal sphincter; and on delta cells.

Specific antagonists to both receptors have been developed and have proven useful for studying physiology. It is likely that these antagonists have a therapeutic role in the future.

Biological Actions of CCK

The following are the major biological actions of CCK:

1. Stimulation of pancreatic enzyme secretion. CCK is the principal mediator of food-stimulated pancreatic secretion. The action is complex and involves intrapancreatic cholinergic mechanisms. Intrapancreatic CCK is also involved in the mediation of vagal stimulation of pancreatic secretion.

2. Gallbladder contraction. CCK is the primary stimulant of gallbladder contraction and acts partly by releasing acetylcholine from cholinergic neurons within the wall of the gallbladder.

3. Delay of gastric emptying. Regulation of gastric emptying is a physiological action of CCK, probably indi-

rect, resulting from activation of afferent sensory neurons.

4. Peristaltic reflex. CCK is a cotransmitter, in conjunction with acetylcholine, of the peristaltic reflex.

5. Colonic motility. CCK is an inhibitor of colonic motility.

6. Gastric acid. CCK inhibits gastric acid secretion, probably through the release of somatostatin.

7. Insulin and pancreatic polypeptide. CCK initiates the release of insulin and pancreatic polypeptide.

8. Satiety. CCK initiates the sensation of satiety.

SECRETIN

Secretin was the first peptide hormone to be identified. Its discovery inaugurated the beginning of modern endocrinology as we know it. In 1902, Bayliss and Starling showed that perfusion of the small intestine with acid released a circulating substance that stimulated pancreatic juice flow.[7] This first demonstration of a circulating humoral substance dealt a severe blow to the tenet of *nervism* upheld by Pavlov and his students.[8] In 1968, secretin was purified and subsequently sequenced.[9]

Distribution

Secretin is secreted by S cells located predominantly in the duodenum and proximal jejunum. As far as is known, secretin is found only in these cells and has not been shown to be present in neural tissue. In this sense, it is a classical hormone.

Structure and Synthesis

Secretin is a linear peptide containing 27 amino acid residues. It is structurally similar to glucagon, VIP, GIP, growth hormone-releasing factor (GHRF), PHI, pituitary cyclase-activating polypeptide (PCAP), and calcitonin gene-related peptide (CGRP). The secretin gene is composed of four exons spanning 813 base pairs, and the entire secretin sequence is encoded in a single exon. A precursor secretin consisting of the secretin molecule plus a 41-amino acid C-terminal extension is first produced, from which the secretin is cleaved. While the S-17 C-terminal fragment retains activity, the full 27-amino acid sequence is required for full potency.

Release of Secretin

Secretin is released by acid in the duodenum. The pH threshold for secretin release is 4.5. Fat is another potent releaser of secretin. Oleate releases secretin but triglycerides do not. Bile in the duodenum releases secretin, while pancreatic juice inhibits its release. Vagal stimulation does not release secretin, while somatostatin and metenkephalin inhibit its release.

Receptors and Postreceptor Signaling

The secretin receptor has been cloned and is similar to the receptors of VIP, calcitonin, and parathyroid hormone (PTH). They are all G protein-coupled, 7-transmembrane receptors. Secretin binding to its receptor activates adenylate cyclase, and cAMP serves as the second messenger.

Biological Actions of Secretin

Secretin has several major biological actions:

1. Pancreatic bicarbonate secretion. The most important action of secretin is stimulation of ductal cells to secrete water and bicarbonate. Small doses of secretin also potentiate the action of CCK to stimulate pancreatic enzyme release.
2. Biliary secretion. Secretin stimulates bile acid-independent bile flow.
3. Pancreatic growth. Secretin has only minimal trophic action on pancreatic growth but potentiates the trophic effects of CCK.
4. Gastric acid secretion. Secretin is an inhibitor of gastric acid secretion.
5. Gastric pepsin secretion. Secretin stimulates the secretion of gastric pepsin.
6. Chloride, sodium, and bicarbonate secretion. Secretin stimulates chloride secretion and inhibits sodium and bicarbonate secretion in the intestine.
7. Inhibition of gastrin release. Secretin is a weak inhibitor of food-stimulated gastrin release. In patients with ZES, it has the paradoxical effect of significantly increasing the release of gastrin, a phenomenon that is the basis for the secretin test in the diagnosis of gastrinoma.
8. Gastric emptying of solids. Secretin inhibits gastric emptying of solids.

VASOACTIVE INTESTINAL POLYPEPTIDE

Vasoactive intestinal polypeptide (VIP) was discovered in 1970 by Said and Mutt, while they were screening extracts of gut and lung for vasodilator activities.[6] VIP belongs to the secretin family of peptides.

Distribution

VIP is found in neurons throughout the GI tract. The same neurons also contain PHI. In pancreatic and salivary neurons, VIP is colocalized with acetylcholine. VIP-containing neurons are abundant in the enteric nervous system and its ganglia. In the anal sphincter, it is colocalized with NO synthase. VIP neurons project to the circular smooth muscle of the gut and are particularly numerous in the sphincters of the GI tract.

Structure and Synthesis

VIP is a 28-residue basic peptide. The gene for VIP was cloned from human neuroblastoma and contains seven exons, of which five contain coding sequences separately for VIP, PHI and signal sequence.

Release of VIP

Because VIP is a locally acting neuropeptide, plasma concentrations are low unless excessive VIP is being secreted by a vipoma. However, elevated levels of VIP are present in the venous outflow of the gut in response to luminal fat and HCl, electric stimulation of extrinsic nerves, and in response to distension or stroking of the mucosa.

Receptors and Postreceptor Signaling

The VIP receptor has been cloned and has a molecular weight of 48.8 kDa. The VIP receptor binds VIP and PACAP with equal affinity but binds secretin with lower affinity. PHI acts via the VIP receptor. The VIP receptor is also a G-protein-coupled, 7-transmembrane receptor. Like the secretin receptor, it is adenylate cyclase linked, with cAMP acting as the second intracellular messenger.

Biological Actions of VIP

The major biological actions of VIP include:

1. Secretory action. VIP stimulates intestinal secretion and pancreatic water and bicarbonate secretion.
2. Somatostatin release. Both VIP and PHI release somatostatin from delta cells in the stomach. This mechanism probably explains its inhibitory effect on gastric acid secretion.
3. Motility effects. VIP is a powerful relaxant of smooth muscle and is responsible for the descending inhibition of the peristaltic reflex; the receptive relaxation of the stomach; and the relaxation of the lower esophageal, pyloric, ileocecal and anal sphincters. Its muscle-relaxing effect appears to take place in cooperation with NO.
4. Mucosal blood flow. VIP increases mucosal blood flow.

GLUCAGON FAMILY OF PEPTIDES

The glucagon family of peptides consists of pancreatic glucagon and enteroglucagons. The latter are a group of peptides produced in the intestine by differential processing of the same glucagon gene as the one present in pancreatic alpha cells. The enteroglucagons include glicentin, oxyntomodulin, glucagon-like peptide (GLP-1) and GLP-2.

Distribution

Pancreatic glucagon is secreted by the alpha cells of the pancreatic islets. Enteroglucagons are released by the L cells, endocrine cells in the small intestinal mucosa.

Structure and Synthesis

The structure of the preproglucagon gene consists of six exons and five introns. Separate exons encode the signal peptide and each of the glucagon sequences. Proglucagon is formed first and in the pancreas is processed to form glucagon. In the small intestine, post-translational processing is accomplished by enzymes to produce glicentin, GLP-1, GLP-2, and oxyntomodulin. Pancreatic glucagon is a 29-amino acid peptide. Glicentin is the largest molecule, consisting of 69 amino acid residues. Oxyntomodulin, also known as enteroglucagon, is a 37-amino acid peptide, consisting of the glucagon molecule with an 8-amino acid extension at the C terminus. GLP-1 corresponds to proglucagon 78–107 amide. GLP-2 is proglucagon 126–158 and does not appear to have much biological action.

Release of Glucagon and GLP

Glucagon is released from the A cells of the pancreas in response to hypoglycemia and catchelomines. Enteroglucagons are released from the intestine by an ordinary mixed meal, digestible fat and carbohydrates. Enteroglucagon, also released by GRP, GIP, and substance P, is inhibited by somatostatin.

Receptors and Postreceptor Signaling

Two important receptors have been identified and cloned. One is the glucagon receptor, which binds not only glucagon but also oxyntomodulin. The second is the GLP-1 receptor, which does not bind glucagon. Both are G protein-coupled, adenylate cyclase-activating, 7-transmembrane receptors with cAMP serving as the second messenger.

Biological Actions of the Glucagon Family of Peptides

The different peptides of the glucagon family have different biological actions, as follows:

1. Pancreatic glucagon. Glucagon has general biological and metabolic actions that include glycogenolysis, lipolysis, gluconeogenesis, and ketogenesis. Other actions include the inhibition of: intestinal motility and absorption, pancreatic exocrine secretion, gastric acid secretion, and pentagastrin-stimulated lower esophageal sphincter pressure. Relaxation of the sphincter of Oddi and stimulation of hepatic bile flow are additional actions.

2. GLP-1. The most biologically active glucagon gene product made in the intestine, GLP-1 stimulates insulin release and inhibits pancreatic glucagon release. It is thus an important incretin. GLP-1 inhibits pentagastrin-stimulated gastric acid secretion and is a strong inhibitor of gastric emptying. It also inhibits pancreatic exocrine secretion. It stimulates the release of somatostatin. GLP-1 is an important enterogastrone and inhibitor of pancreatic secretion.

3. Oxyntomodulin and glicentin. Oxyntomodulin is a weak stimulator of insulin release, but glicentin has no such action. Glicentin is a weak inhibitor of gastric acid and pancreatic secretion, while oxyntomodulin is equipotent to GLP-1. Enteroglucagon has trophic action on small intestinal mucosa and may be responsible for the adaptive intestinal hypertrophy seen after massive small bowel resection. Tumors that produce enteroglucagon cause giant small intestinal villi.

GASTRIN-RELEASING PEPTIDE OR BOMBESIN

The amphibian analogue of the mammalian gastrin-releasing peptide (GRP), bombesin, was isolated from frog skin by Erspamer and colleagues.[10] It is a general stimulant of gastrointestinal peptide release, analogues to somatostatin's function as a paninhibitor.

Distribution

GRP is found in neurons of the enteric nervous system in the stomach, intestines, and pancreas but not in endocrine cells.

Structure and Synthesis

GRP is a 27-amino acid peptide. The human GRP gene contains three exons and two introns.

Release of GRP

Vagal stimulation releases GRP into the gastric venous outflow, and vagal release of gastrin is mediated through GRP. GRP is also released by gastric distention and luminal nutrients, suggesting that it may play a role in the release of gastrin by these stimuli.

Receptors and Postreceptor Signaling

Three bombesin receptors have been cloned, one of which has high affinity for GRP. The receptor belongs to the G protein superfamily. Activation of GRP receptors increases inositol triphosphate and intracellular calcium.

Biological Actions of GRP

The major biological actions of GRP include the following:

1. Release of gastrin and other GI peptides. GRP is an important mediator of vagal stimulation of gastrin and inhibition of somatostatin, as well as of gastrin release in response to luminal stimulants. GRP also stimulates release of CCK and several other GI peptides.

2. Stimulation of the pancreas. GRP stimulates pancreatic exocrine and endocrine secretion.

3. Mitogenic effects. GRP and bombesin stimulate division of various cell lines and may stimulate growth of small-cell lung cancer. Chronic exogenous administration of GRP in the rat increases antral G cell proliferation.

4. Motility. GRP has an excitatory effect on GI smooth muscle. The motor response of the gastric antrum to vagal stimulation is mediated by GRP.

SOMATOSTATIN

Guillemin and Schally isolated somatostatin from sheep hypothalamus in 1973, and, in 1977, they were awarded the Nobel Prize for their discovery.[11]

Distribution

Somatostatin is present in endocrine cells—known as the D or delta cell—throughout the mucosa of the gastrointestinal tract and in the islets of Langerhans in the pancreas. It is also widely distributed in the central nervous system, the autonomic nervous system, and the enteric nervous system.

Structure and Synthesis

Somatostatin exists in two biologically active forms, somatostatin-14 and somatostatin-28, so designated because of the number of amino acid residues they contain. The human somatostatin gene is located on chromosome 3. The predicted precursor of 116 amino acids contains the somatostatin-28 sequence at its carboxyl terminus. Somatostatin-28 is cleaved from prosomatostatin, and somatostatin-14 is enzymatically derived from somatostatin-28 with the actions of an endopeptidase and aminopeptidase. In the stomach, somatostatin-14 may be formed directly from prosomatostatin. Somatostatin gene expression studies have shown that chronic alkalinization and GRP reduce somatostatin mRNA in the antrum, while prolonged fasting increases it.

Release of Somatostatin

Feeding releases both somatostatin-14 and somatostatin-28 from the gastrointestinal tract. Fat and protein are stronger releasers than carbohydrates. Insulin hypoglycemia and isoproterenol release somatostatin from both the pancreas and the gastrointestinal tract.

In the antrum, somatostatin is released by food, adrenergic nerves, CGRP, and acidification of the lumen. Antral acidification, the primary mechanism by which gastrin release is turned off, is accomplished through release of somatostatin from delta cells, and results in inhibition of G cells. Vagal stimulation inhibits somatostatin release through both atropine-sensitive muscarinic nerves and GRP release.

Receptors and Postreceptor Signaling

At least five somatostatin receptors have been cloned. The multiplicity of the somatostatin receptors gives rise to diverse signal transduction mechanisms. Both forms of somatostatin bind to SSTR-1, SSTR-2, and SSTR-3, but somatostatin-28 binds preferentially to SSTR-2 and somatostatin-14 to SSTR-5. The receptors belong to the G-protein-coupled, 7-transmembrane family of receptors, but in different tissues, different G proteins are implicated. The long-acting somatostatin analogue octreotide binds with high affinity to SSTR-2, -3 and -4, but not to SSTR-1 and -5.

Biological Actions of Somatostatin

Somatostatin is a pan-inhibitor of gastrointestinal endocrine and exocrine secretion and has variable effects on motility:

1. Inhibition of hormone and neurotransmitter secretion. Somatostatin inhibits the release of acetylcholine and of all GI peptides.

2. Inhibition of exocrine secretion. Somatostatin inhibits gastric secretion of acid, pepsin, and ECL-cell histamine. It inhibits pancreatic enzyme and bicarbonate secretion as well as the bile salt-independent bicarbonate secretion in bile. It also inhibits intestinal water and electrolyte secretion.

3. Motility. Its effect on motility is variable. While it stimulates the early phase of gastric emptying, somatostatin inhibits the late phase. While it simulates distal intestinal migrating motor complexes, it inhibits those in the gastroduodenum. It inhibits ileal and gallbladder contraction.

4. Nutrient absorption. Somatostatin is an inhibitor of nutrient absorption in the intestine.

5. Tissue responses. Through its antitrophic action on tissues, somatostatin inhibits tissue response to growth factors.

6. Blood flow. It inhibits splanchnic blood flow.

7. Sensation. GRP has an antinociceptive effect and causes decreased rectal sensation.

GASTRIC INHIBITORY POLYPEPTIDE

Gastric inhibitory polypeptide (GIP) was isolated by Brown et al. from impure porcine CCK by its inhibitory effect on acid secretion.[12] Subsequently, the peptide was found to be more important for its insulin-releasing action and was renamed glucose-dependent insulinotropic peptide.

Distribution

GIP is produced by K cells, primarily in the duodenum and jejunum.

Structure and Synthesis

A linear peptide of 42 amino acid residues, GIP is structurally related to glucagon. The human GIP gene consists of six exons, with GIP being coded mainly in exon 3.

Release of GIP

GIP is released by oral but not by intravenous glucose and by emulsified fat and amino acids.

Receptors and Postreceptor Signaling

The GIP receptor has been cloned and is a G-protein-coupled, adenylate cyclase-activating, 7-transmembrane receptor.

Biological Actions of GIP

The major biological actions of GIP include the following:

1. Inhibition of gastric acid secretion. GIP inhibits pentagastrin-stimulated acid secretion from denervated gastric pouches. This inhibitory action can be reversed by cholinergic agonists. The acidic inhibitory effect in humans is relatively weak, and GIP is not considered a major enterogastrone.
2. Intestinal secretion. GIP inhibits intestinal secretion of water and electrolytes.
3. Stimulation of insulin release. Probably the most important action of GIP, insulin release is considered physiologic. The insulinotropic action of GIP occurs only when the blood glucose level is raised to 125 mg/dL or higher. GIP also stimulates insulin release from isolated rat islets in a glucose-dependent manner.
4. Simulation of somatostatin release. GIP releases somatostatin from the gastric fundus and antrum. The gastrin inhibitory action in antral mucosa in organ culture is reversed by somatostatin antibody.

SUBSTANCE P

Substance P (SP) was the first gut peptide to be isolated. This was accomplished in 1931 by Von Euler and Gaddum.[13] It is an 11-amino acid peptide belonging to the tachykinin family, which includes calcitonin gene-related peptide (CGRP), neurokinin A, neurokinin B, physalaemin, kassinin, and eledoisin.

Distribution

SP is present in the central nervous system. In the GI tract, it is found in both small-diameter spinal afferent neurons and in the neurons of the ENS. SP neurons are present in myenteric plexus and enter the circular muscle. The C fibers that contain SP are thought to be sensory neurons and can be lesioned with the sensory neurotoxin capsaicin.

Receptor and Postreceptor Processes

Three receptor subtypes have been characterized: NK_1, NK_2, and NK_3. The NK_1 receptor is the preferred receptor for SP. These receptors are G-protein-coupled, 7-transmembrane spanning receptors. When activated, cytosolic inositol triphosphate and calcium are elevated.

Biological Actions of SP

SP and the other tachykinins have several biological actions, including:

1. Pain. SP mediates central transmission of pain.
2. Neurogenic inflammation. SP and the other tachykinins regulate neurogenic inflammation (vasodilatation and plasma extravasation) in the gut, airways, skin, and joints.
3. Motility action. Orad contraction of the peristaltic reflex (Figure 5.11) is mediated by SP and related peptides. Excitation of smooth muscle occurs directly and through the release of acetylcholine from neurons of the myenteric plexus.
4. Secretion. SP stimulates salivary and intestinal secretion.
5. Vasodilation. These peptides are potent vasodilators.
6. Sensory innervation. SP mediates sensory innervation of the gut.

CALCITONIN GENE-RELATED PEPTIDE

Calcitonin gene-related peptide (CGRP) is a 37-amino acid peptide produced by alternative processing of the glucagon gene in neural tissues. It is a member of the tachykinin family.

Distribution

CGRP is widely distributed in the gut, both in sensory afferent C fibers and in the neurons of the ENS. Like SP,

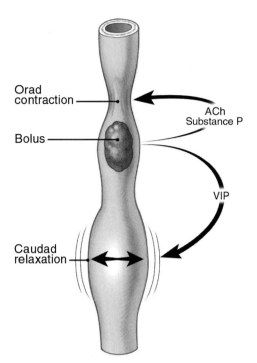

FIGURE 5.11. The peristaltic reflex. When a bolus of food distends the intestine, two reflex arcs are activated: Proximally, neural release of ACh and substance P causes contraction; while distally, peptidergic neurons release VIP, leading to relaxation of the intestinal musculature. The effect is to propel the bolus of food distally.

CGRP fibers are present in myenteric plexus, circular smooth muscle, around submucosal blood vessels and in the mucosa of the gut. CGRP is also present in the CNS.

Structure and Synthesis

The alternative processing that produces CGRP from the calcitonin gene is shown in Figure 5.12. The CGRP so produced is α-CGRP (or CGRP-I). A second CGRP, β-CGRP (or CGRP-II) is also produced from a gene that does not encode CGRP. The spinal afferent neurons express α-CGRP, but both α- and β-CGRP are found in the CNS and in the gut. CGRP is a 37-amino acid residue peptide.

Release of CGRP

CGRP is released by the sensory neurotoxin capsaicin. Low doses of capsaicin stimulate CGRP release, but in high doses, capsaicin destroys spinal afferent neurons. Little information exists on the release of CGRP during normal digestion.

Receptors and Postreceptor Signaling

The CGRP receptor is a G protein-coupled, 7-transmembrane receptor that predominantly activates adenylate cyclase. The CGRP receptor has recently been cloned.

Biological Actions of CGRP

The major biological actions of CGRP include:

1. Sensory neurotransmission along with SP.
2. Gastric mucosal protection (cytoprotection).
3. Release of somatostatin.
4. Powerful vasodilatory action.
5. Potent inhibition of gastric acid secretion, probably through release of somatostatin.
6. Relaxation of gastric smooth muscle and inhibition of gastric emptying.

PANCREATIC POLYPEPTIDE FAMILY

Three peptides comprise the pancreatic polypeptide (PP) family: PP, peptide YY (PYY), and neuropeptide Y (NPY).

Distribution

The islets of Langerhans, particularly in the head of the pancreas, are the major site of production of PP. No PP release occurs after total pancreatectomy. PYY cells are located in the ileal and colonic mucosa.

Structure and Synthesis

PP, PYY, and NPY each contain 36 amino acid residues, and each have 18 amino acid identities. The PP gene contains four exons and three introns. Prepropancreatic polypeptide contains 95 amino acids.

Release of PP

PP is released by protein meals and cholinergic reflexes. The basal level increases with each myoelectric motor

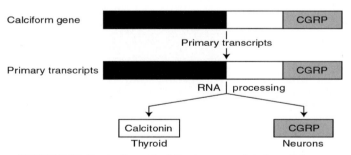

FIGURE 5.12. Production of calcitonin gene-related peptide (CGRP) from the calcitonin gene. The calcitonin gene contains within it the structure of not only calcitonin but also that of another peptide, which came to be known as calcitonin gene-related peptide. Post-translational processing in the thyroid produces calcitonin. In neurons in the gastrointestinal tract, however, post-translational processing results in CGRP.

complex (MMC). PP is also released by intravenous amino acids and vagal simulation which occurs during sham feeding or insulin hypoglycemia. Oleic acid and glucose also release PP but to a smaller degree than amino acids. Atropine pretreatment abolishes PP release in response to vagal simulation. GRP (bombesin) is a potent stimulant of PP release. Adrenergic and dopaminergic stimulation also releases PP.

PYY is released by a mixed meal and oleic acid, but there is no evidence that the vagus nerve releases PYY. Postprandial PYY release is prolonged and lasts 5 to 6 h.

Receptors and Postreceptor Processes

At least three receptors have been cloned for PP, PYY, and NPY. They are typical G-protein-coupled, 7-transmembrane receptors.

Biological Actions of the PP Family

The major biologic actions of the PP family include:

1. Gastric acid secretion. PP is a weak stimulant of acid, but PYY is a potent inhibitor of acid and pepsin.
2. Pancreatic secretion. Both PP and PYY are potent inhibitors of pancreatic protein and bicarbonate secretion.
3. Biliary motility. PP relaxes the gallbladder and stimulates choledochal sphincter tone.
4. Gastrointestinal motility. PP increases motility in the stomach and intestine and accelerates gastric emptying and intestinal transit. PYY inhibits gastric emptying and the propagation of the interdigestive MMC; it also delays intestinal transit of food.
5. Vascular effects. Both PYY and NPY are intestinal and cerebral vasoconstrictors and raise systemic arterial pressure.

NEUROTENSIN

Neurotensin is a tridecapeptide that was isolated from a side fraction of the purification of SP from bovine hypothalamus.

Distribution

Neurotensin is found in N cells, endocrine cells in the ileal mucosa. N cells are of the open type and have microvilli. Small quantities of neurotensin are found in jejunum, stomach, duodenum, and colon. Neurotensin is also found in the nerves of the ENS and in the brain.

Structure and Synthesis

Neurotensin is released by oleic acid, and fats are the potent releasers of the peptide. Neurotensin release in humans is abolished by ileal resection. In monolayer culture, epinephrine and bombesin release neurotensin, and somatostatin inhibits its release.

Biological Actions of Neurotensin

The major biological actions of neurotensin include:

1. Vasodilation, cyanosis, increased capillary permeability, and systemic hypertension.
2. Hypoinsulinemia, hypoglycemia, hyperglucagonemia, and release of histamine.
3. Inhibition of pentagastrin-stimulated gastric acid and pepsin (i.e., a strong enterogastrone).
4. Stimulation of pancreatic bicarbonate and protein secretion.
5. Inhibition of gastric emptying.
6. Increased esophageal, intestinal, and colonic motility.

CLINICAL SIGNIFICANCE OF GASTROINTESTINAL PEPTIDES

Gastrointestinal peptides have clinical significance in three areas, including: (1) peptide-secreting tumors (apudomas), (2) use in diagnosis and imaging, and (3) use in therapy.

APUD CONCEPT AND THE DIFFUSE NEUROENDOCRINE SYSTEM

Before describing the clinical significance of peptides and peptide-secreting tumors, this section briefly discusses the

inception of the seminal concepts of APUD and the diffuse neuroendocrine system (DNES).

In 1968, Anthony Pearse (Hammersmith Hospital, London, England, UK) described the endocrine cells in the pancreas and the gastrointestinal tract as deriving from the embryonic neural crest and sharing certain histochemical characteristics.[14] The shared characteristics included amine precursor uptake and presence of the enzyme decarboxylase, which can act on the amine precursors to convert them into amines and peptides, which endocrine cells can secrete. Based on these shared features, Pearse

TABLE 5.4. Diffuse Neuroendocrine System
Central division
Pineal gland
Pituitary gland
Hypothalamus
Peripheral division
Gastroenteropancreatic (GEP)
Ultimobranchial body
Parathyroid
Carotid body
Adrenal medulla
Sympathetics

TABLE 5.6. Tumors of the MEN-1 Syndrome
Parathyroid adenoma (90%)
Islet cell tumor (80%)
Pituitary adenoma (65%)
Carcinoid tumors

coined the acronym APUD and put forth the hypothesis that all cells with APUD characteristics are derived from the neural crest of the embryo.[14]

Subsequently, it was shown that the endocrine cells of the pancreas and the GI tract derive not from the neural crest but from the foregut endoderm of the embryo. Nevertheless, the work of Pearse and others after him did identify a diffuse neuroendocrine system of cells, widely distributed within and outside the central nervous system. The gastroenteropancreatic (GEP) family of endocrine cells forms part of this diffuse neuroendocrine system (DNES). A list of the component parts of the DNES is given in Table 5.4.

PEPTIDE-SECRETING TUMORS (APUDOMAS) OF THE GEP SYSTEM

Tumors arising from cells with APUD characteristics have come to be known as apudomas. A list of the apudomas of the pancreas and GI tract is given in Table 5.5.

Histologically, all these tumors are carcinoid and, as such, it is difficult to distinguish benign from malignant tumors. Most tumors, perhaps more than 66% according to some studies, are malignant and capable of local invasion and metastasis. They are given a particular name (e.g., gastrinoma, insulinoma) because of the predominant immunohistochemically stainable cell and/or peptide secreted. However, any given apudoma may contain more than one endocrine cell and may secrete more than one peptide.

TABLE 5.5. Apudomas of the GEP System
Gastrinoma (Zollinger–Ellison syndrome)
Insulinoma
Glucagonoma
VIPoma
Somatostatinoma
Others

Metastasis is usually to regional lymph nodes and the liver. These tumors can metastasize more diffusely but rarely do so. Even when malignant, apudomas are compatible with long survival. Hence, palliative and symptomatic care is important in the treatment.

Apudomas may occur in the sporadic form or as part of the familial condition known as multiple endocrine neoplasia type 1 (MEN-1). When apudomas occur as part of the MEN-1 syndrome, they tend to be multicentric, contain more than one endocrine cell, and secrete more than one peptide. A secondary peptide often secreted in the MEN-1 syndrome is pancreatic polypeptide (PP).

Tumors frequently seen in the MEN-1 syndrome are given in Table 5.6. Those most frequently associated with islet cell tumors include parathyroid adenoma and pituitary adenoma. The most common pituitary adenoma in MEN-1 syndrome is prolactinoma.

Gastrinoma or Zollinger-Ellison Syndrome

In 1955, Drs. Zollinger and Ellison reported on two patients with severe, intractable and complicated peptic ulcer disease (PUD) in association with a tumor in the pancreas.[15] Astutely, they suggested that the pancreatic tumor was responsible for the peptic ulcer, and the syndrome now bears their names. The terms Zollinger–Ellison syndrome (ZES) and gastrinoma syndrome are used synonymously. The essentials of ZES are summarized in Table 5.7.

Incidence

ZES is rare, occurring in about 1 in 1,000,000 of the population. Its incidence in individuals with PUD has been estimated at 1 in 1000 and, in those with ulcer recurrence following an ulcer-reducing surgical procedure, 1 in 50.[16] ZES occurs in two forms, sporadic and familial. The sporadic form accounts for 70% to 80% of all cases. The familial form occurs as part of the MEN-1 syndrome, is transmitted as an autosomal dominant trait, and is due to LOA on chromosome 11.

Secretory Products

ZES is caused by hypersecretion of gastrin from the tumor. Gastrin is secreted in several molecular forms, including G-34, G-17, and G-13. Indeed, these molecular forms of gastrin were first purified from metastatic gastrinoma in the liver. In addition to gastrin, the tumor may elaborate

TABLE 5.7. Essentials: Gastrinoma or Zollinger-Ellison Syndrome

Incidence
Rare: 1:1,000,000 in U.S. population
Estimated 1:1000 in PUD; 1:50 in recurrent ulcer following ulcer surgery
Two forms:
- Sporadic form accounts for 70%–80% of cases
- Familial form (autosomal dominant) associated with MEN-1 syndrome due to LOA on chromosome 11

Clinical picture (see Table 5.8)
PUD sometimes severe and intractable
Diarrhea and increased intestinal motility due to acid in small intestine
Associated tumor in duodenum or pancreas

Etiology
Hypersecretion of gastrin from tumor causes acid hypersecretion
Other effects include:
- Oxyntic mucosa thickening
- ECL-cell hyperplasia
- Infiltrating carcinoid tumors of the stomach
- Thickening of duodenal mucosa

Diagnosis
History
- Recurrent ulcer despite surgery
- PUD associated with diarrhea
- Multiple ulcers in unusual locations
- Family history of gastrinoma or other neuroendocrine tumors
Elevated plasma gastrin levels
Positive secretin test
Ratio of basal to maximal acid secretion >0.6
Radiologic findings
- Giant gastric folds
- Marked gastric hypersecretion causing barium flocculation
- Dilated and edematous duodenum
- Ulcers in the jejunum
- Evidence of intestinal hypermotility
MEN-1 syndrome must be ruled out

Tumor localization
Preoperative
- Abdominal ultrasound
- Endoscopic ultrasound
- CT scan
- Secretin or calcium angiography
- ^{125}I-octreotide
- Transhepatic venous sampling
Intraoperative
- Complete exploration
- Intraoperative ultrasound
- Duodenotomy and eversion

Treatment
In the absence of hepatic metastases: Surgical exploration and resection
In the presence of hepatic metastases: Long-term PPI therapy
Advanced disease: Chemotherapy, debulking procedures

Abbreviations: CT, computerized tomography; ECL, enterochromaffin-like; MEN-1, multiple endocrine neoplasia type 1 syndrome; PPI, proton pump inhibitor; PUD, peptic ulcer disease.

other peptides, the most common being pancreatic polypeptide (PP). The secretion of PP occurs most commonly when the tumor is part of the MEN-1 syndrome.

The primary effect of hypergastrinemia is acid hypersecretion. In addition, however, long-term hypergastrinemia has important trophic actions, including:

1. Increased thickening of oxyntic mucosa can occur, due to parietal cell and mucous neck cell hyperplasia.

2. ECL cell hyperplasia may occur. It is often simple but can occasionally become micronodular, even adenomatous or dysplastic. Dysplastic hyperplasia is precarcinoid and may progress to the development of infiltrating carcinoid tumors of the stomach. The incidence of small gastric carcinoids in ZES is 3% but increases to 13% when associated with MEN-1 syndrome.

3. Increased thickening of duodenal mucosa may occur due to crypt cell hyperplasia.

Gastrin is also trophic to colonic mucosa. A potential but unproven consequence of long-term hypergastrinemia may be growth and/or development of colonic polyps and carcinoma. Epidemiologic studies of long-term hypergastrinemia, however, do not support association with colonic neoplasia in humans.

Site of Tumor

Prior to the mid-1980s, it was believed that most gastrinomas arose in the pancreas. With the advent of better imaging techniques and more careful exploration for duodenal gastrinoma, it is now known that 40% to 50% of all gastrinomas arise in the duodenum. Most of the remainder develop in the pancreas, but 1% to 5% of tumors are found only in lymph nodes. The latter observation has provoked a debate as to whether these lymph node gastrinomas are primary or secondary arising from a small primary in the pancreas or duodenum that cannot be identified. Similarly, a few gastrinomas have been found in the liver without any evidence of a primary tumor anywhere. Again, are these hepatic primary tumors? The answer is unknown.

Clinical Features

ZES is characterized by a pentad of clinical features (Table 5.8).

TABLE 5.8. ZES Pentad of Clinical Features

Peptic ulcer disease
Diarrhea
Acid hypersecretion (BAO/MAO ≥0.6)
Basal hypergastrinemia (>2 times normal)
Positive secretin test (rise in plasma gastrin to twice basal level)

PEPTIC ULCER DISEASE   Only rarely has ZES been diagnosed in the absence of PUD. Prior to the advent of radioimmunoassay for gastrin, improved imaging techniques, and greater general awareness—all of which have allowed earlier diagnosis—ZES ulcers tended to be in unusual locations (e.g., jejunum, esophagus), multiple, associated with florid x-ray evidence of gastric and duodenal mucosal growth, and associated with clinical complications of ulcer. In recent years, however, PUD seen in ZES has become increasingly indistinguishable from that seen with ordinary duodenal ulcer.

DIARRHEA   Diarrhea, a common feature, is caused by high acid load into the small intestine, causing mucosal irritation and inactivation of pancreatic lipase and brush-border enzymes. Gastrin in high doses also causes increased motility and leads to more rapid intestinal transit time. When diarrhea is due to ZES, the stools have an acid pH, as opposed to the alkaline pH associated with VIPoma. In about 5% to 10% of cases, diarrhea has been the presenting symptom of ZES.

ACID HYPERSECRETION   A most significant finding in ZES is the presence of basal acid hypersecretion. Not only is there an absolute increase in basal acid output (BAO)—sometimes as high as 20 to 40 mEq/h—but the proportion of basal acid secretion to maximal acid output (MAO) in response to histamine or pentagastrin is also increased. The BAO-to-MAO ratio is frequently greater than 0.6. The absolute MAO is also increased as a result of parietal cell hyperplasia and may occasionally reach 60 mEq/h or more.

BASAL HYPERGASTRINEMIA   Often basal plasma gastrin levels are elevated several times above normal. The absolute level of basal gastrin, although it varies from laboratory to laboratory, is normally about 100 pg/ml. In ZES, one may encounter fasting plasma gastrin levels of 500 to 1000 pg/ml or even considerably higher. Basal hypergastrinemia may be due to other causes, particularly achlorhydria or long-term therapy with proton pump inhibitors (PPIs). Achlorhydria as a cause can be easily eliminated by measuring gastric acid secretion. When patients have been on long-term PPI therapy, it is necessary to discontinue the drug for at least 2 weeks before repeating measurements of plasma levels.

POSITIVE SECRETIN TEST   The secretin test has emerged as one of the best tests to establish the diagnosis of ZES. Secretin is administered as a bolus intravenous injection (2 U/kg), and plasma gastrin levels are typically measured at 1, 2, 5, 15, and 30 minutes. In normal subjects, patients with ordinary PUD, and those with hypergastrinemia due to causes other than gastrinoma, intravenous secretin administration either decreases or does not change basal plasma gastrin levels. In ZES, however, a paradoxical rise in plasma gastrin occurs. A secretin test is considered positive if the basal (presecretin) plasma gastrin level doubles, usually an elevation of about 200 pg/ml.

Diagnosis

Diagnosis is established with the patient's medical history, plasma gastrin measurement, a positive secretin test, and presence of typical radiological findings.

ZES should be suspected clinically in high-risk patients. These include patients with ulcer recurrence despite seemingly adequate surgical operation; PUD associated with diarrhea; multiple ulcers or ulcers in abnormal locations; and those associated with a family history of gastrinoma, other neuroendocrine tumors or, in particular, MEN-1 syndrome. In this group of patients, the plasma gastrin level should be determined in the fasting state. Fasting plasma gastrin levels may need to be repeated on three separate days. In patients suspected of having achlorhydria, gastric acid secretory studies (BAO and MAO) may be needed. Otherwise, a secretin test may be sufficient.

A positive secretin test establishes the diagnosis. False positive results are few. The best description of the radiological manifestations of ZES remains that provided by Zollinger and his colleagues.[17] These include giant gastric folds, marked gastric hypersecretion causing the barium to flocculate, dilated and edematous duodenum, the presence of multiple ulcers or an ulcer in the jejunum, and evidence of intestinal hypermotility (Figure 5.13). The best test to establish a positive diagnosis, however, is the secretin test. Once the diagnosis is established and acid hypersecretion has been controlled by PPI therapy, tumor localization studies are begun.

TUMOR LOCALIZATION   The various techniques available for preoperative localization of the tumor have been discussed and are summarized in Table 5.9. In gastrinoma, CT scan and MRI are useful only when the tumor is 2 cm or larger in diameter. A duodenal gastrinoma may occasionally be seen on endoscopy, but this is rare. Endoscopic ultrasound is proving to be an excellent method to demonstrate a tumor in the pancreas. Paradoxically, it does not seem to be as sensitive in detecting duodenal gastrinoma. Selective abdominal angiogram is useful in only 25% of patients. Secretin angiography, however, has identified 80% to 90% of tumors in the experience of National Institutes of Health (NIH) investigators.[18] Radionucleotide scan with ^{125}I-octreotide may be positive in 40%–50% of patients. Portal venous sampling is rarely used because it is a highly interventional study with a yield of 40% or less.

When the diagnosis is established and preoperative tumor localization studies have been negative, a final technique for localizing tumor is surgical abdominal exploration. Operative localization encompasses three procedures.

Surgical Exploration   Thorough surgical exploration of the abdomen is performed following complete mobilization of the duodenum and pancreas. The liver, pancreas,

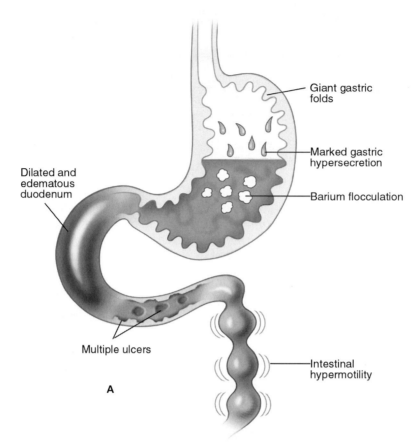

FIGURE 5.13. (A) Radiological manifestations of ZES in barium swallow studies may include giant gastric folds, marked gastric hypersecretion causing the barium to flocculate, dilated and edematous duodenum, presence of ulcer(s) in the jejunum, and evidence of intestinal hypermotility. (B) The upper GI series and small bowel examination in a patient with ZES demonstrate typical findings, including large gastric folds, an edematous and narrowed duodenum (large arrowhead), and thickened jejunal folds (small arrows). (Courtesy of Henry I. Goldberg, MD.) (C) The contrast-enhanced CT scan in a patient with ZES shows multiple metastatic nodules in both lobes of the liver, as well as a fluid-filled stomach with a markedly thickened gastric wall and the hypertrophic rugae typical of gastrinoma. Abbreviations: CT, computerized tomography; ZES, Zollinger-Ellison syndrome. (Reprinted from Orloff SL, Debas HT. Advances in the management of patients with Zollinger-Ellison syndrome. Surg Clin North Am 1995;75:514, with permission from Elsevier.)

and duodenum should be carefully palpated. The lesser sac, the suprahepatic and subhepatic spaces, the roots of the small and large intestine, and the paraaortic region should be carefully examined.

Ultrasound Examination Intraoperative ultrasound examination of the liver, the entire pancreas, duodenum, and lesser sac is performed.

Duodenal Exploration If no tumor is localized using the preceding techniques, attention is focused on the duodenum. Endoscopic transillumination of the duodenum can be helpful, especially if performed early, before the duodenum is traumatized by palpation. The most important technique, however, is longitudinal duodenotomy, including eversion and inspection of the duodenal mucosa and palpation of the opened duodenal walls between fingers. The success of these maneuvers to localize a duodenal gas-

trinoma can be summarized as follows: closed exploration and palpation, 50%; intraoperative ultrasound, 40%; endoscopic transillumination, 80%; and duodenotomy and eversion, 90% to 100%. The success of duodenal exploration has not only increased the incidence with which duodenal gastrinomas are localized, but it has also significantly decreased the incidence of nonlocalizable tumors.

RULING OUT MEN-1 SYNDROME MEN-1 syndrome is seen in 25% to 30% of patients with ZES. As mentioned earlier, when gastrinomas occur in association with MEN-1 syndrome, they tend to be multiple and may be associated with other neuroendocrine tumors of the pancreas and carcinoid tumors in the stomach. Parathyroid and pituitary adenomas, if present, require treatment. Once the diagnosis of gastrinoma is established, MEN-1 syndrome should be excluded. Insulinomas may be ruled out by performing fasting plasma glucose levels; determination of the

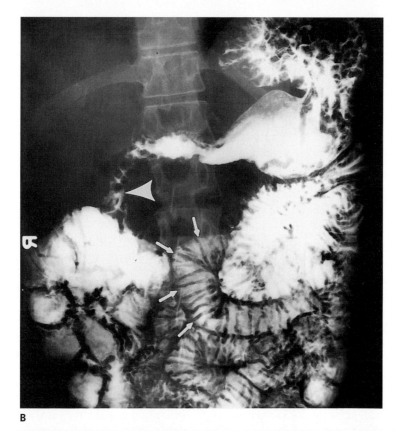

B

C

FIGURE 5.13. *Continued*

TABLE 5.9. Success Rate of Tumor Localization Studies

Study	Gastrinoma	Insulinoma
Abdominal ultrasound	30%	20%
CT scan	40%	24%
Angiography	25%	60%–80%
Secretin angiography	80%	—
Endoscopic ultrasound	high[1]	high
[125]I-octreotide	40%	60%
Transhepatic venous sampling	45%	60%

[1]More successful in localizing pancreatic gastrinoma than duodenal gastrinoma.
Abbreviation: CT, computerized tomography.

plasma insulin level is rarely required. Parathyroid adenomas are ruled out by showing normal levels of ionized calcium in the blood and/or by measuring plasma PTH by radioimmunoassay. The most common pituitary adenoma seen in the MEN-1 syndrome is prolactinoma. Plasma levels of prolactin should be determined. CT of the skull or plain x-rays of the sella turcica are alternative methods for identifying pituitary tumor.

Indications for Surgery

An algorithm for the management of ZES is given in Figure 5.14. Surgical exploration with intent to resect the tumor is indicated in two clinical situations. First, when the tumor is localized preoperatively, and liver metastasis has been ruled out by CT or MRI, surgical removal of the tumor is indicated. Second, when all preoperative attempts at tumor localization fail, abdominal exploration is indicated because a significant number of resectable tumors, particularly in the wall of the duodenum, will be found. When hepatic secondary tumors are seen on CT/MRI, whether or not the primary tumor is localized, nonsurgical treatment with long-term PPI therapy is indicated.

Operative Procedure

Abdominal exploration can be done through either a vertical midline or bisubcostal incision. The thorough exploration technique required has been described above. Even when the primary tumor is identified, full exploration including intraoperative ultrasonography should be undertaken. Clearly, if a tumor is identified in the pancreas or elsewhere outside the duodenum, duodenotomy is unnecessary.

The goal of surgery is curative excision of the tumor. When the tumor is in the distal body or tail of the pancreas, distal pancreatectomy is indicated. If possible, an attempt should be made to preserve the spleen. Tumors in the head of the pancreas are often treated with local excision, which usually means shelling out the lesion. An alternative approach is pancreaticoduodenectomy. Although the latter is a better operation for cancer, the associated

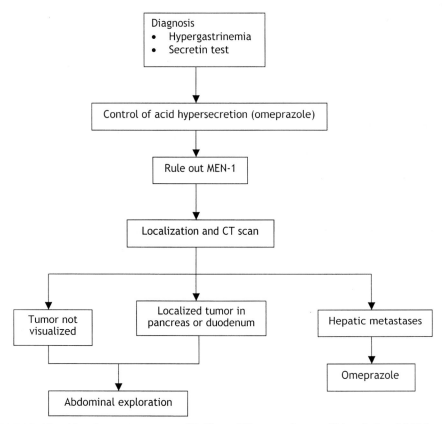

FIGURE 5.14. Algorithm for management of Zollinger-Ellison syndrome. *Abbreviation*: MEN-1, multiple endocrine neoplasia type 1.

mortality and morbidity rates and the relatively benign course of malignant gastrinoma usually make local excision preferable. Large tumors or those deep within the head of the pancreas, however, require pancreaticoduodenectomy.

Duodenal gastrinomas are excised with a margin of normal duodenum around them. Because most recurrences following this procedure occur locally either in the lymph nodes or in the duodenum itself, some surgeons have suggested that duodenal gastrinomas should be treated with pancreaticoduodenectomy. This approach has not been widely accepted. A tumor found in a lymph node, without any apparent primary site in the pancreas or duodenum, is locally resected. Paradoxically, this type of tumor has the best prognosis after resection. A solitary hepatic tumor should also be excised if this can be readily accomplished with wedge resection.

If previously undetected hepatic secondary tumors are found during the operation, palliative resection of the primary tumor is useful, provided this can be performed simply and expeditiously.

Palliative Therapy

Palliative therapy is indicated when acid hypersecretion becomes difficult to control with PPI therapy or when rapid tumor growth occurs. Available methods include octreotide treatment, systemic chemotherapy with 5-fluorouracil and streptozotocin, hepatic artery chemoembolization, and surgical debulking procedures.

Insulinoma

Insulinomas occur almost exclusively within the pancreas. They are small tumors, 95% of which are less than 2 cm in diameter. Ninety percent of insulinomas are benign. They are associated with the MEN-1 syndrome in 5% of patients. Insulinoma is well described in most textbooks of surgery and endocrinology; only the salient points of the disease are covered here. The essentials of insulinoma are summarized in Table 5.10.

Incidence

Insulinomas are rare, although they occur with slightly higher frequency than gastrinoma.

Secretory Product

Proinsulin, insulin, and C peptide are the secretory products of this tumor. C peptide is cleaved from proinsulin to liberated insulin. The presence of elevated levels of C peptide in patients with hyperinsulinism excludes factitious hyperinsulinism as the diagnosis.

Site of Tumor

Insulinomas occur almost exclusively within the pancreas and are distributed equally between the head, body, and tail of the organ. Occasionally, more than one insulinoma is found, most frequently in association with MEN-1 syndrome.

Clinical Features

Symptoms of hypoglycemia develop insidiously, and patients often harbor these tumors for several years before seeking medical attention. The symptoms are both central (neuropsychiatric) and peripheral. Central symptoms include mental obtundation, dizziness, weakness, seizures, and even loss of consciousness. Neuropsychiatric symptoms occur in 30% to 40% of patients. Peripheral symptoms are caused by catecholamine response to hypoglycemia and include anxiety attacks, sweating,

TABLE 5.10. Essentials: Insulinoma

Incidence
  Rare, occur almost exclusively in pancreas
  Small, with 95% <2 cm
  Benign in 90% of cases
  Associated with MEN-1 syndrome in 5% of cases
  Tumor secretes proinsulin, insulin, and C peptide

Clinical picture
  Symptoms of hypoglycemia develop insidiously over time
  Central (neuropsychiatric) symptoms in 30%–40% of cases
  ■ Mental obtundation
  ■ Dizziness
  ■ Weakness
  ■ Seizures or loss of consciousness
  Peripheral symptoms caused by catecholamine response
  ■ Anxiety attacks
  ■ Sweating
  ■ Tremors
  ■ Palpitation
  ■ Hunger

Diagnosis
  Whipple's triad
  ■ Hypoglycemic symptoms on fasting
  ■ Blood glucose levels below 50 mg/dL during symptoms
  ■ Rapid relief of symptoms with glucose intake
  Factitious hyperinsulinism ruled out by measuring proinsulin and C peptide

Tumor localization
  CT and MRI scans may be useful
  Endoscopic ultrasound, octreotide scan, selective angiogram, or transhepatic venous sampling may be helpful
  Exploratory laparotomy and intraoperative ultrasound locate 90% of tumors when other methods fail

Treatment
  Curative excision of the tumor is the goal of surgery
  Distal pancreatectomy if tumor is located in body, tail
  Local excision preferred if tumor is located in head of pancreas
  Pancreaticoduodenectomy required for large or deep tumors in the head
  Palliative therapy indicated when tumor is malignant and extensive hepatic or lymph node metastases exist (octreotide, chemotherapy)

Abbreviations: CT, computerized tomography; MEN-1 syndrome, multiple endocrine neoplasia type 1 syndrome; MRI, magnetic resonance imaging.

tremors, palpitation, and hunger. These patients not infrequently gain weight and become obese because they learn that they can abort hypoglycemic symptoms by eating.

Diagnosis

The cornerstone of diagnosis is the Whipple's triad, which includes: (1) hypoglycemic symptoms on fasting, (2) blood glucose levels below 50 mg/dl during the symptomatic period, and (3) rapid relief of symptoms with oral or intravenous intake of glucose. Plasma levels of both insulin and glucose should be concurrently determined at several different times, preferably during a period of 24-h fasting. Plasma insulin levels are elevated to above 5 µU/ml and, more importantly, the insulin-to-glucose ratio is abnormal (>0.4). The single most important condition that must be differentiated is factitious or self-administered hyperinsulinism. The latter diagnosis is readily excluded by demonstrating elevation in plasma levels of proinsulin and C peptide, which indicates endogenous hyperinsulinism. Preoperatively, symptoms are best controlled with the use of subcutaneous octreotide.

Tumor Localization

Because insulinomas are small, frequently 1 cm or less in diameter, imaging techniques such as ultrasonography, CT, or MRI were once unlikely to localize the tumor. However, with continued improvements in these techniques, especially MRI and CT scanning (Figure 5.15), it is sometimes possible to visualize insulinomas without having to resort to endoscopic ultrasound, ^{125}I-octreotide

scan, and selective angiogram. In some cases, transhepatic venous sampling for insulin assay helps to indicate the region of pancreas where the tumor is located. Transhepatic venous sampling technique is useful in about 60% of cases.

When preoperative localization studies fail, exploratory laparotomy and intraoperative ultrasonography is necessary. The pancreas is completely mobilized and carefully palpated inch by inch. The combination of palpation and intraoperative ultrasound localize 90% of tumors. What should be done when no tumor can be found on complete preoperative and intraoperative evaluation? Although some surgeons advocate blind distal pancreatectomy, this author does not support this practice. Instead, particularly in patients with severe symptoms, intraoperative blood sampling along the entire length of the splenic vein and in the superior mesenteric vein may help locate the tumor. If rapid intraoperative insulin assay is not available, the abdomen should be closed to await the results of insulin assay.

Operative Procedure

The patient's blood glucose level is maintained at or above 100 mg % by glucose infusion. A separate intravenous line should be inserted in case administration of 50% glucose in water becomes necessary. Some studies have demonstrated that perioperative octreotide treatment reduces the incidence of postoperative pancreatic complications.[19] This practice is probably wise.

The pancreas is explored through a vertical, midline, or bilateral subcostal incision. The duodenum and pancreatic head are completely mobilized. The lesser sac is

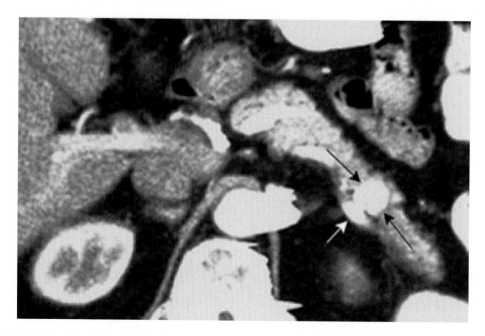

FIGURE 5.15. This contrast-enhanced CT scan of the abdomen shows a normal pancreas containing a small, brightly enhanced insulinoma (black arrows) located adjacent to the splenic vein (white arrow). *Abbreviation*: CT, computerized tomography. (Courtesy of Henry I. Goldberg, MD.)

opened through the gastrocolic omentum and the entire pancreas exposed to the hilum of the spleen. The pancreas is carefully inspected visually and then meticulously palpated. The tumor may be visible on the surface of the pancreas. At other times, it may only be palpable within the substance of the pancreas. Because two or more tumors may be present, the surgeon should not stop evaluation when one tumor is found.

Intraoperative ultrasonography is indispensable and should always be performed. Insulinomas in the body and head are removed by shelling out. Those in the tail can also be locally excised, but if there is any suspicion of multicentricity, distal pancreatectomy is preferred. Following successful excision of the tumor, the blood glucose level rises within 15 to 20 minutes, unless perioperative octreotide has been given. A lesser sac drainage system is established in the event that a pancreatic fistula develops postoperatively. In such cases, octreotide treatment will be needed.

Palliative Therapy

Palliative therapy may become necessary when an insulinoma is malignant and extensive hepatic or lymph node metastases exist. Symptoms can usually be controlled with octreotide therapy. When this is not possible, alternative treatments such as chemotherapy (5-fluoruracil and streptozotocin), hepatic chemoembolization, and even palliative (debulking) resection must be considered.

TABLE 5.11. Essentials: Glucagonoma

Incidence
    Rare tumor, usually located in the pancreas
    Tumors tend to be bulky
    Over 70% incidence of malignancy
    Secretory product: glucagon

Clinical features
    Symptoms due to catabolic effect of glucagon
    ■ Distinctive necrolytic migratory dermatitis, often the first manifestation
    ■ Stomatitis
    ■ Anemia
    ■ Malnutrition
    ■ Diabetes of a characteristically mild form

Diagnosis
    Characteristic subepithelial necrosis on biopsy from affected skin
    Elevated plasma glucagon (>150 pg/mL)
    Bulky tumor frequently localized by ultrasound, CT, MRI

Treatment
    Subcutaneous octreotide injection to control symptoms
    Goal of surgery is complete tumor excision if possible
    Debulking facilitates medical control of symptoms
    Palliative therapy with octreotide, chemotherapy

Abbreviations: CT, computerized tomography; MRI, magnetic resonance imaging.

Glucagonoma

Glucagonoma is a rare glucagon-secreting tumor arising almost exclusively from the pancreas. Tumors tend to be bulky and the incidence of malignancy is probably over 70%. The essentials of glucagonoma are summarized in Table 5.11.

Secretory Product

The secretory product is the hormone glucagon.

Clinical Features

The glucagonoma syndrome is characterized by necrolytic migratory dermatitis, stomatitis, anemia, malnutrition, and diabetes. The dermatitis is so characteristic that the syndrome is often first diagnosed by dermatologists. Most of these clinical features of the disease are due to the catabolic effects of the hormone glucagon. The diabetes is characteristically mild.

Diagnosis

Diagnosis is based on demonstrating characteristic subepithelial necrosis in skin biopsy from affected areas and an elevated plasma glucagon level (>150 pg/ml). Because the tumors tend to be bulky, imaging techniques such as ultrasound, CT, and MRI are frequently successful in localizing the tumor.

Treatment

Preoperatively, symptoms can be controlled well using subcutaneous octreotide injections (50 mg tid). The goal of surgery is complete tumor excision either by local resection or, when appropriate, by pancreatectomy. When curative resection is impossible, as much of the tumor as possible should be removed. Debulking procedures significantly increase the ability to control symptoms with drug therapy.

Palliative Therapy

Palliative therapy is similar to that described for gastrinoma and insulinoma.

VIPoma

In 1958, Verner and Morrison described the association of a pancreatic tumor with severe watery diarrhea.[20] The syndrome then came to be known as the Verner–Morrison syndrome. Much later, it was discovered that the tumor causing the syndrome was a VIP-secreting tumor, hence the term VIPoma. Other names that have been used to describe the VIPoma syndrome are pancreatic cholera, and the WDHA (watery diarrhea, hypokalemia, achlorhydria) syndrome. The tumor is malignant in over two-thirds of cases. The essentials of VIPoma are summarized in Table 5.12.

Incidence

VIPoma is a rare tumor, occurring with about half the frequency of gastrinoma.

Secretory Products

The main secretory product is vasoactive intestinal polypeptide (VIP). Nearly all symptoms of the disease can be attributed to an excess of VIP. PHI, a peptide derived from the same precursor as VIP, may also be found in the tumor. The tumor may also secrete PP, usually when it occurs as part of the MEN-1 syndrome.

Site of Tumor

Nearly 70% of these tumors occur in the pancreas. The remainder are usually located in the retroperitoneum, particularly in children. In children, the VIP-secreting tumor that causes this syndrome is a ganglioneuroblastoma.

Clinical Features

All the clinical features are due to an excess of VIP and include:

WATERY DIARRHEA Diarrhea is a major symptom, often in excess of one liter per day. The stools are isoosmotic, alkaline, and have a high potassium content. The diarrhea persists despite long periods of fasting and leads to contraction of extracellular fluid space and often, as a result, to hypercalcemia.

HYPOKALEMIA Large losses of potassium in the stool result in hypokalemia, which causes fatigue, listlessness, and EKG changes.

ACHLORHYDRIA Achlorhydria, or hypochlorhydria, occurs because VIP inhibits gastric acid secretion. Achlorhydria and alkaline stool distinguish this syndrome from ZES, which is characterized by acid hypersecretion and acid stools.

VASOMOTOR SYMPTOMS Flushing and attacks of hypotension may be present, particularly at times of VIP surge. VIP is a potent vasodilator.

MEN-1 SYNDROME MEN-1 syndrome occurs in about 20% of cases.

Diagnosis

The diagnosis is based on:

1. Demonstrating that the diarrhea is secretory and occurs despite fasting and that the stools are isoosmotic and alkaline.
2. Demonstrating elevated plasma VIP levels greater than 200 pg/mL.
3. Excluding MEN-1 syndrome with measurements of blood glucose levels, PTH levels, prolactin levels, and pituitary x-rays, if necessary.

TUMOR LOCALIZATION These tumors tend to be large and often localizable by ultrasound, CT or MRI. Radionuclide scan with ^{125}I-octreotide may be useful, as is endoscopic ultrasonography. If these tests are negative, selective abdominal angiogram may be required.

MEDICAL TREATMENT Symptomatic control is readily accomplished by subcutaneous octreotide injections

---

TABLE 5.12. Essentials: VIPoma

Incidence
  Rare, about half as frequent as gastrinoma
  Nearly 70% of tumors occur in pancreas
  Malignant in over two-thirds of cases

Clinical picture
  Pancreatic tumor with severe watery diarrhea
  Tumor secretes vasoactive intestinal polypeptide (VIP), causing:
  ■ Watery diarrhea, often leading to hypercalcemia
  ■ Hypokalemia from potassium loss, causing fatigue and EKG changes
  ■ Achlorhydria (hypochlorhydria) due to VIP's inhibition of gastric acid secretion
  ■ Vasomotor symptoms (i.e., flushing, hypotension)
  ■ MEN-1 syndrome in about 20% of cases

Diagnosis
  Diarrhea is secretory, occurs despite fasting
  Stools are isoosmotic and alkaline (vs. the acid stools of ZES)
  Elevated plasma VIP levels (>200 pg/ml)

Tumor localization
  Large tumors often localized by ultrasound, CT or MRI
  Radionuclide scan and endoscopic ultrasound may be useful
  Selective abdominal angiogram may be required

Medical treatment
  Subcutaneous octreotide to control symptoms
  Correction of dehydration and hypokalemia
  Octreotide and/or chemotherapy for multiple liver metastases

Surgical treatment
  Surgical excision is the definitive approach
  Distal pancreatectomy for lesions in body and tail of pancreas
  Enucleation or pancreaticoduodenectomy for lesions in head
  Wedge resection for single liver metastasis

Palliative treatment
  Debulking procedures when curative resection is impossible
  Chemotherapy for rapid tumor growth or retractable symptoms

Abbreviations: CT, computerized tomography; EKG, electrocardiogram; MEN-1 syndrome, multiple endocrine neoplasia type 1 syndrome; MRI, magnetic resonance imaging; ZES, Zollinges–Ellison syndrome.

(50 to 150 mg tid). Dehydration and hypokalemia must be corrected. If the CT scan shows multiple liver metastases, octreotide therapy may need to be continued indefinitely, with the addition of chemotherapy at the appropriate time.

SURGICAL TREATMENT Surgical excision is the definitive form of therapy. Lesions in the body and tail of the pancreas are best resected with distal pancreatectomy. Small lesions in the head may be amenable to enucleation; otherwise, pancreaticoduodenectomy is required. Single liver metastasis should be removed with wedge resection.

PALLIATIVE TREATMENT Debulking procedures are useful when curative resection is impossible. Chemotherapy, either systemic or regional by hepatic chemoembolization, is necessary if rapid tumor growth occurs or symptoms become difficult to control with octreotide. Streptozotocin and 5-fluoruracil are commonly used.

Somatostatinoma

Somatostatin-producing tumors are rare, with fewer than 200 cases reported in the literature. Nearly all reported tumors have been malignant. The essentials are summarized in Table 5.13.

Secretory Product

Tumors may secrete both somatostatin-14 and somatostatin-28; larger forms of somatostatin are frequently extracted from tumor tissue. Other peptides such as adrenocorticotropic hormone (ACTH) may also be produced.

TABLE 5.13. Essentials: Somatostatinoma

Incidence
  Rare, with fewer than 200 cases reported
  Almost always in the pancreas
  Nearly all tumors are malignant
Clinical features
  Somatostatin is the secretory product responsible for the
    triad of symptoms
  ■ Gallstone formation due to inhibition of CCK release
    leading to gallbladder stasis
  ■ Mild diabetes due to inhibition of insulin and glucagon
  ■ Steatorrhea due to inhibition of pancreatic enzyme
    secretion
Other possible features
  Weight loss
  Low acid secretion
  Delayed gastric emptying
Treatment
  Surgical excision preferred
  Cholecystectomy required
  Chemotherapy if the tumor is unresectable

Clinical Features

A triad of symptoms characterizes the syndrome:

1. Mild diabetes. Diabetes arises because somatostatin inhibits both insulin and glucagon release.
2. Steatorrhea. Maldigestion and malabsorption of fat occur because somatostatin is a potent inhibitor of pancreatic enzyme secretion.
3. Gallstones. Gallstones are characteristic because somatostatin inhibits gallbladder contraction, both by direct action and by inhibition of CCK release from the duodenum.
4. Other symptoms. Weight loss can be a prominent symptom. Low acid secretion and delayed gastric emptying may also occur.

Site of Tumor

In nearly all reported cases, the tumor has arisen from the pancreas.

Treatment

Surgical excision is the treatment of choice. Cholecystectomy is required. If the tumor is unresectable, chemotherapy is needed.

Carcinoid Tumors

Carcinoid tumors are the most common of the GEP tumors. The essential features and treatment are summarized in Table 5.14.

Secretory Product

Carcinoid tumors may secrete a variety of products. The most common secretory product is 5-hydroxtryptamine (serotonin), which is thought to mediate the diarrhea. Other secretory products include vasoactive amines (e.g., bradykinin), substance P, and neurotensin. All are vasoactive and probably contribute to the nongastrointestinal symptoms.

Sites of Tumor

The most common sites are the appendix and distal ileum. They also occur in the stomach (see Chapter 2), the jejunum, pancreas, and rectum.

Clinical Features

Symptoms are both gastrointestinal and nongastrointestinal. Carcinoid tumors have a well-known association with fibrosis, which is responsible for tricuspid valve insufficiency, shortening of the mesentery of the small intestine, and acute kinking of the bowel and consequent bowel obstruction.

TABLE 5.14. Essentials: Carcinoid Syndrome

Incidence
Most common GEP tumor, often nonfunctioning
Secretes a variety of products (i.e., 5-hydroxtryptamine, vasoactive amines, substance P, neurotensin)
Full-blown carcinoid syndrome in only 5%
Tumors most common in appendix and distal ileum, but also in stomach, jejunum, pancreas and rectum

Clinical features
Gastrointestinal symptoms
- Diarrhea
- Colicky abdominal pain
- Loud borborygmi
- Bowel obstruction that may present as acute appendicitis
- Bleeding in rare cases
Extragastrointestinal symptoms due to hepatic metastases or tumor drainage directly into lumbar veins
- Flushing and wheezing
- Right-sided congestive heart failure due to tricuspid valve insufficiency

Diagnosis
Readily made in full-blown carcinoid syndrome
Requires measurement of serotonin and urinary 5-HIAA
Radioimmunoassay measurement of neurotensin and SP helpful
Incidental discovery of carcinoid tumor during other surgery (e.g., appendicitis)

Tumor localization
Difficult
Barium swallow and follow-through examination of intestine
Fluoroscopy of small intestine with barium
CT for hepatic metastases
Laparotomy definitive when tumor is not otherwise localized

Symptom control
Diarrhea and other symptoms controlled by octreotide
Steroid therapy less effective

Operative treatment
Small intestine tumors require resection to prevent bowel obstruction, metastasis
Careful not to over-resect mesentery foreshortened by scarring
Appendiceal carcinoids require appendectomy or right hemicolectomy
Palliative hepatic resection useful if major lobectomy can be avoided
Regional or systemic chemotherapy
Long-term octreotide therapy for effective relief of symptoms
No evidence that somatostatin therapy shrinks tumor

Abbreviations: CT, computerized tomography; GEP, gastroenteropancreatic; 5-HIAA, 5-hydroxy-indol acetic acid; SP, substance P.

GASTROINTESTINAL SYMPTOMS Diarrhea, colicky abdominal pain, and loud borborygmus are features of the carcinoid syndrome. At times, the tumor may cause obstruction and present as acute appendicitis or small bowel obstruction. Bleeding is a rare symptom.

EXTRAGASTROINTESTINAL SYMPTOMS The most common of these are flushing and wheezing due to vasoactive substances released by the tumor. Right-sided congestive heart failure may also be seen as a consequence of tricuspid valve insufficiency. These complications arise when the products of tumor secretion escape hepatic degradation and reach the systemic circulation. This occurs when there are hepatic metastases or when retroperitoneal tumors drain directly into lumbar veins.

Diagnosis

The diagnosis is readily made when a full-blown picture of the carcinoid syndrome is present. Often, however, the picture is only partial, with diarrhea as the presenting symptom. In these cases, serum levels of serotonin, and urinary 5-hydroxy-indol acetic acid (5-HIAA)—the metabolic product of serotonin—should be measured, preferably during an attack. These substances can also be measured after provocation with pentagastrin, which stimulates the release of serotonin and other secretory products from the tumor. In some instances, it is useful to measure plasma levels of neurotensin and SP by radioimmunoassay. Most commonly, the diagnosis of carcinoid tumor is made during surgery for appendicitis, small bowel obstruction, or for some unrelated condition.

Tumor Localization

Tumor localization may be extremely difficult. Barium swallow and follow-up examination of the intestine or fluoroscopy of the small intestine with introduction of barium through a nasojejunal tube may occasionally show the tumor. Capsule video endoscopy has recently been used successfully in localizing tumors in the small intestine. CT helps determine whether hepatic metastases are present. Often laparotomy is the definitive way to localize the tumor.

Symptom Control

Diarrhea and the other symptoms of the carcinoid syndrome are effectively controlled by subcutaneous administration of octreotide (50–150 mg tid), which is much more effective than steroid therapy in controlling symptoms.

Operative Treatment

All carcinoid tumors in the small intestine should be resected because they might eventually obstruct the bowel or metastasize. Care must be taken in bowel resection, especially when mesenteric lymph nodes are involved. The mesentery may be foreshortened due to scarring, and care must be taken not to resect it too extensively because of the danger of inadvertently causing short bowel syndrome.

Appendiceal carcinoids present special management challenges. Most are adequately treated with appendectomy. A right hemicolectomy may be required under three circumstances:

1. When the appendiceal carcinoid is 2 cm or larger.
2. When it is located at the base of the appendix.
3. When mesenteric lymph node spread is present.

Palliative Treatment

Palliative resection of large metastases in the liver is useful if this can be accomplished without major lobectomy. Otherwise, regional or systemic chemotherapy is used. Long-term octreotide therapy provides effective symptomatic relief. There is no evidence that somatostatin therapy shrinks the tumor.

Other Tumors

Several other rare tumors of the GEP system have been reported, including:

1. PPoma. This tumor of the pancreas secretes PP, which produces no symptoms. Consequently, these tumors may be considered nonfunctional unless PP is measured.
2. GRFoma. This tumor secretes growth hormone-releasing factor and causes acromegaly.
3. ACTHoma. This tumor secretes ACTH and causes Cushing's syndrome.
4. Neurotensinoma. This tumor secretes neurotensin and causes diarrhea, hypotension, flushing, cyanosis, and hypokalemia.

DIAGNOSTIC USES OF GI PEPTIDES

Several GI peptides are useful in the diagnosis of disease, as adjuncts in radiology and endoscopy and in radionuclide imaging including in vivo receptor imaging.

Provocative Testing

Radioimmunoassay techniques have allowed for easier diagnosis of peptide-secreting tumors, which often demonstrate elevated levels of the peptide or peptides secreted. When the diagnosis is equivocal, some GI peptides are effectively used in provocative tests:

Secretin Test

The secretin test was described earlier as the most specific test for ZES. A bolus intravenous administration of secretin (2 U/kg) causes paradoxical elevation in plasma gastrin levels only when a gastrinoma is the cause of hypergastrinemia. An elevation of 100 pg/mL over the basal level is considered positive.

Pentagastrin Provocative Test

Pentagastrin, a synthetic analogue of gastrin, when given by intramuscular injection (2 μg/kg), causes discharge of secretory products from carcinoid tumors. Following pentagastrin administration, diagnostic elevation in circulating serotonin or urinary 5-HIAA may occur. The pentagastrin provocative test is an important diagnostic

maneuver in patients with MEN-2 syndrome, where release of calcitonin is stimulated.

Uses in Radiology and Endoscopy

Glucagon is used to relax the duodenum for detailed contrast studies. Glucagon has replaced the use of local anesthetic to cause duodenal ileus for examination. Glucagon is also useful in intraoperative cholangiography in order to relax the sphincter of Oddi, allowing contrast to enter the duodenum. When dye will not enter the duodenum, this test distinguishes between spasm and a stone at the terminal end of the common bile duct as the cause. The use of glucagon also helps in cannulation of the papilla in performing endoscopic retrograde cholangiopancreatography (ERCP).

Use in Radionuclide Imaging and Radioreceptor Studies

^{125}I-octreotide, the labeled long-acting analogue of somatostatin, helps to localize peptide-secreting tumors. Some 50% to 60% of gastrinomas, insulinomas, VIPomas, and carcinoids have a sufficiently high density of somatostatic receptors that they can be visualized with a gamma camera after administration of labeled octreotide. ^{125}I-octreotide could also be given immediately preoperatively, and the pancreas and retroperitoneum can be scanned by a hand-held gamma camera to localize peptide-secreting tumors at operation.

^{125}I-octreotide binding to tissue in biopsy specimens can provide useful information about the responsiveness of the tumor to somatostatin therapy.

THERAPEUTIC USES OF GI PEPTIDES

The best-established peptidomimetic therapy in the GI tract is the use of octreotide in controlling symptoms caused by peptides secreted from apudomas. The beneficial action of octreotide arises from its ability to inhibit both the release of peptides from tumors and their action on target cells. A large body of experience now exists to show that octreotide therapy is effective in controlling diarrhea and flushing in over 80% of patients with VIPomas and carcinoids. Octreotide is also effective in controlling the dermatitis of glucagonoma in most patients. It controls the symptoms of insulinoma in about 60% of patients. In all these cases, while improvement in symptoms is accompanied by a drop in the circulating level of peptide, improvement is greater than can be inferred from the decrease in peptide release. This is, of course, because somatostatin inhibits the action of whatever peptide is released.

Although somatostatin does possess antitrophic action in vitro, its use in vivo has not been associated with decrease in tumor size to any significant degree.

Bombesin (GRP) is a potent growth factor in small cell lung cancer. Monoclonal antibodies to bombesin have been used in treatment of patients with this tumor, and significant tumor regression has been observed. Powerful CCK and gastrin receptor antagonists have been developed. It is likely that these may, in the future, have therapeutic application.

CGRP is important in mediating gastric mucosal cytoprotection and in preventing stress- and NSAID-related ulcers. These actions of CGRP are likely to be applied in therapeutic strategies in the future.

Peptide Growth Factors in the GI Tract

Several peptides play an important role in regulating proliferation in gastrointestinal mucosa (Table 5.15). These peptides are important in the regulation of mucosal cell and mesenchymal cell proliferation, fetal development, regeneration of mucosal defects or organs, and in angiogenesis. Some may also play a role as autocrine growth factor for human colon cancer.

Depending on the proximity of their release to the target cell, they may be autocrine (controlling the cell that

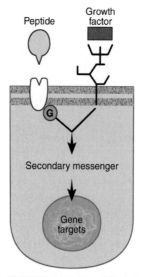

Ligand	EGF, TGFβ IGF, FGF, HGF
Receptors	Transmembrane proteoglycan
Secondary messengers	cAMP, cGMP, IP3, Calcium
Transcription factors	Jun, fos, erg, e-myc NFKβ

FIGURE 5.16. Simplified depiction of the actions of peptide growth factors. Binding of growth factors to specific transmembrane proteoglycan receptors results in the release of second messengers (cAMP, cGMP, IP3, calcium), which activate nuclear transcription factors (jun, fos, erg, e-myc, NFKβ). The nuclear transcription factors then mediate cell growth.

produces them), paracrine (reaching the target cell by diffusing through interstitial tissue), or endocrine (reaching the target cell via the circulation). Key to the mechanism of their action is ligand-receptor binding. Generally, two receptor types mediate their function: transmembrane receptors or extracellular proteoglycan side chains of different receptors. Signaling mechanisms include adenylate cyclase-generated cAMP, the inositol pathway and calcium, and the products of protein kinase C. Ultimately, they must modulate cellular proliferation through the alteration of transcription of various genes. Figure 5.16 provides a highly simplified depiction of these processes.

All these peptides exert growth effects outside the GI tract except the trefoil peptides, which seem to be specific to the GI tract. Trefoil peptides have two functions: In basal circumstances they play a role in mucus stabilization; when an acute injury occurs, they are rapidly upgraded and stimulate the repair process, particularly epithelial restitution. The effects on epithelial cells are closely integrated with effects in extracellular matrix, and each may have a regulating effect on the other.

Recently, a novel gastric hormone, ghrelin, has been shown to be an endogenous ligand for the growth hormone secretagogue receptor (GHSR) that can stimulate growth hormone release. Ghrelin is somatotrophic, orexigenic, and adipogenic and thus plays a role in the regulation of growth and energy balance.

TABLE 5.15. Peptide Growth Factors of the Gastrointestinal Tract

Peptides	Growth Effects

EGF family
  EGF
  TGF-α
  HB-EGF
	Increased cell proliferation
	Increased insulin synthesis
	Increased food intake
	Angiogenesis

TGFβ Family	Inhibition of cell proliferation Production of collagen, fibronectin, laminin Increased insulin synthesis

IGF Family
  IGF-I
  IGF-II
	Stimulation of cell proliferation and mucosal growth
	Autocrine growth of human colon cancer
	Fetal growth of GI tract
	Autocrine growth of human colon cancer

FGF Family
  bFGF
  aFGF
	Neovascularity
	Proliferation of fibroblasts
	Post-mucosal injury repair

Hepatocyte growth factor	Liver regeneration Renal development Epithelial and mesenchymal cell migration
Others Hematopoietic stem cell factors	Integration of leukocyte production
PDGF	Mitogen for fibroblasts and mesenchymal cells
Trefoil peptides	Regulation of mucosal proliferation

Abbreviations: aFGF, acid fibroblast growth factor; bFGF, basic fibroblast growth factor; EGF, epidermal growth factor; HB-EGF, heparin-binding EGF; HGF, hepatocyte growth factor; IGF, insulin growth factor; PDGF, platelet-derived growth factor; TGF, transforming growth factor.

REFERENCES

1. Edkins JS. On the chemical mechanism of gastric secretion. *Proc R Soc Lond B Biol Sci* 1905;76:376.
2. Komorov SA. Gastrin. *Proc Soc Exp Biol Med* 1938;38:514–516.

3. Gregory RA, Tracy HJ. The constitution and properties of two gastrins extracted from hog antral mucosa. *Gut* 1964;5:103–117.

4. Ivy AC, Oldberg E. A hormone mechanism for gallbladder contraction and evacuation. *Am J Physiol* 1928;86:599–613.

5. Harper AA, Raper HS. Pancreazymine, a stimulant of the secretion of pancreatic enzymes in extracts of the small intestine. *J Physiol* 1943;102:115–123.

6. Mutt V, Jorpes JE. Structure of porcine cholecystokinin-pancreozymin. 1. Cleavage with thrombin and with trypsin. *Eur J Biochem* 1968;6:156–162.

7. Bayliss WM, Starling EH. The mechanism of pancreatic secretion. *J Physiol (Lond)* 1902;28:325–353.

8. Bayliss WM, Starling EH. Croonian Lecture. The chemical regulation of the secretory process. *Proc R Soc Lond (Biol)* 1904; 73:310–332.

9. Mutt V, Jorpes JE, Magnusson S. Structure of porcine secretin. The amino acid sequence. *Eur J Biochem* 1970;15:513–519.

10. Erspamer V, Erspamer GF, Inselvini M, et al. Occurrence of bombesin and alytesin in extracts of the skin of three European discoglossid frogs and pharmacological actions of bombesin on extravascular smooth muscle. *Br J Pharmacol* 1972;45:333–348.

11. Brazeau P, Vale W, Burgus R, et al. Hypothalamic polypeptide that inhibits the secretion of immunoreactive pituitary growth hormone. *Science* 1973;179:77–79.

12. Brown JC, Pederson RA, Jorpes E, et al. Preparation of highly active enterogastrone. *Can J Physiol Pharmacol* 1969;47: 113–114.

13. Von Euler US, Gaddum JH. An unidentified depressor substance in certain tissue extracts. *J Physiol (Lond)* 1931;72:74–87.

14. Pearse AG. Common cytochemical and ultrastructural characteristics of cells producing polypeptide hormones (the APUD series) and their relevance to thyroid and ultimobranchial C cells and calcitonin. *Proc R Soc Lond B Biol Sci* 1968;170:71–80.

15. Zollinger RM, Ellison EH. Primary peptic ulceration of the jejunum associated with islet cell tumors of the pancreas. *Ann Surg* 1955;142:709–728.

16. Debas HT. Clinical significance of gastrointestinal hormones. *Adv Surg* 1988;21:157–187.

17. Zollinger RM, Ellison EC, O'Dorisio TM, et al. Thirty years' experience with gastrinoma. *World J Surg* 1984;8:427–435.

18. Doppman JL, Jensen RT. Localization of gastroenteropancreatic tumours by angiography. *Ital J Gastroenterol Hepatol* 1999; 31(Suppl 2):S163–166.

19. Halloran CM, Ghaneh P, Bosonnet L, et al. Complications of pancreatic cancer resection. *Dig Surg* 2002;19:138–146.

20. Verner JV, Morrison AB. Islet cell tumor and a syndrome of refractory watery diarrhea and hypokalemia. *Am J Med* 1958; 29:374–380.

SELECTED READINGS

Ahlman H, Nilsson. The gut as the largest endocrine organ in the body. *Ann Oncol* 2001;12 Suppl 2:S63–S68.

Beinfeld MC. An introduction to neuronal cholecystokinin. *Peptides* 2001;22:1197–1200.

Debas HT. Gastroenteropancreatic endocrine tumors. *The Regulatory Peptide Letter.* Ann Arbor, MI: MedPub Inc.; 1988;1:1–6.

Debas HT. Neuroendocrine tumors of the pancreas: management. *Pract Gastroenterol* 1997;21:38–45.

Degen L, Matzinger D, Drewe J, et al. The effect of cholecystokinin in controlling appetite and food intake in humans. *Peptides* 2001;22:1265–1269.

Dockray GJ. Varro A, Dimaline R, et al. The gastrins: their production and biological activities. *Annu Rev Physiol* 2001;63: 119–139.

Drucker DJ. Gut adaptation and the glucagon-like peptides. *Gut* 2002;50:428–435.

Evangelista S. Involvement of tachykinins in intestinal inflammation. *Curr Pharm Des* 2001;7:19–30.

Hokfelt T, Pernow B, Wahren J. Substance P: a pioneer amongst neuropeptides. *J Intern Med* 2001;249:27–40.

Li ML, Norton JA. Gastrinoma. *Curr Treat Options Oncol* 2001;2: 337–346.

Lindstrom E, Chen D, Norlen P, et al. Control of gastric acid secretion: the gastrin-ECL cell-parietal cell axis. *Comp Biochem Physiol A Mol Integr Physiol* 2001;128:505–514.

Martinez C, Abad C, Delgado M, et al. Anti-inflammatory role in septic shock of pituitary adenylate cyclase-activating polypeptide receptor. *Proc Natl Acad Sci USA* 2002;99:1053–1058.

Rozengurt E, Walsh JH. Gastrin, CCK, signaling, and cancer. *Annu Rev Physiol* 2001;63:49–76.

Sandstrom O, El-Salhy M. Ontogeny and the effect of aging on pancreatic polypeptide and peptide YY. *Peptides* 2002;23:263–267.

Scarpignato C, Pelosini I. Somatostatin analogs for cancer treatment and diagnosis: an overview. *Chemotherapy* 2001;47(Suppl 2): 1–29.

Ukkola O, Poykko S. Ghrelin, growth and obesity. *Ann Med* 2002;34:102–108.

Upp JR Jr, Singh P, Townsend CM Jr, et al. Clinical significance of gastrin receptors in human colon cancers. *Cancer Res* 1989; 49:488–492.

Wick MR, Graeme-Cook FM. Pancreatic neuroendocrine neoplasms: a current summary of diagnostic, prognostic, and differential diagnostic information. *Am J Clin Pathol* 2001;115 Suppl:S28–S45.

6

Liver

The liver is the only organ in the abdomen without which life cannot be sustained. The liver is a master organ for its role in metabolism, excretion, and synthesis. In surgical practice, its importance lies not only in the surgical management of treatable liver disorders such as end-stage liver disease but also in sustaining adequate function to enable the conduct of all anesthesia and all surgical procedures and to maintain blood coagulability and hemostasis.

SURGICAL ANATOMY

EMBRYOLOGY

The liver, the biliary tree, and the pancreas develop from a diverticulum of the foregut of the 3-mm embryo. This diverticulum has three buds. The caudal bud forms the pancreas, the cranial bud gives rise to the liver, and the middle bud forms the gallbladder. The ventral bud begins as a hollow tube but soon becomes a solid mass within which biliary ducts form by a process of canalization. The hepatocytes line small biliary canaliculi, which drain into larger ducts and then into the lobar ducts. The lobar ducts, in turn, drain into the right and left hepatic ducts.

SEGMENTAL ANATOMY

Traditionally, the insertion into the liver of the falciform ligament was thought to divide the liver into a right and a left lobe. In 1981, Couinaud provided a more accurate description of the segmental anatomy of the liver (Figure 6.1).[1] The true division into a right and a left lobe lies in the main lobar fissure, an oblique plane passing from the gallbladder fossa anteriorly to the bed of the inferior vena cava posteriorly (Cantile's line). Thus, the portion of the liver between the main lobar fissure and the falciform ligament represents the medial segment of the left lobe, while the traditional left lobe is the lateral segment of the true (i.e., anatomic) left lobe. A right segmental fissure divides the right lobe into anterior and posterior segments.

BILE DUCT ANATOMY

Each of the nine segments of the liver is drained by a segmental duct. In the right lobe, the ducts of the right anterior and right posterior segments join to form the right hepatic duct. In the left lobe, the segmental ducts of the medial and lateral segments unite to form the left hepatic duct. The right and left hepatic ducts join at the hilum of the liver to form the common hepatic duct.

BLOOD SUPPLY

The vasculature of the liver has three important components, that is, the hepatic artery, the portal vein, and the hepatic venous system.

Hepatic Artery

The common hepatic artery is a branch of the celiac axis. After giving off the right gastric and gastroduodenal arteries, it ascends to the liver in the hepatoduodenal segment, where it usually lies to the left of the common bile duct and anterior to the portal vein. In 17% of individuals, the right hepatic artery originates not from the celiac axis but from the superior mesenteric artery. The hepatic artery branches into the cystic artery and, at the hilum of the liver, divides into a left and a right hepatic artery. The hepatic arteries carry oxygenated blood and provide 25% of the total blood supply to the liver.

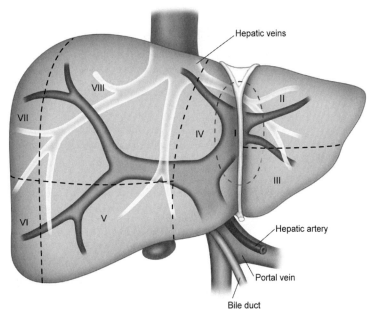

FIGURE 6.1. Segmental anatomy of the liver, based on Couinaud.[1]

Portal Vein

The portal vein accounts for 75% of the blood supply of the liver, but its blood has an oxygen saturation of only 60%. The portal vein originates from the confluence of the superior mesenteric and splenic veins, posterior to the neck of the pancreas. It reaches the liver in the hepatoduodenal ligament, where it lies behind the common bile duct and hepatic artery. In the porta hepatis, the portal vein divides into right and left branches, which continue to their respective hepatic lobes. The portal vein possesses no valves.

Hepatic Venous System

Knowledge of the hepatic venous system anatomy is crucial to the performance of hepatic lobectomy. Venous blood from hepatic lobules drains into the sinusoids and then into the central veins. Central veins join to form sublobular veins and then collecting veins. Collecting veins coalesce to form three major hepatic veins (Figure 6.2):

1. The right hepatic vein, which drains all of the posterior segment and part of the anterior segment of the right lobe.

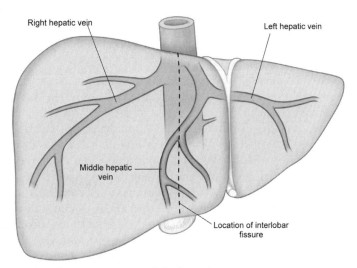

FIGURE 6.2. Anatomy of the hepatic venous system.

2. The middle hepatic vein, which drains the inferior area of the medial and anterior portions of the two lobes.
3. The left hepatic vein, which drains the entire area to the left of the umbilical fissure.

Hepatic venous pressure is approximately 8 mm Hg; total blood flow through the hepatic veins is approximately 1500 mL/min/1.73 m^2 of body surface.

LYMPHATIC DRAINAGE

A significant portion of the lymphatic drainage of the liver collects in the subcapsular area, from which it passes in lymphatic channels through the diaphragm and suspensory ligaments of the liver into the posterior mediastinal nodes. A smaller portion of the lymphatic drainage either accompanies the hepatic veins or drains to the porta hepatis along the portal venous system.

NERVE SUPPLY

The liver has a rich sympathetic nerve supply derived from ganglia T-7 to T-10. The parasympathetic innervation is derived from the hepatic branch of the anterior vagus nerve and from the celiac branch of the posterior vagus nerve. From the celiac ganglia, both sympathetic and parasympathetic fibers travel to the liver in the adventitia of the hepatic arteries.

PHYSIOLOGY OF THE LIVER

The major functions of the liver include metabolism, bile formation, inactivation and excretion, reticuloendothelial system, and liver regeneration.

METABOLISM

The liver plays an important role in the metabolism of carbohydrates, lipids, and proteins.

Carbohydrate Metabolism

A key function of the liver is to maintain normal blood glucose levels. Between meals, it exports 10 g of glucose per hour. Several hepatic processes are important in carbohydrate metabolism:

1. Glycogen storage. All hexose sugars that do not enter the glycolytic pathway are converted into glycogen and stored. Insulin promotes glucose storage as glycogen.
2. Glycogenolysis. In times of hypoglycemia, glycogen is converted into glucose by the action of catecholamines and/or glucagon to rapidly restore blood glucose. This requires the enzyme glucose-6-phosphatase. Absence of the enzyme causes glycogen storage diseases.
3. Glycolysis. This is the process by which glucose is phosphorated to enter Krebs cycle, which generates high-energy phosphates and lactate.
4. Gluconeogenesis. This is the reverse of glycolysis, by which glucose is synthesized from lactate/pyruvate and amino acids.

Lipid Metabolism

Lipoprotein complexes absorbed from the gut are captured by the cathrin-coated pits of hepatocytes and internalized. The lipid thus taken up into the hepatocyte may be used for one of two purposes:

1. Secretion into the space of Disse as very low density lipoprotein (VLDL) or low density lipoprotein (LDL) or
2. Generation of fatty acids and acetyl-coenzyme A (acetyl CoA).

Protein Synthesis

Most plasma proteins except immunoglobulins are synthesized by the hepatocyte. These plasma proteins include albumin, transferrin, and lipoproteins. Also synthesized by the hepatocytes is the group of peptides involved in the coagulation cascade. These include Factors II, VII, IX, and X. Only Factor VIII, the anti-hemophiliac factor, is produced not by hepatocytes but in vascular endothelium. The liver also produces fibrinogen and antiplasmin. Thus, liver failure can lead to hypoprothrombinemia, which, when severe, can lead to fibrinolysis and disseminated intravascular coagulopathy (DIC).

BILE FORMATION

Albumin-bound bilirubin is carried into the hepatocyte, where it is made water soluble by the addition of glucuronide, and catalyzed by uridine diphosphonucleotide glucuronyl transferase (UDPGT). The soluble bilirubin is transported into the bile canaliculus. The hepatocyte also oxidizes cholesterol to form cholic acid and chenodeoxycholic acid, two primary bile acids that are important in micelle formation. The rate of formation of these bile acids is governed by the enterohepatic circulation, with the return of bile salts acutely stimulating the production of bile, that is, bile salt-dependent bile secretion. Cholesterol and lecithin are also secreted in the bile. Bile acids and lecithin form micelles, which carry cholesterol in micellar core, thus solubilizing it and preventing its deposition as stone. An additional substance released into the bile by the hepatocytes is immunoglobulin A. The bile delivered by the hepatocyte into the bile canaliculi is isotonic. The epithelium of the bile ductules adds bicarbonate to the bile under the influence of secretin and VIP.

INACTIVATION AND EXCRETION

The liver is an important organ for inactivating drugs and toxins, which are then excreted into the bile. Because the liver is also important for drug metabolism, dosage of any drug must be adjusted in treating liver disease. In addition, some drugs may inhibit the hepatic enzymes needed to metabolize other drugs, a problem that may cause dangerous drug interactions. An example is the combination of Coumadin® and the H_2-receptor antagonist cimetidine. Cimetidine inhibits P-450 and, in turn, inhibits the degradation of Coumadin®. This can precipitate hemorrhage.

RETICULOENDOTHELIAL SYSTEM FUNCTION

The reticuloendothelial system (RES) of the liver is thought to function as an important filtration system, removing bacteria and endotoxin that may be translocated from the gut. Kupffer cells are thought to remove as much as 99% of bacteria from portal blood. The RES also inactivates small gastrointestinal peptides and amines, thus protecting the systemic circulation. The carcinoid syndrome develops when this hepatic degradation of amines is bypassed, allowing them to enter the systemic circulation.

HEPATIC REGENERATION

The liver has remarkable regenerative capacity, as evidenced after major liver resection or hepatocyte destruction by toxins or viral hepatitis. The capacity of the liver to regenerate permits the use of the right lobe for liver transplantation. The major hepatic growth factors important in regeneration include epidermal growth factor (EGF), transforming growth factor-α (TGF-α) and the hepatocyte growth factor (HGF). For these growth factors to initiate growth, a certain amount of liver must be resected (70% in rats) or a certain number of hepatocytes must be destroyed. Once this condition is present, TGF-α or HGF induce the crucial transcription factors of c-jun and NFK-β.

PATHOPHYSIOLOGY

CIRRHOSIS

Liver injury from several causes may lead to hepatic fibrosis and cirrhosis. The process has been studied best in alcoholic liver disease. Approximately 10% of alcoholic patients will develop cirrhosis. The central mechanism of fibrosis involves stimulation of the perisinusoidal or stellate cells, which reside in the space of Disse. The stellate cell becomes actively proliferative and changes into a myofibroblast-like cell that produces collagen. Collagen deposition causes perisinusoidal fibrosis. The known stimulants for the stellate cell include acetaldehyde, products of lipid peroxidation, and TGF-β. Once stellate cells are activated, they produce TGF-β.

Other types of cirrhosis include: (1) postnecrotic cirrhosis, which may follow liver destruction by viral infection or toxins; (2) biliary cirrhosis, which results from prolonged biliary obstruction; (3) cirrhosis associated with hemochromatosis, due to iron load; and (4) cirrhosis associated with Wilson's disease, due to abnormal copper metabolism.

In all types of cirrhosis, it is necessary to have criteria for assessing hepatic functional reserve, the most common of which are those promulgated by Child (Table 6.1).

FULMINANT LIVER FAILURE

Fulminant liver failure is an emergency characterized by rapid development of severe hepatocellular dysfunction,

TABLE 6.1. Child's Classification of Hepatic Functional Reserve

Level of Function	Class A	Class B	Class C
Serum bilirubin (mg/dL)	<2	2–3	>3
Serum albumin (g/dL)	>3–5	3–3.5	<3
Ascites	None	Medically controlled	Poorly controlled
Neurological signs	None	Minimal	Severe or coma
Nutrition	Excellent	Good	Poor

encephalopathy, cerebral edema, and coma. Jaundice and coagulopathy are important manifestations. The most common causes are drugs and hepatotropic viruses. The drug that most commonly causes liver failure is acetaminophen in doses of 4g or more per day. Other associated drugs include halothane, sulfonamides, phenytoin, isoniazid, and valproic acid. The most important viral causes are hepatitis A and B. Fulminant liver failure can also be caused by acute ischemia and primary graft nonfunction during liver transplantation.

Major complications of fulminant liver failure include hypoglycemia, cerebral edema, sepsis, hemorrhage from coagulopathy or stress ulceration, hypotension, and respiratory and renal failure. Renal failure may occur as a result of hypovolemia, hepatorenal syndrome, or acute tubular necrosis.

Management includes:

1. Blood glucose and intracranial pressure monitoring and treatment.
2. Surveillance for infection and immediate antibiotic therapy when detected.
3. Avoidance of benzodiazepines and sedatives.
4. H_2-receptor antagonist therapy.
5. Monitoring of coagulation and administration of vitamin K, platelets, and fresh frozen plasma; monitoring and normalizing hemodynamic parameters.
6. Mechanical ventilation and hemofiltration or renal dialysis when necessary.

With intensive medical care, the high mortality rate of fulminant liver failure has improved modestly. Only liver transplantation, however, has allowed the salvage of patients with irreversible fulminant hepatic failure. As a bridge to recovery or liver transplantation, other devices have been used, including bioartificial liver devices, nonhuman liver, and hepatocyte transplantation. All of these bridge treatments are now experimental.

HEPATORENAL SYNDROME

Hepatorenal syndrome (HRS), defined as renal failure in the setting of cirrhosis or severe liver disease but in the absence of intrinsic renal disease, is characterized by intense vasoconstriction in the renal cortex. The incidence of HRS in cirrhosis with ascites has been reported to range from 18% to 35%.[2]

The pathogenesis of HRS is believed to be peripheral arterial vasodilatation due to nitric oxide, glucagon, substance P, CGRP, and insulin; it leads to reduction of effective circulating volume. Decreased renal perfusion leads to increased renal vascular resistance as well as sodium and water retention involving the renin-angiotensin-aldosterone mechanism, the sympathetic nervous system, vasopressin, endothelin, and leukotriene E_2.

TABLE 6.2. Essentials: Portal Hypertension

Primary Causes	Location	Disorder
	Prehepatic	Portal vein thrombosis
	Intrahepatic	Cirrhosis
	Posthepatic	Hepatic vein/IVC thrombosis
Primary Complications	Disorder	Treatment Options
	Acute variceal hemorrhage	Endoscopic sclerotherapy or ligation
		Pharmacologic (pitressin, somatostatin)
		Balloon tamponade
		TIPS
		Emergency portocaval shunt
	Recurrent variceal hemorrhage	Endoscopic obliteration of varices
		Portocaval shunt
		Distal splenorenal shunt
		Mesocaval shunt
		TIPS and liver transplantation
	Ascites	Medical therapy (low sodium diet, spironolactone)
		Peritoneovenous shunt
		TIPS
		Side-to-side portocaval shunt
		Liver transplantation

Abbreviations: IVC, inferior vena cava; TIPS, transjugular intrahepatic portasystemic shunt.

PORTAL HYPERTENSION

Portal hypertension arises when portal venous pressure exceeds hepatic venous pressure by 8mm Hg. Normal portal vein pressure is 7 to 10mm Hg. In portal hypertension, portal pressure averages about 20mm Hg but can occasionally rise to 50mm Hg or greater. The portal vein has no valves; therefore, any increase in portal pressure is reflected back to the tributaries, causing varices at all sites of portasystemic anastomosis. The essentials of portal hypertension are summarized in Table 6.2.

Pathogenesis of Portal Hypertension

Portal pressure can rise due to: (1) increased resistance within the portal circulation and (2) increased portal blood flow. Worldwide, the most common cause of portal hypertension is schistosomiasis, with the exception of North America, where alcoholic cirrhosis is the most common cause. Causative factors are classified and listed in Table 6.3.

TABLE 6.3. Causative Factors of Portal Hypertension

Increased resistance to flow
  Prehepatic
- Portal vein thrombosis
- Splenic vein thrombosis
- Cavernous transformation of portal vein
- Congenital atresia of portal vein
  Hepatic
- Cirrhosis
    Alcoholic
    Postnecrotic
    Biliary
    Hemochromatosis
- Schistosomiasis
- Acute alcoholic liver disease
  Posthepatic
- Budd-Chiari syndrome
    Hepatic vein thrombosis
    Inferior vena cava thrombosis
- Constrictive pericarditis

Increased portal blood flow
- Traumatic arterioportal venous fistula
- Splanchnic arteriovenous fistula

Increased Resistance

Increased resistance may be caused by prehepatic, hepatic, or posthepatic factors.

PREHEPATIC CAUSES Portal vein thrombosis is common in children due to umbilical vein sepsis. In adults it is rare but may be caused by malignancy, pancreatitis, or as a consequence of pylephlebitis. While portal vein thrombosis may cause portal hypertension, liver function is usually maintained and ascites is uncommon. Splenic vein thrombosis occurs in the course of pancreatitis or is caused by neoplasms. The resulting hypertension is located in the venous bed drained by the splenic vein (left-sided portal hypertension), which leads predominately to gastric varices.

HEPATIC CAUSES Cirrhosis and schistosomiasis are the primary causes. Resistance to flow is caused by intrahepatic obstruction, which may be predominantly presinusoidal, sinusoidal or postsinusoidal (Figure 6.3). Obstruction often occurs at more than one level. Presinusoidal obstruction, which takes place at the presinusoidal level, causes increased portal pressure proximal to the sinusoids and normal or decreased sinusoidal pressure. When the block is postsinusoidal, however, both sinusoidal and presinusoidal (portal) pressures rise. Increased sinusoidal pressure leads to the formation of large amounts of lymph, causing ascites. Thus, ascites is not a major feature of presinusoidal block—or even of sinusoidal block—but is prominent when the obstruction is either postsinusoidal or in the hepatic vein.

Schistosomiasis causes predominantly presinusoidal block, but alcoholic and postnecrotic cirrhosis cause both sinusoidal and postsinusoidal block.

POSTHEPATIC CAUSES Budd–Chiari syndrome is a rare disorder resulting in hepatic vein thrombosis. In some patients the cause is unknown. In many patients, however, there is associated polycythemia vera or a history of oral contraceptive use. Constrictive pericarditis (e.g., tuberculosis) can also cause the syndrome.

Increased Portal Blood Flow

The primary cause of increased hepatopetal flow resulting in elevated portal pressure is the formation of arteriovenous fistulas between the hepatic artery and portal vein or between the splenic artery and splenic vein. The main cause of arteriovenous fistula formation is trauma, including operative trauma. Another cause of increased hepatopetal flow is increased splenic blood flow due to Banti's syndrome or other conditions associated with splenomegaly.

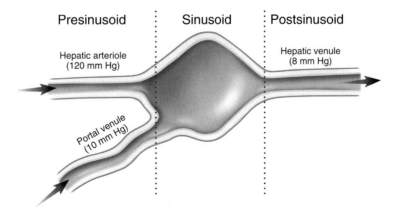

FIGURE 6.3. Hepatic causes of portal hypertension and ascites.

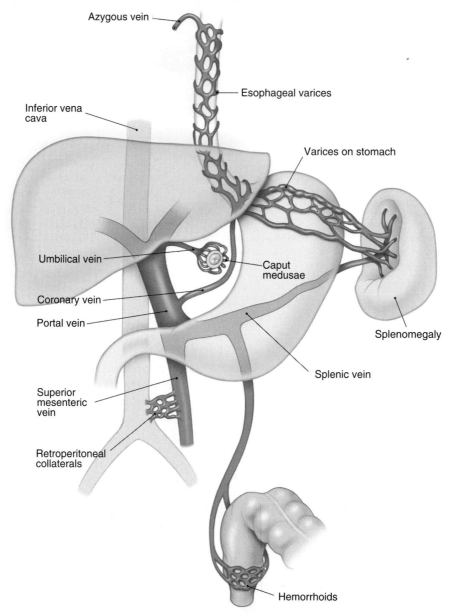

Azygous vein

Esophageal varices

Inferior vena cava

Varices on stomach

Umbilical vein

Caput medusae

Coronary vein

Portal vein

Splenomegaly

Superior mesenteric vein

Splenic vein

Retroperitoneal collaterals

Hemorrhoids

FIGURE 6.4. The major sites of portasystemic anastomosis, where varices can develop as collaterals between the portal and systemic circulations.

Consequences of Portal Hypertension

Clinically significant consequences of portal hypertension include varices, splenomegaly, ascites, encephalopathy, and hepatic coma.

Formation of Varices

Varices develop as collaterals between the portal and systemic circulations (Figure 6.4). The major sites of portasystemic anastomosis include the lower end of the esophagus (esophageal varices), the umbilical vein (caput medusa), the hemorrhoidal plexus (hemorrhoids), and retroperitoneal collaterals through lumbar veins (retroperitoneal varices).

Collateral formation is different in prehepatic and hepatic portal hypertension. In prehepatic hypertension, collaterals form in the diaphragm and in the hepatogastric and hepatocolic ligaments. They form to bypass the obstruction in the portal vein and carry blood to the liver; in other words, they are hepatopetal. In hepatic causes of portal hypertension, however, the collaterals serve to decompress the liver by carrying blood away from it, that is, they are hepatofugal. Hepatofugal flow tends to create esophageal and gastric varices. Bleeding from esophageal varices is a major complication of portal hypertension. Less commonly, bleeding can also occur from hemorrhoids.

Portal Hypertensive Gastropathy

This complication results from venous congestion in the gastric wall, resulting in engorged, friable mucosa, which can lead to indolent bleeding from the stomach.

Splenomegaly

Portal hypertension causes splenomegaly through engorgement of the intrasplenic vascular spaces. Splenomegaly results in sequestration and destruction of blood elements by immune mechanisms. The process, known as hypersplenism, causes leukopenia (WBC <4000/mm^3) and thrombocytopenia (platelet count <100,000 mm^3). Although the spleen is always enlarged in hypersplenism, there is no correlation between spleen size and degree of hypersplenism, indicating the importance of immune destruction in the process.

Ascites

Postsinusoidal and hepatic venous obstruction lead to increased hepatic lymph formation. The increased lymph formed extravasates into the peritoneal cavity through the liver capsule (Figure 6.5). An important contributing factor to the formation of ascites is the presence of hypoalbuminemia as a result of hepatocellular damage. A third important factor is retention of sodium and water due to increased secretion of adrenocortical hormones. Ascites does not occur in prehepatic portal hypertension.

Encephalopathy and Hepatic Coma

Portasystemic encephalopathy—which occurs in patients with marked decrease in hepatic function—is due largely to hyperammonemia, increased levels of γ-aminobutyric acid (GABA), and false neurotransmitters. Hence, it rarely occurs in extrahepatic portal hypertension. Hyperammonemia is due to both impaired liver function and hepatic bypass through portasystemic collaterals. Normally, all the ammonia produced in the gut is deactivated in the liver by conversion into urea.

The neuropsychiatric manifestations of encephalopathy include altered consciousness, depressed motor activity, and decreased deep tendon reflexes. A characteristic sign is the *liver flap*, that is, when the patient, with arm outstretched, wrist extended, and fingers straight, exhibits repeated involuntary flexions of the wrist and fingers.

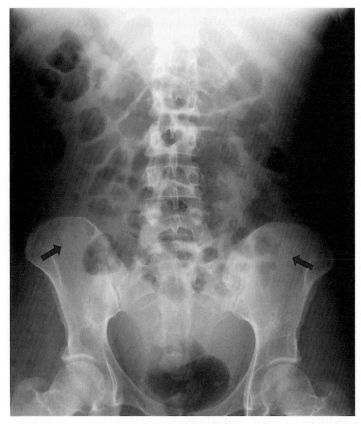

FIGURE 6.5. In portal hypertension, ascites is caused by discharge of increased hepatic lymph into the peritoneal cavity through the liver capsule. This supine x-ray shows large and small bowel gathered in the center of the abdomen with ascites fluid appearing as a gray background occupying both flanks (arrows). (Courtesy of Henry I. Goldberg, MD.)

As the condition worsens, delirium gives way to stupor, then coma. Electroencephalogram (EEG) is a sensitive way to detect encephalopathy. In hepatic coma, blood levels of ammonia are frequently elevated to 125 μg/dL or more.

Encephalopathy may be worsened and hepatic coma precipitated by severe variceal hemorrhage, which leads to decreased liver blood flow, and increased ammonia formation from blood in the GI tract due to action of gut flora.

MANAGEMENT: PORTAL HYPERTENSION

Portal hypertension is an important condition that requires team management by gastroenterologists, radiologists, and surgeons. Variceal hemorrhage and intractable ascites are the usual reasons for surgical treatment. Over the years, surgeons have developed several ingenious ways of decompressing portal hypertension. Recently, the availability of liver transplantation as an option for definitive treatment has resulted in the use of radiological or surgical procedures that leave the portal vein intact to treat acute variceal hemorrhage.

ACUTE VARICEAL HEMORRHAGE

Esophageal varices may develop without causing bleeding, but 25% to 35% of patients with esophageal varices will eventually bleed (Figure 6.6).[3] Variceal hemorrhage is responsible for approximately 25% to 30% of deaths in patients with cirrhosis.[4] Most commonly, the varices that rupture are within 2 to 3 cm of the gastroesophageal junction. Bleeding may be minor or massive. Massive bleeding has a 50% mortality rate when associated with severe liver dysfunction. Approximately 50% to 60% of patients with esophageal varices bleed from a cause other than the varices.[3] Nevertheless, patients with esophageal varices will often have the stigmata of chronic liver disease, including jaundice, ascites, splenomegaly, spider nevi, gynecomastia, and testicular atrophy. The management is discussed below and depicted in Figure 6.7.

Investigations

Helpful investigations in acute variceal hemorrhage include laboratory studies, endoscopy, radiological studies, and duplex ultrasonography.

Laboratory Studies

Liver function test results are nearly always abnormal and include elevated bilirubin and depressed serum albumin levels. These findings—combined with the presence or absence of ascites and neurological and nutritional disorders—must be used to determine the patient's hepatic functional reserve according to Child's criteria (see Table 6.1). The hemogram and coagulation profile should be determined. If the presence of hepatoma is suspected, serum alpha protein and a CT scan may be required.

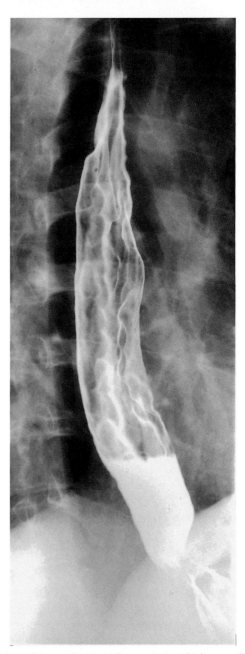

FIGURE 6.6. This esophagram demonstrates thick wavy linear structures in the body of the esophagus, representing varices. (Courtesy of Henry I. Goldberg, MD.)

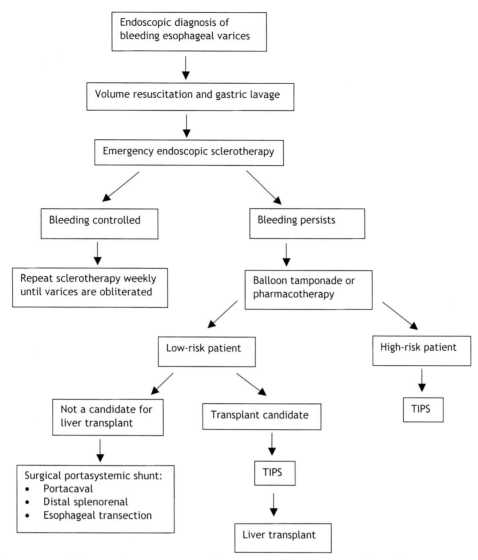

FIGURE 6.7. Decision tree for management of acute variceal hemorrhage. *Abbreviation*: TIPS, transjugular intrahepatic portasystemic shunt.

Endoscopy

Esophagogastroduodenoscopy, the most important investigation to identify the cause of bleeding, should be performed as soon as hemodynamic stability is restored. Large, tortuous submucosal varices may be seen. The bleeding varix may be visible. If no bleeding is seen from the varices, the absence of a bleeding lesion in the stomach and duodenum strongly suggest variceal hemorrhage. Patients with cherry red spots and red wale markings on large thin-walled varices are likely to bleed from varices.

Radiology

Barium swallow is of little investigative use in variceal hemorrhage, but it is often on barium swallow that the presence of varices is detected.

Duplex Ultrasonography

Doppler duplex ultrasonography is useful in defining portal venous anatomy, patency of the portal vein, and the presence of splenomegaly. This study is more useful preoperatively than during acute hemorrhage.

Treatment

Treatment of acute variceal hemorrhage requires resuscitation, prevention of encephalopathy, and control of bleeding.

Resuscitation and Prevention of Encephalopathy

Rapid hemodynamic resuscitation and oxygen administration are important to prevent further deterioration of hepatocellular function. Central venous or pulmonary artery pressure as well as urine output monitoring may be required. The patient may have or may develop encephalopathy and obtundation. Should these conditions become a problem, the airway should be controlled quickly to prevent aspiration, and mechanical ventilation should be instituted. Saline solutions should be avoided and potassium chloride given as soon as adequate urine output is established. Parenteral vitamin K should also be given. Measures to prevent encephalopathy should be instituted early, including protection of hepatic function by prompt hemodynamic resuscitation, administration of oxygen, evacuation of blood from the gastrointestinal tract (using nasogastric lavage, magnesium sulfate, enemas), and luminal acidification of the gut (using lactulose) and reduction of gut flora using neomycin.

Control of Bleeding

Acute bleeding may be controlled by endoscopic sclerotherapy, balloon tamponade, radiological measures, or emergency surgery:

Endoscopic sclerotherapy. Injection of a sclerosant (e.g., 5% sodium morrhuate or 5% ethanol amine oleate) into either the varices or the paravariceal mucosa may control acute hemorrhage. Obliteration of varices usually requires repeated endoscopic sclerotherapy at weekly intervals for 3 or more weeks. Endoscopic sclerotherapy has emerged as the best initial technique to control hemorrhage. However, it has significant complications, including recurrent bleeding from mucosal ulceration in 20% of patients, esophageal stricture in up to 15%, pleural effusion, and, rarely, esophageal perforation.

Endoscopic variceal ligation. Also known as variceal banding, endoscopic variceal ligation (EVL) is safer than sclerotherapy but more difficult to perform. The varices are grasped serially and elastic O-rings applied to the base of each, much as is done in hemorrhoid banding.

Pharmacologic control. Vasopressin and glypressin and either somatostatin or the long-acting somatostatin analogue, octreotide, may stop bleeding by reducing portal pressure. Vasopressin lowers portal pressure by causing splanchnic arterial vasoconstriction, while octreotide acts

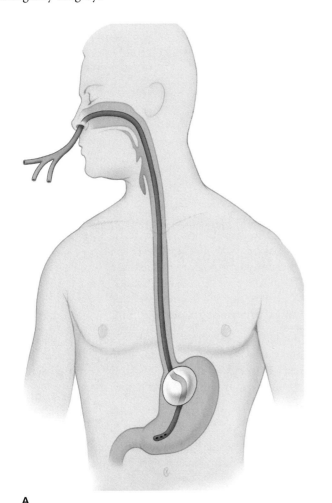
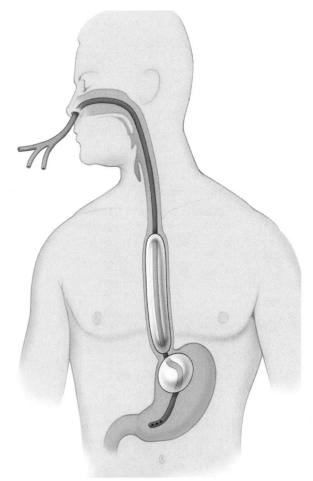

A   B

FIGURE 6.8. The Sengstaken–Blakemore tube is indicated to control bleeding when endoscopic sclerotherapy is unavailable or fails. (A) The device creates a tamponade by putting traction on an inflated gastric balloon (B); the esophageal balloon is inflated only if the gastric balloon fails to get bleeding under control. (Adapted from Greenfield L, ed. Surgery: Scientific Principles and Practice. 2nd ed. Philadelphia: Lippincott-Raven; 1997.)

Table 6.4. Proper Use of the Sengstaken–Blakemore Tube

Pre-insertion
- Assess need for nasogastric intubation
- Apply topical anesthesia to nasal passage
- Evacuate stomach of blood
- Label gastric and esophageal tubes

Insertion
- Through nostril is preferred
- Insert tube well into stomach
- Inflate gastric balloon to 250 ml of air
- Pull gastric balloon snugly to gastroesophageal junction
- Plain abdominal x-ray to check placement
- Insert #14 Salem into esophagus and apply suction
- If bleeding is controlled, no need to inflate esophageal balloon
- If bleeding is not controlled, inflate esophageal balloon to 25–45 mm Hg
- Chest and abdominal x-rays to check position of balloons

Follow-up
- 24–h/day nursing supervision
- Tape scissors to head of bed to cut tubes in case of respiratory difficulty
- Serial hematocrit levels every 6 h
- Deflate balloons in 24 h but leave tube in situ for additional 24 h
- Remove tube if no bleeding occurs in 24 h

Source: Reprinted with permission from Rikker, Goldsmith, eds. Practice and Surgery. Philadelphia: Harper & Row, 1981.

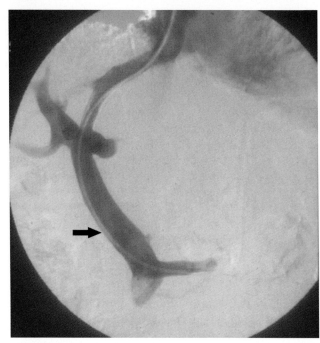

FIGURE 6.9. Transjugular intrahepatic portasystemic shunt (TIPS) procedure. This subtraction angiogram shows a catheter entering the liver in the hepatic vein and passing through the metallic stent into the portal vein (arrow). (Courtesy of Henry I. Goldberg, MD.)

on the venous side by inhibiting the release and action of vasodilators. Vasopressin has an efficacy of only 50%; it has the potential to reduce coronary blood flow and cause myocardial infarction. Nitroglycerin has been used concomitantly to block the coronary vasospastic effects. Glypressin is an analogue with fewer side effects. Somatostatin and octreotide are initially given as an intravenous bolus of 250 μg/hr or 50 to 100 μg/hr, respectively. In controlled trials, somatostatin therapy resulted in control of bleeding in 63% compared to 46% with vasopressin.[5]

Balloon tamponade. Use of the Sengstaken–Blakemore tube (Figure 6.8) to control bleeding is indicated when endoscopic sclerotherapy fails or is not available. Balloon tamponade provides effective and immediate control of bleeding but must be used under strict protocol as outlined in Table 6.4. Bleeding is usually controlled by applying traction on the inflated gastric balloon. The esophageal balloon is inflated only if the gastric balloon fails to control the bleeding. The most common complication is aspiration and aspiration pneumonia. The most dreaded complications, both of which are rare, are migration of the esophageal balloon to obstruct the airway and esophageal perforation.

The balloon(s) is(are) deflated after 24 h but kept in place for another 24 h in the event bleeding recurs. Balloon tamponade controls bleeding in over 90% of patients, but rebleeding after balloon deflation occurs in some 25%.[6]

Radiologic control. Two techniques have been used to control bleeding radiologically: percutaneous, transhep-

atic obliteration of varices by selective gel foam embolization into individual collaterals and transjugular intrahepatic portasystemic shunt (TIPS). Because of the success of TIPS, percutaneous transhepatic obliteration is now rarely used.

TIPS accomplishes intrahepatic portasystemic shunting using a flexible, expandable metal stent (Wall stent). The stent is introduced over a guidewire after an intrahepatic track is formed between the hepatic and portal veins using a balloon catheter (Figure 6.9). Once the stent is in place, portal pressure falls rapidly so that the portal vein to inferior vena caval pressure gradient is less than 12 mm Hg, the threshold below which varices rarely bleed.

Complications occur in about 10%, but life-threatening bleeding from puncture of the liver capsule occurs in only approximately 1% to 2%.[7] Encephalopathy develops frequently. Randomized clinical trials have shown that the rebleeding rate after TIPS is consistently lower than the rate following endoscopic sclerotherapy, while mortality rates are comparable.[7]

The best indication for using TIPS is failure of endoscopic sclerotherapy in patients who are candidates for liver transplantation. In this case, TIPS serves as a bridge to transplantation. It may also be the best option in Child C patients who have failed sclerotherapy. The major concern with TIPS is long-term stenosis or occlusion. In the most experienced centers, TIPS patency has been maintained in 90% of patients over a 2-year follow-up period by performing TIPS revisions on an outpatient basis when necessary.[8]

Emergency surgical treatment. Failure to control hemorrhage nonoperatively or recurrence of hemorrhage within 48h is an indication for expeditious operation. Three surgical techniques are available: emergency portasystemic shunt, esophageal transection, and variceal ligation.

Several factors must be considered in selecting the procedure, including the patient's Child's class, the candidacy of the patient for liver transplantation, and the surgeon's experience. Patients who are Child's class A or B are not candidates for liver transplantation, while Child's C patients may be. Whenever a patient is judged to be a candidate for liver transplantation, procedures that violate the porta hepatis or portal vein should be avoided. In this case, the remaining choices are then direct variceal ligation, stapled esophageal transection, or mesocaval H-graft. Even here, however, the procedure of choice, if available, is TIPS. In Child's A or B patients, the most expeditious operation is emergency portacaval shunt. If bleeding can be controlled with balloon tamponade, however, a selective distal splenorenal shunt may be possible.

1. Portasystemic shunt. Performed either as an end-to-side portacaval or an H-mesocaval shunt, emergency portacaval shunt is 95% successful in controlling bleeding (Figure 6.10). Mortalities rates are similar to endoscopic sclerotherapy. In an NIH-funded prospective randomized clinical trial comparing emergency portacaval shunt and endoscopic sclerotherapy in unselected patients with variceal hemorrhage, the 30-day survival was equal at about 50%.[9]

2. Esophageal transection. Esophageal transection is accomplished using an end-to-end stapler to transect and reanastomose the distal esophagus (Figure 6.11). In so doing, the procedure disconnects the portal circulation from the systemic circulation, and the doughnut of esophagus excised removes segments of the varices. Unfortunately, bleeding will recur as varices reform.

3. Variceal ligation. Performed by the thoracic or abdominal approach, variceal ligation involves opening the distal esophagus and oversewing the varices individually with suture. The procedure is now rarely performed.

Prevention of Recurrent Hemorrhage

In acute variceal hemorrhage that has been successfully controlled nonoperatively, the goal is to prevent further hemorrhage. Available methods include pharmacotherapy, obliteration of varices by endoscopic sclerotherapy, and surgery.

PHARMACOTHERAPY Nonselective β-blockade with propranolol has been shown to reduce the likelihood of recurrent bleeding by 30%.[10] Unfortunately, the drug requires strict compliance, its effect on individual patients is inconsistent, and it reduces cardiac output. Conse-quently, this therapy has to date not proven to be a long-term option.

ENDOSCOPIC OBLITERATION OF VARICES Long-term results indicate that this procedure is effective in only 40% to 60% of patients and that it decreases the mortality rate of acute variceal hemorrhage by 25%.[11] The advent of this form of therapy has reduced the incidence of shunt surgery. Nevertheless, endoscopic sclerotherapy is associated with a high rate of long-term mortality because of recurrent hemorrhage.

SURGERY: SHUNT PROCEDURES Total shunts or selective shunts can be used to prevent recurrent hemorrhage. All shunt procedures reduce the rebleeding rate to less than 10%, but this success comes at the price of a high mortality rate (5%–20%) and an increased incidence of encephalopathy.[12] In general, the incidence of encephalopathy in selective distal splenorenal shunt is 50% of that seen in nonselective shunts.

In selecting the procedure, the distal splenorenal shunt is the first choice. When it cannot be performed, either mesocaval or end-to-side portacaval shunt is selected. Central splenorenal shunt is now rarely performed, as is side-to-side portacaval shunt.

Total shunts. Total procedures include end-to-side or side-to-side portacaval shunt and mesocaval shunts. End-to-side portacaval shunt provides effective and long-lasting protection from rebleeding. The side-to-side shunt is usually reserved for treating Budd–Chiari syndrome and ascites. The incidence of encephalopathy after portacaval shunt is 20% to 40% with nonselective shunts and 10% to 20% with selective shunts.[13]

Mesocaval shunt is accomplished by interposing a segment of vein or prosthetic graft between the superior mesenteric vein and the inferior vena cava. Mesocaval shunts that use grafts of 12 to 20mm result in total diversion of portal flow. If the shunt is limited to 8mm, portal liver flow is preserved and the incidence of encephalopathy is significantly reduced.

Selective shunts. The distal splenorenal (Warren) shunt is accomplished by anastomosing the distal end of the transected splenic vein to the side of the left renal vein, then transecting the coronary vein, the right gastroepiploic vein, and the veins in the splenocolic ligament. The operation is complex, requires special expertise, and is contraindicated in several situations, including too great a distance between the splenic and renal veins to permit anastomosis, previous splenectomy, and ascites. Distal splenorenal shunt is not an effective treatment for ascites. With time, this selective shunt becomes less selective as new collaterals form.

Liver Transplantation

Liver transplantation not only resolves the problem of varices, but it restores normal liver function. Unfortunately, the

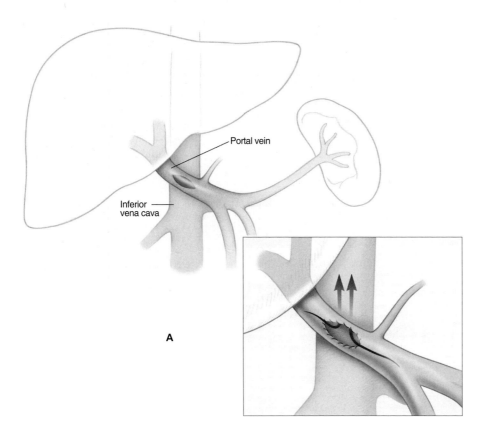

Portal vein

Inferior
vena cava

A

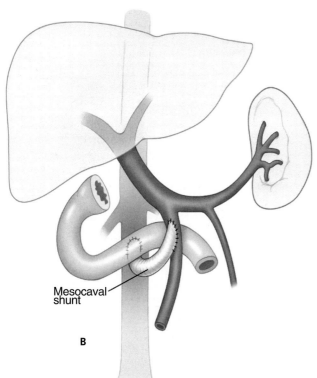

Mesocaval
shunt

B

FIGURE 6.10. Emergency portacaval shunt is effective in control-ling bleeding by decompressing the portal system flow into the inferior vena cava and other lower-pressure systems. A number of procedures can by used, including (A) end-to-side portacaval shunt and (B) H-mesocaval shunt.
Continued on next page

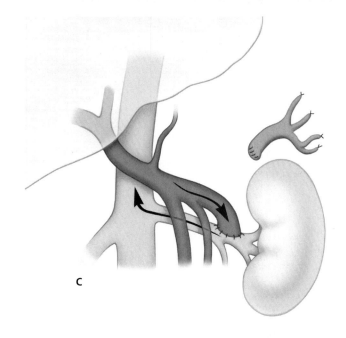

C

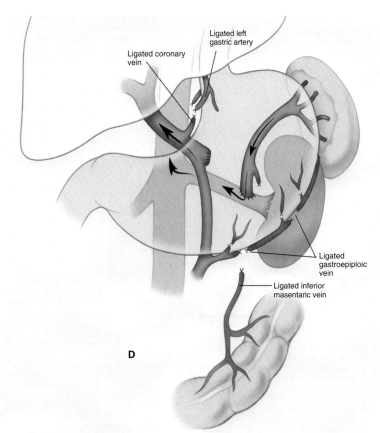

Ligated left
gastric artery

Ligated coronary
vein

Ligated
gastroepiploic
vein

Ligated inferior
masentaric vein

D

FIGURE 6.10. *Continued*
The H-mesocaval shunt may be either proximal
(C) or distal, also known as the Warren shunt (D).
(Adapted from Greenfield L, ed. Surgery: Scien-
tific Principles and Practice. 2nd ed. Philadelphia:
Lippincott-Raven; 1997.)

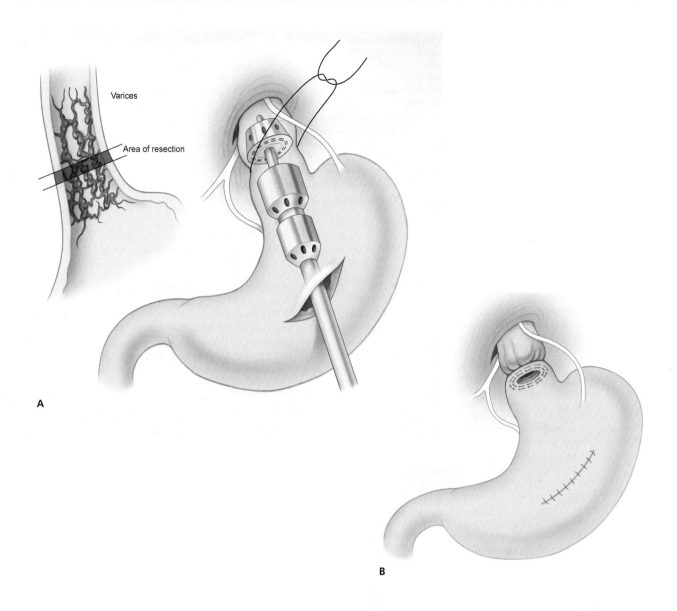

FIGURE 6.11. Esophageal transection. (A and B) An end-to-end stapler is used to transect and reanastomose the distal esophagus to remove segments of the varices and disconnect the portal circulation from the systemic circulation. (Adapted from Greenfield L, ed. Surgery: Scientific Principles and Practice. 2nd ed. Philadelphia: Lippincott-Raven; 1997.)

scarcity of donor organs makes liver transplantation a less viable option. Acute alcoholic patients and drug users are not candidates. It is also difficult to justify liver transplantation to treat varices when end-stage liver disease is not present. In such cases, either selective shunts or the TIPS procedure may be used.

ASCITES

Ascites can be a major problem in patients with portal hypertension, especially in those with Budd–Chiari syndrome and postsinusoidal portal hypertension. As ascites

develops, relative deficit of circulating volume occurs. Patients with abdominal wall hernias—particularly umbilical hernias—have the additional risk of spontaneous perforation.

Medical Therapy

Medical therapy has a large measure of success in treating ascites, but some patients must be treated surgically. More than 90% of patients can be treated satisfactorily with medical therapy, including sodium restriction (to a maximum of 2–3 g/day) and spironolactone therapy (100–400 mg/day). Other diuretics (e.g., furosemide, hydrochlorothiazide) may also be used, but they can cause hypokalemia, which can precipitate or aggregate encephalopathy. Hence, spironolactone is the diuretic of first choice. Intermittent large-volume paracentesis and colloid administration are also effective.

Surgical and Radiologic Therapy

Approximately 5% to 10% of patients will develop diuretic-resistant ascites. Therapeutic options include peritoneovenous shunt, TIPS, side-to-side portacaval shunt, or liver transplantation.

Peritoneovenous Shunt

A shunt with a one-way valve is placed under local anesthesia between the peritoneal cavity and the superior vena cava or right atrium. The transfer of fluid from the peritoneum into the bloodstream reverses most of the pathophysiological factors that produce ascites or are caused by it. Circulating volume and cardiac output are restored. Plasma levels of renin, aldosterone, and antidiuretic hormone become normal, and renal function improves. Despite the simplicity of the procedure, the peritoneovenous shunt is associated with complications in 40% to 50% of patients. The most common complications are sepsis, disseminated intravascular coagulopathy, and shunt

occlusion. Mortality rates of approximately 25% have also been reported, but these rates represent the seriousness of the underlying liver disease.[14] Controlled trials have shown that peritoneovenous shunt does not improve survival.[14]

TIPS

TIPS, increasingly replacing peritoneovenous shunt in the treatment of resistant ascites, is rapidly effective, but long-term results are not encouraging because of the higher rate of encephalopathy and liver failure. Of course, in patients with end-stage liver disease, TIPS serves as an excellent bridge to liver transplantation.

Side-to-side Portocaval Shunt

When ascites is associated with variceal bleeding, side-to-side portocaral shunt is indicated. Even then, the advent of TIPS has made surgical shunts less common except in treating the Budd–Chiari syndrome.

Liver Transplantation

Liver transplantation is indicated as a definitive procedure in selected patients when ascites is associated with end-stage liver disease.

MANAGEMENT: LIVER ABSCESS

Abscess of the liver may be caused by bacteria, fungi, or ameba. In surgical practice, the most important of these are bacterial and amebic abscesses (Table 6.5 and Figure 6.12).

BACTERIAL ABSCESS

Bacterial liver abscess may develop as a result of hematogenous spread from biliary tract infection or extension from adjacent septic focus. Hematogenous spread from acute appendicitis and diverticulitis was common prior to the advent of antibiotics. The abscess may or may not be preceded by infection of the portal vein (pylephlebitis). Both aerobes and anaerobes are usually involved as a polymicrobial infection. The most common aerobes are *Escherichia coli, Klebsiella pneumoniae, Pseudomonas, Proteus, Enterococcus, and Streptococcus pyogenes.* The most common anaerobic organisms are bacteroides and streptococci. Bacterial abscesses tend to be multiple and are often found in both lobes. They present in a subacute fashion with fever, with chills developing later. Mild jaundice may be present, and about a third of patients will complain of right upper quadrant pain.

AMEBIC ABSCESS

Amebiasis is endemic in several parts of Africa, Southeast Asia, Mexico, and South America. In North America, the infection may be acquired either from travels to these regions or from individuals who acquired amebiasis in these parts of the world. Outside the body, *Entameba histolytica* exists in trophozoite or cyst forms. In infection, amebic cysts enter the gastrointestinal tract and, in the colon, become trophozoites, which invade the mucosa and result in typical flask-shaped ulcers. From there, the organism is transported via the portal circulation to the liver, where the amebic abscess forms.

Amebic abscesses present more acutely than bacterial abscesses. An antecedent history of bloody diarrhea is obtained in only 10% of cases. Fever can be high and is often intermittent. Moderate jaundice may also be present.

Investigations

Laboratory and radiological studies can help determine the causative factors.

TABLE 6.5. Essentials: Liver Abscess	
Bacterial abscess	
Causes	*Escherichia coli*
	Klebsiella
	Pseudomonas
	Proteus
	Enterococcus
	Streptococcus pyogenes
Symptoms	Fever and chills
	Jaundice
	RUQ pain
Treatment	Broad-spectrum antibiotics (6 weeks)
	Percutaneous drainage (unilocular abscess)
	Surgical drainage
Amebic abscess	
Cause	*Entamoeba histolytica*
Symptoms	High fever
	Jaundice
	Antecedent bloody diarrhea (10%)
Diagnosis	Serologic (hemagglutination, complement fixation, ELISA)
	US or CT-guided aspiration ("anchovy paste")
Treatment	Medical (metronidazole)
	Surgical drainage (rarely)

Abbreviations: CT, computerized tomography; ELISA, enzyme-linked immunosorbent assay; RUQ, right upper guadrant; US, ultrasonography.

Laboratory Studies

A high level of leukocytosis is usually present. Anemia is frequent in bacterial abscesses. Serum bilirubin is usually normal, but alkaline phosphatase is frequently elevated. Blood cultures are positive in 50% of patients and are more likely to be positive if obtained while the patient is experiencing chills.

In amebic abscess, the laboratory findings are indistinguishable from those of bacterial abscess. Specific diagnosis may be obtained from serologic tests, including hemagglutination, complement fixation, indirect fluorescent antibody assays, enzyme-linked immunosorbent assay (ELISA), countercurrent immunoelectrophoresis, and agar gel diffusion. Aspiration of amebic abscesses is performed as a last resort. If done, the result is typical "anchovy paste" aspirate.

Radiologic Studies

Ultrasonography is the initial imaging test of choice. CT is more accurate but also more expensive. Ultrasonographic or CT-guided aspiration of abscess may be done for Gram stain, culture, and sensitivity studies.

Treatment

Medical therapy is usually adequate and differs for bacterial and amebic abscesses. Surgery may be required in special circumstances.

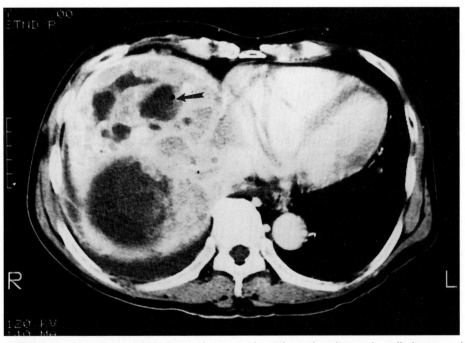

FIGURE 6.12. Liver abscess. This CT scan shows one large (arrow) and several small abscesses, the margins of which are irregular in contour; one contains an air bubble due to bacterial infection (tiny black opaque dot). The irregular contour and shape of these lesions are typical of infection or tumor and help distinguish them from hepatic cysts. (Courtesy of Henry I. Goldberg, MD.)

Bacterial Abscess

Patients should be placed on broad-spectrum antibiotics (usually a combination of an aminoglycoside, metronidazole, and ampicillin) given intravenously. This regimen will cover the most common offending bacteria and may be changed later when the results of culture and sensitivity are obtained.

Multiple liver abscesses are treated with intravenous antibiotics for 2 weeks followed by oral antibiotics for 6 weeks. Streptococcal abscess may require as long as 6 months of treatment. Large single abscesses are best treated with antibiotics and percutaneous catheter drainage. Surgical drainage is reserved for cases in which catheter drainage either fails or is technically impossible. Surgery is also indicated when an underlying disease (e.g., cholangitis, cholecystitis) must be treated with an operation.

Amebic Abscess

Metronidazole, the treatment of choice, is given in doses of 750 mg tid either orally or intravenously. A second oral amebicide (e.g., diloxanide) is usually added. Surgical drainage may be necessary if bacterial superinfection is present.

MANAGEMENT: LIVER CYSTS

CONGENITAL CYSTS

Solitary Cysts

Unilocular cysts are rare but can sometimes attain large size (Figure 6.13). They have a serous lining and must be differentiated from cystadenomas, which have cuboidal epithelial lining and are premalignant. Solitary cysts are usually discovered incidentally, but they might produce clinical symptoms if they (1) attain large size, causing dull ache and mass, and (2) become infected, a very rare occurrence.

Large and symptomatic cysts are best treated laparoscopically. The cyst is unroofed and the cavity filled with omentum. Rarely, the cyst may communicate with the biliary tree. This may be detected preoperatively but is readily determined by aspirating the cyst fluid. If there is communication with the biliary tree, the cyst should be drained into the intestine by Roux-en-Y cyst-jejunostomy.

Multiple Cysts

Multiple cysts occur in polycystic disease, which affects the liver, kidney, and spleen. The disease is congenital with autosomal dominant inheritance but occurs in adults. A nonlethal polycystic disease occurs in children as a result of autosomal recessive inheritance. Polycystic liver disease rarely requires surgical treatment.

ECHINOCOCCUS (HYDATID) CYST

Two types of hydatid cyst exist, the unilocular cyst caused by *Echinococcus granulosus* and the alveolar type caused by *Echinococcus multilocularis*. Approximately 70% are single cysts, and the right lobe is affected in 85% of cases. The cysts have a double membrane, contain colorless alkaline fluid on the inner side of the membrane, and are usually found to have numerous daughter cysts. The fluid may be highly allergenic and can precipitate anaphylaxis if spilled intraperitoneally (Table 6.6).

Over two-thirds of patients present with a palpable mass, abdominal pain, and tenderness. If intrabiliary rupture occurs, biliary colic, jaundice, and urticaria result. Patients may also have emesis or pass feces containing hydatid membrane. When cysts are secondarily infected, the typical picture of liver abscess emerges with fever, chills, and hepatic tenderness. Spontaneous intraperitoneal rupture may lead to anaphylactic shock.

Complications

The complications of hydatic cysts are:

1. Intrabiliary rupture, which occurs in 5% to 10% of cases.
2. Intraperitoneal rupture, which is uncommon but may lead to the formation of new cysts in the peritoneal cavity.
3. Secondary bacterial infection, leading to abscess formation and death of the scolices.
4. Transdiaphragmatic extension into the pleural cavity.

Investigations

Useful tests in echinococcal liver cysts include laboratory studies, skin testing, and radiologic studies.

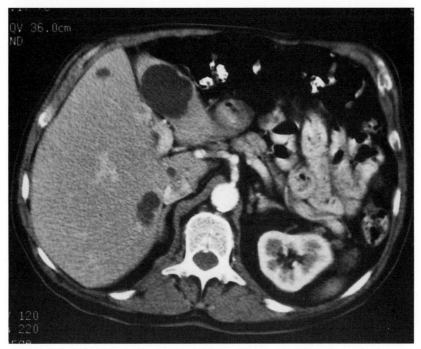

FIGURE 6.13. Hepatic cyst. This CT scan shows one large and three small cysts in the liver, all characterized by thin walls, smooth margins, and homogeneous low density. (Courtesy of Henry I. Goldberg, MD.)

Laboratory Studies

A blood test will reveal eosinophilia in less than 30% of patients. The indirect agglutination test is positive in 85% of patients. The complement fixation test is less sensitive.

Skin Test

The Casoni skin test is positive in approximately 90% of cases of hydatid cysts. A positive Casoni test persists in patients for years after an initial infection.

Radiologic Testing

Ultrasound or CT scan will show the cyst. The CT scan may show multiple septa, even daughter cysts, and sometimes a calcified shadow (Figure 6.14).

Treatment

Large symptomatic cysts are treated laparoscopically or with open surgery. The steps in operative management include:

1. Isolation of the cyst from the peritoneal cavity to minimize spillage of cyst fluid.
2. Aspiration of the cyst as completely as possible, exercising caution as cyst fluid is often under pressure.
3. Instillation into the cyst cavity of a scolecocidal agent such as hypertonic saline or alcohol.
4. Excision of the hydatid cyst by separating the cyst from the liver along a cleavage plane between the germinal layer and adventitia.
5. Alternatively, the cyst may be removed by liver resection or, when extensive, it may be marsupialized and filled with omentum.

TABLE 6.6. Essentials: Echinococcus (Hydatid) Cyst

Most common in
- Australia
- South America
- Greece

Causes
- *Echinococcus granulosus* or *E. multilocularis*
- Intermediary hosts: sheep, pigs, cattle

Clinical presentation
- Palpable mass
- Pain
- Fever and chills if secondary infection

Diagnosis
- Eosinophilia in 30%
- Positive indirect agglutination test in 85%
- Positive Casoni skin test in 90%
- Imaging shows cyst with daughter cysts, calcification

Treatment
- Surgical excision of cyst
- Prevent peritoneal spillage (anaphylaxis)
- Occasionally liver resection

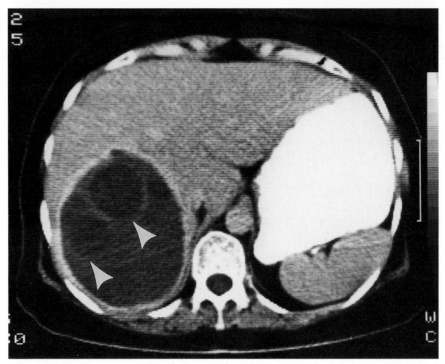

FIGURE 6.14. Echinococcus cysts of the liver. This CT scan shows a single large cyst containing two smaller daughter cysts (arrows), typical of cysts caused by *Echinococcus granulosa*. (Courtesy of Henry I. Goldberg, MD.)

MANAGEMENT: BENIGN NEOPLASMS OF THE LIVER

Benign liver tumors are less common than malignant tumors, from which they must be distinguished. These lesions are often found incidentally at laparotomy or during ultrasonographic or radiologic investigation of other hepatobiliary disease. Most commonly, they are asymptomatic, but occasionally they may produce complications of hemorrhage and necrosis.

HEMANGIOMA

The most common benign lesion, hemangiomas, are of two types: small capillary hemangiomas or cavernous hemangiomas. The former tend to be small, multiple, and asymptomatic (Figure 6.15). Cavernous hemangiomas, on the other hand, can attain a large size and are usually solitary. They are more common in women and may enlarge during pregnancy, suggesting dependency on female sex hormones. They are not known to undergo malignant degeneration.

Most hemangiomas are asymptomatic. When symptoms occur, they are usually nonspecific, consisting of vague abdominal pain and fullness. Rarely, they may cause acute pain or rupture, causing intra-abdominal hemorrhage. Occasionally, they may cause obstruction of the biliary tract, resulting in jaundice. They are rarely palpable and may cause a bruit.

Investigations

Ultrasonography will show hyperechoic lesions. CT is the most useful examination for showing well-delineated hypodense lesions (Figure 6.16). When intravenous contrast is injected during CT, the periphery of the lesion is enhanced and pooling of the dye will occur. The CT findings are often sufficient to distinguish the lesion from hepatocellular carcinoma. MRI gives similar accuracy to CT.

Angiography is rarely indicated but produces a characteristic cotton wool appearance with the filling of large vascular spaces. Needle biopsy should not be performed. If biopsy is considered necessary, the lesion should be examined laparoscopically and biopsy obtained only if the lesion does not appear to be a hemangioma. It is usually better to remove the lesion in its entirety if the diagnosis is difficult.

Treatment

When lesions are found incidentally and are asymptomatic, no therapy is needed. Instead, the patient is simply

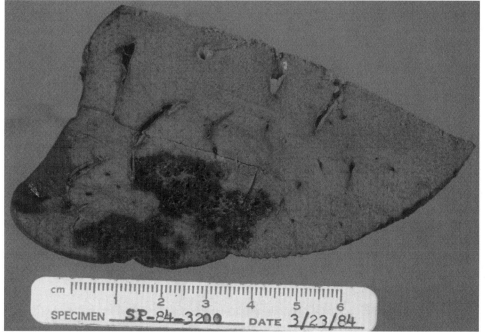

A

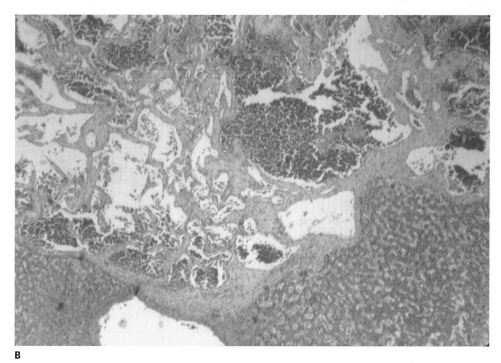

B

FIGURE 6.15. Hemangioma of the liver. Gross appearance of a fixed specimen shows a multifocal hemangioma (A). Microscopic examination demonstrates wide vascular channels lined with flat endothelial cells (B). (Courtesy of Linda D. Ferrell, MD.)

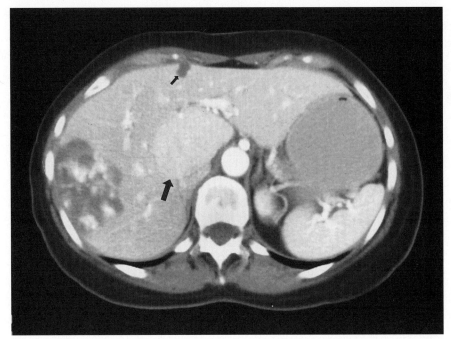

FIGURE 6.16. This CT scan using an intravenous contrast agent shows a large hypodense lesion at the periphery of the liver, with several puddles of dense contrast material seen in the periphery of the lesion. This is a characteristic appearance for cavernous hemangioma. Incidentally noted is a small cyst at the margin of the liver (small arrow) and a large hyperdense lesion in the center of the liver, which was proven by biopsy to be focal nodular hyperplasia (large arrow). (Courtesy of Henry I. Goldberg, MD.)

reassured and informed that large cavernous hemangiomas have been followed for many years without evidence of complication. Surgical resection can usually be performed safely but is indicated only if the patient is symptomatic or the diagnosis uncertain. Wedge resection may suffice, but formal hepatic lobectomy may be required. Hepatic artery ligation and embolization therapy are less effective than surgical resection and are rarely recommended.

HEPATIC ADENOMA

The risk of presenting with this benign hepatocellular neoplasm occurs mostly in women 30 to 50 years of age. A history of oral contraceptive use is present in 90% of women who develop the tumor; risk increases with the duration and strength of the oral contraceptive used. The reported incidence of 3 to 4 per 100,000 of oral contraceptive users who have taken the contraceptive beyond 2 years has been significantly reduced with the administration of low estrogen contraceptives. Typically, the tumor is solitary and smooth-surfaced. Malignant degeneration can occur, but its incidence is not known (Table 6.7).

Investigations

Ultrasonography usually shows a solid tumor, but computerized tomography provides better definition. An isotope scan shows the tumor as a filling defect. Angiography will show a hypervascular lesion. Needle biopsy is apt to precipitate hemorrhage because of the hypervascularity of the lesion. When hepatocellular carcinoma cannot be excluded, laparoscopic evaluation is useful, and biopsy can then be obtained under direct vision.

Treatment

Asymptomatic patients with lesions less than 6 cm in diameter can be treated conservatively if, after discontinuing contraceptive therapy, the tumor regresses. All symptomatic patients and those with asymptomatic tumors larger than 6 cm are best treated by hepatic resection. Patients with intra-abdominal hemorrhage may be preoperatively palliated with angiographic embolization, but early surgical resection is the definitive approach.

TABLE 6.7. Essentials: Hepatic Adenoma

Demographics
- Benign neoplasm common in women 30–50 years old
- History of contraceptive use in 90%

Clinical presentation
- Abdominal pain in 40%
- Incidentally found in 30%
- Palpable mass in 30%
- Spontaneous hemorrhage in 20%

Diagnosis
- Computerized tomography: Solid tumor
- Isotope scan: Shows as filling defect
- Angiogram: Hypervascular lesion
- Biopsy: Only under vision (laparoscopy)

Treatment
- Lesion <6 cm: Discontinue contraceptive drugs
- Lesion >6 cm: Hepatic resection

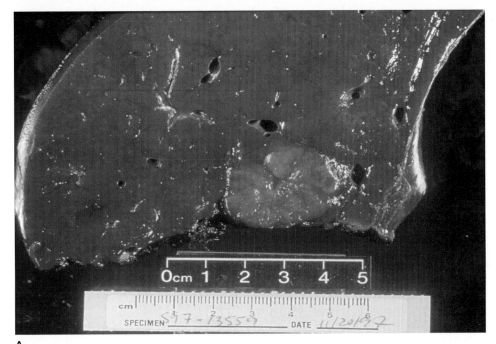

A

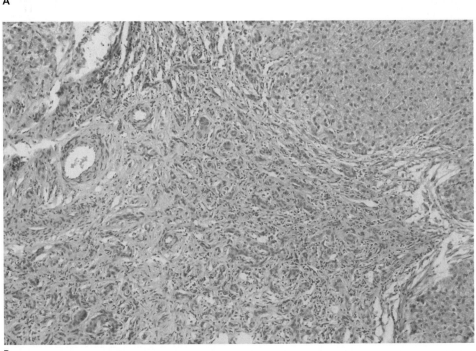

B

FIGURE 6.17. Gross appearance of benign focal nodular hyperplasia. (A) A 3-cm-diameter lesion typical of focal nodular hyperplasia shows central fibrosis. (B) Histologically, nodules of liver and bile ductular proliferation are seen within a fibrous stroma. (Courtesy of Linda D. Ferrell, MD.)

FOCAL NODULAR HYPERPLASIA

Because most focal nodular hyperplasia (FNH) occurs in women of the same age group as adenomas, diagnostic differentiation may be difficult (Figure 6.17).

Unlike hepatic adenoma, FNH neither bleeds nor undergoes malignant transformation. Most patients have no symptoms, but mild and episodic pain may be present. Spontaneous bleeding may rarely occur.

Investigations

Ultrasound and computerized tomography fail to show the lesion in detail because it is isodense. Angiogram will show a typical sunburst hypervascular lesion. Deep biopsy is necessary to reach the central scar, which is diagnostic. Otherwise, the liver parenchyma is normal.

Treatment

Treatment is not usually necessary. Occasionally, the lesion is resected if it causes significant pain or ruptures.

MISCELLANEOUS BENIGN LESIONS

Other benign tumors include bile duct adenoma and hamartoma. Occasional mesenchymal hamartomas may grow into large masses in children and may require resection.

MANAGEMENT: MALIGNANT PRIMARY LIVER NEOPLASMS

The most common malignant primary tumors are hepatocellular carcinoma (HCC) or hepatoma and cholangiocarcinoma. HCC arises from the hepatocytes and cholangiocarcinoma from the epithelium of the intrahepatic biliary tract. Although the causes of these two types of primary liver cancer are not known, several etiological associations are evident (Table 6.8). A mixed form, hepatocholangioma, has also been described but is very rare. In children, hepatoma has malignant cells that resemble fetal hepatocytes. The tumor, referred to as hepatoblastoma, occurs almost exclusively in the first 3 years of life. Primary malignant tumors can also arise from the stroma of the liver (i.e., sarcoma), but these are rare.

HEPATOCELLULAR CARCINOMA

Uncommon in North America but endemic in sub-Saharan Africa, China, and Southeast Asia, hepatocellular carcinoma (HCC) is five times more common in men (Table 6.9) than in women. The peak incidence in endemic regions is the third and fourth decades, but the peak incidence in North America is in the fifth and sixth decades.

TABLE 6.8. Primary Liver Cancer: Etiological Associations

Hepatocellular carcinoma
- Viral infections
    Hepatitis B (HB$_5$Ag seropositivity)
    Hepatocellular carcinoma (7% of cases)
- Mycotoxins (e.g., aflatoxin)
- Iron overload (primary hemochromatosis)
- Steroids (androgenic, anabolic, contraceptives)
- Tyrosinemia type 1
- Cirrhosis (alcoholic and others)

Cholangiocarcinoma
- Primary sclerosing cholangitis
- Ulcerative colitis
- Clonorchis sinensis
- α_1-tripsin deficiency

TABLE 6.9. Essentials: Hepatocellular Carcinoma

Principal causes
  Hepatitis B (HBsAg seropositivity)
  Hepatitis C

Diagnosis (often late)
  Clinical
  - Pain, weight loss, jaundice
  - Mass, bruit
  - Rapid deterioration of liver function
  Laboratory
  - Abnormal LFT (30%–40%)
  - HBsAg seropositivity (50%)
  - Elevated AFP (30% U.S., 80% Africa)
  Imaging
  - MRI to assess hepatic vein invasion
  Biopsy
  - Risk of bleeding
  - Laparoscopic biopsy under vision safest

Treatment
Resection or transplantation only chance of cure
Criteria for respectability
  - Tumor removable by local excision or lobectomy
  - Adequate functional reserve in residual liver
  - No hepatic or portal vein invasion
  - No metastases or extrahepatic extension
Criteria for transplantation
  - Three or fewer lesions
  - Less than 5 cm in diameter
  - Presence of cirrhosis
Prognosis
  - Resectability rate 20%
  - Five-year survival after curative resection: 33%–64%
  - Five-year survival after transplantation: 19%–70%
  - Average survival in unresectable disease: 4 months

Abbreviations: AFP, alpha-fetoprotein; LFT, liver function test; MRI, magnetic resonance imaging.

Early recognition is difficult because symptoms and signs develop late. Abdominal pain, weight loss, and jaundice are the most common symptoms. In patients with known cirrhosis, development of HCC may be manifested by rapid deterioration of liver function. Physical examination may reveal hepatomegaly and ascites. A bruit is heard in the liver in about 10% of patients. Occasionally, patients present acutely, either with fever and pain or with massive intraperitoneal hemorrhage. Rarely, patients may present with paraneoplastic syndromes, most commonly hypoglycemia, hypercalcemia, and polycythemia.

Pathogenesis and Pathology

The principal causative factor of HCC is chronic hepatitis B virus (HBV) infection. Seropositivity for HBsAg is associated with the highest incidence of HCC. In some countries, HCC is commonly associated with hepatitis virus infection. Other conditions associated with the development of HCC include alcoholic cirrhosis, hemochromatosis, and α_1-anti-trypsin deficiency. At one time, thorotrast was used as a contrast material for radiological studies, and some 20 years later, a high incidence of HCC was seen in these patients studied with thorotrast. Vinyl chloride is hepatotoxic and a chemical carcinogen that can cause HCC. Aflatoxin, produced by the aspergillus group of fungi, contaminates grain in Africa and China and is thought to act as a carcinogen.

HCC can produce a tumor, which can be either a single mass, multinodular (Figure 6.18), or a diffuse infiltrative type. By the time of diagnosis, metastasis has occurred in over two-thirds of patients. The most common sites of metastasis are the nodes at the liver hilum and the celiac axis. The tumor may invade the capsule and spread transcoelomically in the peritoneal cavity. Metastasis can also occur in the lungs.

Investigations

In addition to laboratory and radiological testing, laparoscopy and liver biopsy may be required to arrive at a definitive diagnosis.

Laboratory Studies

Abnormal liver function tests (hyperbilirubinemia and/or elevated serum alkaline phosphatase) will be present in 30% to 40% of patients. About half of these will be HBsAg-positive. Alpha-fetoprotein (AFP) will be elevated in some 75% of patients with HCC in Africa but only in 30% of patients in the U.S. and Europe.

Radiological Studies

A variety of imaging techniques will show the tumor, including CT, MRI, and scintiscan (Figure 6.19). MRI has the advantage of detecting extension into hepatic veins. On angiography, hepatomas appear as hyper-vascular lesions supplied primarily by the hepatic artery. Chest x-ray may show elevated right diaphragm, pleural effusion, and sometimes, pulmonary metastasis. The chief value of ultrasonographic examination is that it will distinguish a solid from a cystic tumor, but it is not as sensitive as CT or MRI. Ultrasound Doppler studies, however, are useful in assessing the patency of the portal vein, hepatic vein, and inferior vena cava.

Laparoscopy and Liver Biopsy

CT-guided percutaneous core biopsy can establish the diagnosis. Since HCC is hypervascular, the risk of bleeding is high. Hence, laparoscopy and biopsy under vision is preferable.

Treatment: Definitive Surgical Options

Unfortunately, only about 20% of patients meet the criteria for surgical treatment. The outlook is, therefore, dismal, except in those with early lesions amenable to surgical treatment. The only definitive treatment options are complete tumor resection or total hepatectomy and liver transplantation. Patients with unresectable tumor live, on average, 4 months.

Hepatic Resection

Great regenerative capacity allows resection of up to 85% of the liver, as long as the remaining organ is normal. Two limiting factors are extent of tumor within the liver and extent of cirrhosis in residual liver. The criteria for resection, therefore, are:

1. The entire tumor with a 1-cm margin of normal liver can be removed by local excision, lobectomy, or trisegmentectomy.
2. Residual parenchyma must provide adequate liver function. Thus, if the residual liver is cirrhotic, liver reserve may be inadequate.
3. Hepatic and portal vein invasion must be absent.
4. Extrahepatic extension and distant metastases must also be absent.

Intraoperative ultrasound and anatomic-based resection have improved the adequacy of this procedure and lowered operative mortality to approximately 5%. After curative resection, which is possible in less than 20% of patients, the 5-year survival rate varies from 33% to 64%.[15] The best prognosis is associated with lesions <3 cm in diameter and an absence of cirrhosis.

TYPES OF RESECTION Several types of liver resection techniques are possible, including wedge resection, seg-

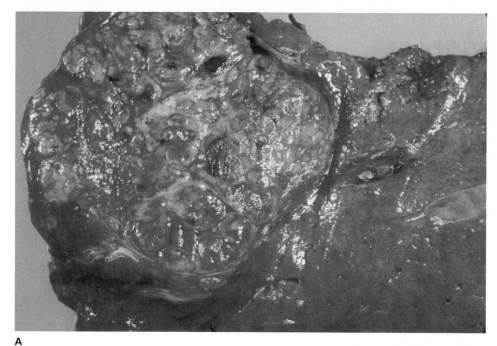

A

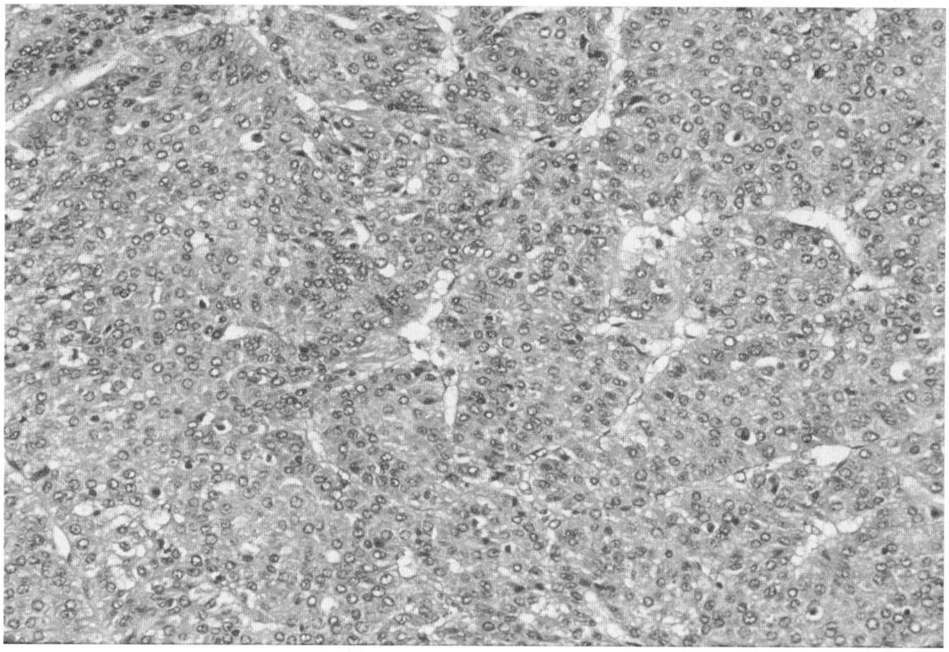

B

FIGURE 6.18. Hepatoma. (A) A large, partially encapsulated, multinodular hepatoma with areas of hemorrhage involving much of the right lobe (B). Microscopically, tumor cells are arranged in a tra-becullar pattern with broad plates, sometimes giving the impression of floating islands. (Courtesy of Linda D. Ferrell, MD.)

FIGURE 6.19. CT and MRI are the most commonly used techniques for imaging hepatoma. (A) CT scan of the liver of a patient with a known hepatoma in the right posterior portion of the liver (arrows) was obtained 70 sec after injection of intravenous contrast material. (B) The same area pictured 25 seconds after contrast injection not only shows the dominant lesion but three smaller lesions (arrows) in the left lobe that ruled out the option of performing resection in this patient. (C) The dual-phase CT scan is designed specifically to uncover vascular tumors. MRI is equally sensitive in detecting the large hepatoma (arrow). (Courtesy of Henry I. Goldberg, MD.)

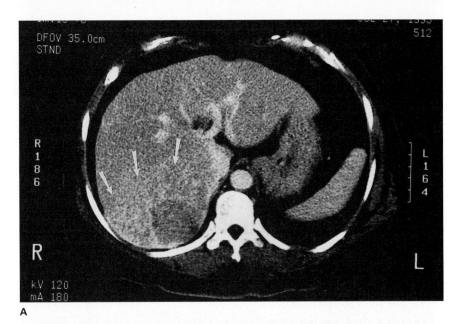

A

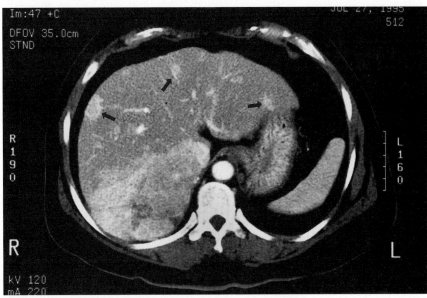

B

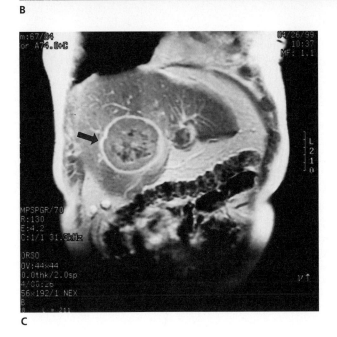

C

Types of hepatic resection

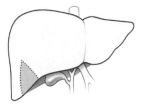
Wedge resection

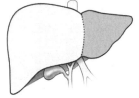
Left lateral segmentectomy

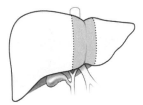
Left medial segmentectomy

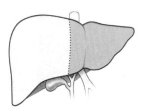
Total left hepatic lobectomy

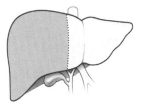
Right hepatic lobectomy

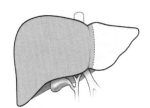
Extended right hepatectomy AKA trisegmentectomy

FIGURE 6.20. Hepatic resections. The type of liver resection performed depends on the type and extent of the pathology. (Adapted with permission from Schwartz SI, ed. Principles of Surgery. 6th ed. New York: McGraw-Hill, Inc., Health Professions Division, 1994.)

mentectomy, lobectomy, and trisegmentectomy (Figure 6.20). The selection of one approach over another depends on the type and extent of the pathology. The usual operations performed for HCC are hepatic lobectomy or trisegmentectomy:

Wedge resection. Benign tumors superficially located in the liver are amenable to wedge resection that involves removal of less than one segment of liver. The procedure usually requires little mobilization of the liver and no anatomic plane dissection. Resection is usually accomplished with electrocautery and bleeding controlled by heavy mattress sutures using #1 absorbable suture.

Segmentectomy. This operation requires anatomic plane dissection along the lines of Couinaud. The simplest segmental resection is *left lateral segmentectomy*, also known as *left hepatic lobectomy*. An alternate procedure, *left medial segmentectomy*, is a more complicated approach

requiring dissection along the main interlobar fissure in the right and left segmental fissure.

Hepatic lobectomy. In hepatic lobectomy, all liver tissue to one side of the main interlobar fissure is removed, either all tissue to the left in a *left hepatic lobectomy* or all tissue to the right in a *right hepatic lobectomy*. In either case, full mobilization of the liver is required (see below).

Trisegmentectomy. Also known as *extended right hepatectomy*, trisegmentectomy involves removing the right lobe as well as the medial segment of the left lobe. This procedure can be considered only when the hepatic parenchyma in the left lateral segment is normal.

TECHNIQUE OF LIVER RESECTION Several steps are involved in performing liver resection:

1. *Incision.* Either a long midline incision or a large right subcostal incision can be used. If necessary, either can be extended into medial sternotomy (Figure 6.21).

2. *Mobilization.* Key to major liver resection is adequate mobilization of the liver by dividing ligamentous attachments. The type of resection to be performed determines the degree of mobilization required (Figure 6.22).

3. *Portal dissection.* Dissection of the hepatoduodenal ligament allows accurate application of a noncrushing clamp, should the Pringle maneuver be required at any time in the course of the operation (Figure 6.23).

4. *Intraoperative ultrasound.* Intraoperative ultrasound provides precise identification of the size of the tumor and its relationship to major ducts and vessels, particularly the hepatic veins. Hence, resection margins and avoidance of the unintended hepatic venous injury can be planned before embarking on the parenchymal dissection.

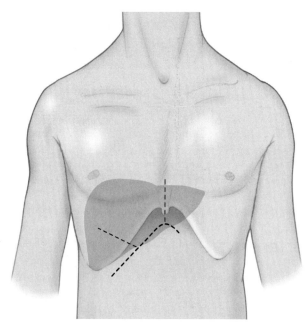

FIGURE 6.21. Surgical incision for liver resection. A modified chevron incision is often used. If necessary, the incision can be extended up into the chest, either as a median sternotomy or right lateral thoracotomy.

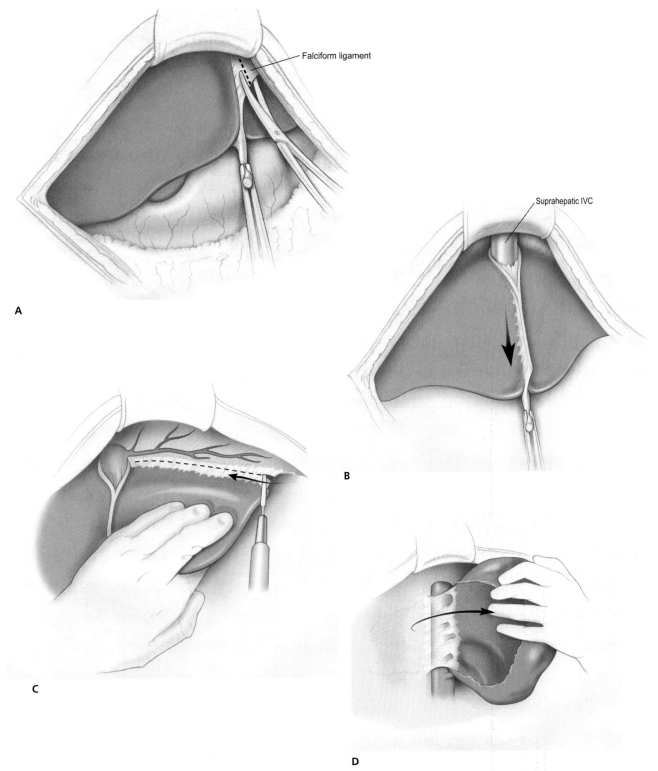

FIGURE 6.22. Mobilization of the liver. The extent to which the liver must be mobilized depends on the type of resection to be performed. (A–C) Trisegmentectomy requires complete liver mobilization, which involves division of the triangular and coronary ligaments, the ligamentum teres and the falciform ligament. (D) The liver is then rotated to the left and posterior attachments are dissected to expose the inferior vena cava and hepatic veins as they enter it. (Adapted from Blumgart LH, ed. Surgery of the Liver and Biliary Tract. 3rd ed. London: W.B. Saunders Company Ltd.; 2000.)

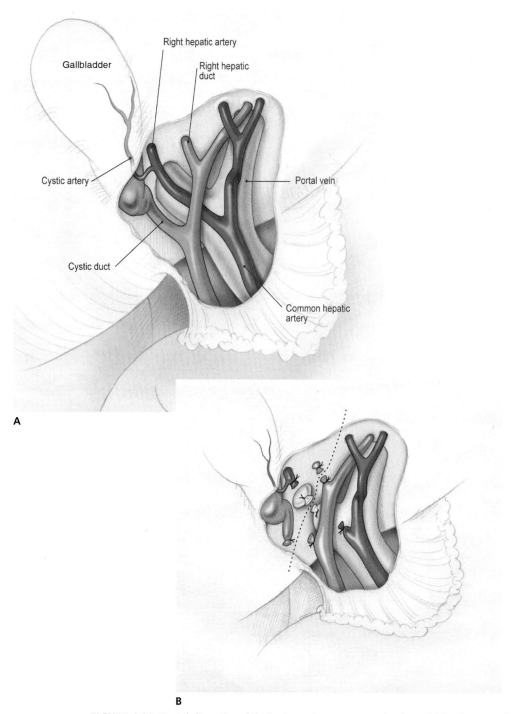

FIGURE 6.23. Portal dissection. (A) The hepatic artery, portal vein and bile duct are dissected in the hepatoduodenal ligament. (B) Dissection is carried to the liver parenchyma so that the right and left divisions of these structures can be identified and, if possible, encircled individually with tape before subsequent division between ligatures.

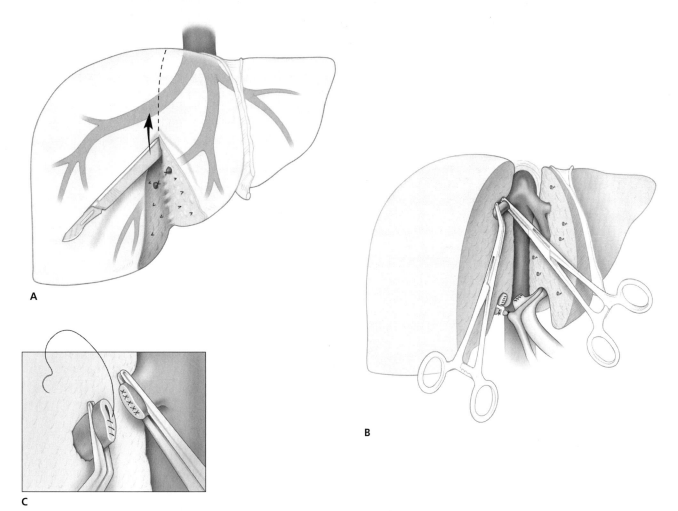

FIGURE 6.24. Parenchymal and hepatic vein dissection. (A) The relevant vascular structures in the porta hepatis are clamped and the liver capsule incised along the surgical plane with scalpel or electrocautery. The surgical plane is developed by blunt dissection using the scalpel handle or by finger fracture technique. Vessels and bile ductal structures are clamped as they are encountered and individually ligated (B). At the conclusion of the hepatic parenchymal division, the right, middle, and left hepatic veins can be isolated and the appropriate vein divided between vascular clamps and (C) the proximal end closed with continuous suture. (Adapted from Warren KW, Jenkins RL, Steele GD, Jr. Atlas of Surgery of the Liver, Pancreas and Biliary Tract. Norwalk, CT.: Appleton & Lange; 1991.)

5. *Parenchymal dissection* (Figure 6.24). Several other techniques may be used to aid in parenchymal dissection, including electrocautery, water-jet dissection, and ultrasonic dissector. The procedure described above uses the technique of *selective inflow control*. *Total inflow control* by the Pringle maneuver may also be used but requires inflow restoration for several minutes every half hour to avoid warm ischemic injury to the liver.

6. *Hepatic vein division.* The intrahepatic dissection is continued posteriorly until the major hepatic veins are identified. Those draining the portion of the liver to be removed are doubly ligated in continuity and divided; care must be taken not to damage the venous drainage of the portion of the liver that is to be left behind. Now, the portion of liver to be excised is completely freed and removed. At this point, any clamps previously applied on the vessels in the porta hepatis are unclamped and the cut surface of the liver examined for any bleeding. Bleeders are individually controlled and ligated. When all bleeding has stopped, the raw surface of liver is covered with omentum.

Another technique used for major hepatic resection is *total vascular isolation* of the liver, in which total inflow is controlled and the inferior vena cava is clamped below and above the liver. Total vascular isolation is safe for up to 60 minutes and is appropriate only for technically demanding cases in which hepatic vein dissection is complicated by pathology in that region of the liver.

7. *Drainage.* Two large closed sump drains are inserted, one posteriorly in the right subphrenic space and the other more anteriorly, close to the porta hepatis.

1. *Functional complications.* Patients who undergo 50% or more resection may develop metabolic complications:

a. *Hypoglycemia* may occur when the remaining liver cannot provide adequate glycogenolysis. It can be prevented by administering 10% glucose solution intravenously and frequently monitoring blood glucose levels.

b. *Hypoalbuminemia* may require administration of albumin but is rarely serious.

c. *Coagulopathy* may occur because of inadequate synthesis of prothrombin, fibrinogen, and factor ix. Prothrombin time should be monitored and vitamin K administered intravenously if prothrombin time is prolonged.

d. *Hyperbilirubinemia* and AST and LDH elevation may occur but are temporary and resolve in 3 to 5 days.

2. *Postoperative hemorrhage.* The incidence of hemorrhage is significantly reduced by ensuring meticulous hemostatis during the operation. Occasionally, significant postoperative bleeding requires control angiographically or with reoperation.

3. *Sepsis.* Subphrenic or perihepatic abscess may develop, causing fever and leukocytosis. These abscesses are usually successfully treated by percutaneous drainage.

4. *Stress ulcer.* Upper gastrointestinal bleeding from stress ulcer is now very rare because of the prophylactic use of histamine H_2-receptor antagonists and antacids.

Total Hepatectomy and Liver Transplantation

Liver transplantation is emerging as a viable option in patients with lesions of less than 5 cm in size, three or fewer lesions, and with associated cirrhosis, which renders partial hepatectomy risky. Recently reported studies indicate 5-year survival of 19% to 70%.[16] Favorable prognostic factors are tumor size of 5 cm or less, unicentric tumors, absence of vascular invasions, presence of pseudocapsulae, and low histologic grade. In one report by Mazzaferro et al.,[17] the 4-year survival for single nodules less than 5 cm or fewer than three nodules each less than 3 cm in size was 92%.

Palliative Therapy

When curative resection or transplantation are not possible a number of palliative therapeutic modalities are available.

1. Transarterial chemoembolization with doxorubicin may be helpful because the blood supply of HCC is derived from the hepatic artery. A 1-year survival rate of 40% to 50% has been achieved.[18]
2. Hepatic artery ligation can be performed to produce tumor necrosis and may be combined with chemoembolization.

3. Percutaneous ethanol injection may lead to partial regression.
4. Cryosurgery with liquid nitrogen may help shrink the tumor.
5. Systemic chemotherapy is particularly useful in children with hepatoblastoma, in which subsequent resection might achieve very high cure rates of 80% to 90%.[19]

CHOLANGIOCARCINOMA

The incidence of cholangiocarcinoma in patients is about 5% of the incidence of HCC. Its incidence is much higher in areas of the world where chronic infestation of liver flukes (*Clonorchis sinensis* and *Opisthorchis viverrini*) occurs in the biliary tree (i.e., Thailand, Hong Kong, and Canton Province of China). Other conditions associated with cholangiocarcinoma are sclerosing cholangitis and α_1-antitrypsin deficiency. While the symptoms and signs are similar to those of HCC, jaundice is more common and more severe. The picture is one of progressive obstructive jaundice.

Investigations

Liver function studies show a mixture of obstructive and hepatocellular abnormality. AFP is infrequently elevated. CT and ultrasound show the tumor. Hepatic angiography reveals a tumor that is not hypervascular, and the branches of the hepatic artery are diminished in number and size because of the associated fibrosis that occurs. Endoscopic retrograde cholangiopancreatography (ERCP) or transhepatic cholangiography are useful localizing techniques.

Treatment

Resection is rarely possible because the lesion is diagnosed late. Similarly, the tumor is unresponsive to radiotherapy or chemotherapy. Resection of hilar tumors is discussed separately in Chapter 7.

METASTATIC NEOPLASMS OF THE LIVER

The liver is a common site for metastatic cancer. Metastatic cancer accounts for 95% of all neoplasms in the liver. The liver represents the first hematogenous filter of tumor cells spread from abdominal organs via the portal vein. Thus, it is a frequent site of metastasis from the pancreas, stomach, and small and large intestine. Secondary spread to the liver can also occur via the systemic circulation, and common primary tumors that metastasize there are breast, lung, kidney, ovary, and uterus.

The clinical picture is usually dominated by that of the primary neoplasm. Since liver metastasis represents advanced malignancy, patients frequently exhibit weight loss, anorexia, and fatigue. The liver lesions, however, may be painful and become palpable on abdominal examination. Jaundice is a rare symptom.

Investigations

Abnormal liver function is seen in more than 50% of patients. Elevated alkaline phosphatase is more common than elevated bilirubin levels. CT, ultrasound, or MRI will show the lesion. MRI is the superior imaging modality because it provides information about venous invasion. Needle biopsy can be obtained under CT or ultrasound guidance, at laparoscopy, or laparotomy.

Treatment

In ninety percent of patients with liver metastases, the disease will have spread to other organs. Only nonsurgical palliative therapy can be offered to these patients. In some, presence of multiple lesions precludes surgical treatment, and in others, the known aggressive biological behavior of the primary makes consideration of surgical treatment of liver secondaries futile. Hence, secondaries from the esophagus, stomach, pancreas, lung, and usually breast and liver are not considered for surgical extirpation.

Patients with colorectal primary neoplasms have been shown to benefit most from resection of hepatic metastasis. Even here, fewer than 5% of patients are candidates for liver resection. Patients who should be considered for removal of hepatic secondaries include those with:

1. No extrahepatic disease.
2. A single metastatic tumor or not more than three or four lesions.
3. A time lapse of 1 year from colectomy or proctectomy.
4. Duke B stage of primary tumor.

Other patients who may be candidates for resection of hepatic metastases are those with carcinoid syndrome and other neuroendocrine tumors. Hepatic resection may be limited to wedge resection or may involve hepatic lobectomy (see Figure 6.20).

Outcome

Some 25% of patients with colorectal cancer who meet the criteria for resection of hepatic metastasis will live 5 years after resection.[20] Patients who undergo palliative liver resection for the carcinoid syndrome or for other malignant neuroendocrine tumors (e.g., VIPoma, insulinoma) experience significant improvement of their symptoms and are more successfully managed postoperatively pharmacologically with octreotide.

REFERENCES

1. Couinaud C. Controlled hepatectomies and exposure of the intrahepatic bile ducts: anatomical and technical study. Paris, France: self-published; 1981.
2. Iwatsuki S, Stieber AC, Marsh JW, et al. Liver transplantation for fulminant hepatic failure. *Transplant Proc* 1989;21(1 Pt 2): 2431–2434.
3. Matloff DS. Treatment of acute variceal bleeding. *Gastroenterol Clin North Am* 1992;21:103–118.
4. D'Amico G, Pagliaro L, Bosch J. The treatment of portal hypertension: a meta-analytic review. *Hepatology* 1995;22:332–354.
5. Hwang SJ, Lin HC, Chang CF, et al. A randomized controlled trial comparing octreotide and vasopressin in the control of acute esophageal variceal bleeding. *J Hepatol* 1992;16:320–325.
6. Panes J, Teres J, Bosch J, et al. Efficacy of balloon tamponade in treatment of bleeding gastric and esophageal varices. Results in 151 consecutive episodes. *Dig Dis Sci* 1988;33:454–459.
7. Crecelius SA, Soulen MC. Transjugular intrahepatic portosystemic shunts for portal hypertension. *Gastroenterol Clin North Am* 1995;24:201–219.
8. Fillmore DJ, Miller FJ, Fox LF, et al. Transjugular intrahepatic portosystemic shunt: midterm clinical and angiographic follow-up. *J Vasc Interv Radiol* 1996;7:255–261.
9. Orloff MJ, Orloff MS, Orloff SL, et al. Three decades of experience with emergency portacaval shunt for acutely bleeding esophageal varices in 400 unselected patients with cirrhosis of the liver. *J Am Coll Surg* 1995;180:257–272.
10. Henderson JM, Barnes DS, Geisinger MA. Portal hypertension. *Curr Probl Surg* 1998;35:379–452.
11. Stiegmann GV, Goff JS, Michaletz-Onody PA, et al. Endoscopic sclerotherapy as compared with endoscopic ligation for bleeding esophageal varices. *N Engl J Med* 1992;326:1527–1532.
12. Langer B, Taylor BR, Mackenzie DR, et al. Further report of a prospective randomized trial comparing distal splenorenal shunt with end-to-side portacaval shunt. An analysis of encephalopathy, survival, and quality of life. *Gastroenterology* 1985;88:424–429.
13. Rikkers LF, Sorrell WT, Jin G. Which portosystemic shunt is best? *Gastroenterol Clin North Am* 1992;21:179–196.
14. Stanley MM, Ochi S, Lee KK, et al. Peritoneovenous shunting as compared with medical treatment in patients with alcoholic cirrhosis and massive ascites. Veterans Administration Cooperative Study on Treatment of Alcoholic Cirrhosis with Ascites. *N Engl J Med* 1989;321:1632–1638.
15. Lai EC, Fan ST, Lo CM, et al. Hepatic resection for hepatocellular carcinoma. An audit of 343 patients. *Ann Surg* 1995;221: 291–298.
16. Simonetti RG, Liberati A, Angiolini C, et al. Treatment of hepatocellular carcinoma: a systematic review of randomized controlled trials. *Ann Oncol* 1997;8:117–136.
17. Mazzaferro V, Regalia E, Doci R, et al. Liver transplantation for the treatment of small hepatocellular carcinomas in patients with cirrhosis. *N Engl J Med* 1996;334:693–699.
18. Liu CL, Fan ST. Nonresectional therapies for hepatocellular carcinoma. *Am J Surg* 1997;173:358–365.
19. Reynolds M, Douglass EC, Finegold M, et al. Chemotherapy can convert unresectable hepatoblastoma. *J Pediatr Surg* 1992;27: 1080–1084.

20. Ohlsson B, Stenram U, Tranberg KG. Resection of colorectal liver metastases: 25-year experience. *World J Surg* 1998;22: 268–277.

SELECTED READINGS

Anatomy

Bismuth H. Surgical anatomy and anatomical surgery of the liver. *World J Surg* 1982;6:3–9.

Couinaud C. Surgical anatomy of the liver. Several new aspects. *Chirurgie* 1986;112:337–342.

Physiology

Dixon JL, Ginsberg HN. Hepatic synthesis of lipoproteins and apolipoproteins. *Semin Liver Dis* 1992;12:364–372.

Mammen EF. Coagulation defects in liver disease. *Med Clin North Am* 1994;78:545–554.

Meier PJ. Molecular mechanisms of hepatic bile salt transport from sinusoidal blood into bile. *Am J Physiol* 1995;269(6 Pt 1): G801–G812.

Nathanson MH, Boyer JL. Mechanisms and regulation of bile secretion. *Hepatology* 1991;14:551–566.

Pilkis SJ, Granner DK. Molecular physiology of the regulation of hepatic gluconeogenesis and glycolysis. *Annu Rev Physiol* 1992;54:885–909.

Rothschild MA, Oratz M, Schreiber SS. Serum albumin. *Hepatology* 1988;8:385–401.

Steer CJ. Liver regeneration. *FASEB J* 1995;9:1396–1400.

Portal Hypertension

Collins JC, Rypins EB, Sarfeh IJ. Narrow-diameter portacaval shunts for management of variceal bleeding. *World J Surg* 1994;18: 211–215.

Klein AS, Sitzmann JV, Coleman J, et al. Current management of the Budd–Chiari syndrome. *Ann Surg* 1990;212:144–149.

Langer B, Taylor BR, Mackenzie DR, et al. Further report of a prospective randomized trial comparing distal splenorenal shunt with end-to-side portacaval shunt. An analysis of encephalopathy, survival, and quality of life. *Gastroenterology* 1985;88: 424–429.

Millikan WJ Jr, Warren WD, Henderson JM, et al. The Emory prospective randomized trial: selective versus nonselective shunt to control variceal bleeding. Ten year follow-up. *Ann Surg* 1985;201:712–722.

Patch D, Sabin CA, Goulis J, et al. A randomized, controlled trial of medical therapy versus endoscopic ligation for the prevention of variceal rebleeding in patients with cirrhosis. *Gastroenterology* 2002;123:1013–1019.

Resnick RH, Chalmers TC, Ishihara AM, et al. A controlled study of the prophylactic portacaval shunt. A final report. *Ann Intern Med* 1969;70:675–688.

Rikkers LF, Jin G. Emergency shunt. Role in the present management of variceal bleeding. *Arch Surg* 1995;130:472–477.

Stanley MM, Ochi S, Lee KK, et al. Peritoneovenous shunting as compared with medical treatment in patients with alcoholic cirrhosis and massive ascites. Veterans Administration Cooperative Study on Treatment of Alcoholic Cirrhosis with Ascites. *N Engl J Med* 1989;321:1632–1638.

Terblanche J, Kahn D, Bornman PC. Long-term injection sclerotherapy treatment for esophageal varices. A 10-year prospective evaluation. *Ann Surg* 1989;210:725–731.

Liver Abscess

Donovan AJ, Yellin AE, Ralls PW. Hepatic abscess. *World J Surg* 1991;15:162–169.

Huang CJ, Pitt HA, Lipsett PA, et al. Pyogenic hepatic abscess. Changing trends over 42 years. *Ann Surg* 1996;223:600–609.

Echinococcus (Hydatid) Cyst

Khuroo MS, Wani NA, Javid G, et al. Percutaneous drainage compared with surgery for hepatic hydatid cysts. *N Engl J Med* 1997;337:881–887.

Lewall DB. Hydatid disease: biology, pathology, imaging and classification. *Clin Radiol* 1998;53:863–874.

Xynos E, Pechlivanides G, Tzortzinis A, et al. Hydatid disease of the liver. Diagnosis and surgical treatment. *HPB Surg* 1991;4: 59–67.

Benign Neoplasms of the Liver

Belli L, De Carlis L, Beati C, et al. Surgical treatment of symptomatic giant hemangiomas of the liver. *Surg Gynecol Obstet* 1992;174: 474–478.

Ishak KG, Rabin L. Benign tumors of the liver. *Med Clin North Am* 1975;59:995–1013.

Lise M, Feltrin G, Da Pian PP, et al. Giant cavernous hemangiomas: diagnosis and surgical strategies. *World J Surg* 1992;16:516–520.

Ros PR, Li KC. Benign liver tumors. *Curr Probl Diagn Radiol* 1989;18:125–155.

Shortell CK, Schwartz SI. Hepatic adenoma and focal nodular hyperplasia. *Surg Gynecol Obstet* 1991;173:426–431.

Hepatocellular Carcinoma and Cholangiocarcinoma

DeMatteo RP, Fong Y, Blumgart LH. Surgical treatment of malignant liver tumours. *Baillieres Best Pract Res Clin Gastroenterol* 1999;13:557–574.

Dmitrewski J, El-Gazzaz G, McMaster P. Hepatocellular cancer: resection or transplantation. *J Hepatobiliary Pancreat Surg* 1998; 5:18–23.

Gores GJ. Early detection and treatment of cholangiocarcinoma. *Liver Transpl* 2000;6(6 Suppl 2):S30–S34.

Khan SA, Davidson BR, Goldin R, et al. Guidelines for the diagnosis and treatment of cholangiocarcinoma: consensus document. *Gut* 2002;51 Suppl 6:VI1–9.

Lau WY, Leow CK, Li AK. Hepatocellular carcinoma. *Br J Hosp Med* 1997;57:101–104.

Nagorney DM, Gigot JF. Primary epithelial hepatic malignancies: etiology, epidemiology, and outcome after subtotal and total hepatic resection. *Surg Oncol Clin North Am* 1996;5:283–300.

Nair S, Shiv Kumar K, Thuluvath PJ, et al. Mortality from hepatocellular and biliary cancers: changing epiderniological trends. *Am J Gastroenterol* 2002;97:167–171, Erratum in: *Am J Gastroenterol* 2002;97:2484, *Am J Gastroenterol* 2002;97:1280.

Sakon M, Nagano H, Nakamori S, et al. Intrahepatic recurrences of hepatocellular carcinoma after hepatectomy: analysis based on tumor hemodynamics. *Arch Surg* 2002;137:94–99.

Slakey DP. Radiofrequency ablation of recurrent cholangiocarcinoma. *Am Surg* 2002;68:395–397.

Tsao JI, DeSanctis J, Rossi RL, et al. Hepatic malignancies. *Surg Clin North Am* 2000;80:603–632.

Varnholt H, Weimann A, Wittekind C, et al. Intrahepatic cholangiocarcinoma. *J Am Coll Surg* 2002;194:550–551.

Metastatic Neoplasms of the Liver

Cady B, Stone MD, McDermott WV Jr, et al. Technical and biological factors in disease-free survival after hepatic resection for colorectal cancer metastases. *Arch Surg* 1992;127:561–569.

Langer B, Gallinger S. The management of metastatic carcinoma in the liver. *Adv Surg* 1995;28:113–132.

Registry of Hepatic Metastases. Resection of the liver for colorectal carcinoma metastases: a multi-institutional study of indications for resection. *Surgery* 1988;103:278–288.

Hepatic Resection

Bismuth H, Dennison AR. Segmental liver resection. *Adv Surg* 1993;26:189–208.

Emre S, Schwartz ME, Katz E, et al. Liver resection under total vascular isolation. Variations on a theme. *Ann Surg* 1993;217:15–19.

Fan ST, Lo CM, Liu CL, et al. Hepatectomy for hepatocellular carcinoma: toward zero hospital deaths. *Ann Surg* 1999;229:322–330.

Launois B, Jamieson GG. The importance of Glisson's capsule and its sheaths in the intrahepatic approach to resection of the liver. *Surg Gynecol Obstet* 1992;174:7–10.

Taniguchi H, Takahashi T, Shioaki Y, et al. Vascular inflow exclusion and hepatic resection. *Br J Surg* 1992;79:672–675.

7

Biliary Tract

Management of biliary tract disease constitutes an important segment of gastrointestinal surgery. Patients recovering from biliary tract surgery once accounted for a significant number of inpatients on the surgical wards. The advent of minimally invasive surgery and advances in both interventional endoscopy and interventional radiology has changed all this. Following laparoscopic cholecystectomy and endoscopic sphincterotomy and removal of common duct stones, most patients now are admitted for only 24 to 48 h or need not be admitted at all. Nonetheless, the incidence of biliary tract surgery has not decreased.

EMBRYOLOGY AND ANATOMY

The biliary tree and liver develop from a diverticulum of the embryonic foregut at approximately 18 days of gestation. Between the fourth and fifth weeks, the diverticulum consists of a solid cranial portion and a hollow caudal portion. The solid cranial portion differentiates into the liver with the development of hepatocytes and intrahepatic bile ducts, while the hollow caudal portion gives rise to the gallbladder, the extrahepatic bile ducts, and the ventral pancreas (Figure 7.1).

GALLBLADDER

In the adult, variability in the anatomy of the biliary tree is more the norm than the exception. The gallbladder (GB) is a pear-shaped organ (50 ml volume) consisting of the fundus, corpus, infundibulum, and neck, which tapers into the cystic duct. Its wall is made up of smooth muscle encased in fibrous tissue. The mucosa is made up of columnar epithelial cells with tight junctions and microvilli suited for absorption. The cystic duct connects the GB to the common bile duct (CBD) and contains the spiral valve of Heuser, which provides a measure of resistance to outward flow.

COMMON BILE DUCT

The left and right hepatic ducts form the common hepatic duct. The cystic duct entrance into the common hepatic duct represents the beginning of the CBD, which then runs inferiorly toward the duodenum in the free edge of the lesser omentum to the right of the hepatic artery and anterior to the portal vein. The CBD passes behind the first part of the duodenum and then courses within the pancreas to enter the second part of the duodenum. The CBD is about 7 cm long and less than 1 cm wide when assessed intraoperatively with the naked eye or with a choledochogram. When seen by ultrasonography, however, normal CBD width should be less than 0.7 cm. The mucosa is cuboidal epithelium, and the wall of the CBD is fibrous tissue with small amounts of smooth muscle.

CHOLEDOCHAL SPHINCTER COMPLEX OR SPHINCTER OF ODDI

The entrance of the CBD into the second portion of the duodenum is oblique and surrounded by the choledochal sphincter complex, which controls bile flow into the duodenum in a manner that is coordinated with GB contraction. The choledochal sphincter complex or sphincter of Oddi (Figure 7.2) is composed of several portions:

1. The choledochal sphincter, comprised of a compact area of circular muscle around the intramural part of the duct.
2. The pancreatic duct sphincter, present in about one-third of individuals.

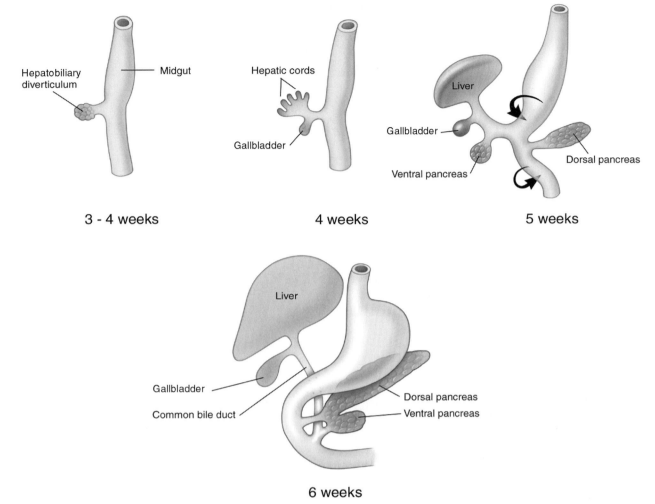

Hepatobiliary diverticulum — Midgut

3 - 4 weeks

Hepatic cords

Gallbladder

4 weeks

Liver

Gallbladder

Ventral pancreas

Dorsal pancreas

5 weeks

Liver

Gallbladder

Common bile duct

Dorsal pancreas

Ventral pancreas

6 weeks

FIGURE 7.1. Embryologic development of the biliary tree.

3. The sphincter of the ampulla, the grouping of longitudinal and circular muscles around the ampulla of Vater.
4. The duodenal wall surrounding the intramural CBD.

ANOMALIES OF THE BILIARY TREE

Gallbladder

Congenital absence of the GB is rare (0.03% in autopsy studies). Also rare are the duplication of the GB with single or double cystic duct, a GB that is abnormal in location, and a left-sided GB. Not uncommonly, it is partially intrahepatic and completely intrahepatic in rare cases.

Cystic Duct

In three out of four individuals, the cystic duct enters the CBD at right angles. In the remainder, it may run parallel to the CBD for variable distances or enter the CBD on the left by passing either in front of or behind it (Figure 7.3).

Ducts of Luschka

Small bile ducts may drain directly from the liver into the GB. The significance of these ducts of Luschka lies in their ability to cause postcholecystectomy bile leak or biloma if they are unrecognized and not ligated.

Common Bile Duct

Congenital cystic anomalies may affect the entire biliary tract. These rare anomalies are of three types:

1. Cystic dilation of the entire CBD (choledochal cyst).
2. Localized cystic malformation of a portion of the CBD, usually distally.
3. Diffuse fusiform dilation of the CBD.

Biliary Atresia

Congenital biliary atresia involves both the intra- and extrahepatic biliary tree. It is estimated to occur in

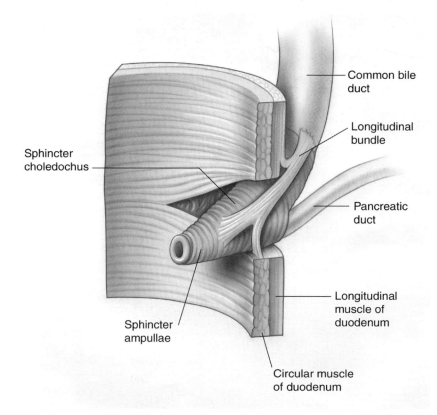

Common bile
duct

Longitudinal
bundle

Pancreatic
duct

Sphincter
choledochus

Longitudinal
muscle of
duodenum

Sphincter
ampullae

Circular muscle
of duodenum

FIGURE 7.2. Anatomy of the choledochal sphincter. The complex structure of the choledochal sphincter is made up of the choledochal sphincter, the pancreatic duct sphincter, the sphincter of the ampulla, and the duodenal wall surrounding the intramural common bile duct. (Adapted from Netter FH. Icon Learning Systems Atlas of Human Anatomy, Ciba-Geigy, 1989. All rights reserved.)

1:20,000 live births and is associated with malformations in other organs.

Blood Supply

The GB is supplied by the cystic artery, a branch of the right hepatic artery in 95% of individuals and located in the triangle of Calot. Rarely, the cystic artery may originate from the gastroduodenal artery. There may also be two cystic arteries, with one often originating from the right hepatic and the other from the left hepatic or gastroduodenal artery (Figure 7.4).

Nerve Supply

The GB receives extrinsic innervation from both the sympathetic and the vagus nerves. Sympathetic innervation is from the celiac axis and distributed on the adventitia of arteries. Vagal innervation is largely from the hepatic branches of the right vagus, but some vagal innervation is also distributed in the gastrohepatic omentum from the celiac axis. The vagal fibers are cholinergic and peptidergic. The intrinsic innervation (analogous to the enteric nervous system) is a network of nerves in the wall of the gall bladder that utilize a variety of neurotransmitters, chief among which are cholinergic and peptidergic.

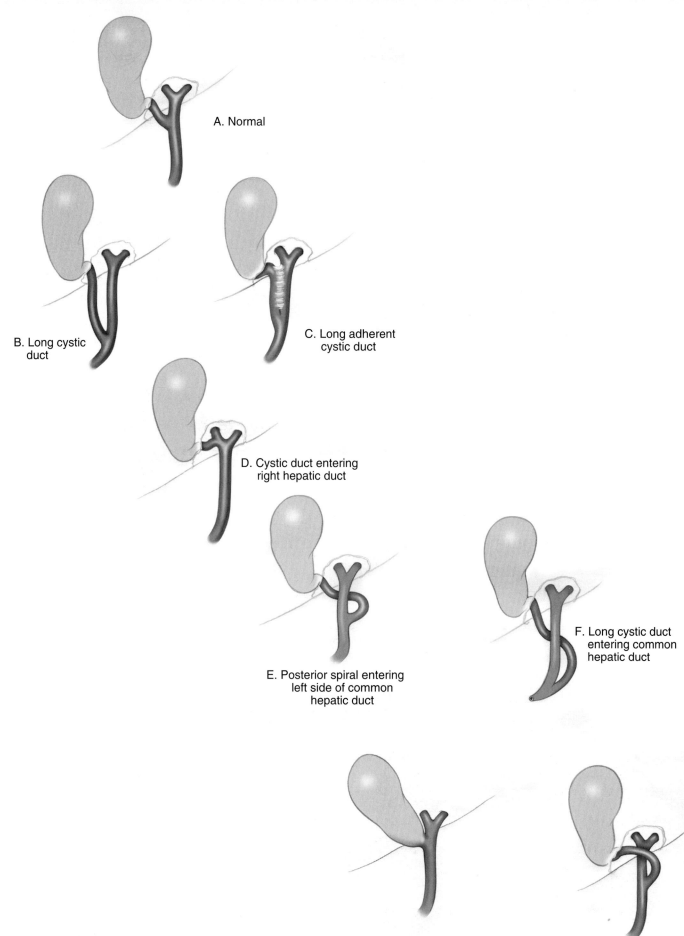

A. Normal

B. Long cystic duct

C. Long adherent cystic duct

D. Cystic duct entering right hepatic duct

E. Posterior spiral entering left side of common hepatic duct

F. Long cystic duct entering common hepatic duct

G. Absent cystic duct

H. Anterior spiral entering common hepatic duct on left side

FIGURE 7.3. (A–H) Congenital abnormalities of the cystic duct. (Adapted with permission from Schwartz SI: Principles of Surgery. New York: McGraw-Hill, 1994:1369.)

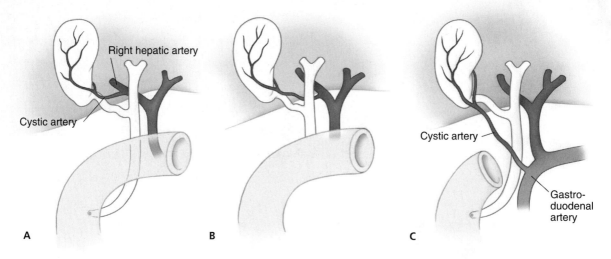

Right hepatic artery origin

Gastroduodenal artery origin

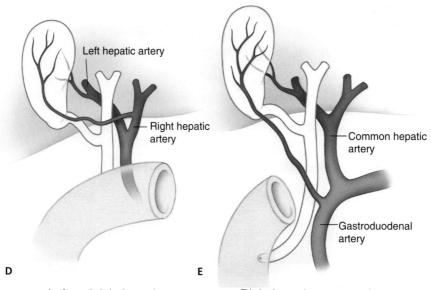

Left and right hepatic
artery origins

Right hepatic artery and
gastroduodenal artery origins

FIGURE 7.4. (A–E) Anomalies of the cystic artery.

PHYSIOLOGY

GALLBLADDER

The gallbladder has absorptive, secretory, and motor functions.

Absorption

Bilirubin metabolism and bile formation have been described in detail in Chapter 5. Bile flows from the liver into the extrahepatic ducts. With the choledochal sphincter contracted, bile is directed into the GB via the cystic duct. The main functions of the GB in this regard are to store and concentrate bile during fasting for delivery to the CBD and to the duodenum on demand during eating. The gallbladder's capacity is 40 to 50 ml, but the liver produces about 600 ml of bile daily. Because of the significant absorptive ability of the GB, biliary pressure is kept low. The GB concentrates bile tenfold by absorbing sodium chloride and water. The mechanism of absorption across the GB mucosa is due to electroneutral sodium-coupled chloride transport.

Secretion

The GB secrets mucus at about 20 ml/h. In hydrops of the GB, this colorless secretion comprises white bile.

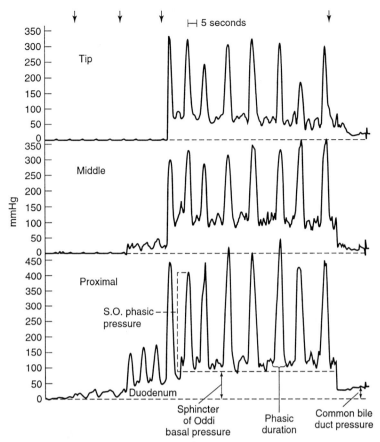

FIGURE 7.5. Manometric profile of the sphincter of Oddi obtained during station pullthrough tracing of a triple-lumen catheter. (Adapted from Feldman M, Sleisenger MH, Scharschmidt BF, eds. Schlesinger & Fordtran's Gastrointestinal and Liver Disease: Pathophysiology, Diagnosis, and Management, 6th ed. Philadelphia, PA: WB Saunders, 1998:933, with permission from Elsevier Science.)

Motor Function

During fasting, the GB does not simply fill up passively, but undergoes rhythmic contractions that exchange concentrated bile with dilute bile. During eating, however, the GB undergoes major contraction coordinated with relaxation of the sphincter of Oddi, thus delivering into the duodenum concentrated bile required for digestion. The major stimulus for gallbladder contraction is the hormone cholecystokinin (CCK), released from the duodenum by the stimulation of fat and acid. The contractile action of CCK on GB muscle appears to be mediated through activation of intrinsic cholinergic neurons. Other mediators of GB contraction are cholinergic reflexes (antrocholecystic, enterocholecystic) and the intestinal peptide motilin.

Relaxation of the GB muscle is mediated through VIP and nitric oxide.

CHOLEDOCHAL SPHINCTER OR SPHINCTER OF ODDI

Manometric studies in humans show a 5-mm zone of resting high pressure that is 5 to 10 mm Hg greater than CBD pressure. On top of this resting pressure, phasic, high-pressure antegrade contractions occur (Figure 7.5). Bile flow into the duodenum requires relaxation of the sphincter of Oddi, which is mediated via VIP and nitric oxide. CCK, cholinergic stimulation, and glucagon also relax the sphincter.

PATHOPHYSIOLOGY

GALLSTONE FORMATION

Gallstones are the most common cause of biliary tract disease. Gallstones are composed of cholesterol, bilirubin, and calcium. Gallstones in the West are primarily choles-

terol stones. Pigment stones are often associated with hemolytic disease and are prevalent in areas endemic to hemolytic anemia and malaria. The major factors involved in gallstone formation are listed in Table 7.1.

Cholesterol Stones

Cholesterol and other lipids in the bile are not water soluble but have to be kept solubilized to prevent them from deposition as stone. The ingenious mechanism of solubilization depends on transporting cholesterol in the lipophilic core of micelles. The structure of a micelle is shown in Figure 7.6. Bile salts and lecithin are amphoteric and aggregate to form a lipophilic core that carries cholesterol, while their water-soluble ends are arranged peripherally at the circumference of the micelle. The maximal ability of the micelles to carry cholesterol is called the critical micellar concentration (Figure 7.7). When the critical micellar concentration is exceeded, a metastable phase is reached at which cholesterol does not precipitate due to vesicular phase in bile. Beyond this, cholesterol molecules precipitate by first aggregating together and then forming crystals. A high calcium content in the bile favors cholesterol precipitation. Cholesterol supersaturated bile from patients with gallstones forms cholesterol crystals more easily than that from individuals with no gallstones. This observation suggests that other substances (e.g., apo-AI, mucus, and other bile proteins) also play a role in gallstone formation.

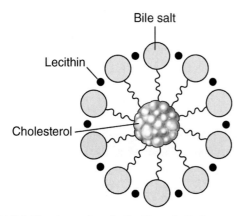

FIGURE 7.6. Structure of a micelle. The micelle is an aggregation of bile salts and lecithin with a lypophyllic core that carries the water-insoluble cholesterol.

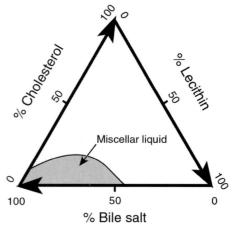

FIGURE 7.7. Tricoordinate phase diagram for determination of cholesterol saturation index. The shaded area represents micellar liquid in which cholesterol remains solubilized. Beyond this, cholesterol molecules precipitate to form crystals.

In addition to cholesterol saturation, other conditions that favor gallstone formation include stasis, bacterial infection, rate of water and electrolyte absorption, estrogen therapy, and pregnancy.

Pigment Stones

Pigment stones account for 10% to 25% of gallstones in the U.S.[1] They are black in appearance, composed primarily of calcium bilirubinate, and 50% of them are radiopaque. The incidence of pigment stones is high in Japan and in countries endemic to malaria and hemolytic diseases.[1] Primary choledocholithiasis is usually due to pigment stones. The major event in the formation of pigment stones is an increase in unconjugated bilirubin in the bile. An important factor is the presence of bacteria, which deconjugate bilirubin using the enzyme β-glucosidase, phospholipase A, and others. Pigment stones contain bacteria or bacterial skeletons in 90% of cases. Other factors in bile that favor deconjugation are the presence of calcium carbonate and phosphate, suggesting defective alkalinization of bile.

BILIARY COLIC

Attacks of colicky right-upper quadrant (RUQ) pain, often radiating to the right infrascapular region, are caused by intermittent obstruction of the cystic duct by a gallstone. This clinical syndrome is the most common manifestation of gallstones. The attack often follows ingestion of food, which contracts the gallbladder and impacts a stone in the cystic duct. The cystic duct obstruction is temporary, lasting from a few minutes to several hours, and is roughly coincident with the duration of pain. Presumably, the stone falls back into the gallbladder, relieving the obstruction. Because no significant inflammatory process ensues, tachycardia, fever, or leukocytosis are uncommon. Simi-

TABLE 7.2. Spectrum of Clinical Pathology in Cholecystitis

Acute Cholecystitis
  Acalculous
  Calculous
   ▪ Nonperforated
   ▪ Perforated
       Localized: Pericholecystic abscess
       Free: Bile peritonitis
   ▪ Cholecystenteric fistula: Gallstone ileus
   ▪ Empyema
   ▪ Emphysematous

Chronic Cholecystitis
  Uncomplicated
  Mucocele

larly, jaundice or significant liver dysfunction does not occur.

CHOLECYSTITIS

Cholecystitis or inflammation of the gallbladder has many forms. The spectrum of clinical pathology is summarized in Table 7.2.

Acute Calculous Cholecystitis

Acute cholecystitis usually results from a gallstone impacted in Hartmann's pouch, obstructing the neck of the GB. The result is distension of the gallbladder, resulting in concentration of bile, which causes subserosal inflammation with edema and thickening of the GB wall.

Mucosal hemorrhage and ulceration are common. The obstructing stone and ensuing inflammation may also cause ischemic necrosis of the neck of the GB and may result in thrombosis of the cystic artery, leading to gangrenous cholecystitis. The process is almost always complicated by secondary bacterial infection. Transmural necrosis may lead to perforation and pericholecystic abscess (Figure 7.8). Free perforation and bile peritonitis are rare but may occur in the immunocompromised patient. Rarely, the gallstone in Hartmann's pouch may erode into adjacent bowel, usually the duodenum, to cause cholecystoenteric fistula and gallstone-induced small bowel obstruction (gallstone ileus).

The local inflammatory process is accompanied by systemic manifestations including tachycardia, fever, and leukocytosis. Jaundice and mild liver dysfunction occur infrequently. Hyperbilirubinemia is always mild (<3 mg%).

Empyema of the Gallbladder

Occasionally, the GB lumen becomes filled with frank pus (Figure 7.9). The patient becomes acutely toxic, with spiking high fever, chills, and marked leukocytosis. Why some patients develop empyema as a complication of acute cholecystitis is unknown.

Acute Emphysematous Cholecystitis

This is a rare form of acute cholecystitis in which anaerobic infection of the GB develops, causing formation of gas

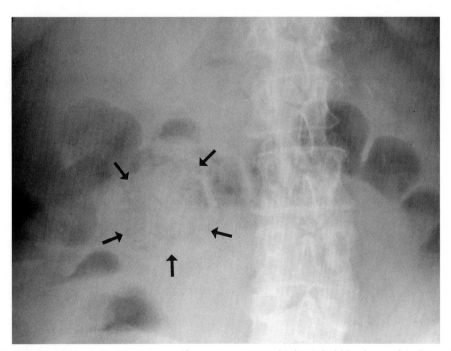

FIGURE 7.8. Pericholecystic abscess is manifest on x-ray as multiple air bubbles (arrows) indicating air both within and surrounding the inflamed gallbladder. (Courtesy of Henry I. Goldberg, MD.)

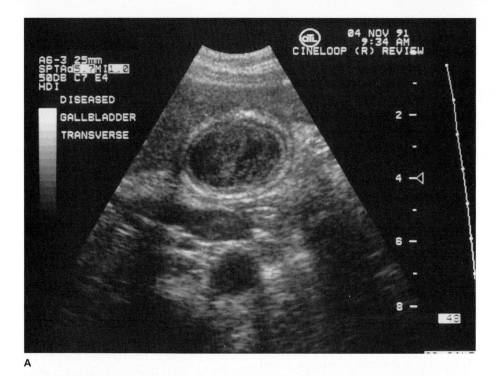

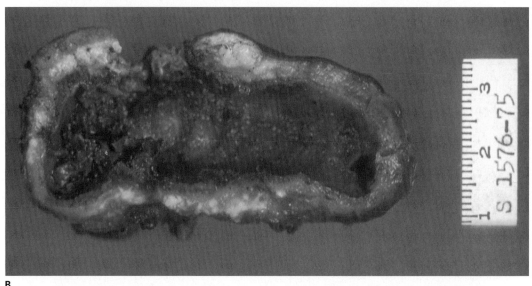

FIGURE 7.9. Empyema of the gallbladder. (A) The ultrasound shows complex echoes within the gall-bladder caused by the presence of pus and a greatly thickened wall due to acute cholecystitis. (B) The gross cut section of empyema demonstrates distention with pus and marked thickening of the wall. (Courtesy of Linda D. Ferrell, M.D., and Henry I. Goldberg, MD.)

within the lumen and gallbladder wall (Figure 7.10). This complication is more likely to occur in patients with diabetes. The anaerobic bacteria involved may be clostridia, anaerobic streptococci, or gas-forming *Escherichia coli.*

Acute Acalculous Cholecystitis

Approximately 5% of patients with acute cholecystitis have no gallstones. This condition is frequently associated with other major systemic insults resulting from multiple trauma, sepsis, major burn, or multiple organ failure.

Acalculous cholecystitis may also occur postoperatively, usually immediately upon the resumption of oral feeding. The exact pathophysiological mechanisms are unknown. The hypotheses include hypoperfusion or ischemia of the GB and primary bacterial invasion (*Escherichia coli,* clostridia and rarely *Salmonella typhi*). In postoperative patients and in those on TPN with prolonged fast, sludge is often found within the lumen. It is possible that in these cases of prolonged stasis, contraction of the GB leads to obstruction of the cystic duct from accumulated sludge. The essential features are summarized in Table 7.3.

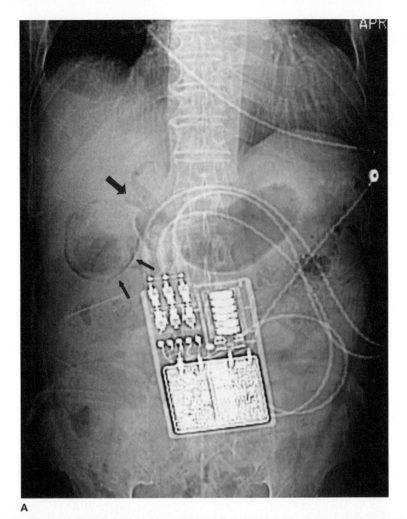

A

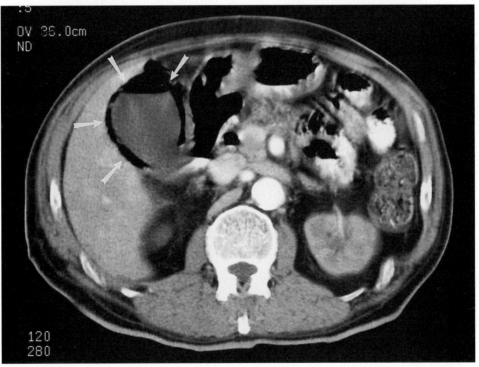

B

FIGURE 7.10. Acute emphysematous cholecystitis. (A) The plain abdominal x-ray shows a large gas bubble within the gallbladder lumen, surrounded by a linear streak of air (arrows) in the GB wall. Air is also present in the biliary tree (large arrow). The metallic device is a dorsal column stimulator. (B) The CT scan shows an air-fluid level in the gallbladder and air in the wall of the gallbladder (arrows). (Courtesy of Henry I. Goldberg, MD.)

TABLE 7.3. Essentials: Acute Acalculous Cholecystitis

Incidence
- 5% of all acute cholecystitis

Clinical setting
- Multiple organ failure, shock
- Major trauma, major burn
- TPN
- Postoperative

Clinical picture
- Abdominal pain in 90%–100%
- Fever in 65%–70%
- Leukocytosis in 85%
- Abnormal liver function in 82%

Diagnosis: ultrasound
- Thickened gallbladder wall (>3.5 cm)
- Distended gallbladder (hydrops)
- Gallbladder sludge
- Submucosal edema
- Pericholecystic fluid

Treatment options
- Laparoscopic cholecystostomy/cystectomy
- Percutaneous cholecystostomy

Abbreviation: TPN, total parenteral nutrition.

Chronic Cholecystitis

Gallstones may cause chronic inflammation of the wall of the GB. The symptoms are chronic, intermittent, mild to moderate pain, intolerance to fatty foods, and intermittent nausea or vomiting. The inflammatory process involves infiltration of the mucosa and submucosa by chronic inflammatory cells, and the formation of crypts in the mucosa known as Rokitansky–Aschoff sinuses.

Mucocele of the Gallbladder

Chronic obstruction of the gallbladder may sometimes cause chronic rather than acute inflammation, with preservation of the secretory epithelium of the GB. Over a period of time, the lumen becomes filled with a clear or slightly milky fluid due to the mucous secretion of the epithelium. Mucocele of the gallbladder may attain large size and present as a right abdominal mass.

OBSTRUCTIVE JAUNDICE

Intrahepatic obstructive jaundice was discussed in Chapter 6. This section focuses on extrahepatic obstructive jaundice. The latter may be caused by gallstones, tumor, or benign stricture (Table 7.4).

Most commonly, stones found in the CBD are produced in the GB and enter the CBD through the cystic duct. Approximately 15% of patients with cholelithiasis have stones in the CBD (choledocholithiasis). On rare occasions, however, in conditions of prolonged stasis or infection, stones can form primarily in the CBD. Obstruc-tive jaundice is usually caused by a stone obstructing the ampulla of Vater. Gallstones impacted in the neck of the gallbladder or cystic duct can obstruct the CBD by extrinsic compression causing obstructive jaundice. This rare phenomenon is known as Mirizzi's syndrome.

Tumors that can cause obstructive jaundice may arise from the CBD, the head of the pancreas or the periampullary region. Tumors of the gallbladder and metastatic neoplasm in the hilum of the liver can cause obstructive jaundice by extrinsic compression. Benign strictures can also cause obstructive jaundice, and may be the result of operative injury of the CBD or sclerosing cholangitis.

Obstruction of the CBD leads to proximal dilatation. The CBD may dilate to 1.0 to 2.5 cm in diameter. The resultant liver dysfunction typically includes conjugated hyperbilirubinemia and elevated alkaline phosphatase, with normal or slightly elevated levels of hepatocellular enzymes. Longstanding obstruction of the CBD can cause biliary cirrhosis, a process that takes many years to develop. The more urgent and dreaded complication of obstructive jaundice is cholangitis, sometimes referred to as ascending cholangitis or suppurative cholangitis.

Cholangitis

Cholangitis arises from secondary infection within an obstructed bile duct. Approximately 90% of cases are due to choledocholithiasis. Cholangitis occurs in only 15% of obstructions caused by a neoplasm. The bacteria most commonly cultured from the bile are *E. coli*, *Klebsiella* organisms, pseudomonas, *Proteus* organisms, enterococci, *Clostridium perfringens* and *Bacteroides fragilis.* Anaerobes are cultured in 15% of cases. In 1877 Charcot described a triad of symptoms characteristic of cholangitis including upper abdominal pain, fever with chills, and jaundice.[2] Charcot's triad is present in about three-fourths of patients with cholangitis. In more severe cases, known as suppurative cholangitis, two additional clinical findings become important: septic shock and mental obtundation. The chills that are characteristic of suppurative cholangitis are due to septicemia and endotoxemia. Blood cultures

TABLE 7.4. Causes of Extrahepatic Obstructive Jaundice

Gallstones
- Choledocholithiasis
- Mirizzi's syndrome

Benign strictures
- Operative trauma
- Sclerosing cholangitis

Neoplasms
- Common bile duct cancer
- Cancer of head of pancreas
- Ampullary cancer
- Invasive gallbladder cancer
- Metastatic tumor

taken during chills are more likely to be positive. The essentials of cholangitis are summarized in Table 7.5.

Biliary Pancreatitis

This topic is discussed in detail in Chapter 4.

Gallstone Ileus

Any gallstones that can pass into the duodenum through the sphincter of Oddi are not large enough to obstruct the bowel. Larger stones can cause small bowel obstruction by entering the intestine through a cholecysto-enteric fistula. This complication is seen most commonly in elderly patients. Symptoms of acute cholecystitis may precede symptoms of bowel obstruction, but acute intermittent bowel obstruction is often the first symptom. The gallstone causes intermittent obstruction as it travels down the intestine by lodging in narrowed segments of the small intestine (e.g., duodenojejunal flexure, areas narrowed by adhesions) until it finally lodges in the ileocecal sphincter. Initial proximal small bowel obstruction is followed by distal small bowel obstruction. Colicky pain, vomiting, abdominal distension, and dehydration are the clinical features. Imaging studies may show not only typical small bowel obstruction but also gas in the biliary tract (Figure 7.11).

Rarely, a gallstone may enter the gastrointestinal tract through either a cholecystogastric or cholecystocolic fistula. The essentials of gallstone ileus are summarized in Table 7.6.

Sclerosing Cholangitis

Primary sclerosing cholangitis may occur without any identifiable cause or associated condition. Two-thirds of cases, however, occur in association primarily with inflammatory bowel disease. Some cases are associated with systemic fibrosing conditions or with autoimmune disorders. The incidence of sclerosing cholangitis in chronic ulcerative colitis is approximately 2.4% to 4%, with the highest incidence occurring in pancolitis. The pathogenesis is unknown. Autoimmune causes are most commonly believed to be involved, but other factors that have been considered include enterohepatic toxins and portal bacteremia, viral infections [e.g., cytomegalovirus (CMV)], and *Cryptococcus neoformans.* A genetic component is suggested by the familial occurrence of primary sclerosing cholangitis and ulcerative colitis, and by the association of the disease with certain human leukocyte histocompatibility antigens (B8 and DR3). Secondary sclerosing cholangitis may be caused by toxic agents (e.g., formaldehyde, hypertonic saline injected into echinococcal cysts, absolute alcohol), ischemia associated with allograft rejection, and even operative trauma.

The affected bile ducts are thickened and narrowed. The thickening is due to fibrosis in the duct wall. The disease is often segmental, but sometimes the entire CBD may be affected. Occasionally, the gallbladder may be involved. Extrahepatic disease is often associated with intrahepatic sclerosing cholangitis. Cholangiography is often diagnostic and shows multifocal stricture in both extra- and intrahepatic ducts. The strictures are often short, with more proximal dilatation causing a beaded appearance (Figure 7.12). Complications of sclerosing cholangitis include obstructive jaundice, biliary stones, cholangitis, biliary cirrhosis, and cholangiocarcinoma. The incidence of cholangiocarcinoma in sclerosing cholangitis is about 4% to 10% and carries a particularly poor prognosis. The essentials of sclerosing cholangitis are summarized in Table 7.7.

Recurrent Pyogenic Cholangitis

Formerly referred to as Oriental cholangiohepatitis, this disease is endemic in Asian countries. It is characterized by intra- and extrahepatic bilirubin stones that cause chronic obstruction and dilatation of the biliary tract with recurrent attacks of septic cholangitis. The gallbladder is usually free of disease. Recurrent pyogenic cholangitis is being seen more and more in the U.S. in the migrant population from Southeast Asia. Several etiological hypotheses have been put forward, including parasitic infection with *Clonorchis sinensis,* indolent bacterial infection, and protein malnutrition. With recurrent sepsis, not only biliary dilatation but also several focal strictures form. The formation of intrahepatic stones is also a feature. Symptoms include chronic abdominal pain, intermittent

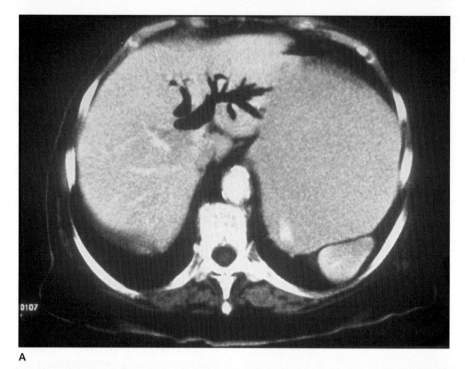

A

B

FIGURE 7.11. Gallstone ileus as manifest on CT scan. (A) Air in the biliary tree is a result of a cholecystoduodenal fistula due to a gallstone. (B) In the second scan, a gallstone (black arrow) partially obstructs a jejunal loop of bowel; collapsed segments of bowel (small arrows) can be seen beyond the site of obstruction. (Courtesy of Henry I. Goldberg, MD.)

TABLE 7.6. Essentials: Gallstone Ileus

Definition

Bowel obstruction due to passage of large stone into small intestine through cholecystoduodenal fistula

Clinical picture
- Intermittent attacks of small bowel obstruction preceding complete obstruction of distal small intestine
- Biliary tract symptoms may or may not be present

Radiologic diagnosis
- Mechanical small bowel obstruction
- Air in biliary tree

Treatment
- Nasogastric suction and fluid and electrolyte resuscitation
- Prompt operation
    Removal of stone by enterotomy proximal to site of obstruction
    Search for other stones in transit
    Closure of enterotomy
    No attempt to take down fistula or perform cholecystectomy

TABLE 7.7. Essentials: Sclerosing Cholangitis

Causes unknown
- Two-thirds associated with IBD
- Autoimmune
- Enterohepatic toxins
- Portal bacteremia, viremia
- Genetic: Human histocompatibility; antigens (B_8, DR_3)

Pathology
- Segmental fibrosis and stricture of bile ducts with dilatation of intervening duct segment (beaded appearance)
- May affect intra- as well as extrahepatic ducts

Complications
- Obstructive jaundice
- Biliary stones
- Cholangitis
- Biliary cirrhosis
- Cholangiocarcinoma (4%–10%)

Treatment
- Medical: immunosuppression (corticosteroids, azothyoprine)
- Interventional: endoscopic/transhepatic stenting
- Surgical
    Resection of CBD and hepaticojejunostomy
    Colectomy for associated ulcerative colitis

Abbreviations: CBD, common bile duct; IBD, inflammatory bowel disease.

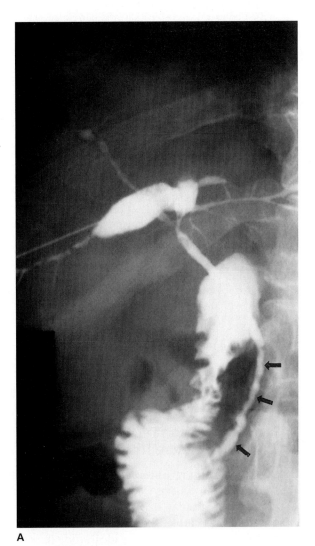

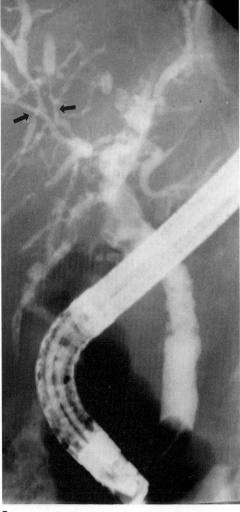

A

B

FIGURE 7.12. Cholangiography is often diagnostic in primary sclerosing cholangitis. (A) The percutaneous THC shows a beaded appearance in the common bile duct (arrows). (B) The ERCP demonstrates a normal caliber common duct but short strictures in intrahepatic ducts (arrows). (Courtesy of Henry I. Goldberg, MD.)

obstructive jaundice, and, occasionally, frank septic cholangitis. Because the cause is not understood, the treatment is to try to clear the common bile duct and prevent further obstruction by creating a wide anastomosis between the common duct and the GI tract, either with choledochoduodenostomy or choledochojejunostomy. Because recurrent obstruction is possible after either of these procedures, easy subsequent access to the CBD should be created for endoscopic or percutaneous intervention. CBD obstruction after choledochoduodenostomy can be managed endoscopically by introducing a basket through the wide stoma. When the initial operative treatment is choledochojejunostomy, the distal end of the cut jejunum is brought out on the abdominal wall as a stoma and choledochojejunostomy is performed some 6 to 8 inches distally. This procedure allows access to the CBD through the jejunal stones.

CLINICAL MANAGEMENT

IMAGING STUDIES OF THE BILIARY TRACT

During the last 25 years, the most revolutionary advances in imaging of the biliary tract have occurred, which have significantly improved both diagnosis and interventional approaches in biliary tract disease. During that period, ultrasonography increasingly improved to become the standard screening test for gallstone disease, virtually replacing the old standard imaging techniques of oral cholecystogram, intravenous cholangiogram, and scintigraphy. In addition to ultrasonography, the most important imaging studies include magnetic resonance cholangiopancreatography (MRC), endoscopic retrograde cholangiopancreatography (ERCP), transhepatic cholangiography (THC), computed tomography (CT), and intraoperative cholangiography (IOC). The essentials of biliary tract imaging are listed in Table 7.8.

Ultrasonography

Abdominal ultrasonography (Figure 7.13) is noninvasive and has sensitivity and specificity rates of 90% to 95% in the diagnosis of cholelithiasis. In this regard, it is superior to CT. It is not as good, however, in demonstrating stones in the common bile duct (CBD). It can accurately measure the CBD diameter, which, on ultrasonography is normally 6 to 7 mm, with anything larger indicating abnormal dilatation. When a patient presents with typical signs and symptoms of biliary colic or acute cholecystitis, ultrasound is often the only preoperative imaging study required, unless jaundice is associated.

Ultrasonography is also possible via probes introduced through endoscopes or laparoscopic trocars. Endoscopic ultrasound is particularly useful in preoperative screening of the CBD. Laparoscopic ultrasound is becoming increasingly useful for assessing the CBD during cholecystectomy but has not replaced intraoperative cholangiography, particularly when the need arises to accurately demonstrate bile duct anatomy during a difficult operation. Duplex ultrasound is very useful in identifying masses and the presence of neoplasms in the bile ducts or portal veins.

TABLE 7.8. Essentials: Biliary Tract Imaging
Oral cholecystogram, intravenous cholangiogram   ■ Of historic interest
Ultrasonography   ■ Best initial study   ■ Diagnostic in acute cholecystitis   ■ Demonstrates bile duct dilatation   ■ Can be used laparoscopically and endoscopically
Magnetic resonance cholangiography   ■ Excellent evaluation of bile ducts and pancreatic duct   ■ Diagnostic in bile duct tumors   ■ Safe in pregnancy
Endoscopic retrograde cholangiopancreatography (ERCP)   ■ Excellent evaluation of biliary and pancreatic systems   ■ Most useful in pathology of distal common bile duct   ■ Permits biopsy and brushing   ■ Facilitates papillotomy, choledocholithotomy, stenting, and nasobiliary drainage   ■ 0.5%–1.0% complication rate
Transhepatic cholangiography (THC)   ■ Most useful in pathology of proximal common bile duct   ■ Permits percutaneous biliary drainage, stenting, and biopsy
Computed tomography (CT)   ■ Most useful in evaluation of tumors   ■ Spiral CT provides three-dimensional image
Hepatic iminodiacetic acid (HIDA) scan   ■ Useful in diagnosis of selected patients with acute cholecystitis or CBD obstruction

Magnetic Resonance Cholangiopancreatography

Rapidly becoming one of the most important imaging studies of the biliary tract, magnetic resonance cholangiopancreatography (MRC) is noninvasive, requires no contrast, and poses no risk of radiation (Figure 7.14). These properties make it the ideal study in pregnancy and

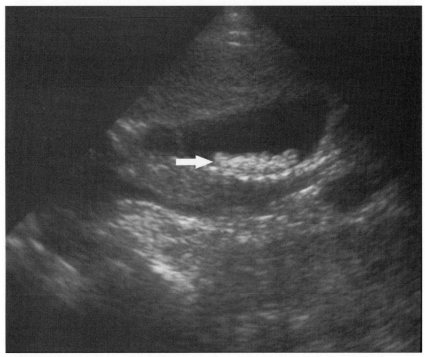

FIGURE 7.13. Abdominal ultrasonography is the most useful screening study for biliary tract disease, especially in stone disease. The ultrasonogram shows several stones (arrow) in the dependent portion of the gallbladder in a patient with clinical features of an early cholecystitis. The gallbladder wall is not yet thickened as in Figure 7.9. (Courtesy of Henry I. Goldberg, MD.)

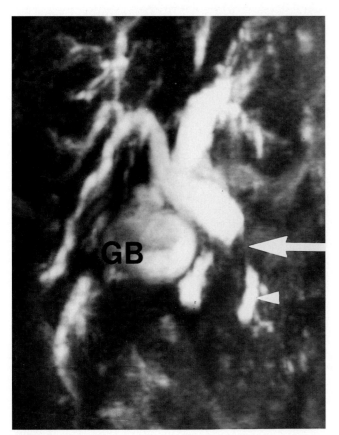

FIGURE 7.14. The magnetic resonance cholangiopancreatography (MRC) scan shows a stricture of the common bile duct (large arrow) with a normal distal common duct (arrowhead). The bile ducts proximal to this malignant stricture are dilated. *Abbreviation*: GB, gallbladder. (Courtesy of Henry I. Goldberg, MD.)

in clinical situations where use of contrast increases the risk of renal failure. Because fluid (e.g., bile, pancreatic juice) shows as white, MRC images of the biliary tract and pancreatic duct are as good or nearly as good as those obtained with ERCP or transhepatic cholangiography. Magnetic resonance can also be used to perform angiography in the evaluation of complex disease or for planning surgery. Magnetic resonance angiography (MRA) is extremely fast, enabling 3D imaging and excellent visualization of strictures in both the arterial and venous phases. It is likely that in the future, MRC and MRA may replace the other imaging studies now in greater use.

Endoscopic Retrograde Cholangiopancreatography

Endoscopic retrograde cholangiopancreatography (ERCP) has represented a major advance in diagnosis and therapy of the biliary tract and has had significant impact on the treatment of choledocholithiasis and cholangitis (Figure 7.15). Its major advantage over other imaging studies is that treatment (e.g., papillotomy, choledocholithotomy, stenting) can be provided at the same time. It is an invasive procedure with complications of perforation and pancreatitis of 0.5% to 1%.

ERCP is most important in the management of retained stones (Figure 7.16), ampullary and distal CBD tumors, cholangitis, and biliary pancreatitis. Retained stones can be extracted after papillotomy. In ampullary

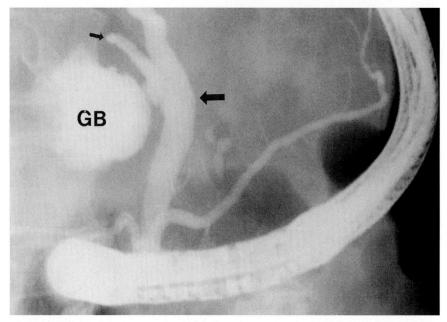

FIGURE 7.15. This endoscopic retrograde cholangiopancreatography (ERCP) scan demonstrates a normal common bile duct (large arrow), cystic duct (small arrow) and gallbladder (GB). (Courtesy of Henry I. Goldberg, MD.)

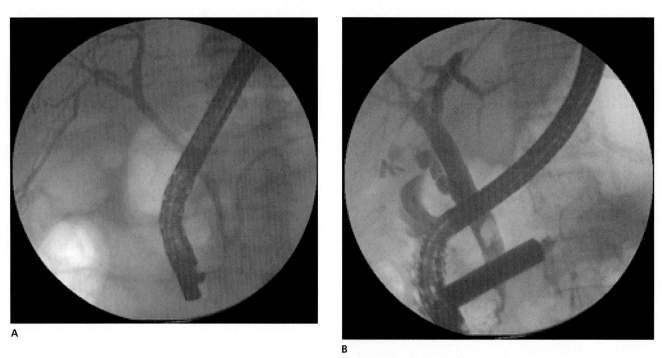

A

B

FIGURE 7.16. (A) Normal endoscopic retrograde cholangiopancreatography (ERCP) scan shows the biliary tree and pancreatic duct in a patient who previously underwent cholecystectomy. (B) The ERCP scan in another patient shows a dilated common bile duct containing a large stone. (Courtesy of John P. Cello, MD.)

and distal CBD tumors, tissue for histological diagnosis can be obtained by biopsy or brushing. In suppurative cholangitis, ERCP can be used to rapidly decompress the CBD by papillotomy or by the placement of nasobiliary drain. It converts a life-threatening condition that once required emergency surgery to one that can be treated by elective operation. In severe biliary pancreatitis, early ERCP and sphincterotomy have been shown to reduce mortality tenfold.[3] In the future, it is likely that MRC will replace ERCP as the most common diagnostic imaging study for the CBD, but ERCP will continue to be important as an interventional therapeutic procedure.

Transhepatic Cholangiography

Excellent imaging of both the intra- and extrahepatic biliary tract can be obtained with percutaneous transhepatic injection of dye into a biliary radical in the liver (Figure 7.17). Transhepatic cholangiography (THC) and ERCP are complementary in imaging the CBD, with THC being more useful for proximal lesions and ERCP for distal lesions. While these therapeutic uses of the transhepatic approach will continue to be important, MRC is increasingly replacing THC as the diagnostic imaging study in hilar lesions.

Computed Tomography

The most important use of computed tomography (CT) in biliary tract disease is in the evaluation of tumors and biliary pancreatitis. As indicated earlier, ultrasound provides cheaper, noninvasive, and more accurate assessment of stone disease. CT is superior, however, in the diagnosis and staging of neoplasms in the biliary tract. Spiral CT has significantly improved the usefulness of the study (Figure 7.18).

Hepatobiliary Scintigraphy

The most useful application of hepatobiliary scintigraphy is to ascertain biliary tree patency. Radionuclide agents (e.g., ^{99m}Te) administered intravenously are excreted by the

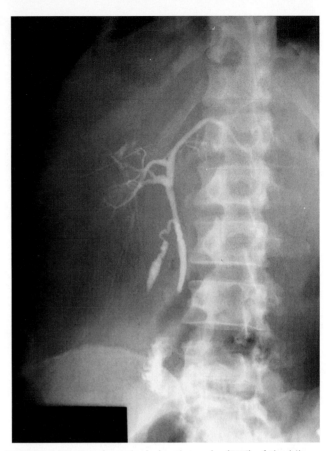

FIGURE 7.17. Transhepatic cholangiography (THC) of the bile duct. THC is useful for imaging the common bile duct and proximal lesions of the biliary tract, inserting drains or stents, and for biopsy of lesions. This cholangiogram shows a normal unobstructed biliary tract. (Courtesy of Henry I. Goldberg, MD.)

hepatocytes into the biliary tract. Failure of the GB to opacify some 60 minutes after injection provides strong presumptive evidence that the cystic duct is obstructed and, in the presence of relevant clinical symptoms, strongly suggests the diagnosis of acute cholecystitis. Hepatic iminodiacetic acid (HIDA) scanning diagnoses acute cholecystitis with 98% accuracy (Figure 7.19). When obstruction at the distal CBD is present, the biliary tract and the GB may be visualized without any opacification of the duodenum.

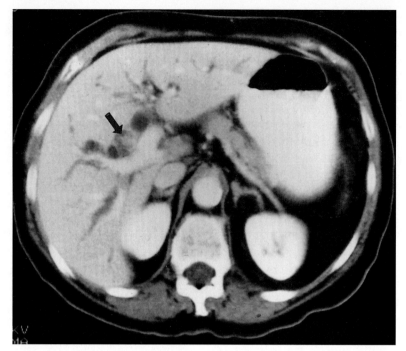

FIGURE 7.18. Spiral CT is superior to ultrasound in diagnosis and staging of neoplasms in the biliary tree. This CT scan shows dilated intrahepatic bile ducts radiating to the proximal common hepatic duct, which is abruptly cut off (arrow). A subtle cholangiocarcinoma is present. (Courtesy of Henry I. Goldberg, MD.)

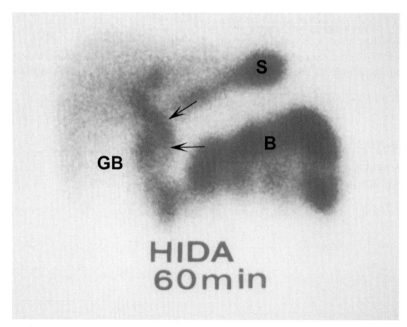

FIGURE 7.19. This HIDA scan was taken 60 minutes after injection of the radionuclide. The common hepatic and bile ducts are shown (arrows), but no filling of the gallbladder (GB) has occurred. HIDA has entered the small bowel (B) and refluxed into the stomach (S). (Courtesy of Henry I. Goldberg, MD.)

ASYMPTOMATIC CHOLELITHIASIS

Silent gallstones may be discovered incidentally during imaging studies or abdominal exploration. Long-term followup studies show that only 10% to 20% of individuals with silent gallstones develop symptoms, most commonly biliary colic.[4] Fewer than 3% develop acute cholecystitis, and fewer than 1% die from gallstone complications.[4] A study comparing prophylactic cholecystectomy with no treatment showed that surgery decreased expected survival slightly.[1] It is now generally agreed that asymptomatic gallstones should be managed conservatively, even in diabetic individuals, who seem to have an increased risk for developing symptoms. It is prudent, however, to perform cholecystectomy in most patients with asymptomatic gallstones in the course of abdominal surgery for other indications. This recommendation is particularly important in patients who have diabetes, large stones, or calcified gallbladder, because they all have a slightly increased risk of complications from asymptomatic gallstones.

BILIARY COLIC

Typically, pain in biliary colic is felt in the right upper quadrant (RUQ) of the abdomen and often radiates to the back in the right infrascapular region. The pain may last from minutes to hours and often follows ingestion of a meal, particularly one with a large fat content. Nausea and vomiting may be present, but fever and abdominal tenderness are not.

Investigations

Abdominal ultrasound is the simplest and best diagnostic tool and shows stones in the gallbladder, usually with minimal gallbladder wall thickening or pericholecystic fluid. Fever or leukocytosis are absent in most cases. Liver function tests and serum amylase are usually normal.

Treatment

The standard treatment is early laparoscopic cholecystectomy. Once surgery is scheduled, the patient is advised to adhere to a low-fat diet. Analgesia is required only during the acute attack. In early pregnancy, conservative management with a low-fat diet is appropriate, and this approach may succeed in postponing cholecystectomy until after delivery. Otherwise, cholecystectomy may be required and performed safely during the second half of the second trimester or in the third trimester if symptoms worsen or if acute cholecystitis develops.

ACUTE CHOLECYSTITIS

The characteristic symptoms are RUQ pain, nausea, vomiting with mild fever, and leukocytosis. The pain typically radiates to the right infrascapular region in the back. Abdominal examination elicits RUQ tenderness, perhaps guarding, and sometimes a mass due to omentum surrounding an inflamed gallbladder. A positive Murphy's sign is typically elicited: Palpation in the subhepatic region at the time of deep inspiration causes arrest of inspiration as the inflamed gallbladder and surrounding tissue descend to the examiner's touch. Clinical jaundice is rarely present. If the patient appears toxic and has a high fever, a complication must be suspected, either gangrenous cholecystitis, perforation of the gallbladder, or empyema.

Investigations

Hemogram shows low-grade leukocytosis with a shift to the left. Liver function tests are usually normal but may sometimes show low-grade elevation of the bilirubin (<2 mg%) and even minor elevation in liver enzymes. Serum amylase is typically normal. Ultrasound is the best way to confirm the diagnosis (Figure 7.9A). The typical findings are: (1) stones in the gallbladder (Figure 7.13), (2) thickening of the gallbladder wall, and (3) pericholecystic fluid collection. The ultrasonographer is also able to elicit Murphy's sign by pressing the transducer into the RUQ.

Treatment

The diagnosis is usually readily confirmed. The patient requires analgesia. A nasogastric tube should be inserted if the patient is vomiting. The patient should be hydrated quickly and broad-spectrum antibiotics should be administered intravenously. Laparoscopic cholecystectomy should be performed without too much delay. In the past, patients with acute cholecystitis were treated conservatively until inflammation resolved, and then elective cholecystectomy was performed. Six randomized trials have compared this delayed treatment with prompt cholecystectomy within 1 to 10 days in 1019 patients.[5] Complication rates were 21.0% for early and 16.5% for late cholecystectomy. The corresponding mortality rates were 0.2% and 1.8%, respectively. As a result of these studies, it is now recommended that cholecystectomy be performed within 24 to 48 h of establishing the diagnosis. The early treatment strategy returns patients to their normal lives much more quickly, particularly if the cholecystectomy is done laparoscopically.

When cholecystectomy for acute cholecystitis becomes technically difficult because of severe inflammation, excessive bleeding, or difficulty in safely identifying the cystic and bile ducts, the preferred procedure is tube cholecystostomy and drainage of the right upper quadrant. All the stones in the gallbladder should be removed if possible. The patient usually recovers rapidly, and elective cholecystectomy can be scheduled in 3 to 6 months. In the very elderly patient, if cholangiogram through the cholecystostomy tube shows no residual stones either in the gallbladder or in the CBD and dye flows freely through the cystic duct, no further surgery may be required. Such decisions must be highly individualized.

CHRONIC CHOLECYSTITIS

Chronic cholecystitis is difficult to diagnose. The symptoms are vague abdominal pain, often occurring postprandially. When the course is punctuated with clear-cut episodes of biliary colic, the diagnosis is easier. Ultrasonography shows cholelithiasis without evidence of acute inflammation. If other conditions can be excluded, the treatment is laparoscopic cholecystectomy. It must be pointed out that some 10% to 15% of these patients develop postcholecystectomy syndrome.

ACALCULOUS CHOLECYSTITIS

Because acalculous cholecystitis (AC) most often occurs in the setting of critical illness or postoperatively, the diagnosis may be difficult. Undiagnosed and untreated, AC has a high mortality rate. The clinical signs are right upper quadrant pain, tenderness, and fever, but they are not always present. Pain and/or tenderness are seen in only 70% and fever in less than 66% of patients. Tenderness may be present more diffusely in the upper abdomen rather than localized to the right upper quadrant.

Investigations

Laboratory Tests

Leukocytosis with a shift to the left is found in approximately 85% of patients. Liver function test results are abnormal in approximately 80% of cases.

Imaging Studies

Abdominal ultrasound is the best initial imaging study and should be performed whenever the diagnosis is suspected. The three major diagnostic criteria are: (1) thickening of the gallbladder wall exceeding 3 to 5 mm, (2) distention (hydrops) of the gallbladder, and (3) presence of sludge within the gallbladder.

Other secondary diagnostic criteria include subserosal edema, pericholecystic fluid, and positive ultrasonographic Murphy's sign. Ultrasound has more than 90% sensitivity and specificity. CT examination is necessary only if ultrasonography is negative. HIDA scan has a 30% to 50% false–positive error rate. The error rate is reduced somehow by the use of morphine cholecystography, in which intravenous morphine is used to contract the sphincter of Oddi to promote gallbladder filling. The gallium or [111]Indium leukocyte scan is used infrequently. A positive test shows a doughnut pattern of uptake in the inflamed GB wall.

Treatment

Early diagnosis and early treatment are essential to reduce mortality. Open cholecystectomy in these very ill patients is associated with a 30% mortality rate.[6] This observation led to the introduction of percutaneous cholecystostomy or percutaneous transhepatic cholecystostomy, both of which lead to rapid improvement in most patients. The problem arises when the gallbladder wall is gangrenous or when a complication of the procedure (e.g., hemorrhage, bile leak) occurs. At present, the optimum treatment is laparoscopic cholecystostomy or cholecystectomy. In the desperately ill patient without gangrenous cholecystitis, laparoscopic cholecystostomy is preferred. When the patient is not so critically ill or when gangrene is present, laparoscopic cholecystectomy is the treatment of choice.

TECHNIQUES OF GALLBLADDER SURGERY

Laparoscopic Cholecystectomy

Laparoscopic cholecystectomy (LC) is now the standard procedure for calculous gallbladder disease. This minimally invasive approach has dramatically reduced postoperative pain, length of hospital stay, and the patient's return to active life. The mortality rate is less than 0.2% and similar to that of open cholecystectomy.[7] The morbidity rate at over 7% and bile duct injury rate at about 0% to 4% are higher than for open cholecystectomy.[7]

Relative contraindications for LC include previous upper abdominal surgery, severe obesity, pregnancy, and acute cholecystitis. As LC has become established, none of these conditions absolutely contraindicate performing LC. On the other hand, significantly greater technical difficulty may be encountered, and the surgeon should have low resistance to converting the procedure to open surgery. Mean conversion rate for all LC is almost 5% but can be as high as 7% to 10% in the above circumstances.

LC is performed under general anesthesia. A nasogastric tube and bladder catheter are introduced. Pneumoperitoneum is created using a Veress needle or a Hassan cannula. Trocar placement for performing LC is shown in Figure 7.20. After adequate insufflation is achieved to 18 cm of water using nitrous oxide, a periumbilical trocar is placed for the introduction of the laparoscope. Then, three other trocars are placed while the site of peritoneal puncture done with each trocar is directly viewed through the laparoscope. The assistant stands on the right of the patient, the surgeon on the left, and the camera operator between the patient's legs.

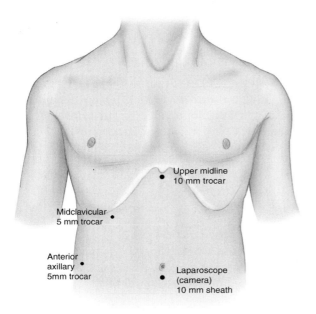

FIGURE 7.20. Trocar placement in laparoscopic cholecystectomy.

The gallbladder fundus is grasped with a forceps and the assistant elevates it toward the left shoulder. Another forceps grasps Hartmann's pouch and retracts it laterally. This move is critical to open the triangle of Calot. The surgeon then dissects the cystic artery and cystic duct as it leaves the gallbladder. The cystic duct is traced down to its entrance into the CBD. Once these structures are identified, the cystic artery and duct are clipped and divided, and the GB is dissected off from the liver bed toward the fundus.

While this infundibular technique of cholecystectomy is the most popular, some surgeons consider it unsafe because the cystic artery and duct, and the CBD, common hepatic duct, and right hepatic duct cannot be identified with enough confidence to reduce the possibility of damage to near zero. Strasberg et al. have advocated that, once the structures thought to be the cystic duct and cystic artery are identified, dissection should be carried out from the fundus down to the infundibulum.[7] Only after the GB is removed is it then optimally safe to divide the cystic artery and duct. Whenever there is any doubt about the anatomy, an operative cholangiogram should be obtained through the cystic duct or the gallbladder. Routine cholangiogram is advocated by some and not performed by most.

Placement of a drain in the right subhepatic space is not usually necessary. The nasogastric tube and urinary catheter are removed at the end of the procedure. Most patients stay overnight in the hospital, but increasingly patients are being discharged home on the day of operation. On average, the mean return to work period is 6 days.

Open Cholecystectomy

The incisions and exposure techniques used in open chole-cystectomy are illustrated in Figure 7.21. The most common incisions used are right subcostal or midline.

Less commonly, transverse, right paramedial, or the Kehr incisions may be used.

After general anesthesia is administered, a nasogastric tube and urinary catheter are inserted and the abdomen opened. Following general abdominal exploration, the gallbladder and CBD are exposed. Any omental adhesions to the gallbladder fundus are divided, and the gallbladder is lifted off the transverse colon. The hepatic flexure and stomach are packed away laterally. If the gallbladder is tensely distended, it may be decompressed by inserting a suction cannula through a stab wound using a purse-string suture. The fundus and the Hartmann pouch are then clasped with a hemostat and a long forceps, respectively. Key to obtaining adequate exposure are: (1) retraction of the gallbladder upward and laterally using the two forceps, (2) retraction of the liver upwards and slightly to the left using a sponge-covered Deaver retractor, and (3) retraction of the distal CBD and duodenum inferiorly by the assistant's left hand.

The dissection begins at the triangle of Calot, which is opened by laterally retracting Hartmann's pouch and upwardly displacing the liver. The cystic artery normally crosses the triangle of Calot and courses up onto the gallbladder, where it starts to divide. Inferior retraction of the CBD and lateral retraction of Hartmann's pouch brings into prominence the cystic duct. Silk sutures (2–0) are applied around the cystic artery and cystic duct, but the structures are left undivided. The safest procedure is now to dissect the gallbladder down from fundus to infundibulum. When this dissection is completed, the gallbladder is free and remains attached by the cystic duct and cystic artery. These structures can now be divided safely between ligatures of 2–0 silk. The cystic duct is divided 3 to 5 mm from its junction with the CBD.

If an operative cholangiogram is to be performed, it is best to do it after the gallbladder is completely removed

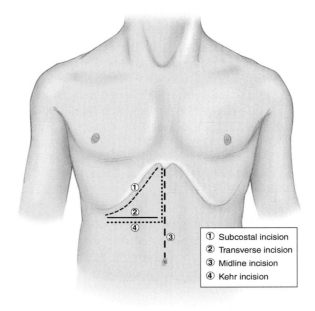

① Subcostal incision
② Transverse incision
③ Midline incision
④ Kehr incision

FIGURE 7.21. Choice of incisions for open cholecystectomy.

from the liver with the cystic duct intact. A catheter can easily be inserted into the cystic duct near its junction with the gallbladder.

The primary disadvantage of the fundus-to-infundibulum dissection technique is that more blood oozes because the cystic artery has not been ligated. This disadvantage is more than compensated for by the safety of the procedure, which makes an inadvertent division of the CBD, common or right hepatic ducts virtually impossible. Most surgeons place a closed drainage catheter in the infrahepatic space, but this practice is not always necessary.

Cholecystostomy

Cholecystostomy can be performed either laparoscopically or with the open technique. In either case, a pursestring suture is applied to the fundus of the gallbladder, and a catheter (e.g., #16 Foley) is introduced through a stab wound within the pursestring suture. The pursestring suture is securely tied after the balloon of the Foley catheter is inflated and pulled up to the stab wound. It is wise to suture the gallbladder fundus to the peritoneum after the catheter is exteriorized through a stab wound in the abdominal wall. The subhepatic space is routinely drained with closed catheter suction.

Unusual Treatment Circumstances

The inflammatory response, particularly near the junction of the cystic and common hepatic ducts, may be so intense that the cystic duct cannot be identified. If so, the choices are to perform cholecystostomy and close, or to start dissection from the fundus downward to see if the anatomy can be better delineated to enable safe division of the cystic duct. If not, cholecystostomy should be performed.

In severe acute cholecystitis with gangrene of the fundus and body, the cystic duct and artery may not be identifiable because of the inflammatory response. In this case, it may be feasible to perform partial cholecystectomy, remove all calculi from the remaining portion of the gallbladder and close the remnant over a Foley catheter using a pursestring suture. The Foley should be passed through the abdominal wall before it is inserted into the gallbladder remnant. The pericholecystic area should always be drained with a suction catheter.

OBSTRUCTIVE JAUNDICE DUE TO STONES

The main symptom of stones in the CBD is obstructive jaundice. This is often associated with pain, which tends to be upper midline in distribution and aggravated by eating. Intermittent, painful jaundice is usually due to stones and not carcinoma. The dreaded complications are cholangitis and pancreatitis, which are discussed elsewhere. The patient may or may not have had cholecystectomy previously.

Investigations

Liver functions tests show direct hyperbilirubinemia and elevated alkaline phosphatase with minimal or no abnormality of hepatocellular function. The ultrasonogram shows a dilated CBD (>6mm diameter) and sometimes stones within the duct (Figure 7.13). More definitive evaluation of the CBD is provided by either MRC or ERCP. Although MRC is noninvasive, ERCP provides the additional advantage of performing sphincterotomy and removing common duct stones.

Treatment

Choledocholithotomy

Common bile duct stones may be removed with ERCP, laparoscopy, or open surgery. The essentials of treatment are summarized in Table 7.9.

ERCP

Endoscopic sphincterotomy and removal of common duct stones using forceps, baskets, or balloons has proven safe and effective. It has a mortality rate of 0.5% to 1.0% and a morbidity rate of 8% to 10%. It is primarily indicated in the following conditions:

1. Retained stones or stones developing in the CBD after previous cholecystectomy.
2. Severe biliary pancreatitis, where therapeutic ERCP within the first few days of attack has reduced the incidence of mortality to a tenth of what it was.
3. Severe ascending cholangitis, where the patient is extremely ill and the CBD can be decompressed quickly.
4. Planned operation in a patient with stones in both gallbladder and CBD, in which preoperative clearing of the

---

TABLE 7.9. Essentials: Treatment of Choledocolithiasis

Gallbladder intact
- Preferred approach: Laparoscopic cholecystectomy and choledocolithotomy
- Alternatives if laparoscopic choledocolithotomy is unsuccessful
  Open choledocolithotomy
  Postoperative removal by ERCP

Gallbladder previously removed
- Preferred approach: Endoscopic papillotomy and choledocolithotomy
- Alternatives:
  If preferred approach is unsuccessful, open CBD exploration and choledocolithotomy
  If stone cannot be removed via choledocolithotomy, duodenotomy, and sphincteroplasty

Too many CBD stones
- End-to-side Roux-en-Y choledocojejunostomy
- Choledocoduodenostomy

Abbreviation: CBD, common bile duct; ERCP, endoscopic retrograde cholangiopancreatography.

CBD by ERCP allows laparoscopic cholecystectomy and operative cholangiogram to be done without the need to explore the CBD.

Laparoscopic CBD Exploration and Choledocholithotomy

The experienced laparoscopist can explore the CBD and remove stones through the cystic duct or after choledochotomy at the time of laparoscopic cholecystectomy. Choledochoscopy can also be performed, allowing direct examination of the extrahepatic biliary tract. The safety and success rate of laparoscopic choledocholithotomy is directly related to the experience of the surgeon and must not be attempted by the person who performs laparoscopy infrequently.

The procedure is indicated:

1. When, in the course of laparoscopic cholecystectomy, stones are discovered in the CBD, a situation that obtains in 10% to 15% of cases.
2. When preoperative ERCP has failed to cannulate the ampulla in patients known to have CBD stones.

Open CBD Exploration

It is imperative that every biliary tract surgeon maintain his or her ability to perform open exploration of the CBD. Clearly, the frequency with which this operation is performed has declined as more and more CBD stones are removed by ERCP or laparoscopically. However, the procedure is still the gold standard by which the successes, failures, and morbidity and mortality of other techniques must be judged.

The procedure is performed either in conjunction with open cholecystectomy or, in the patient with retained stones, after previous cholecystectomy, especially where ERCP has failed and the laparoscopic approach is either not available or deemed too difficult because of adhesions. The approach is usually through a right subcostal or midline incision. In patients who still have their gallbladder, cholecystectomy is first performed and identification of the CBD is not difficult. In patients who have had prior cholecystectomy, however, careful dissection of the structures in the subhepatic fossa is required. The CBD is normally to the right of the common hepatic artery and anterior to the portal vein. When a structure that resembles the CBD is identified, it is confirmed by aspiration of bile with a 21-gauge needle on a syringe. The CBD is then dissected and a suitable place for choledochotomy chosen. The best location is just distal to the entrance of the cystic duct but in the supraduodenal part of the structure. Two stay sutures of 3–0 silk are applied to the anterior wall, and the duct is opened between the sutures for about 2 cm.

At times, stones are immediately visible and can be removed by irrigation. Some surgeons prefer to perform choledochoscopy early, others later. One simple procedure to follow is to start by irrigating the CBD, both below and above the incision, using a red rubber catheter (#10 or

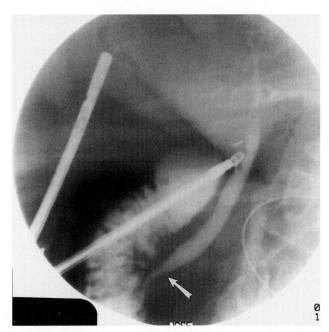

FIGURE 7.22. This intraoperative cholangiogram, performed during a laparoscopic cholecystectomy, shows a normal common bile duct and common hepatic duct. It is often difficult to fill the intrahepatic ducts with contrast when the sphincter of Oddi relaxes, as it does here (arrow). (Courtesy of Henry I. Goldberg, MD.)

#12). The maneuver may result in removing all or most of the floating stones. Next, a biliary Fogarty catheter is passed distally and, if possible, into the duodenum. The balloon is inflated and pulled snug against the ampulla. The balloon is then deflated slowly as it is pulled up through the sphincter. As soon as the give is felt, the balloon is inflated, pulled up and out of the choledochotomy. If this procedure is unsuccessful after two or three attempts, stone forceps and/or Dormia baskets are used. Several applications of these procedures alternated with liberal saline irrigation may be required. The proximal extrahepatic biliary tract must also be explored both by balloon catheter and stone forceps, if necessary.

It is helpful to know before exploration how many stones there are, but even after removing the expected number of stones, completion cholangiogram and/or choledochoscopy is essential (Figure 7.22). When the CBD has been satisfactorily cleared of stones, the choledochotomy is closed after inserting a T-tube. The closure is accomplished with absorbable 4–0 sutures, ensuring that the T-tube is not kinked inside the duct. The transverse portion of the T-tube often needs to be bivalved or the inferior half excised to facilitate its removal from the duct when the time comes. A closed suction-drain is placed in the right subhepatic fossa.

POSTOPERATIVE CARE OF THE T-TUBE The T-tube is allowed to drain freely into a bag. The amount of drainage decreases with time. A T-tube cholangiogram may be obtained safely after postoperative day 7. If no residual stones are seen and dye flows freely into the duodenum, the T-tube is clamped. It is unclamped only if the patient develops pain; otherwise, it is kept clamped until its removal in the office at about 3 weeks, when a well-formed tract has developed. If a retained stone had been identified, it can be removed through this T-tube tract.

Unusual Circumstances

IMPACTED STONES In some cases, impacted stones may be located at the distal end and cannot be removed from above. The prudent thing to do in this case is to open the second portion of the duodenum over the ampulla and perform sphincterotomy to remove the stone either from below or by dislodging it upwards. The technique of sphincterotomy is depicted in Figure 7.23. The other alternative is intraoperative or postoperative ERCP.

TOO MANY STONES When stones are too numerous to extract, the prudent procedure is to perform either a choledochoduodenostomy or Roux-en-Y choledochojejunos-

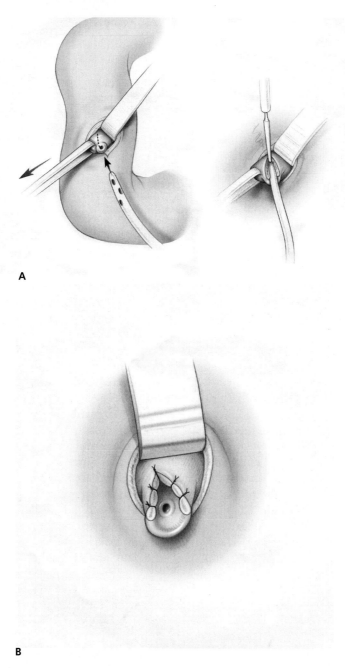

FIGURE 7.23. Dislodgement of impacted stone in GB via sphincterotomy. (A) Open sphincterotomy is accomplished via duodenotomy and the sphincter is incised at 11 o'clock. (B) The open edges are then kept open by interrupted sutures. (Adapted from Blumgart LH. Surgery of the Liver and Biliary Tract, 2nd ed. New York: Churchill Livingstone, 1994:846–847.)

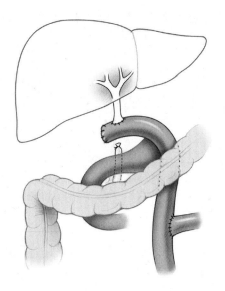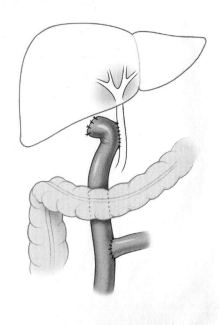

FIGURE 7.24. End-to-side or side-to-side Roux-en-Y choledochojejunostomy.

tomy (Figure 7.24). The choice depends on anatomy, age and condition of the patient. An end-to-side Roux-en-Y choledochojejunostomy is preferred, since it has a lower long-term incidence of stricture or cholangitis. A side-to-side Roux-en-Y choledochojejunostomy should not be performed because it is associated with development of the sump syndrome, in which the distal portion of the CBD acts as a collection vestibule for debris and infection.

GIANT STONE IN THE CBD   On occasion, a large stone wedged in the CBD cannot be moved up or down. Two techniques may be used in conjunction with one another or with a T-tube to address this problem:

1. Stone fragmentation by extracorporeal short-wave lithotripsy (ESWL) has been effective in fragmenting stones in over 90% of 56 patients in a multicenter trial.[2]
2. Stone dissolution with chemicals such as monooctanoin and MBTE has been used successfully to dissolve stones when topically applied. The efficacy and associated risks of MBTE are less well known than those of monooctanoin.

When a T-tube is in place in the management of these giant stones, ESWL can be used to fragment the stones, with subsequent dissolution through octanoic acid infusion into the T-tube or extraction using a Dormia basket through the T-tube tract.

CHOLANGITIS

The disease occurs with a spectrum of severity. In mild or moderate disease, the predominant symptoms are abdominal pain, fever and chills, and jaundice. These three symptoms coexist as Charcot's triad in only 60% of patients. In severe cholangitis, constituting about 5% of all cases of cholangitis, the patient may demonstrate Reynold's pentad of symptoms, which include Charcot's triad plus septic shock and mental obtundation. RUQ or epigastric tenderness is common.

Investigations

Laboratory Tests

Leukocytosis with a shift to the left occurs in most patients, as does hyperbilirubinemia and elevated serum levels of aspartate aminotransferase (AST), alanine aminotransferase (ALT), and alkaline phosphatase. The presence of leukopenia carries a poor prognosis. Bilirubin levels vary from a mean of 6.6 mg% in calculous disease to over 15 mg% when the cause is malignant obstruction. The serum amylase level is elevated in about one-third and often suggests benign calculous disease as the cause. Blood cultures should be obtained, particularly during attacks of fever and chills.

Imaging Studies

Abdominal ultrasound may show a dilated CBD (>6 mm), but cholangiography—either transhepatic (THC) or ERCP—is necessary to establish the diagnosis and the cause of obstruction. Diagnostic cholangiography should be postponed until fever resolves and should be done only under systemic antibiotic coverage. Both PTH and ERCP can be used to provide internal or external drainage of the biliary tract. When calculous disease or distal CBD obstruction is suspected, ERCP is preferred because it facilitates performance of endoscopic papillotomy, which may provide temporary or permanent relief.

Treatment

Supportive therapy consists of nasogastric suction, intravenous fluids, intravenous broad-spectrum antibiotics, and vitamin K to correct any subclinical coagulopathy. Antibiotics that cover both Gram-negative and anaerobic bacteria should be given. A popular initial choice is a combination of ampicillin, an aminoglycoside, and metronidazole. Subsequently, the choice of antibiotics is determined from the results of culture and sensitivity studies. Good response to antibiotic therapy occurs in approximately 85% to 90%, permitting the performance of definitive treatment on an elective basis. In those 10% to 15% of patients who fail to improve, bile duct decompression is urgently needed. Endoscopic papillotomy and nasobiliary drainage (alone or in combination) are preferable to emergency surgical exploration of the CBD. In a prospective, randomized trial, Fan et al. demonstrated that endoscopic decompression has lower morbidity (34% vs. 66%, p <0.05) and mortality (10% vs. 32%, p <0.03) rates than surgical exploration.[3]

Patients initially treated endoscopically on an urgent basis or those who had a good response to medical therapy require subsequent definitive treatment, depending on what the urgent procedure was and whether or not they still have a gallbladder. Patients who have had nasobiliary drainage alone and prior cholecystectomy may be definitively treated with elective ERCP and endoscopic papillotomy. Those who still have a gallbladder with calculous disease may be treated with endoscopic papillotomy and subsequent laparoscopic cholecystectomy or with laparoscopic cholecystectomy and common duct exploration. Open cholecystectomy and common duct exploration may be necessary on rare occasions.

In patients who are critically ill from toxic cholangitis in whom endoscopic drainage is technically not possible, common duct decompression may be obtained by either the percutaneous transhepatic route or laparoscopically. When cholangitis is associated with malignant obstruction, the appropriate palliative or curative procedure is required once the acute cholangitis is treated. When the patient has an inoperable tumor, the common duct may be drained via an internal stent placed either with ERCP or transhepatically. Such stents may require repeated replacement because of blockage with sludge.

GALLSTONE ILEUS

Acute, intermittent attacks of small bowel obstruction over several days are the dominant clinical presentation of gallstone ileus. A history suggestive of acute cholecystitis may or may not be present. The picture is initially that of high small bowel obstruction associated with abdominal pain and frequent vomiting but successively becomes that of middle and lower small bowel obstruction as the stone moves distally to lodge at the ileocecal valve. These intermittent attacks of small bowel obstruction may last a few

to several days and, by the time the patient presents, significant dehydration and electrolyte imbalance may have occurred. As a result, the patient, who is often elderly, may be critically ill.

Investigations

Laboratory Tests

A high hematocrit level may be present as a result of dehydration. Depending on how severe the high small bowel obstruction has been, electrolyte imbalance may be present with hypokalemia and metabolic alkalosis.

X-ray Studies

Definitive diagnosis may be established by plain abdominal films, which show mechanical small bowel obstruction with air-fluid levels and air in the biliary tree (Figure 7.11).

Treatment

Nasogastric suction is initiated, the fluid and electrolyte imbalance rapidly corrected, and surgery performed to relieve the obstruction. The steps in the operation include:

1. Identification of the obstructing stone at the ileocecal valve.

2. Removal of the stone through an enterotomy performed in healthy ileum at a point proximal to the site of obstruction, which may be bruised and edematous.

3. Running the small bowel back to the region of the cholecystoduodenal fistula to look for additional large stones, in transit or in the gallbladder, which, if present, are milked distally and removed through the enterotomy.

4. Closure of the enterotomy in two layers.

5. No attempt to take down the cholecystoduodenal fistula or perform cholecystectomy.

In most patients, no further treatment of the biliary tract disease is necessary. In some patients, because of persistent biliary tract symptoms, cholecystectomy is necessary. If at the time of cholecystectomy a fistula is still present, it needs to be taken down and the duodenum closed in two layers.

BILIARY PANCREATITIS

This topic is covered extensively in Chapter 4 under the section entitled *Acute Pancreatitis.*

BILIARY TRACT INJURY

The mechanisms by which laparoscopic biliary tract injury may occur are described in Table 7.10. Injuries vary from relatively simple bile leak from the gallbladder bed to incomplete or complete transection of the CBD, right hepatic duct, or common hepatic duct. A useful clinical classification of laparoscopic biliary tract injury from

TABLE 7.10. Classification of Causes of Laparoscopic Biliary Injuries

Misidentification of bile ducts as cystic duct
- Common hepatic duct
- Aberrant right hepatic duct

Technical causes
- Failure to securely occlude cystic duct
- Plane of dissection too deep on liver bed
- Injudicious use of thermal energy
- Tenting injury of cystic duct
- Injudicious use of clips
- Improper technique of ductal exploration

Strasberg and colleagues[7] is given in Figure 7.25 and Table 7.11. As is evident from the classification, not all injuries lead to biliary stricture. Postoperatively, biliary tract injury may become clinically manifest within days, weeks, or months.

Strictures

Benign Biliary Strictures

Most benign strictures of the extrahepatic bile ducts are due to iatrogenic injury, with 95% due to operative trauma. The incidence of operative injury of the bile ducts rose rapidly with the general adoption of laparoscopic chole-cystectomy in the late 1980s and early 1990s. Since then, the incidence has declined significantly as laparoscopic techniques have improved and experience has increased, but the incidence of operative bile duct injury at present is still higher than in the prelaparoscopic era. Other causes of benign stricture include sclerosing cholangitis, chronic pancreatitis, and blunt or penetrating abdominal trauma. The management algorithm is shown in Figure 7.26.

Postoperative Bile Duct Strictures

Most bile duct injuries occur as a result of operations on the GB or CBD. When surgery for complicated duodenal ulcer disease was common, the CBD was occasionally inadvertently divided or sutured during difficult gastrectomy or suture-control of a bleeding duodenal ulcer in cases where the first portion of the patient's duodenum had been significantly foreshortened by scarring. Because, at present, most injuries occur in the course of laparoscopic cholecystectomy, the following discussion focuses on this mechanism of injury.

Bile duct injuries during cholecystectomy are due to either misidentification of structures or errors of technique. Either the CBD or the right hepatic duct may be misidentified as the cystic duct and divided. A common error is to retract the infundibulum of the gallbladder vertically upwards. This maneuver aligns the cystic duct with the CBD, and the latter structure is mistaken for the cystic duct. This is especially so in young women and when the CBD is small. In other situations, the right hepatic duct or common hepatic duct may be entered through the gallbladder bed. Errors of technique include excessive bleed-ing and misuse of cautery. The application of clips to control bleeding when the ductal anatomy is not clearly visible is another cause of injury. Aberrant bile ducts may be inadvertently divided.

Postoperative leak from inadvertent bile duct injury must be distinguished from bile leak caused by small accessory ducts in the bed of the gallbladder or a slipped ligature of the cystic duct.

Clinical Presentation

Early Presentation

Patients with bile leak usually present symptoms early, either because of excessive bile in suction drainage or because of accumulation of bile in the subhepatic space (biloma), which may cause malaise, pain, and fever within days of the operation. Bile leak may occur from accessory bile ductules in the bed of the gallbladder, from slipped cystic duct ligature, or from partial or complete transection of the CBD, the right hepatic duct, or the common hepatic duct. Acute free biliary peritonitis is rare.

Late Presentation

When the common bile duct is mistaken for the cystic duct and is transected, it is usually transected both distally and proximally to the cystic duct. If both ends are ligated, no bile leak occurs. Although most of these patients present with progressive elevation of bilirubin and jaundice, usually within weeks, it may take months for the situation to be fully recognized. The diagnosis of traumatic stricture of the bile ducts is established in approximately 70% within 6 months and over 80% within 12 months. Occasionally, the diagnosis is made 2 to 5 years after surgery.

Management

Postoperative Bile Leak

When no drain is present, the diagnosis of bile leak should be suspected in the patient who develops malaise, RUQ pain, and fever. An ultrasonogram of the subhepatic space shows the presence of bile collection, which is readily drained with a percutaneously introduced catheter. Next, the leak site must be identified. If bile drainage subsides rapidly, no further investigation may be necessary. Introduction of contrast material through the drain catheter can sometimes identify the site of leakage. Otherwise, the best diagnostic technique is ERCP. Further management depends on three possible ERCP findings:

1. If the biliary tract is intact without evidence of injury or bile leak, the presumptive evidence is that leakage is from the gallbladder bed. The only treatment required is to continue catheter drainage until the drainage subsides.

2. If the biliary tract is intact but the cystic duct is leaking, the treatment is endoscopic stenting of the bile duct and continued drainage of the subhepatic space. The cystic duct closes with time.

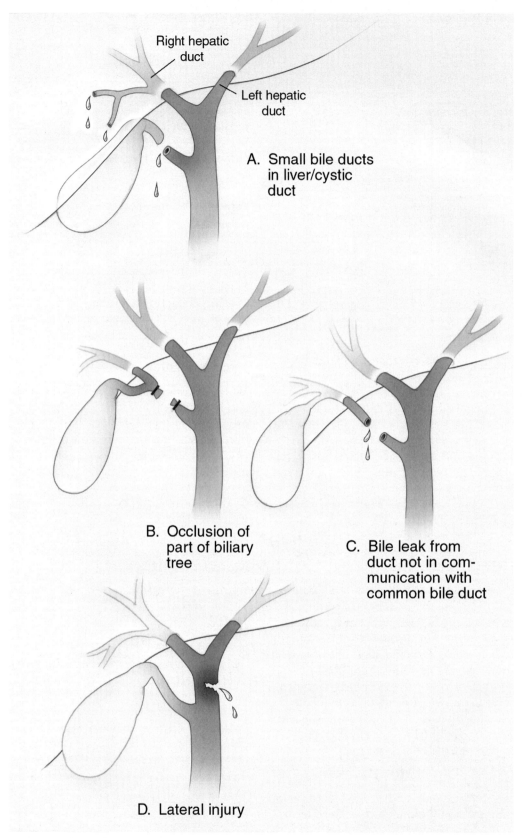

Right hepatic
duct

Left hepatic
duct

A. Small bile ducts
   in liver/cystic
   duct

B. Occlusion of
   part of biliary
   tree

C. Bile leak from
   duct not in com-
   munication with
   common bile duct

D. Lateral injury

FIGURE 7.25. Strasberg's classification of laparoscopic injuries to the biliary tract shows injuries Type A to E. The E injuries are subdivided according to the Bismuth classification. Type A injuries originate from small bile ducts that are entered in the liver bed or from the cystic duct. Type B and C injuries almost always involve aberrant right hepatic ducts. Type A, C, D, and some E injuries may cause bilomas or fistulas. Type B and other type E injuries occlude the biliary tree and bilomas do not occur. (Adapted with permission from Strasberg SM, Hertl M, Soper NJ. An analysis of the problem of biliary injury during laparoscopic cholecystectomy. J Am Coll Surg 1995;180:101–125.)

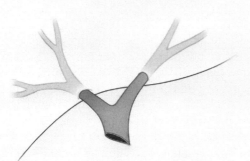

E₁ --Excision less than 2 cm

E₂ --Excision greater than 2 cm

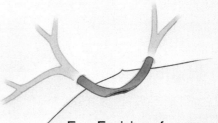

E₃ --Excision of common hepatic duct

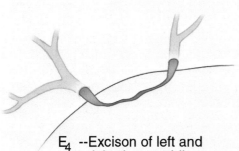

E₄ --Excison of left and right ducts at hilum

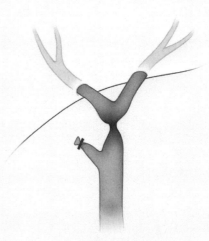

E₅ --Combined common hepatic duct and aberrant right duct injury

FIGURE 7.25. *Continued*

3. If the common bile duct or the right hepatic duct has been transected, the key steps are to ensure adequate drainage of bile leak and to control sepsis with broad-spectrum antibiotics. Besides external drainage of the subhepatic space, internal biliary drainage by the percutaneous transhepatic route may be necessary. Once this is accomplished, surgery may be planned electively at a later date.

When a patient presents late after surgery, diagnosis of bile duct stricture is established first by ultrasonography, which shows dilated intrahepatic bile ducts and no visualization of the CBD. The next most useful investigation is THC,

which accurately establishes the site of injury. It is crucial that the patient be covered with broad-spectrum antibiotics prior to THC and that, if possible, the procedure not be done in the presence of cholangitis. The transhepatic route may also be used to decompress the biliary tract with a catheter.

Surgical Repair

Immediate Intraoperative Repair

Partial transection of the bile duct can be repaired primarily using fine absorbable sutures. Closed drainage of

TABLE 7.11. Classification by Strasberg and colleagues of Laparoscopic Injury Biliary Tract

Type A: Bile leak from minor bile ducts in continuity with common bile duct
- Cystic duct leaks
- Leaks from liver bed (ducts of Luschka)

Type B: Occlusion of part of the biliary tract
- Occlusion of aberrant right hepatic duct

Type C: Bile leak from duct not in communication with common bile duct
- Transection of aberrant right hepatic duct

Type D: Lateral injury to extrahepatic bile ducts
- May involve common hepatic duct, right or left hepatic duct

Type E: Circumferential injury of major bile ducts
- E_1: Excision of common hepatic duct <2 cm
- E_2: Excision of common hepatic duct >2 cm
- E_3: Total excision of common hepatic duct
- E_4: Excision of common hepatic duct and left and right hepatic ducts
- E_5: Combined common hepatic duct and aberrant right hepatic duct injury

Source: Reprinted with permission from Strasberg SM, Hertl M, Soper NJ. An analysis of the problem of biliary injury during laparoscopic cholecystectomy. J Am Coll Surg 1995;180:101–125.

the subhepatic space should be instituted. Depending on the extent of laceration, T-tube drainage of the CBD may be required.

When the common duct is completely transected, primary repair has a high failure rate, even when the surgeon feels the anastomosis can be done without tension. The safest procedure is a Roux-en-Y hepaticojejunostomy, primarily with mucosa-to-mucosa anastomosis using fine absorbable sutures. Optical magnification is useful, particularly when the bile duct is small.

Delayed Elective Repair

Critical in elective repair of established stricture are an experienced surgeon and accurate anatomic definition of injury preoperatively. This is especially true in high hilar injuries when the remnant hepatic duct is short or absent, necessitating separate anastomosis of both the left and right hepatic ducts to the Roux-en-Y jejunal limb. When an adequate length of the common hepatic duct is not available, long-term stenting of the biliary-enteric anastomosis is necessary.

SCLEROSING CHOLANGITIS

In sclerosing cholangitis, progressive fatigue, pruritus, and jaundice develop insidiously over 2 to 3 years. In some patients, the diagnosis is made incidentally due to blood tests or ERCP. Physical examination is either negative or demonstrates hepatosplenomegaly and jaundice. The histopathology shows replacement of bile ducts by dense scarring, sometimes referred to as the disappearing duct syndrome (Figure 7.27).

Investigations

Laboratory Tests

Alkaline phosphatase is usually elevated twofold or higher. Serum bilirubin and transaminase levels are mildly increased. Increased levels of circulating immune complexes and immunoglobulin M (IgM) are seen in 80% and 50% of patients, respectively. Antineutrophil cytoplasmic antibody with a distinct perinuclear pattern (pANCA) is present in over 80%. Serum copper levels are elevated in 49% of patients and ceruloplasmin levels in 71%.

Radiologic Assessment

Cholangiography—by the transhepatic route, ERCP or MRC—is diagnostic. ERCP and MRC are the preferred methods. Both intra- and extrahepatic ducts are involved, particularly the hepatic duct bifurcation. The typical findings are multifocal strictures, which are short (1–2 cm), alternating with slightly dilated ducts, giving a beaded appearance (Figure 7.12). The incidence of cholangiocarcinoma is as high as 10%. Other imaging techniques such as ultrasound, CT, or scintigraphy are not as useful as ERCP and MRC.

Treatment

Medical Treatment

All fat-soluble vitamins (A, D, E, and K) must be replaced. Pruritus is treated with cholestyramine, activated charcoal, phenobarbital, and ursodeoxycholic acid. Medical treatment of the primary disease involves immunosuppression with corticosteroids and/or azathioprine.

Surgical Therapy

Biliary stricture may be managed by endoscopic bile duct dilatation or stenting, but severe cases of extrahepatic stricture require resection and hepaticojejunal Roux-en-Y reconstruction. Any associated intrahepatic strictures can be managed by percutaneous insertion of silastic stents. The incidence of cholangiocarcinoma in ducts with sclerosing cholangitis is 7% to 15%. Resection of the involved common bile duct reduces this risk. Surgical proctocolectomy may be required for associated ulcerative colitis, but the procedure does not control sclerosing cholangitis.

For advanced disease with liver failure, the treatment of choice is liver transplantation. The 1- and 2-year actuarial survival rates are over 88%.[8] The recurrence rate of primary sclerosing cholangitis is low. An interesting question, for which a definitive answer does not exist, is whether post-transplantation immunotherapy increases the incidence of carcinoma in patients who have associated ulcerative colitis. It is probably prudent to perform total proctocolectomy in patients with a history of ulcerative colitis of 15 years or longer.

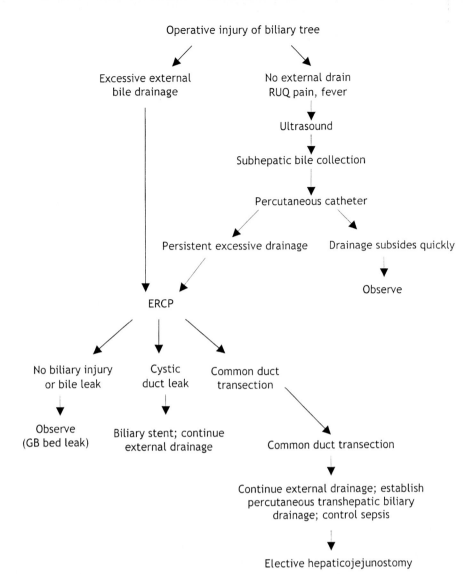

FIGURE 7.26. Management algorithm for biliary tract injury. *Abbreviations*: ERCP, endoscopic retrograde cholangiopancreatography; GB, gallbladder; RUQ, right upper quadrant.

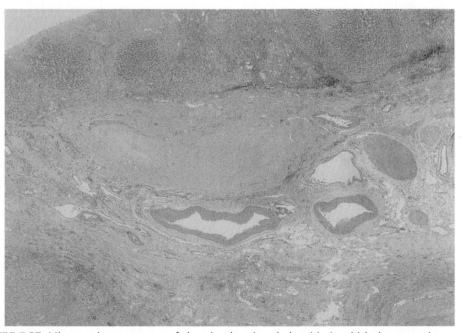

FIGURE 7.27. Microscopic appearance of chronic sclerosing cholangitis, in which dense scarring replaces bile ducts, sometimes referred to as the disappearing duct syndrome. (Courtesy of Linda D. Ferrell, MD.)

RECURRENT PYOGENIC CHOLANGITIS

Over 85% of patients with recurrent pyogenic cholangitis are under 50 years of age, and associated malnutrition and low socioeconomic status are common. Approximately 25% of patients have *Clonorchis sinensis* ova in their stool. Another 13% to 20% have ascariasis. The most common clinical presentation is that of Charcot's triad: RUQ pain, fever and chills, and jaundice. Attacks are intermittent and may occur from every week to every several months. Severe attacks can lead to septic shock and death. Approximately 20% of patients have hepatomegaly and 9% a palpable gallbladder. Chronic acalculous cholecystitis has been reported in as many as 40% of patients.

Investigations

Laboratory Studies

The findings are those of obstructive jaundice with high alkaline phosphatase. Leukocytosis and eosinophilia may be present, and blood culture may be positive for gram-negative organisms and anaerobes.

Imaging Studies

Ultrasound is useful if there are dilated ducts but not as useful as ERCP or THC. CT scan may demonstrate duct dilatation, hepatic atrophy, and intraductal stones (Figure 7.28). About 80% of cases have stones, both intrahepatically and extrahepatically. These stones are the pigment type. The most distinctive features are biliary strictures, most commonly hilar stricture involving the left hepatic duct, followed by common duct stricture. Typically, strictures occur at several levels, with some dilatation of the duct between levels, giving a beaded appearance. Intrahepatic biliary stricture is common, particularly in the left system. Hepatic abscess, hepatic fibrosis, and atrophy may also be present.

Treatment

The principles of surgical treatment are to achieve adequate drainage, remove as many stones as possible, and create biliary-enteric anastomoses to allow other stones to empty out and provide ready future access to the biliary tract.

The surgical techniques used include Roux-en-Y hepaticojejunostomy, with the proximal end of the Roux limb brought out in the RUQ as a fistula or a wide choledochoduodenostomy to allow endoscopic intubation of the CBD when needed (Figure 7.29). Occasionally, the left hepatic lobe may be severely abscessed or severely atrophied enough to require resection.

Reoperation is required in approximately 75% of patients unless the biliary tree can be accessed through a jejunal fistula or choledochoduodenostomy to facilitate removal of recurrent stones endoscopically. The mortality rate, which is related to duration of disease and number of reoperations, is 5% in 5 to 10 years and 12.5% in 10 to 20 years.[9]

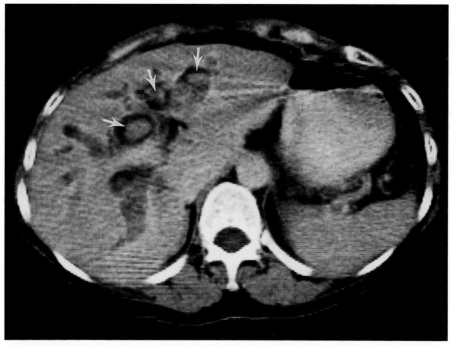

FIGURE 7.28. Recurrent pyogenic cholangitis. This CT scan illustrates some of the common features, including dilated intrahepatic ducts and stones or debris in several ducts (arrows). (Courtesy of Henry I. Goldberg, MD.)

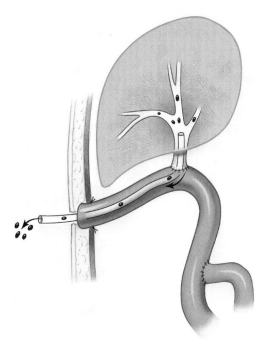

FIGURE 7.29. Roux-en-Y hepaticojejunostomy for oriental cholangiohepatitis. The end of the Roux limb is brought out to the abdominal wall to provide subsequent access in the event of recurrent stones.

NEOPLASMS OF THE BILIARY TRACT

Neoplasms of the intrahepatic ducts and of the hilum of the liver were discussed in Chapter 6. This section discusses carcinomas of the gallbladder and the extrahepatic bile ducts.

Carcinoma of the Gallbladder

Carcinoma of the GB is the fifth most common malignancy in the gastrointestinal tract and has a dismal prognosis. The incidence is highest in Israel, Bolivia, Chile, and in native Americans in the southwestern United States.[10] The disease occurs most commonly in people over the age of 65 years. The etiology is unknown, but the pattern of distribution among native Indians in both North and South America suggests a strong genetic cause. Gallstones, closely associated with gallbladder cancer, are found in 70% to 90% of patients with cancer. But gallbladder cancer is seen in only 0.5% to 3.0% of patients with gallstones, while the incidence increases to 20% when the gallbladder is calcified or porcelain. The incidence of GB cancer in cholelithiasis is not high enough to justify prophylactic cholecystectomy in asymptomatic patients. Histologically, the tumor is adenocarcinoma, most often scirrhous. In 15% of patients, the tumor is papillary. The spread is locoregional to the lymphatics. Direct invasion of the liver, duodenum, or stomach occurs frequently.

Clinical Picture

Most gallbladder cancers are found incidentally at the time of cholecystectomy for gallstones. The tumor may represent a polypoid mass or diffuse thickening of the gallbladder wall (Figure 7.30), or it may have spread extensively to lymph nodes or invaded adjacent organs. If symptoms are present preoperatively, they are indistinguishable from those due to gallstones, although weight loss, anorexia, and jaundice in the absence of choledocholithiasis may be suggestive of the diagnosis.

Treatment

When the lesion is resectable, cholecystectomy is the treatment of choice, with or without regional lymph node dissection and wedge excision of the liver at the GB fossa. More radical operations have been recommended, but there are no data to justify them. Often the tumor is advanced at the time of surgery and resection is not possible. Occasionally, the presence of cancer is detected postoperatively by the pathologist in the gallbladder specimen. What should be done? No data exist to definitively indicate that reoperation is indicated to perform lymphadenectomy and limited hepatic resection. The approach, however, appears reasonable unless the tumor is only intramucosal, in which case the patient has been adequately treated with cholecystectomy alone. The prognosis is grim, with a 5-year survival rate of less than 15%.[11]

Extrahepatic Bile Duct Tumor or Cholangiocarcinoma

Primary bile duct tumors are usually adenocarcinomas involving the common hepatic or common bile ducts. They may involve the bifurcation of the hepatic duct (hilar); the proximal, middle or distal third; or the ampullary region (Figure 7.31). These tumors are more common in patients with ulcerative colitis and sclerosing cholangitis. Tumors at the hepatic hilum present a greater surgical challenge and are often unresectable.

The classic presentation is progressive, painless jaundice, pruritus, anorexia, and weight loss. RUQ or deep epigastric discomfort is often present. Hepatomegaly may be present, but the tumor itself is rarely palpable. When the tumor involves the distal common bile duct with a patent cystic duct, an enlarged gallbladder may be palpable (Courvoisier's sign). Malignant bile duct obstruction may be complicated by cholangitis, but the incidence is not high except following ERCP or THC when prophylactic antibiotic coverage has not been used.

Investigations

LABORATORY FINDINGS The serum bilirubin level is generally markedly elevated (>10 mg/dl), as is the alkaline phosphatase. Hepatocellular dysfunction, if present, is minimal.

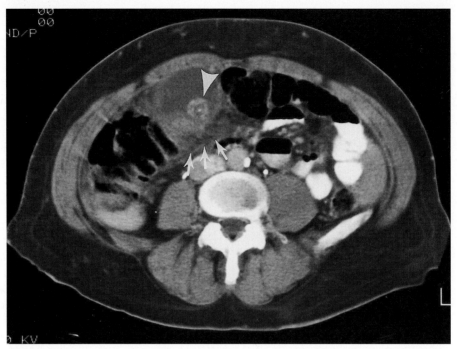

FIGURE 7.30. Carcinoma of the gallbladder. The CT scan shows a calcified stone in the gallbladder (arrowhead) and a soft tissue mass in the gallbladder wall (small arrows) due to gallbladder carcinoma. (Courtesy of Henry I. Goldberg, MD.)

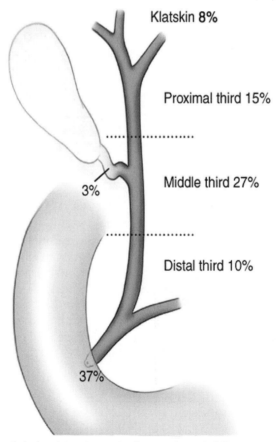

Klatskin 8%

Proximal third 15%

3%

Middle third 27%

Distal third 10%

37%

FIGURE 7.31. Distribution of cholangiocarcinoma in the extrahepatic biliary tract. (Adapted from Blumgart LH. Surgery of the Liver and Biliary Tract, 2nd ed. New York: Churchill Livingstone, 1994.)

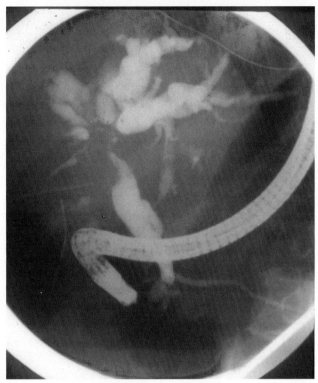

FIGURE 7.32. The ERCP shows a cholangiocarcinoma at the junction of the right and left hepatic ducts, known as a Klatskin tumor. Notice marked enlargement of intrahepatic ducts, particularly of the left system. (Courtesy of John P. Cello, MD.)

IMAGING STUDIES Ultrasound, usually performed as the first imaging study, shows dilated intra- and extrahepatic ducts depending on tumor location. Ultrasound examination, however, rarely provides adequate information about the primary pathology. MRC has emerged as the best noninvasive imaging technique (Figure 7.14) and supplants THC. On the other hand, ERCP has the advantage of enabling histological diagnosis from biopsy or brushing. Generally, ERCP is most useful for distal bile duct tumors, while THC is preferred over CT scan for proximal tumors. Preoperative celiac angiography is useful in determining operability by showing whether the portal vein is involved.

Types of Bile Duct Tumors

HILAR CHOLANGIOCARCINOMA OR KLATSKIN TUMOR In hilar cholangiocarcinoma, also known as Klatskin tumor, the resectability rate is less than 20% (Figure 7.32). Nonetheless, all patients should undergo surgical exploration unless inoperability has been established by imaging studies. At exploration, the tumor is not resectable if any of the following circumstances are found: (1) presence of peritoneal metastasis; (2) invasion of adjacent structures; (3) invasion of portal vein, left and right portal veins, or hepatic arteries; and (4) presence of tumor within second-order biliary radicles of both hepatic lobes.

PROXIMAL AND MIDDLE THIRD EXTRAHEPATIC BILE DUCT When resectable, these tumors are amenable to excision of the hepatic and common ducts and Roux-en-Y hepaticojejunostomy (Figure 7.33).

DISTAL THIRD BILE DUCT AND PERIAMPULLARY LESIONS The resectability rate for these lesions is greater than 50%, and the surgical treatment of choice is pancreaticoduodenectomy, either of the pylorus-sparing type or the classic Whipple resection. Five-year survival rates of 30% to 49% have been reported for periampullary cholangiocarcinoma after curative pancreaticoduodenectomy.[12]

Treatment

The essentials of treatment are listed in Table 7.12. Treatment varies by type of tumor, and surgical procedure depends on tumor location. Hilar lesions present the greatest surgical challenge and the worst outcome.

RESECTION FOR CURE Extent of resection depends on the portion of the proximal extrahepatic biliary system involved. The modified Bismuth–Corlett classification of hilar tumors provides a useful anatomic guide for the required resection (Figure 7.34). Type I and II tumors may be removed without the need to perform hepatic resection. Biliary-enteric anastomosis can be accomplished between either the hepatic duct (Type I) or the right and left hepatic ducts (Type II) and a Roux limb of the jejunum. Type III lesion, if resectable, requires either right (IIIA) or left (IIIB)

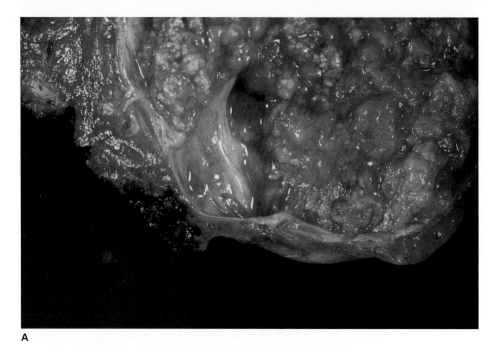

A

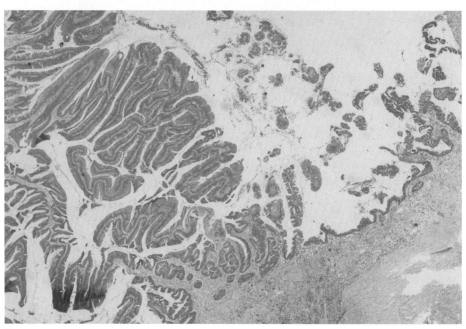

B

FIGURE 7.33. (A) Gross appearance of a large intraductal papillary cholangiocarcinoma of the common bile duct. (B) Microscopically, papillary projection of the tumor is evident. The appearance contrasts with the usual manifestation of cholangiocarcinoma, in which extensive fibrosis is seen with only islands of adenocarcinoma cells. In addition, an intraductal papillary carcinoma may appear large but be attached to the CBD wall through a relatively small pedicle. (Courtesy of Linda D. Ferrell, MD.)

TABLE 7.12. Essentials: Treatment of Bile Duct Tumors

Hilar cholangiocarcinoma (Klatskin tumor)
- Resectability rate: 20%
- Type I and II: Tumor resection with Roux-en-Y hepaticojejunostomy
- Type III: Resection of tumor with left or right hepatectomy, caudate lobectomy and Roux-en-Y hepaticojejunostomy

Carcinoma of proximal and middle third
- Excision of hepatic and common ducts and Roux-en-Y hepaticojejunostomy

Carcinoma of distal third
- Resectability rate: 50%
- Procedures: Pancreaticoduodenectomy
- 5-year survival rate: 20%–60%

Unresectable tumor
- Biliary decompression: Surgical (U-tube) or transhepatic or endoscopic stenting
- Adjuvant therapy: External or local (^{192}Ir wire) radiation
- Chemotherapy of little use

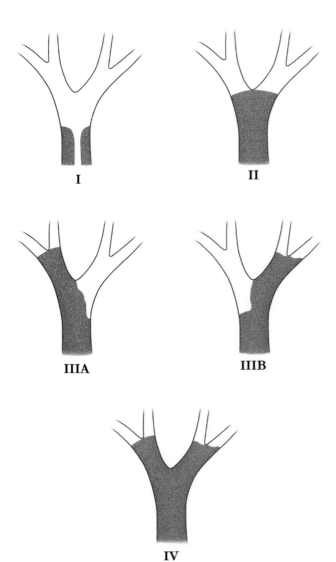

FIGURE 7.34. Bismuth–Corlette classification of hilar tumors. (Adapted with permission from Bismuth H, Nakache R, Diamond T. Management strategies in resection for hilar cholangiocarcinoma. Ann Surg 1992;215:31–38.

hepatic lobectomy for cure (Figure 7.35). Caudate lobe resection may also be required. Some surgeons have performed total hepatectomy and orthotopic liver transplantation after chemoradiation in selected cases.[13] The value of this treatment is unproven.

UNRESECTABLE TUMORS If the tumor cannot be resected, decompression of the biliary tree is required. Several surgical procedures were in use prior to the advent of percutaneous stenting. At the time of surgery, U-tube stenting can be performed. The procedure requires identification of the obstructed left or right hepatic duct system. A silastic tube is placed through the abdominal wall, through the dome of the liver, across the tumor, out of the common bile duct, and through the abdominal wall. The segment of the tube within the bile ducts has multiple perforations. Such tubes tend to be obstructed with sludge but are easily replaceable without operation. Other alternatives, now more commonly used, are placement of stents endoscopically or transhepatically. Endoscopic or transhepatic stenting are equally effective, and selection of one over the other usually depends on the type of expertise available at the institution.

OUTCOME The best 5-year survival rates after curative resection of hilar cholangiocarcinoma have been 30% with an operative mortality of 4%.[5] The 5-year survival after stenting alone is about 5%. Although considerable debate exists about the relative value of surgical and nonsurgical treatment, the only chance of a cure is surgical resection.

ADJUVANT THERAPY Cholangiocarcinoma is resistant to both radio- and chemotherapy. External radiation and local radiation with ^{192}Ir wire have been reported to be of some benefit, and postoperative radiation may reduce recurrence rates.

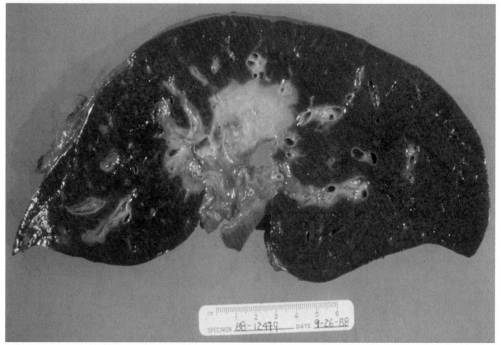

A

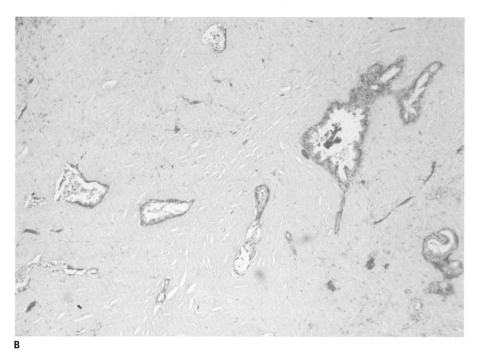

B

FIGURE 7.35. (A) Gross appearance of hilar cholangiocarcinoma at the confluence of the right and left ducts. (B) Microscopically, there is dense stroma, little inflammation, and few isolated tumor cells. (Courtesy of Linda D. Ferrell, MD.)

REFERENCES

1. Trotman BW. Pigment gallstone disease. *Gastroenterol Clin North Am* 1991;20:111–126.
2. Charcot JM. Leçons sur les maladies du foie, des voies biliaires et des reins: faites a la faculté de médecine de paris. Paris: Progrès Médical; 1877:380.
3. Fan ST, Lai EC, Mok FP, et al. Early treatment of acute biliary pancreatitis by endoscopic papillotomy. *N Engl J Med* 1993; 328:228–232.
4. Friedman GD. Natural history of asymptomatic and symptomatic gallstones. *Am J Surg* 1993;165:399–404.
5. Harris HW. Biliary system. In: Norton JA, Bollinger RR, Chang AE, et al., eds. *Surgery: Basic Science and Clinical Evidence.* New York: Springer-Verlag; 2001:566.
6. Werbel GB, Nahrwold DL, Joehl RJ, et al. Percutaneous cholecystostomy in the diagnosis and treatment of acute cholecystitis in the high-risk patient. *Arch Surg* 1989;124: 782–786.

7. Strasberg SM, Hertl M, Soper NJ. An analysis of the problem of biliary injury during laparoscopic cholecystectomy. *J Am Coll Surg* 1995;180:101–125.

8. Ahrendt SA, Pitt HA, Kalloo AN, et al. Primary sclerosing cholangitis: resect, dilate, or transplant? *Ann Surg* 1998;227:412–423.

9. Stain SC, Incarbone R, Guthrie CR, et al. Surgical treatment of recurrent pyogenic cholangitis. *Arch Surg* 1995;130:527–533.

10. Levin B. Gallbladder carcinoma. *Ann Oncol* 1999;10(Suppl 4):129–130.

11. Carriaga MT, Henson DE. Liver, gallbladder, extrahepatic bile ducts, and pancreas. *Cancer* 1995;75(1 Suppl):171–190.

12. Nakeeb A, Pitt HA, Sohn TA, et al. Cholangiocarcinoma. A spectrum of intrahepatic, perihilar, and distal tumors. *Ann Surg* 1996;224:463–475.

13. Urego M, Flickinger JC, Carr BI. Radiotherapy and multimodality management of cholangiocarcinoma. *Int J Radiat Oncol Biol Phys* 1999;44:121–126.

SELECTED READINGS

Anatomy and Physiology

Admirand WH, Small DM. The physicochemical basis of cholesterol gallstone formation in man. *J Clin Invest* 1968;47:1043–1052.

Boyden EA. The anatomy of the choledochoduodenal junction in man. *Surg Gynecol Obstet* 1957;104:641–652.

Csendes A, Burdiles P, Maluenda F, et al. Simultaneous bacteriologic assessment of bile from gallbladder and common bile duct in control subjects and patients with gallstones and common duct stones. *Arch Surg* 1996;131:389–394.

Klein AS, Lillemoe KD, Yeo CJ, et al. Liver, biliary tract and pancreas. In: O'Leary JP, ed. *The Physiologic Basis of Surgery*. Baltimore: Williams & Wilkins; 1993:255–292.

Lindner HH. Embryology and anatomy of the biliary tree. In: Way LW, Pellegrini CA, eds. *Surgery of the Gallbladder and Bile Ducts*. Philadelphia: WB Saunders; 1987:3–15.

Smadja C, Blumgart LH. The biliary tract and the anatomy of biliary exposure. In: Blumgart LH, ed. *Surgery of the Liver and Biliary Tract*. 2nd ed. Edinburgh: Churchill Livingstone; 1994;11–24.

Tierney S, Pitt HA, Lillemoe KD. Physiology and pathophysiology of gallbladder motility. *Surg Clin North Am* 1993;73:1267–1290.

Biliary Tract Imaging

Aronchick CA, Ritchie WG, Kaplan SM, et al. Sincalide-aided ultrasonography of the common bile duct as a predictor of biliary obstruction determined by ERCP and biliary manometry. *Gastrointest Endosc* 1990;36:467–471.

Barish MA, Soto JA. MR cholangiopancreatography: techniques and clinical applications. *AJR Am J Roentgenol* 1997;169:1295–1303.

Blankenberg F, Wirth R, Jeffrey RB Jr, et al. Computed tomography as an adjunct to ultrasound in the diagnosis of acute acalculous cholecystitis. *Gastrointest Radiol* 1991;16:149–153.

Cooperberg PL, Burhenne HJ. Real-time ultrasonography. Diagnostic technique of choice in calculous gallbladder disease. *N Engl J Med* 1980;302:1277–1279.

Magnuson TH, Bender JS, Duncan MD, et al. Utility of magnetic resonance cholangiography in the evaluation of biliary obstruction. *J Am Coll Surg* 1999;189:63–72.

Ohtani T, Kawai C, Shirai Y, et al. Intraoperative ultrasonography versus cholangiography during laparoscopic cholecystectomy: a prospective comparative study. *J Am Coll Surg* 1997;185:274–282.

Parulekar SG, Hillier SA, Adell JA, et al. Color Doppler sonography of the gallbladder wall. *J Ultrasound Med* 1995;14(Suppl):S21.

Paulson EK, Kliewer MA, Hertzberg BS, et al. Diagnosis of acute cholecystitis with color Doppler sonography: significance of arterial flow in thickened gallbladder wall. *AJR Am J Roentgenol* 1994;162:1105–1108.

Robinson BL, Donohue JH, Gunes S, et al. Selective operative cholangiography. Appropriate management for laparoscopic cholecystectomy. *Arch Surg* 1995;130:625–631.

Shaffer EA, Hershfield NB, Logan K, et al. Cholescintigraphic detection of functional obstruction of the sphincter of Oddi. Effect of papillotomy. *Gastroenterology* 1986;90:728–733.

Soto JA, Barish MA, Yucel EK, et al. Magnetic resonance cholangiography: comparison with endoscopic retrograde cholangiopancreatography. *Gastroenterology* 1996;110:589–597.

Stotland BR, Kochman ML. Diagnostic and therapeutic endosonography: endoscopic ultrasound-guided fine-needle aspiration in clinical practice. *Gastrointest Endosc* 1997;45:329–331.

Suarez CA, Block F, Bernstein D, et al. The role of HIDA/PIPIDA scanning in diagnosing cystic duct obstruction. *Ann Surg* 1980;191:391–396.

Zeman RK, Garra BS. Gallbladder imaging: the state of the art. *Gastroenterol Clin North Am* 1991;20:127–156.

Gallstone Disease

Adamek HE, Maier M, Jakobs R, et al. Management of retained bile duct stones: a prospective open trial comparing extracorporeal and intracorporeal lithotripsy. *Gastrointest Endosc* 1996;44:40–47.

Burhenne HJ. Garland lecture. Percutaneous extraction of retained biliary tract stones: 661 patients. *AJR Am J Roentgenol* 1980;134:889–898.

Caprini JA. Biliary stone extraction. *Am Surg* 1988;54:343–346.

Cetta F. The role of bacteria in pigment gallstone disease. *Ann Surg* 1991;213:315–326.

Cotton PB, Kozarek RA, Schapiro RH, et al. Endoscopic laser lithotripsy of large bile duct stones. *Gastroenterology* 1990;99:1128–1133.

Cuschieri A, Berci G. Laparoscopic treatment of common duct stones. In: Cuschieri A. *Laparoscopic Biliary Surgery*. 2nd ed. Oxford; Boston: Blackwell Scientific; 1992:155–169.

Freeman ML, Nelson DB, Sherman S, et al. Complications of endoscopic biliary sphincterotomy. *N Engl J Med* 1996;335:909–918.

Glasgow RE, Visser BC, Harris HW, et al. Changing management of gallstone disease during pregnancy. *Surg Endosc* 1998;12:241–246.

Ikeda S, Tanaka M, Matsumoto S, et al. Endoscopic sphincterotomy: long-term results in 408 patients with complete follow-up. *Endoscopy* 1988;20:13–17.

Kiviluoto T, Siren J, Luukkonen P, et al. Randomised trial of laparoscopic versus open cholecystectomy for acute and gangrenous cholecystitis. *Lancet* 1998;351:321–325.

Larson RE, Hodgson JR, Priestley JT. The early and long-term results of 500 consecutive explorations of the common duct. *Surg Gynecol Obstet* 1966;122:744–750.

Lo CM, Liu CL, Fan ST, et al. Prospective randomized study of early versus delayed laparoscopic cholecystectomy for acute cholecystitis. *Ann Surg* 1998;227:461–467.

Loperfido S, Angelini G, Benedetti G, et al. Major early complications from diagnostic and therapeutic ERCP: a prospective multicenter study. *Gastrointest Endosc* 1998;48:1–10.

Moraca RJ, Lee FT, Ryan JA Jr, et al. Long-term biliary function after reconstruction of major bile duct injuries with hepaticoduodenostomy or hepaticojejunostomy. *Arch Surg* 2002;137:889–894.

Palmer KR, Hofmann AF. Intraductal mono-octanoin for the direct dissolution of bile duct stones: experience in 343 patients. *Gut* 1986;27:196–202.

Perissat J, Huibregtse K, Keane FB, et al. Management of bile duct stones in the era of laparoscopic cholecystectomy. *Br J Surg* 1994;81:799–810.

Proceedings of the NIH Consensus Development Conference on Gallstones and Laparoscopic Cholecystectomy. Bethesda, Maryland, September 14–16, 1992. *Am J Surg* 1993;165:387–548.

Reisner RM, Cohen JR. Gallstone ileus: a review of 1001 reported cases. *Am Surg* 1994;60:441–446.

Rhodes M, Sussman L. Prospective randomized trial of laparoscopic common bile duct exploration versus post-operative ERCP [abstr]. *Gut* 1997;40(Suppl 1):A68.

Saharia PC, Zuidema GD, Cameron JL. Primary common duct stones. *Ann Surg* 1977;185:598–604.

Santucci L, Natalini G, Sarpi L, et al. Selective endoscopic retrograde cholangiography and preoperative bile duct stone removal in patients scheduled for laparoscopic cholecystectomy: a prospective study. *Am J Gastroenterol* 1996;91:1326–1330.

Schwesinger WH, Sirinek KR, Strodel WE 3rd. Laparoscopic cholecystectomy for biliary tract emergencies: state of the art. *World J Surg* 1999;23:334–342.

Stuart SA, Simpson TI, Alvord LA, et al. Routine intraoperative laparoscopic cholangiography. *Am J Surg* 1998;176:632–637.

Targarona EM, Ayuso RM, Bordas JM, et al. Randomised trial of endoscopic sphincterotomy with gallbladder left in situ versus open surgery for common bile duct calculi in high-risk patients. *Lancet* 1996;347:926–929.

Tierney S, Lillemoe KD, Pitt HA. The current management of common duct stones. *Adv Surg* 1995;28:271–299.

Way LW, Admirand WH, Dunphy JE. Management of choledocholithiasis. *Ann Surg* 1972;176:347–359.

Malignancies of the Biliary Tract

Bartlett DL, Fong Y, Fortner JG, et al. Long-term results after resection for gallbladder cancer. Implications for staging and management. *Ann Surg* 1996;224:639–646.

Bismuth H, Nakache R, Diamond T. Management strategies in resection for hilar cholangiocarcinoma. *Ann Surg* 1992;215:31–38.

Burke EC, Jarnagin WR, Hochwald SN, et al. Hilar cholangiocarcinoma: patterns of spread, the importance of hepatic resection for curative operation, and a presurgical clinical staging system. *Ann Surg* 1998;228:385–394.

Jarnagin WR, Fong Y, DeMatteo RP, et al. Staging, resectability, and outcome in 225 patients with hilar cholangiocarcinoma. *Ann Surg* 2001;234:507–519.

Klatskin G. Adenocarcinoma of the hepatic duct at its bifurcation within the porta hepatis: an unusual tumor with distinctive clinical and pathological features. *Am J Med* 1965;38:241–247.

Klempnauer J, Ridder GJ, von Wasielewski R, et al. Resectional surgery of hilar cholangiocarcinoma: a multivariate analysis of prognostic factors. *J Clin Oncol* 1997;15:947–954.

Pitt HA, Dooley WC, Yeo CJ, et al. Malignancies of the biliary tree. *Curr Probl Surg* 1995;32:1–90.

Strasberg SM. Resection of hilar cholangiocarcinoma. *HPB Surg* 1998;10:415–418.

Tsukada K, Hatakeyama K, Kurosaki I, et al. Outcome of radical surgery for carcinoma of the gallbladder according to the TNM stage. *Surgery* 1996;120:816–821.

Weber SM, DeMatteo RP, Fong Y, et al. Staging laparoscopy in patients with extrahepatic biliary carcinoma. Analysis of 100 patients. *Ann Surg* 2002;235:392–399.

Sclerosing Cholangitis

Campbell WL, Ferris JV, Holbert BL, et al. Biliary tract carcinoma complicating primary sclerosing cholangitis: evaluation with CT, cholangiography, US, and MR imaging. *Radiology* 1998;207:41–50.

Goss JA, Shackleton CR, Farmer DG, et al. Orthotopic liver transplantation for primary sclerosing cholangitis. A 12-year single center experience. *Ann Surg* 1997;225:472–481.

Graziadei IW, Wiesner RH, Batts KP, et al. Recurrence of primary sclerosing cholangitis following liver transplantation. *Hepatology* 1999;29:1050–1056.

Lee YM, Kaplan MM. Primary sclerosing cholangitis. *N Engl J Med* 1995;332:924–933.

Martin FM, Rossi RL, Nugent FW, et al. Surgical aspects of sclerosing cholangitis. Results in 178 patients. *Ann Surg* 1990;212:551–556.

Ponsioen CI, Tytgat GN. Primary sclerosing cholangitis: a clinical review. *Am J Gastroenterol* 1998;93:515–523.

Wiesner RH. Liver transplantation for primary biliary cirrhosis and primary sclerosing cholangitis: predicting outcomes with natural history models. *Mayo Clin Proc* 1998;73:575–588.

Congenital Diseases

Asselah T, Ernst O, Sergent G, et al. Caroli's disease: a magnetic resonance cholangiopancreatography diagnosis. *Am J Gastroenterol* 1998;93:109–110.

Dagli U, Atalay F, Sasmaz N, et al. Caroli's disease: 1977–1995 experiences. *Eur J Gastroenterol Hepatol* 1998;10:109–112.

Fieber SS, Nance FC. Choledochal cyst and neoplasm: a comprehensive review of 106 cases and presentation of two original cases. *Am Surg* 1997;63:982–987.

Lipsett PA, Segev DL, Colombani PM. Biliary atresia and biliary cysts. *Baillieres Clin Gastroenterol* 1997;11:619–641.

Miyano T, Yamataka A. Choledochal cysts. *Curr Opin Pediatr* 1997;9:283–288.

Oguchi Y, Okada A, Nakamura T, et al. Histopathologic studies of congenital dilatation of the bile duct as related to an anomalous junction of the pancreaticobiliary ductal system: clinical and experimental studies. *Surgery* 1988;103:168–173.

Stain SC, Guthrie CR, Yellin AE, et al. Choledochal cyst in the adult. *Ann Surg* 1995;222:128–133.

Taylor AC, Palmer KR. Caroli's disease. *Eur J Gastroenterol Hepatol* 1998;10:105–108.

Todani T, Watanabe Y, Narusue M, et al. Congenital bile duct cysts: classification, operative procedures, and review of thirty-seven cases including cancer arising from choledochal cyst. *Am J Surg* 1977;134:263–269.

8

Small and Large Intestine

Digestion of food and absorption of nutrients occurs in the small intestine, the segment of the gastrointestinal tract between the pylorus and the ileocecal valve. While life can be sustained by total parenteral nutrition in the absence of the small intestine, perfect growth and health depend on normal function of this organ.

Although the major function of the colon is reservoir and transport, it also has absorptive and endocrine functions. Some of the most emergent surgical conditions arise from obstruction, perforation, or vascular compromise of the small intestine and colon. The surgeon must treat these conditions adequately, often by resection. In the case of the small intestine, as much of the bowel as possible must be saved; and, in the case of both organs, appropriate conditions for safe anastomosis must be ensured. Not all procedures on the small intestine are performed to treat pathology within it. In some procedures, segments of it are used to replace other organs (e.g., esophagus, ureter). The colon has served a similar function to replace the esophagus. Surgery of the small and large intestine is an important chapter in abdominal surgery.

ANATOMY

EMBRYOLOGY

The small intestine is derived entirely from the midgut of the embryo except for the segment of the duodenum proximal to the ampulla of Vater, which is of foregut origin. The ascending colon and the right half of the transverse colon are also derived from the midgut, while the rest of the colon develops from the hindgut (Figure 8.1). During early fetal life, the small intestine is located in the yolk sac of the embryo. In the tenth week of fetal life, the intestine returns into the abdominal cavity of the embryo and, in so doing, it undergoes a 180° rotation counterclockwise. Because of this rotation, the C-loop of the duodenum faces to the left, and the small intestine fixes obliquely on a mesentery that extends from the right side of L-3 to the left side of L-1.

A number of congenital abnormalities related to malrotation are seen in pediatric surgical practice. On rare occasions, however, intestinal malrotation may not cause problems until adult life and may even be an incidental finding during abdominal operations for other reasons. Other congenital abnormalities of the intestine include strictures, diaphragm formation, duplications, and remnants of the vitelline duct manifesting as a Meckel's diverticulum. Finally, rests of pancreatic tissue in the duodenum and gastric mucosa in a Meckel's diverticulum may occur, and again, these may not be symptomatic until after childhood.

SMALL INTESTINE

The small intestine is about 20 feet long and extends from the pylorus to the ileocecal valve. The absorptive surface, however, is greatly increased by rugal folds and mucosal villus formation. Although it is fixed on a mesentery, as described above, the mesentery is broad based and the small intestine can move freely within the abdominal cavity without becoming obstructed. The mesentery contains one or two vascular arcades in the jejunum, but in the ileum it may contain as many as four or five vascular arcades. The small intestine wall consists of a well-formed serosa as well as a muscular coat made up of an outer longitudinal and inner circular layers, a submucosa, muscularis mucosa, and a mucosal layer.

As a derivative of the midgut, the small intestine receives its blood supply from the superior mesenteric

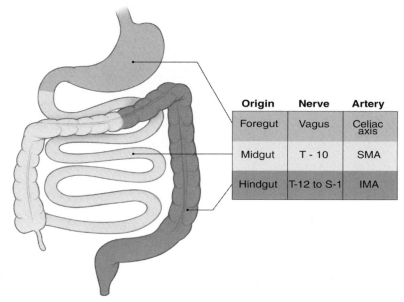

Origin	Nerve	Artery
Foregut	Vagus	Celiac axis
Midgut	T - 10	SMA
Hindgut	T-12 to S-1	IMA

FIGURE 8.1. Embryologic chart and view of the gastrointestinal tract shows the origins and nerve and arterial supply. *Abbreviations*: IMA, inferior mesenteric artery; SMA, superior mesenteric artery.

artery, except for the proximal half of the duodenum, which receives its blood supply from the gastroduodenal artery, a branch of the artery of the foregut, the celiac axis. Venous drainage, which is corresponding, is through the superior mesenteric vein and gastroduodenal veins. The blood supply of the small intestine is depicted in Figure 8.2.

The parasympathetic innervation is derived from the vagus mostly through the celiac branch. The sympathetic innervation, distributed along the adventitia of the arterial supply, derives from the greater and lesser splanchnic nerves. The small intestine is entirely intraperitoneal except for the second, third and fourth portions of the duodenum, which are retroperitoneal.

The absorptive surface of the mucosa is increased many times, first by the formation of finger-like projections called villi and second by the presence of microvilli on the luminal surface of epithelial cells. The villi are covered with a single layer of columnar epithelial cells that includes absorptive, goblet, and endocrine cells, sparsely scattered throughout the layer. While the villi project into the lumen, the crypts of Lieberkühn project into the lamina propria. The crypts have a vital role in cell renewal and secretion (Figure 8.3).

The cells lining the crypts are progenitor, goblet, enterochromaffin (argentaffin), and Paneth. Paneth cells secrete lysozyme and cytokines. The lamina propria, the loose areolar layer between the mucosa and the muscularis mucosa, contains connective tissue, numerous blood vessels and nerves, and several types of cells including lymphocytes, plasma cells, eosinophils, macrophages, and mast cells. Large numbers of lymphatic cells are organized in follicles, known as Peyer's patches, which are found throughout the small intestine and are even more numerous in the ileum. They are thought to play a crucial role in the immune response and immune regulation of the gut.

The submucosa is a connective tissue layer containing blood vessels, lymphocytes, neural plexuses, and the submucosal (Meissner's) ganglia. Outside the submucosa is the muscularis, consisting of an inner circular and outer longitudinal smooth muscle layer. Between these two muscle layers are the myenteric ganglia and the myenteric plexus, an important component of the enteric nervous system that controls motility. Outside the muscularis is a well-developed, relatively less distensible serosal layer. Blood vessels and extrinsic nerves enter and leave the gut wall through the mesentery.

LARGE INTESTINE

The large intestine or colon extends from the ileocecal valve proximally to the retrosigmoid junction distally and is 3 to 5 feet in length. The colon occupies the periphery of the abdominal cavity and is made up of the cecum and ascending colon on the right, the transverse colon, and the descending colon and sigmoid on the left. The splenic flexure is closely related to the spleen and is attached to it by the splenocolic ligament. The right colon has a larger caliber than the left, and the cecum has the largest caliber and is most distensible. The cecum is subject to rupture when it reaches a diameter of 12 cm as a result of complete distal obstruction in the presence of a competent ileocecal valve.

The layers of the colon wall include the mucosa, submucosa, inner circular and outer longitudinal muscu-

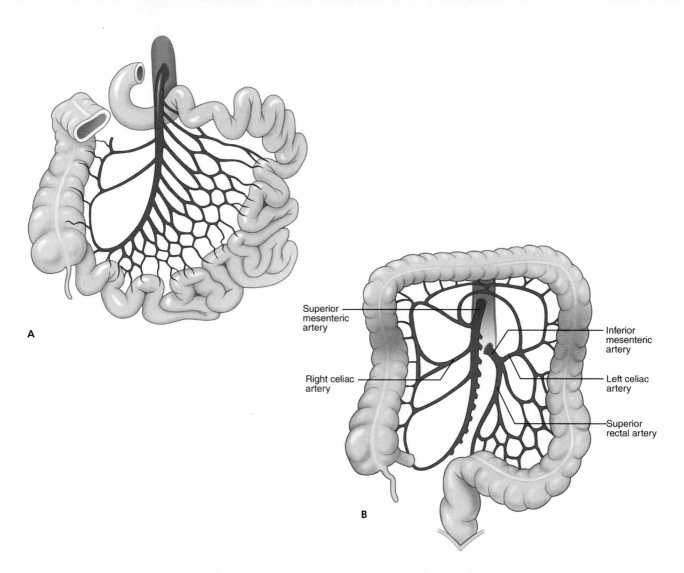

FIGURE 8.2. Arterial blood supply of the (A) small and (B) large intestine from the superior and inferior mesenteric arteries. (Adapted from Schwartz SI, ed: Principles of Surgery, 6th ed. New York: McGraw Hill, 1994:1192.)

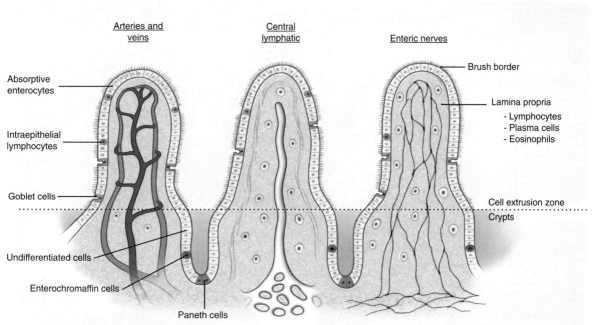

FIGURE 8.3. Anatomy of the small intestinal mucosa, showing the structure of the villi and crypts.

laris, and a serosa. The longitudinal muscle is arranged into three separate bundles called tenia coli. The three teniae are 120° apart around the circumference of the colon. Haustra, or sacculations, are formed because the teniae foreshorten the colon. The serosal surface contains fatty appendages called appendices epiploicae (Figure 8.4).

The cecum is a free intraperitoneal organ, but the ascending colon is partially retroperitoneal up to the hepatic flexure. The transverse colon is draped with the greater omentum, which hangs down from it. The descending colon is fixed to the lateral abdominal wall by a fascia. Where this fascia meets the colon, an avascular plane exists called the line of Tolt, which is incised when the left colon is mobilized.

The superior mesenteric artery supplies the ascending colon and the transverse colon through the ileocecal, right colic, and middle colic branches. The inferior mesenteric artery supplies the ascending colon and the splenic flexure through the left colic branch, and the sigmoid through sigmoid branches. The splenic flexure area is a vascular watershed between the middle colic and left colic arteries and has a more precarious blood supply. As a result, it is susceptible to ischemic disease of the colon. The blood supply of the colon is shown in Figure 8.2.

The arteries to the colon communicate on the mesenteric aspect to form a vascular arcade, which is called the marginal artery of Drummond. The marginal artery enlarges when the superior mesenteric artery becomes occluded, and the entire colon must receive its blood supply in retrograde fashion from the inferior mesenteric artery. Venous drainage follows the arterial supply. Lymphatics from the colonic wall drain into pericolic mesenteric lymph nodes.

ANORECTUM

The rectum and anal canal differ in their embryologic development, both in their type of mucosa and the derivations of their blood and nerve supplies. The rectum, deriving from the terminal portion of the hindgut, is lined with colonic-type mucosa; its principal blood supply comes from the inferior mesenteric vessels. The anal canal derives from the cloaca, and its blood supply is derived from the pudendal vessels. The anal mucosa consists of stratified squamous cells in its distal half and transitional epithelium in its proximal half.

Rectum

The rectum begins at the anorectal junction 3 cm from the anal verge and ends at the retrosigmoid junction just in front of the sacral promontory. The distance from the anal verge to the rectosigmoid junction is 20 cm. The supporting structures of the rectum include the mesorectum posteriorly, the lateral ligaments laterally, and the fascia of Waldeyer and the puborectalis muscle distally (Figure 8.5). The mesorectum fixes the rectum to the anterior surface of the sacrum, which is covered with the presacral plexus of veins.

Blood Supply

Three arterial systems supply the rectum:

1. The superior hemorrhoidal artery, a continuation of the inferior mesenteric artery.
2. The middle hemorrhoidal arteries, branches of the internal iliac arteries running in the lateral ligaments.
3. The inferior hemorrhoidal arteries.

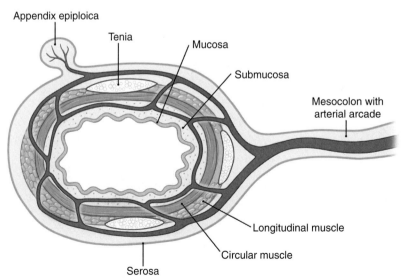

FIGURE 8.4. Cross-sectional anatomy of the colon, showing the location of the three tenia coli. (Adapted from Schwartz SI, ed: Principles of Surgery, 6th ed. New York: McGraw Hill, 1994:1193.)

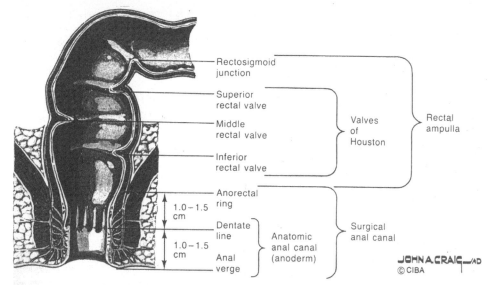

FIGURE 8.5. Anorectal anatomy shows the external and internal anal sphincters. (Adapted from Fry RD, Koduer IJ. Anorectal disorders. Ciba Clinical Symposia 37:6, 1985. Copyright 1985 Ciba-Geigy Corp. Reprinted with permission from Clinical Symposia illustrated by John A. Craig, MD. All rights reserved.)

All three vessels anastomose over the surface of the rectum. Venous drainage is provided via the superior hemorrhoidal veins to the inferior mesenteric veins. The middle and inferior hemorrhoidal veins drain into the internal iliac veins. Several important clinical implications arise from this vascular arrangement:

1. Increased portal pressure is reflected to the hemorrhoidal vessels via the superior hemorrhoidal vein, which lacks valves. This anatomical fact explains the development of hemorrhoids in portal hypertension.
2. If, during rectal mobilization in surgery for rectal cancer, the inferior mesenteric vein is ligated early, a higher number of cancer calls can be recovered from the internal iliac vein.
3. Severely infected hemorrhoids can cause pyelophlebitis, due to septic emboli going up the mesenteric vein.
4. Hematogenous spread to the liver from rectal cancer occurs via the inferior mesenteric vein.

Lymphatic Drainage

Lymphatic drainage of the rectum occurs through the perirectal nodes and then into inferior mesenteric nodes.

Nerve Supply

The nerve supply to the rectum comes from both sympathetic and parasympathetic nerves. The sympathetic innervation is from the thoracolumbar chain and is distributed surrounding the inferior mesenteric artery as a network plexus to the superior hypogastric plexus, just below the aortic bifurcation. The hypogastric plexus gives off the hypogastric nerves that supply the lower rectum, the bladder, and the genitals. Parasympathetic fibers originate from S-2, S-3, and S-4 roots as the nervi erigentes and descend to form the pelvic plexus anterior and lateral to the rectum. These nerves supply the rectum, the internal anal sphincter, prostate, bladder and penis.

Penile erection is mediated by VIP-containing neurons in the parasympathetic nerves, causing vasodilatation, while the sympathetic nerves cause venoconstriction in the corpus callosum, trapping the blood to sustain erection. Thus, damage to either the sympathetic nerves (most often incurred during high ligation of the inferior mesenteric artery) or the parasympathetic nerves (incurred during lateral and periprostatic mobilization of the rectum) can lead to impotence and bladder dysfunction.

The rectum has three spirally arranged mucosal folds called the valves of Houston, two on the left and one on the right, although not every individual has all three valves. These valves are clinically significant because a small tumor can hide behind one and escape detection during sigmoidoscopy unless the area is examined carefully.

Anal Canal

The anal canal is 3 cm long and ends at the anorectal junction, the mucocutaneous junction also referred to as the dentate or pectinate line. Anal crypts and the openings of the anal glands are located at the dentate line. The anal crypts and the openings of the anal glands are located at the distal end of the Columns of Morgagni. The anal canal is pulled anteriorly by the puborectalis, causing it to point towards the umbilicus and form an angle with the rectum (Figure 8.6). The anorectal sphincteric ring is formed by the fusion of the puborectalis and the internal sphincter, the longitudinal muscle, and the muscles of the external sphincter.

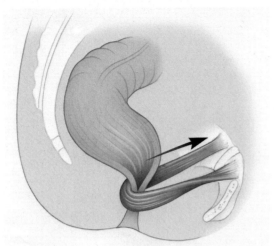

FIGURE 8.6. The puborectalis sling creates an angle between the rectum and the anus that plays an important role in continence. (Adapted from Fleshman JW, et al. In Shackelford's Surgery of the Alimentary Tract, 3rd edition. Philadelphia: WB Saunders, 1991.)

Blood Supply

The anal canal is supplied by the inferior and middle hemorrhoidal arteries and veins.

Lymphatic Drainage

The anal canal mucosa drains into inguinal lymph nodes and then to the external iliac and common iliac lymph nodes.

Nerve Supply

The nerve supply is derived from the inferior rectal and perineal branches of the pudendal nerve. Sensation of heat, cold, pain, and touch is appreciated in the mucosa distal to the dentate line.

PHYSIOLOGY

SMALL INTESTINE

The four key functions of the small intestine are: digestion, absorption, secretion, and motility (transportation).

Digestion

The small intestine is the primary site of digestion of carbohydrate, proteins, and amino acids.

Digestion of Carbohydrate

Carbohydrate digestion begins with the action of salivary amylase, but the complete digestion into monosaccharides occurs in the small intestine by the action of pancreatic amylase and brush border enzymes as shown in Figure 8.7.

Digestion of Fat

The average fat intake in the U.K. and United States is 100 to 150 g/day, although both populations are slowly reducing their fat consumption. Dietary triglycerides contain largely oleate and palmitate as their fatty acids. In addition, 2 to 8 g of phospholipids are ingested daily. The most common phospholipid ingested is lecithin, and the predominant fatty acids are linoleate and arachidonate. Most dietary fat is digested and absorbed in the first half of the jejunum.

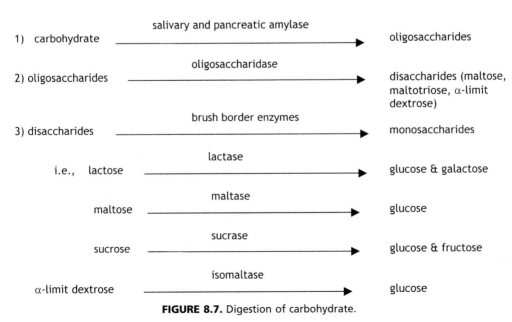

FIGURE 8.7. Digestion of carbohydrate.

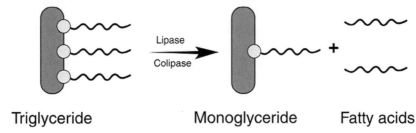

Triglyceride   Monoglyceride   Fatty acids

FIGURE 8.8. Action of lipase and colipase in yielding fatty acids and monoglycerides.

Because fat is not water soluble, an important first step in its digestion is emulsification.

EMULSIFICATION The action of gastric lipase yields fatty acids and diglycerides, which enhance emulsification. The process is further enhanced in the duodenum by bile salts and phsopholipids. The emulsion so produced is then presented to pancreatic lipase.

LIPOLYSIS In the duodenum, the action of lipase and colipase yields fatty acids and monoglycerides as shown in Figure 8.8. Fatty acids and monoglycerides enter bile acid micelles for absorption (see below).

Digestion of Proteins

On the average, 10% to 15% of the energy provided in the Western diet derives from proteins. An average daily consumption is about 70 g. Protein digestion begins in the stomach and is completed in the small intestine.

GASTRIC DIGESTION Gastric digestion is due to the action of pepsin, which is active in acid pH. Proteins are acted upon to produce a mixture of peptides and a small amount of amino acids.

INTESTINAL DIGESTION The main site of protein digestion is the duodenum as a result of the action of pancreatic proteases, which are active in alkaline pH. Trypsinogen and chymotryprisinogen are secreted by the exocrine pancreas and, when they enter the duodenum, the brush-border enzyme enterokinase converts them into the active enzymes trypsin and chymotrypsin. Once trypsin is formed, it promotes this process by autocatalytic action. It also activates other proteases. The active proteases are either endopeptidases (i.e., acting within the structure of the protein) or exopeptidases (i.e., split amino acids off the carboxyl terminus of the protein). Trypsin, chymotrypsin, and lipase are endopeptidases.

The luminal digestion of dietary peptides is summarized in Figure 8.9.

Amino acids are absorbed either as monomers or as dipeptides and tripeptides. Approximately 70% of the products of protein digestions are absorbed as dipeptides or tripeptides. By the time absorbed protein-derived nutrients reach the portal circulation, they are all amino acids, suggesting the importance of peptidase activity in the gut epithelium.

Absorption

Fluid Absorption

On average, approximately 9 L of fluid enter the small intestine daily, either through the pylorus or the sphincter of Oddi. Approximately 2 L consist of ingested fluid; 1 L of saliva; another 2 L of gastric juice; and 4 L of bile, pancreatic juice, and succus entericus. Of this, 4 to 5 L are reabsorbed in the jejunum and 3 to 5 L in the ileum. Thus, about 1 L of fluid enters the colon in a 24-h period. Of this amount, approximately 800 ml are reabsorbed in the colon and 200 ml excreted in the feces.

Absorption of Electrolytes

SODIUM ABSORPTION Sodium is absorbed by both active and passive mechanisms. Sodium is actively cotransported with chloride and nutrients such as glucose in the jejunum and bile salts in the terminal ileum. Cotransport depends on the sodium gradient across the apical mem-

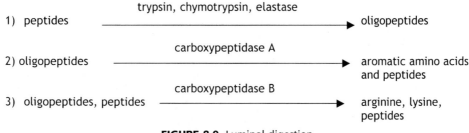

FIGURE 8.9. Luminal digestion.

brane created by the Na⁺K⁺ATPase pump located in the basolateral membrane. Water absorption follows passively to maintain isoosmolality. The sodium-glucose cotransport carrier is the most important clinically. Because this cotransport carrier mechanism is unaffected in most diarrheal states, administration of glucose-salt solution is an important therapeutic strategy to control diarrhea. Another mechanism for sodium absorption is the Na^+-H^+ exchange carrier that permits entry of sodium and chloride into the cell in exchange for hydrogen.

CHLORIDE ABSORPTION The sodium-glucose cotransport mechanism promotes absorption of chloride through a paracellular pathway. In addition, the Na^+-H^+ exchange mechanism permits entry of chloride into the cell in exchange for hydrogen. A third mechanism for chloride absorption is the $Cl^--HCO_3^-$ exchange carrier, in which chloride is absorbed in exchange for HCO_3^-.

POTASSIUM ABSORPTION Potassium is absorbed in exchange for hydrogen.

CALCIUM ABSORPTION Absorption of calcium is regulated by vitamin D and 1,2,5-dihydroxyvitamin D, parathyroid hormone, calcitonin, and a number of calcium-binding proteins.

Absorption of Nutrients

Four types of processes are used for absorption: active transport, passive diffusion, facilitated diffusion, and endocytosis. Active absorption requires transport against an electric or chemical gradient and, therefore, requires energy. Passive diffusion, on the other hand is downhill transport with electric and chemical gradient and requires no energy. Facilitated transport is similar to passive diffusion but requires a carrier-mediated system. Endocytosis, the reverse of exocytosis, is akin to phagocytosis of soluble or particulate substance. This mechanism is used in uptake of antigens.

Various nutrients are absorbed by these different mechanisms as follows:

1. Monosaccharide. The monosaccharide products of carbohydrate digestion are absorbed by active transport.
2. Amino acids. Different mechanisms, both active and passive, are used in the absorption of amino acids.
3. Fatty acids and monoglycerides. The products of triglyceride lipolysis, fatty acids and monoglycerides are absorbed into the cell through micelle formation with bile salts.

Secretion

The intestine secretes water and electrolytes by neurally and humorally controlled mechanisms that are integrated with the mechanisms of absorption. Some secretory mechanisms are active while others are passive. Channels, carriers, and pumps located in the epithelial membrane participate in the process of absorption. Water secretion is inextricably linked to the movement of solutes, but a number of mechanisms are known to stimulate the secretion of water and electrolytes. These include:

Intestinal Distention

Rapid increase in intraluminal pressure stimulates water and chloride secretion into the lumen. This mechanism further contributes to the contraction of the extracellular fluid volume in intestinal obstruction.

Humoral Agents

A large number of endogenous secretagogues stimulate intestinal secretion. These include eicosanoids from the subepithelium, acetylcholine, VIP, and serotonin derived from both extrinsic innervation and from the enteric nervous system (ENS). Additionally, such GI hormones as secretin and gastrin participate. The action of these humoral agents is most pronounced in pathological conditions in which they are produced in abnormally large quantitites, such as carcinoid, VIPoma, or gastrinoma.

Luminal Secretagogues

Bile salts and large-chain fatty acids stimulate intestinal secretion and can, under certain circumstances, cause diarrhea. Bacterial enterotoxin (*Vibrio cholera, Escherichia coli, Salmonella, Campylocacter jejani, Yersina enterocolitica, Clostridium perfringens and C. difficile*) cause diarrhea by stimulating intestinal secretion under pathological conditions.

Motility

Small intestinal motility is regulated through neuroluminal mechanisms. Peristalsis is a coordinated movement that moves intestinal contents aborally. The peristaltic reflex requires descending relaxation of the intestine ahead of the bolus caused by VIP and proximal contraction mediated by acetylcholine and substance P (see Figure 5.11). The small intestine also undergoes segmental contraction in which a portion contracts as a unit. These contractions may cause retropropulsion of intestinal contents or retroperistalsis. Every 90 minutes a wave of contraction starts in the duodenum and sweeps down the small intestine to the colon. This reflex has been called the "housekeeper potential" because it cleanses the small intestine of its contents. It is also called the migrating motor complex or MMC and the peptide motilin is associated with it either as a triggering mechanism or as a secondary phenomenon. Plasma motilin levels are elevated during the MMC. Small intestinal contraction is stimulated by several peptides including substance P, motilin, CCK, gastrin, and gastrin-releasing peptide, but the significance of these peptides in physiological motor function of the intestine is unknown.

LARGE INTESTINE

The large intestine or colon has four functions. They are motility (and reservoir), absorption, secretion, and endocrine.

Motility

Three types of motor activity occur in large intestine function, including segmentation, mass movement, and retrograde peristalsis. Segmentation is the most common motor activity and consists of segmental annular contractions that move intestinal contents short distances in both directions. Mass movement is a strong contractile activity that sweeps across the transverse and descending colon a few times a day. It follows ingestion and may be a response to the gastrocolic reflex. It is the main mechanism by which feces is delivered to the rectum. Retrograde peristalsis begins in the transverse colon and moves proximally into the right colon.

Absorption

Of the 800 ml of water delivered into the colon each day, the colon absorbs 600 ml. Sodium absorption is by electrogenic transport, unaccompanied by cation exchange or anion cotransport. Sodium enters through channels in the apical membrane and is pumped out across the basolateral membrane by $Na^+K^+ATPase$. Approximately 200 to 400 mEq of sodium can be absorbed each day. Chloride is absorbed actively against a concentration gradient in exchange for bicarbonate.

The colon also absorbs short-chain fatty acids, which are formed by bacterial fermentation of carbohydrates and cellulose and absorbed by passive transport. The major short-chain fatty acids are butyrate, acetate, and propionate. It is estimated that daily short-chain fatty acid absorption yields about 540 kcal/day.

Secretion

The colon secretes bicarbonate and potassium. Bicarbonate is secreted in exchange for chloride. Potassium secretion is active.

Endocrine Function

The colon contains L, K, and N cells, which release enteroglucagon, peptide YY (PYY), and neurotensin, respectively. Enteroglucagon is trophic to the small intestinal mucosa, and the colon might participate in regulation of small intestinal mucosal growth. PYY is released from the distal ileum and proximal colon in response to luminal fat and is responsible for the so-called "ileal break," which serves to slow gastric emptying and transport across the small intestine. Neurotensin also inhibits gastric emptying; converts fasting motor complex pattern into the fed pattern; stimulates pancreatic secretion, release of histamine from mast cells, and colon motility; and is a powerful vasodilator. Which of these biological actions are important in normal physiology is unknown.

ANORECTUM

The anorectum demonstrates a coordinated function to both conserve continence and effect defecation.

Continence

Normal anorectal function maintains solid, liquid, and gas continence. The structures responsible for maintaining continence include: (1) the rectum; (2) the internal and external anal sphincters; (3) the pelvic diaphragm, including the puborectalis; and (4) innervation of these structures. When the puborectalis contracts, it pulls the rectum forward, creating a 90° angle between the rectum and anal canal. The puborectalis muscle is believed to be the most important factor in continence. If the puborectalis is intact, division of the internal anal sphincter does not produce severe incontinence.

When feces enter the rectum, the rectum relaxes in accommodation. After a certain point, rectal distension occurs and the internal sphincter relaxes reflexively, but the puborectalis and external anal sphincter contract to prevent defecation.

Defecation

Entrance of a sufficient volume of feces into the rectum stimulates the urge to defecate. The response requires relaxation of the internal sphincter. Defecation is prevented until a squatting position is assumed and the puborectalis muscle and external anal sphincter are voluntarily inhibited. Subsequently, straining and performing a Valsalva maneuver contracts the abdominal muscles and forces the feces out of the anus.

INTESTINAL OBSTRUCTION

Intestinal obstruction may be defined as failure of propulsion of intestinal contents aborally. The condition occurs in many forms in both the small and large intestine (Table 8.1), due to either mechanical obstruction or a motility problem caused by neuromuscular failure or ischemia. Neuromuscular failure is frequently associated with inflammation in the peritoneal cavity or in the retroperitoneum. This type of intestinal obstruction, where the intestinal lumen is not compromised, is also known as adynamic ileus. Pain originating from distension of the intestine, as occurs in bowel obstruction, is initially referred to the embryologic dermatome supplied by the same somatic nerve (Figure 8.10).

TABLE 8.1. Classification of Intestinal Obstruction

Small Intestine
- Mechanical obstruction
    Simple bowel obstruction
    Strangulated bowel obstruction
- Adynamic ileus
- Mesenteric ischemia

Colonic obstruction
- Mechanical obstruction
    Simple obstruction
    Closed-loop obstruction
- Adynamic ileus
- Mesenteric ischemia

Pseudo-obstruction

Small Intestine

Mechanical Obstruction

Mechanical obstruction may be due to luminal causes, intrinsic lesions in the bowel wall, or due to external compression (Table 8.2). Adhesions and hernias account for 75% to 80% of all mechanical small bowel obstruction, adhesions being responsible for 60% to 65%. Obstruction that is caused by an adhesion constricting the bowel at one site is referred to as a simple obstruction, while obstruction at two points causes a closed-loop obstruction. The classic features of small bowel obstruction are summarized in Table 8.3 and the pathophysiology is shown in Figure 8.11.

SIMPLE SMALL BOWEL OBSTRUCTION Simple bowel obstruction usually occurs when an adhesive band compresses and obstructs the bowel at one point. Signs include distention and pain.

Distension Fluid and air accumulate proximal to the obstruction site, leading to progressive dilatation of the proximal bowel and collapse of the distal bowel. Nearly all the air in the dilated bowel is swallowed air, hence the importance of nasogastric aspiration. While the fluid that accumulates in the obstructed bowel (i.e., gastric, biliary, pancreatic juice, succus entericus) is secreted primarily higher up in the gastrointestinal tract, some is due to reflex secretion from the distended bowel itself.

If the obstruction is high in the duodenum or upper jejunum, little or no distension is perceived because the patient will be vomiting and decompressing the

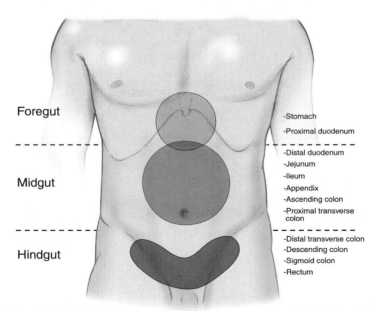

FIGURE 8.10. Sites (shaded areas) of referred pain. Sites of pain in the abdominal wall referred from pathology of different parts of the gastrointestinal tract.

TABLE 8.2. Causes of Mechanical Intestinal Obstruction

	Small Intestine	Colon
Luminal		
	Gallstone ileus	Fecal impaction
	Foreign body	Foreign body
	Worms	
Bowel wall lesions		
	Tumor	Tumor
	Strictures	Strictures
	Intussusception	Diverticular disease
	Radiation enteritis	
Extrinsic compression		
	Adhesions	Volvulus
	Hernias	Extrinsic tumor
	Extrinsic tumor	
	Extrinsic inflammation	

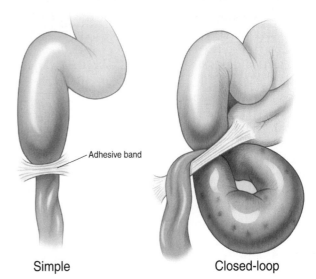

Simple   Closed-loop

FIGURE 8.11. Consequences of simple and closed-loop obstruction by an adhesive band.

obstruction. If the obstruction is more distal, however, abdominal distension occurs, and abdominal x-rays will demonstrate typical air fluid levels and ladder formation. In the latter case, vomiting occurs late, following onset of obstruction and pain. The obstruction may be partial or complete; when partial, less distension is likely and the x-ray will demonstrate gas distal to the point of obstruction.

Pain The pain in simple bowel obstruction is colicky and periumbilical in location; it comes in waves and may be accompanied with audible bowel sounds. The pain is visceral in origin and does not localize to the region affected by the pathology, as happens when the parietal peritoneum is involved.

Fluid and Electrolyte Abnormalities High small bowel obstruction leads to early and severe vomiting, contraction of the extracellular fluid volume, and electrolyte abnor-

malities. The higher the level of obstruction, the more severe these changes become. The electrolyte imbalance at its worst will lead to hypokalemic, hypochloremic metabolic alkalosis similar to that seen in gastric outlet obstruction. Metabolic alkalosis will not occur, however, if significant amounts of pancreatic juice and bile are lost. Indeed, occasionally, a degree of metabolic acidosis may accompany severe dehydration. In low small bowel obstruction, fluid lost into the gut lumen and peritoneal cavity is iso-osmotic. Hence, while contraction of the extracellular space occurs, electrolyte imbalance is rare and appears late when it does occur.

STRANGULATED OBSTRUCTION When the bowel is obstructed at two sites, the segment in between is referred to as the closed segment. This condition is much more serious than simple obstruction because of the risk of volvulus of the obstructed segment and vascular compromise leading to strangulated obstruction. It should always be remembered that proximal to closed-loop obstruction is a simple obstruction (Figure 8.11).

The closed-loop segment undergoes a series of pathophysiological changes leading to vascular compromise. As the closed segment distends, its luminal pressure rises because the serosa is relatively nondistensible. As the luminal pressure increases, first the lymphatic, then the venous drainage of the bowel wall become impaired. In addition, the mesentery of the closed-loop segment is compressed to a variable degree by the adhesive band, leading to edema and thickening of the bowel wall as lymphatic and venous drainage become progressively compromised.

If the obstruction is not relieved, these processes can lead to arterial compromise of the closed-loop segment. Arterial compromise occurs more rapidly and with more catastrophic consequences if the fluid-filled, heavy

TABLE 8.3. Cardinal Features of Small Bowel Obstruction

Simple
- Colicky midabdominal pain
- Nausea and vomiting
- Distension
- Obstipation
- High-pitched bowel sounds with crescendo
- X-ray:
  ➤ Distended small bowel
  ➤ Air-fluid level

Strangulated
- Constant abdominal pain
- Tenderness and rebound tenderness
- Fever, leucocytosis
- X-ray:
  ➤ Thumbprinting
  ➤ Air in bowel wall
  ➤ Air in portal vein radicles
  ➤ Free air if perforated

obstructed segment undergoes rotation or volvulus. The obstruction then becomes a strangulated obstruction.

When strangulated obstruction develops, transmural inflammation leads to peritonitis, and the symptoms and signs change. The pain, instead of intermittent and colicky, becomes constant and more severe. The findings on abdominal examination include tenderness and rebound tenderness, indicating that peritonitis has set in. At times, the obstructed bowel may be palpable. Bowel sounds tend to disappear. Parallel changes may also be seen on abdominal x-ray.

The most significant radiological signal that bowel necrosis has occurred is the presence of air within the bowel wall itself (Figure 8.12). The presence of air within the portal vein is a late sign. Another late development, which must be avoided at all costs, is perforation of the strangulated bowel. If perforation occurs, free air and fluid may accumulate in the peritoneal cavity. The patient develops peritonitis and becomes septic. Septic shock and death will ensue unless the problem is promptly corrected surgically. It is important to note that perforation is not necessary in order for severe sepsis and septic shock to develop.

Following obstruction, bacteria proliferate in the gut lumen. With vascular compromise of the intestinal wall, bacteria and endotoxin invade the peritoneal cavity transmurally, a process referred to as bacterial dislocation.

Adynamic Ileus

When intestinal peristalsis is lost, air and fluid accumulate within the gut lumen. In contrast to mechanical obstruction, air may be present within the entire small and large intestine. Abdominal distension develops, but colicky abdominal pain does not. Any abdominal pain that may be present is likely to be due to the primary pathological process that has caused paralytic ileus.

The causes of adynamic ileus may be abdominal or extra-abdominal. The most frequent abdominal cause is an inflammatory process of the gastrointestinal tract, the pancreas, or the biliary tree (e.g., perforated ulcer, acute appendicitis, acute pancreatitis, acute cholecystitis, ascending cholangitis). Retroperitoneal processes (e.g., acute pyelonephritis, ureteral colic, retroperitoneal hematoma, spinal injury) are also important causes. Extra-abdominal causes include severe systemic sepsis, diabetic ketoacidosis, major burn, severe head injury, and severe inferior myocardial infarction.

Key issues for the clinician are to distinguish adynamic ileus from mesenteric ischemia and to identify the primary cause.

Mesenteric Ischemia

Mesenteric ischemia occurs in acute or chronic forms; it is the acute form that causes acute intestinal obstruction.

The causes of mesenteric ischemia (Table 8.4) are most commonly mesenteric arterial embolism and mesenteric artery thrombosis (Figure 8.13). Frequent causes of mesenteric arterial embolism include atrial fibrillation, postmyocardial infarction mural thrombus, embolism following the use of pump oxygenator during heart-lung bypass, and dislodged atheromas or thrombi during angiography when a catheter is threaded up the aorta into or beyond the mesenteric vessels. Mesenteric artery thrombosis follows atherosclerotic stenosis, usually of the superior mesenteric artery (SMA). Often, the patient may give an antecedent history of intestinal angina. Nonocclusive mesenteric ischemia develops in low-flow states, particularly in patients with low cardiac output and especially when digoxin and/or vasopressors are used. In nonocclusive ischemic states, it is believed that, by mechanisms as yet unknown, a critical drop in mesenteric blood flow causes segmental spasm in secondary and tertiary branches of the SMA.

Although changes are discernible by electron microscope within 10 minutes and by light microscope within 60 minutes of the onset of ischemia, full-thickness infarction of the bowel wall takes about 6 h and sometimes longer to set in. Ischemia causes rapid bacterial proliferation within the lumen. As necrosis occurs, the intestinal wall becomes permeable to luminal bacteria and endotoxin, allowing their entry into the peritoneal cavity. Septicemia and gram-negative bacteremia ensue. Hemorrhage occurs into the lumen, and bloody fluid accumulates in the peritoneal cavity. Massive fluid shifts into the gut lumen and peritoneum cause hemoconcentration, oliguria, and hypotension. Necrosis of the intestinal muscle wall releases creatine phosphokinase (CPK), lactate dehydrogenase (LDH), and glutamic pyruvic transaminase (GPT). These enzymes frequently become elevated in the serum. Also, inorganic phosphate levels rise in the serum and in peritoneal fluid.

Mesenteric venous thrombosis occurs in the setting of portal hypertension, hypercoagulable states, use of contraceptive pills, trauma, or abdominal sepsis. A characteristic feature is the accumulation of large amounts of fluid within the gut wall, within the mesentery, and in the peritoneal cavity (Figure 8.14).

Colonic Obstruction

Mechanical Obstruction

SIMPLE OBSTRUCTION Colon cancer and diverticulitis account for nearly 90% of cases of large intestinal obstruction, with colon cancer alone responsible for 65% to 70% of these.[1] The most frequent site of obstruction from either disease is the sigmoid. Other causes of colon obstruction include inflammatory bowel disease, postanastomotic strictures, benign tumors, and fecal impaction. Simple colonic obstruction occurs only when the ileocecal valve is

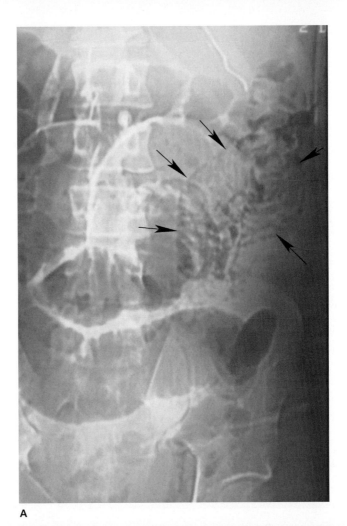

A

B

FIGURE 8.12. Air within the bowel. (A) The supine abdominal x-ray illustrates the presence of streaks of air (arrows) within the wall of small bowel segments that are ischemic as a result of a strangulated small bowel obstruction. Notice the dilated small bowel. (B) The abdominal CT scan in the same patient demonstrates the ischemic segment of bowel with air in the wall (arrows) and contrast material in the lumen. CT is often performed to detect ischemic, strangulated bowel and has a much higher sensitivity than plain x-ray. (Courtesy of Henry I. Goldman, MD.)

TABLE 8.4. Causes of Mesenteric Ischemia

Superior mesenteric artery embolism: 30%
Superior mesenteric artery thrombosis: 25%
Nonocclusive mesenteria ischemia: 5%
Acute mesenteric vein thrombosis: 20%
Miscellaneous: 20%
- Dissecting aortic occlusion
- Trauma
- Collagen vascular disease

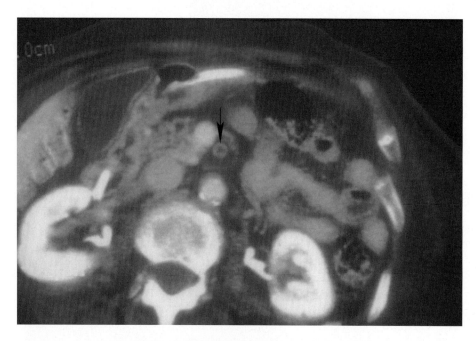

FIGURE 8.13. Mesenteric arterial embolism. The CT scan demonstrates an embolus lodged in the superior mesenteric artery (SMA; arrow) in a patient with atrial fibrillation. CT is the recommended technique to demonstrate SMA embolus or thrombosis. (Courtesy of Henry I. Goldman, MD.)

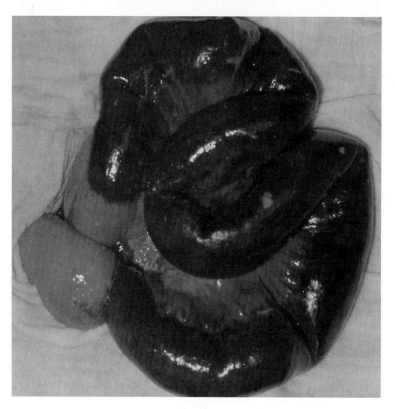

FIGURE 8.14. Recurrent mesenteric venous infarction following previous resection. Notice that the previous anastomosis is one of the demarcation lines. Typically, in venous infarction, both the bowel and the mesentery are edematous. (Courtesy of Theodore Schrock, MD.)

incompetent and coloileal reflux can occur. When the ileocecal valve is competent (see following discussion), a closed-loop obstruction results between the obstructing lesion and the ileocecal valve.

Consequences of simple obstruction of the colon include:

1. Abdominal distension. Distension is usually prominent and involves the lateral aspects of the abdomen. Even in the colon, most of the gas distending the obstructed bowel is derived from swallowed air, although gas produced by bacteria-induced fermentation does contribute.

2. Abdominal pain. Colicky abdominal pain is referred to the suprapubic area (hypogastrium) and is mediated by the T-12 and L-1 nerves.

3. Obstipation. Failure to pass feces and flatus develops with complete colonic obstruction.

4. Vomiting. Vomiting occurs late and is typically feculent. By the time vomiting occurs, distension of the small intestine has also occurred.

CLOSED-LOOP OBSTRUCTION Closed-loop obstruction occurs under three conditions: when complete colonic obstruction occurs in conjunction with a competent ileocecal valve, in sigmoid volvulus, and in cecal volvulus.

Rarely, volvulus of the transverse colon or splenic flexure may occur.

Competent Ileocecal Valve A competent ileocecal valve does not permit colon obstruction to decompress by reflux into the small intestine. As a result, the cecum progressively enlarges from its normal diameter of 10 cm or less. An increase in cecal diameter to 12 cm or more may portend imminent cecal perforation and requires urgent or emergent decompression (Figure 8.15).

Sigmoid Volvulus Three conditions promote sigmoid volvulus: a redundant sigmoid, long sigmoid mesentery with a narrow base, and fecal loading due to chronic constipation. The condition tends to occur in the elderly, in those who are bedridden, and in those receiving psychotropic medication for a psychiatric disorder.

The bowel twists counterclockwise about its long mesentery. A complete twist of 360° leads to occlusion of not only the bowel lumen but also of the vascular pedicle in the mesentery. If the obstruction is not reversed promptly, sigmoid gangrene and perforation ensue. Usually, abdominal distension is very prominent, and colicky suprapubic pain develops. Abdominal films show a single large loop of bowel arising from the pelvis and sometimes reaching the diaphragm (Figure 8.16).

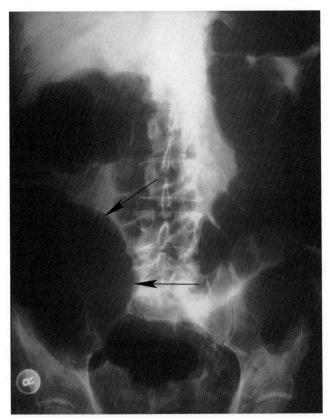

FIGURE 8.15. Large bowel obstruction with cecal dilatation. The x-ray demonstrates a huge cecum (arrows), the result of sigmoid obstruction. The patient noted increasing distention over many hours, and comparison to earlier abdominal films showed that the cecum had increased from 7 cm to 12 cm in diameter. (Courtesy of Henry I. Goldman, MD.)

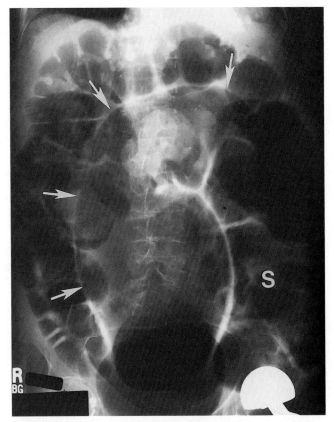

FIGURE 8.16. Sigmoid volvulus. The abdominal x-ray shows a large sigmoid volvulus (arrows) occupying much of the abdomen and pelvis, with distended colon proximally. The volvulus has two limbs, the distal limb (arrows) and the proximal limb (S), forming an inverted U-shape. (Courtesy of Henry I. Goldman, MD.)

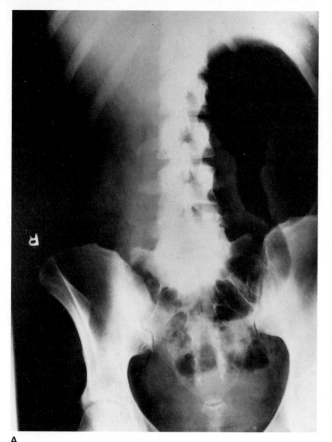

A

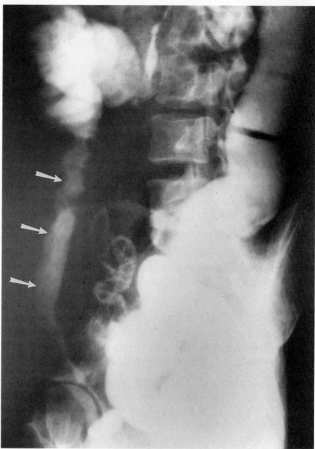

B

FIGURE 8.17. Cecal volvulus. (A) The abdominal x-ray shows a large air collection in the left upper quadrant, with transverse colon gas present. The large air collection is actually the cecum, which has migrated to the left upper quadrant due to a cecal volvulus. (B) The barium enema, taken 4 days later, shows a narrowed cecum and ascending colon (arrows). While the volvulus spontaneously reduced, ischemic changes had already occurred, leading to this appearance of the segment involved in the volvulus. (Courtesy of Henry I. Goldman, MD.)

Cecal Volvulus Cecal volvulus is much less common than sigmoid volvulus, occurring with half the frequency. A predisposing condition is incomplete embryologic fixation of the cecum, which results in hypermobility of the organ. The terminal ileum is also involved in the twisting. The cecum comes to lie in the left upper quadrant, and a closed-loop obstruction occurs (Figure 8.17). Because no twist of the mesentery occurs, vascular obstruction is not a significant problem.

Cecal volvulus causes distal small bowel obstruction proximal to the closed-loop obstruction. Distension and colicky pain develop in the midabdomen. The patient often has a previous medical history of similar but milder attacks.

Pseudo-obstruction

Pseudo-obstruction is profound ileus without evidence of luminal obstruction. Colonic pseudo-obstruction, or Ogilvie's syndrome, is the best known variety, but the disease can also affect the small intestine. Although the cause is unknown, some have suggested sympathetic over-activity based on anecdotal evidence that epidural anesthesia ameliorates the condition. It is likely, however, that the pathophysiology is more complicated and possibly involves abnormalities of the peptidergic enteric nervous system.

Ogilvie's syndrome may follow acute illness, an operation (e.g., hysterectomy), or it might affect patients who are on motility-inhibiting drugs and opiates. Pain is usually not an important symptom, but abdominal distension can be massive and lead to cecal perforation. Cecal dilatation of 12 cm or more should prompt either endoscopic or surgical decompression.

MALABSORPTION SYNDROME

Malabsorption syndrome is caused by a variety of conditions, including maldigestion and as a result of inadequate absorptive surface or primary mucosal absorptive defects, which may be inflammatory, biochemical, genetic, endocrine, or metabolic in nature. Of the numerous causes of malabsorption, those relevant in surgical practice are listed in Table 8.5. The list excludes several disorders of malabsorption, not because they are unimportant, but because they are not usually encountered in surgical practice. These include such conditions as Whipple's disease (due to infection with *Tropheryma whippelii*), celiac sprue (gluten-sensitive enteropathy), tropical sprue (cause unknown), and α-betalipoproteinemia (due to absence of ApoB, which causes defective chylomicron formation).

Maldigestion

Steatorrhea is seen following gastrectomy, in ZES, and in exocrine pancreatic insufficiency. Postgastrectomy steatorrhea is probably due to defective mixing of chyme and pancreatic juice as well as increased intestinal transit time. In ZES, the excessive acid load entering the small intestine inactivates pancreatic lipase and other enzymes. Exocrine pancreatic deficiency is seen primarily in chronic pancreatitis and following major pancreatic resection.

TABLE 8.5. Surgically Relevant Causes of Malabsorption

Maldigestion
- Postgastrectomy steatorrhea
- Pancreatic insufficiency
- Zollinger–Ellison syndrome

Reduced intestinal bile salt
- Blind-loop syndrome
- Ileal resection or disease

Inadequate absorptive surface
- Intestinal resection or bypass
- Chronic mesenteric vascular insufficiency

Primary mucosal defects
- Inflammatory
  ➤ Crohn's disease
  ➤ Radiation enteritis
- Endocrine/metabolic
  ➤ Carcinoid syndrome
  ➤ Hypoparathyroidism
  ➤ Adrenal insufficiency
  ➤ Diabetes mellitus

Important consequences of maldigestion include:

1. Malabsorption of fat, leading to diarrhea with greasy, foul-smelling, and floating stools.
2. Weight loss.
3. Malabsorption of fat-soluble vitamins A, D, E, and K.

In patients with maldigestion, vitamin K deficiency must be corrected with intravenous administration of phytonadione (AquaMEPHYTON®) prior to surgery.

Reduced Intestinal Bile Salt

Reduced intestinal bile salt occurs in the blind-loop syndrome and when the ileum has been resected or severely diseased (e.g., Crohn's ileitis). In the blind-loop syndrome, bacterial overgrowth leads to deconjugation of bile salts, in turn leading to defective micelle formation. The consequences are several and include:

1. Malabsorption of fat and, to a lesser degree, proteins and carbohydrates.
2. Colonic loss of water and electrolytes, due to the stimulating effect of unabsorbed fatty acids entering the colon and leading to diarrhea.
3. Macrocytic anemia due to malabsorption of vitamin B_{12}, which binds to anaerobic bacteria.
4. Hypocalcemia due to the binding of calcium by unabsorbed fatty acids.
5. Enteric hyperoxaluria due to excessive absorption of oxalate from the colon as a consequence of the hypocalcemia, which interferes with formation of insoluble calcium oxalate.
6. Weight loss.

Major resection of the ileum or severe disease in this segment of bowel removes its important absorptive function of fat and vitamin B_{12}.

Inadequate Absorptive Surface

Intestinal resection or bypass and chronic vascular insufficiency lead to malabsorption because of critically reduced absorptive surface. (The short bowel syndrome will be described later.) Intestinal bypass may be performed in the treatment of morbid obesity or heterozygous familial hypercholesterolemia. In the latter, the distal one third of the small intestine is bypassed, interrupting the enterohepatic circulation, and resulting in increasing amounts of cholesterol being converted to bile salts, which are then excreted. Plasma cholesterol levels—particularly LDL cholesterol—fall, resulting in an increased HDL cholesterol ratio in the plasma.

Chronic mesenteric vascular insufficiency leads to general villous atrophy in the small intestine, with loss of absorptive surface and brush-border enzymes. The effect is reduced absorption of all nutrients, leading to severe weight loss.

Primary Mucosal Defects

Malabsorption also occurs when a large segment of the small intestine is damaged by severe Crohn's disease or radiation enteritis. Several endocrine/metabolic disorders can also cause malabsorption, including the carcinoid syndrome, hypoparathyroidism, adrenal insufficiency, and diabetes mellitus.

DIARRHEA

The various causes of diarrhea are given in Table 8.6. Six important categories of causes are recognized, including inflammatory, osmotic, secretory, altered intestinal motility, factitious, and postoperative.

Inflammatory Diarrhea

Inflammatory conditions such as ulcerative colitis, Crohn's disease, and radiation enterocolitis damage the intestinal mucosa and cause diarrhea. Clinical features include fever, abdominal pain, and bloody stools.

TABLE 8.6. Causes of Chronic Diarrhea

Inflammatory
- Ulcerative colitis
- Crohn's disease
- Radiation enterocolitis
- AIDS

Osmotic
- Pancreatic insufficiency
- Short bowel syndrome
- Bacterial overgrowth
- Celiac disease
- Lactase deficiency
- Whipple's disease

Secretory
- ZES
- Carcinoid
- VIPoma
- Medullary thyroid cancer
- Villous adenoma of rectum
- Cholerrhetic diarrhea

Altered intestinal motility
- Inflammatory bowel disease
- Fecal impaction
- Neurologic disease

Factitious
- Laxative abuse

Postoperative
- Postvagotomy
- Dumping syndrome
- Ileoproctostomy

Abbreviations: AIDS, acquired immunodeficiency syndrome; ZES, Zollinger–Ellison syndrome.

Osmotic Diarrhea

Conditions responsible for this type of diarrhea increase the osmotic load in the stool, creating an osmotic gap between the fecal water and plasma. Some conditions—including pancreatic insufficiency, bacterial overgrowth, and short bowel syndrome—increase fatty acid and bile acid concentrations in the stool, typically making it bulky, greasy, and foul smelling. Nutrient deficiencies and weight loss develop. Diarrhea improves with fasting.

Secretory Diarrhea

Secretory diarrhea is most often the result of excessive secretion of peptides by functioning tumors (e.g., ZES, VIPoma). The peptides cause oversecretion of water and electrolytes. There is no osmotic gap between the plasma and fecal water, and the diarrhea does not improve with fasting. The cause of diarrhea in ZES is complex and includes:

1. Large volume acid load into the intestine.
2. Increased small bowel motility because of the action of pharmacologic levels of gastrin.
3. Jejunitis and damage to intestinal mucosa.
4. Inactivation of pancreatic enzymes due to acid pH in the gut lumen.

The secretory products of peptide-secreting tumors and their actions are described in Chapter 4.

Altered Intestinal Motility

Diarrhea can be caused by a number of neurologic conditions that alter intestinal motility, including the early phase of Crohn's disease, and fecal impaction.

Postoperative Diarrhea

Postvagotomy diarrhea and the dumping syndrome are described in detail in Chapter 2. Subtotal colectomy with ileoproctostomy causes diarrhea that tends to improve with time. Approximately 20% to 30% of patients with ileoproctostomy, however, have lifelong diarrhea.

CONSTIPATION

Frequency of defecation varies from individual to individual and may range from two to three times a day, to once every 3 to 5 days. Constipation implies infrequent passage of hard stools. The causes may be metabolic, endocrine, neurologic, mechanical, or drug induced.

Metabolic Causes

Constipation can be caused by hypokalemia, hypercalcemia, and uremia. The exact mechanisms are unknown, but the effects appear to be intestinal smooth muscle repolarization.

Endocrine Causes

Hypothyroidism is the prototypical endocrine cause of constipation. Panhypopituitarism causes constipation, due in part to hypothyroidism. Pregnant women often suffer from constipation, the cause of which may be both hormonal and mechanical.

Neurologic Causes

Constipation is a common feature of a variety of neurologic disorders, including multiple sclerosis and Parkinson's disease. Paraplegic patients and those with stroke also suffer from constipation. Their inactivity and several of the drugs used to treat them contribute to the problem. Patients with psychiatric disorders also suffer from constipation, perhaps for the same reasons.

Mechanical Causes

Constipation may be caused by mechanical obstruction due to tumors, hernias, strictures, and volvulus. Pseudo-obstruction was discussed earlier as a cause of bowel obstruction. Constipation may also be caused by structural abnormalities such as the descending perineum syndrome, rectal prolapse or intussusception, or rectocele.

Drug-induced Constipation

Chronic use of a variety of drugs is associated with constipation. The most common culprits are opiates, psychotropic drugs, antidepressants, aluminum-containing antacids, calcium-channel blockers, antihypertensives, and iron supplements. The mechanisms of action are ill understood.

RADIATION INJURY

The gastrointestinal epithelium, because of its rapid cell turnover rate, is susceptible to radiation injury. When given in weekly fractionated doses not exceeding 200 cGy, a total dose of 4000 cGy is usually well tolerated. The risk of radiation injury increases rapidly beyond that dose, especially beyond 5000 cGy. Radiation injury of the gastrointestinal tract may be acute or delayed.

Acute Radiation Injury

The gastrointestinal mucosa is the site of acute radiation injury, which develops within 3 to 4 days after treatment. Usually, with cessation of therapy, this injury resolves rapidly. Three forms of acute radiation injury may be emphasized:

Gastric Perforation

During or immediately following completion of radiation therapy for large lesions of gastric lymphoma, gastric perforation may occur. This complication occurs when there is transmural involvement with highly radiosensitive lymphoma.

Acute Radiation Enteritis

The rapidly proliferating mucosa of the small intestine, particularly the jejunum, is highly radiosensitive. Symptoms include abdominal pain and diarrhea. The injury is usually self-limited and the mucosa repairs rapidly upon cessation of treatment.

Radiation Proctocolitis

Most commonly associated with pelvic radiation for uterine and cervical cancer and for prostate and bladder cancer. Proctocolitis may also follow adjuvant radiation therapy for rectal cancer. Proctocolitis develops when tissue doses exceed 5000 to 6000 cGy. Symptoms may develop during the course of therapy. The mucosa becomes edematous and hyperemic, accompanied by development of multiple ulcers. Bloody diarrhea and tenesmus indicate more severe damage.

Late Radiation Injury

While acute radiation injury involves primarily the mucosa, late radiation injury is due primarily to injury of small vessels in the submucosa. The vessels undergo progressive proliferative arteritis, leading to vascular obliteration and ischemia and, ultimately, fibrosis and stricture formation. The injury may occur months to years after treatment. In the rectum, radiation endarteritis may produce ischemic mucosal ulceration, bleeding, and tenesmus months to years after completion of therapy. Late radiation enteritis produces a gray, matted small intestine with extensive fibrosis and thickening as well as mucosal ulcerations. As the endarteritis progresses, the ischemic bowel tends to depend on blood supply from adhesions that form. The irradiated bowel therefore tolerates surgical mobilization poorly and is subject to failure of anastomoses and development of fistulas. When an operation must be performed for obstruction caused by radiation enteritis, the overall mortality rate is 25% with a 50% chance that more surgery will be required.[2]

When pelvic irradiation is necessary, several methods are used to reduce damage to the small intestine. These include positioning the patient on the radiotherapy table so that the intestine is displaced out of the pelvis. When a laparotomy precedes radiation, the small bowel may be kept out of the pelvis by the use of omentum or absorbable mesh slings. Following low anterior resection, all attempts are made to approximate the peritoneum over the pelvic floor to prevent the small intestine from being fixed in the pelvic floor.

SHORT BOWEL SYNDROME

The small intestine is about 6 meters in length. Massive small bowel resection implies resection of more than 50% of the bowel, which invariably results in the development of serious malabsorption problems. The reasons for massive small bowel resection in the pediatric population are congenital atresia and necrotizing enterocolitis. In adults, massive resection is most commonly performed for acute mesenteric ischemia, trauma, radiation enteritis, strangulated small bowel obstruction, and radiation enteropathy.

The seriousness of the consequences of massive small bowel resection depend on several factors:

1. Extent of resection. When 2 meters or less of bowel remains following surgery, critical malnutrition will develop.
2. Segment resected. In general, ileal resection is less well tolerated because of ileal function in absorption of fat, bile acids, and vitamin B_{12}. After jejunal resection, the ileum accommodates to take over its function. The reverse is not as true.
3. Preservation of the ileocecal valve. The presence of the ileocecal valve, up to a point, allows for preservation of adequate absorptive function with less remaining intestine.
4. Function. The functional health and adaptability of the remaining intestine determines the extent of recovery of its absorptive function.

Consequences of Massive Small Bowel Resection

Early Physiological Consequences

In the days or weeks following massive small bowel resection, a number of physiological changes occur.

LOSS OF ABSORPTIVE SURFACE Loss of small intestine deprives the bowel of absorptive surface, resulting in loss of water and electrolytes. The results are diarrhea and malabsorption of nutrients, the severity of which depends on the first three factors listed above. When proximal intestine is resected, malabsorption of iron, folate, and calcium occurs. In distal resection, absorption of vitamin B_{12} and bile salts is impaired.

BASAL AND POSTPRANDIAL HYPERGASTRINEMIA While the cause of resection-related hypergastrinemia is unknown, it is thought to arise from two factors: (1) removal of intestinal inhibitors of gastrin release, and (2) loss of intestinal microcirculation, which has an important role in gastrin degradation.

HYPERSECRETION OF GASTRIC ACID Acid hypersecretion, while due partly to hypergastrinemia, is further explained by the loss of enterogastrones, inhibitors of intestinal origin. Acid hypersecretion is time-limited, and normal gastric acid secretion resumes within a few weeks.

ENTEROGLUCAGONEMIA Elevated levels of enteroglucagon are due to increased colonic release of the peptide and serve to stimulate adaptive hypertrophy of the remaining small intestine.

Late Changes

ADAPTIVE CHANGES Hyperplasia of the remaining enterocytes leads to increased cell renewal, lengthening of the villi, and deepening of crypts. This process, which increases the absorptive surface of the small intestine, takes several weeks to months to reach equilibrium. Growth factors that may be involved include enteroglucagon, neurotensin and insulin-like growth factor-1 (IGF-1).

DISRUPTION OF ENTEROHEPATIC CIRCULATION Resection of the ileum disrupts the enterohepatic circulation. The consequences are several:

1. Excessive amounts of bile acids are lost into the colon, where they injure the colonic mucosa. This inhibits water and electrolyte absorption and stimulates excessive water and electrolyte secretion, resulting in diarrhea.
2. Increased hepatic synthesis of bile salts, which leads to even greater losses of bile salts in the stool.
3. Enteric hyperoxaluria occurs when unabsorbed fatty acids bind calcium, making the cation unavailable to form insoluble calcium oxalate. As a result, oxalate remains soluble and available for absorption. Hyperoxaluria develops, leading to formation of oxalate kidney stones.

BACTERIAL OVERGROWTH SYNDROMES

Under normal physiological conditions, several mechanisms prevent bacterial overgrowth in the intestine. One such mechanism is the migrating motor complex (MMC), which, during the fasting state, moves from the duodenum to the ileocecal valve, sweeping away food particles and other intestinal contents. The MMC has been aptly called the "housekeeper potential." Other mechanisms include gastric acid, the secretion of immunoglobulins, and the normal postprandial peristalsis. The concentration of bacteria in the small intestine is estimated at 10^5/ml, with a greater concentration in the ileum and a lower concentration in the jejunum. The ileocecal valve helps prevent reflux of colonic bacteria into the ileum, but the ileocecal valve is not always competent.

Bacterial overgrowth syndromes can be caused by structural or motor abnormalities that favor luminal stagnation. Structural abnormalities include a blind loop, a poorly emptying segment of bowel, strictures, fistulas, and diverticula. Motor abnormalities may be caused by primary failure of the MMC or by conditions such as scleroderma and pseudo-obstruction. Consequences of bacterial overgrowth include:

1. Deconjugation of bile salts, leading to impaired micelle formation and causing fat malabsorption and steatorrhea.
2. Malabsorption of fat-soluble vitamins (A, D, E, K) because of 1.
3. Malabsorption of vitamin B_{12}, leading to megaloblastic anemia.
4. Malabsorption of other nutrients (carbohydrates and proteins).
5. Hypocalcemia due to chelating action of unabsorbed fatty acids.

CROHN'S DISEASE

Crohn's disease (CD) is a granulomatous, transmural inflammation of unknown origin that can affect any part of the GI tract. Although the first case may have been documented by Morgani in 1761, and subsequent reports occurred in the 19th and early 20th century, it is the classic clinical and pathological description by Crohn, Ginzburg, and Oppenheimer from Mount Sinai Hospital in New York that best captured the concept of the disease.[3] Although the small and large intestine and rectum are the most frequent targets, CD can affect the mouth (6% to 9%), the esophagus (<1%), and the stomach and duodenum (1% to 5%). It occurs with equal frequency in both sexes. In Wales, the incidence of CD increased from 0.18 per 100,000 people per year in the 1930s to 8.3 per 100,000 people per year in 1980.[4] The essentials of Crohn's disease are summarized in Table 8.7.

Etiology and Pathogenesis

An interplay of genetic and environmental factors are believed to cause Crohn's disease. No convincing evidence has been provided for an infectious cause.

TABLE 8.7. Essentials: Crohn's Disease

Pathology
- Chronic transmural granulomatous inflammation
- Involvement
  - Small bowel alone: 35%
  - Colon alone: 20%
  - Both small bowel and colon: 45%

Etiology
- Unknown
- *Mycobacterium paratuberculosis* manifest in 66% of tissue cultures

Symptoms
- Diarrhea: 90%
- Abdominal pain: 80%
- Anemia: 33%
- Anorectal disease: 35%–50%
- Arthritis, arthralgia: 20%

Complications
- Bowel osbstruction: 33%
- Enteroenteric fistula: 25%
- Enterocutaneous fistula: 20%
- Enterovesical, enterovaginal fistula: 5%–10%

Environmental Factors

INFECTIOUS AGENTS Two mycobacteria (*Mycobacterium paratuberculosis* and *M. tuberculosis*) have been considered possible etiologic agents because they cause granulomatous inflammation of the gut. Attempts to identify *M. tuberculosis* DNA in affected intestinal tissue by polymerase chain reaction have had varying results. Some investigators have identified such DNA, and CD has been treated with variable success using antimycobacterial drugs.[5] Persistent measles virus and *Yersinia enterocolitica* have also been implicated. No specific viral cause has been identified.

DIET A dietary cause(s) has been suspected because of the finding of several antibodies against food antigens (e.g., milk, baker's yeast) in patients with Crohn's disease. Of course, this finding may simply represent increased permeability to antigens in the diseased bowel.

SMOKING Smoking is an independent risk factor for clinical, surgical, and endoscopic recurrence of CD. Smoking does not have such an adverse effect on ulcerative colitis. CD is twice as common in smokers than in nonsmokers.

Genetic Factors

The risk of developing CD is 30 times higher in siblings of patients with the disease than in normal subjects whose siblings do not have CD.[6] CD is also associated with other genetically determined diseases such as ankylosing spondylitis and tyrosine-positive albinism. A weak correlation with some human leukocyte antigens (HLA) and an inverse correlation with others have been made. Increased levels of haptoglobin type Hp1-I were found in Japanese patients with CD compared with normal subjects.[7] Potentially pathogenetic immune defects that have been identified in individuals with CD [e.g., complement C3-F, increased cytotoxicity against intestinal cell antigen, and epithelial Ca^{++} channels (ECaC)] have been found in unaffected relatives. Using complex familial segregation studies, Mousen et al. have suggested that "CD is an oligogenetically inherited disease with one recessive major gene locus and one modifier gene with a penetrance of 27%."[8]

The most exciting recent contribution of molecular genetics to our understanding of the etiology of CD has been the identification of the NOD2 gene. Genome-wide linkage analysis studies by Hugot and colleagues have identified NOD2 mutations that are present only in patients with CD, suggesting a causal relationship.[9] NOD2 is an intracellular protein with homology to disease resistance (R) genes present in plants.

Immune System

Patients with CD seem to be unable to shut off activation of the gut inflammatory immune responses to luminal bacteria and dietary antigens. Immune dysregulation in CD-affected intestine is suggested by the anatomic distribution of MHC class II antigens in the intestine, which is strikingly similar to the distribution of inflammation of CD. Also, CD epithelial cells inappropriately induce proliferation of T-helper cells, in contrast to normal epithelial cells, which stimulate proliferation of T-suppressor cells. Unopposed T-helper cell proliferation may then nonspecifically induce the cascade of immune activation effects typical of CD.

Psychological Factors

Prospective studies have failed to show that stressful life events precipitate exacerbation of CD. Despite this, successful treatment of patients with CD cannot be provided without attention to psychosocial factors.

Pathology

Anatomic Distribution

CD affects the small intestine alone in 30% to 40% of patients, both small and large bowel in 40% to 55%, and colon only in 15% to 25%. Thus, the small intestine is affected in more than 75% of patients with CD, and the terminal ileum in more than 90% of these. When only the colon is involved, disease tends to primarily involve the distal colon. Perirectal and perianal lesions occur in 33% of patients. In recent years, the incidence of Crohn's disease in the colon has increased. Also, isolated colon lesions are more common in the elderly.[10]

Gross and Microscopic Picture

The involved bowel and its mesentery are thickened, and all layers of the bowel wall are affected (Figure 8.18). Mesenteric fat will be seen creeping onto the serosal surface of the bowel, accompanied by diffuse, nonspecific transmural inflammation (Figure 8.19). Involvement is segmental, with normal intervening portions of bowel. Noncaseating granulomas are present in 50% of cases and may be found in the bowel wall, the mesentery, lymph nodes, or on the peritoneal surface. The inflammatory cells are made up of macrophages, lymphocytes, and plasma cells. As disease progresses, deep transverse and longitudi-

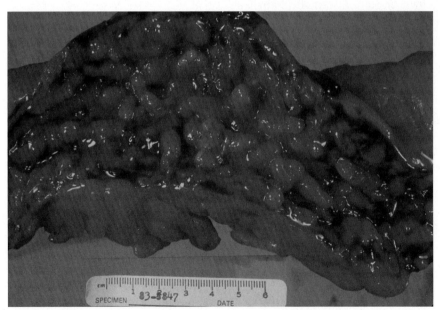

FIGURE 8.18. Crohn's disease. The resection specimen of Crohn's ileitis shows a section of bowel with marked cobblestoning of the mucosa and thickening. (Courtesy of Theodore Schrock, MD.)

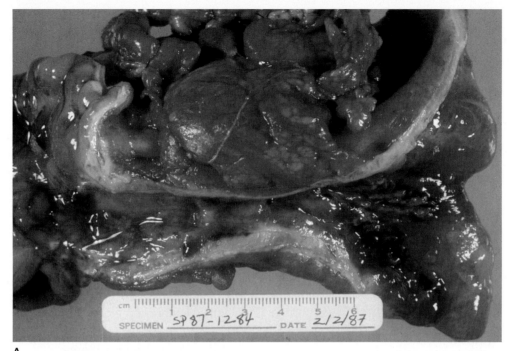

A

B

FIGURE 8.19. (A) The colon resection specimen shows Crohn's disease with thickening and stricture formation. Notice also the transmural character of the process and the fat that creeps to the anterior surface of the colon. (B) Occasionally, a well-formed, noncaseating granuloma may be encountered. (Courtesy of Linda D. Ferrell, MD.)

nal mucosal ulcerations develop, with nodular swelling of the intervening mucosa, giving the characteristic cobblestone appearance. With time, the bowel wall becomes thickened, fibrotic, and stenotic. Burrowing ulcers might form fistulas into adjacent bowel or bladder. Free intestinal perforation is exceedingly rare.

Complications of Crohn's Disease

Three complications are commonly seen in Crohn's disease: obstruction, fistula formation, and extraintestinal manifestations. Hemorrhage and malignancy are less common complications.

Obstruction

CD may cause partial and reversible bowel obstruction or fibrostenotic and fixed irreversible obstruction. In acute Crohn's ileitis, distal small bowel obstruction may be a presenting problem. In longstanding cases, multiple areas of fibrotic stenosis may coexist at different levels of the small intestine.

Fistula Formation

The most common fistulas are into adjacent bowel: ileo-ileal, ileocecal, or ileosigmoid. Less frequently, cologastric or coloduodenal fistulas may form (Figure 8.20). While enteroenteric and even enterocolic fistulas may remain asymptomatic, cologastric or coloduodenal fistulas produce feculent vomiting and diarrhea. Other common types include enterovesical fistulas, which produce recurrent attacks of polymicrobial urinary tract infection and enterovaginal fistulas, which may result in enteric contents discharging from the vagina. Occasionally, enterocutaneous fistulas develop.

Intra-abdominal Abscess

Intraperitoneal abscesses develop frequently. The abscess may sometimes be retroperitoneal, anterior to the psoas muscle, where it may entrap the ureters and cause hydroureter. Intra-abdominal abscesses usually produce fever, sweating, pain, and leukocytosis.

Hemorrhage

Massive hemorrhage is rare, occurring in less than 1% of patients. However, it may be life-threatening, sometimes requiring emergency operation.

Growth Retardation

Crohn's disease retards growth in 15% to 30% of affected children. The combination of chronic inflammation, subclinical sepsis, and malabsorption are contributing factors. Occasionally, failure to thrive is an indication for surgery.

Carcinoma

Carcinoma is not a common complication of CD as it is of ulcerative colitis. Nevertheless, prevalence figures of 0% to 6% for small intestinal cancer and 1% to 4% for colonic cancer have been reported.[11]

Extraintestinal Manifestations

CD has a variety of extraintestinal manifestations that may accompany or even precede the intestinal disease. These include:

1. Dermatological. Associated skin diseases include erythema nodosum, pyoderma gangrenosum, and metastatic Crohn's disease. The latter is an ulcerating skin

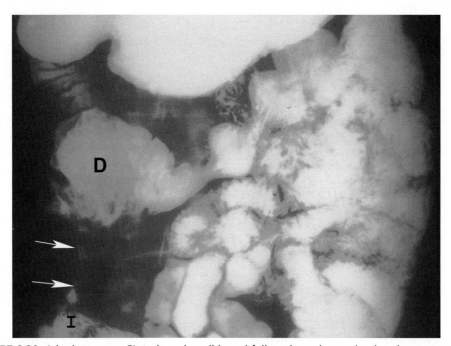

FIGURE 8.20. A barium upper GI study and small bowel follow-through examination demonstrate a duodenal (D)-ileal (I) fistula (arrows) in a patient with Crohn's disease. The duodenal segment is distorted because of the disease, and the fistula is clearly visible because it is surrounded by fat, which effectively prevents the small bowel from obscuring it on x-ray (so-called creeping fat). (Courtesy of Henry I. Goldman, MD.)

lesion, which on biopsy demonstrates granulomatous inflammation.

2. Oral. Oral manifestations include aphthous stomatitis, which on biopsy shows chronic granulomatous inflammation.

3. Ocular. Episcleritis or anterior uveitis may be related to CD.

4. Musculoskeletal. These manifestations include clubbing, ankylosing spondylitis, pelvic osteomyelitis, osteomalacia, and aseptic necrosis. Patients with ankylosing spondylitis exhibit HLA B27 phenotype. Osteomalacia is caused by vitamin D and calcium deficiency due to malabsorption. Aseptic necrosis is less a complication of CD than of steroid therapy.

5. Renal. Kidney stones, typically oxalate stones, are due to enteric hyperoxaluria.

6. Hepatobiliary. Gallstones may occur due to defective enterohepatic circulation of bile salts, which occurs in Crohn's ileitis. Primary sclerosing cholangitis and its complication cholangiocarcinoma occur less commonly in CD than in ulcerative colitis.

7. Amyloidosis. Amyloidosis may occur in longstanding CD.

CHRONIC ULCERATIVE COLITIS

Chronic ulcerative colitis (CUC) is a chronic inflammatory disease of unknown origin that affects the mucosa of the rectum and colon. It was first recognized in 1859 by Samuel Wilks of Guy's Hospital, London,[12] but it was Hawkins in 1909 who gave an excellent description of the disease and its natural history.[13] Subsequently, Sir Arthur Hurst described the sigmoidoscopic appearance and clearly differentiated it from bacillary dysentery.[14]

Epidemiology

Western Europe, North America, and Australia have a high incidence of the disease, varying from 4.3 to 11.3 cases per 100,000.[15] Unlike CD, the incidence of CUC has remained stable. Incidence rates in Eastern Europe, Asia, and South America are tenfold lower.[15] The incidence appears to be high in Ashkenazi Jews and low in black Americans. CUC is a disease of the young, occurring most commonly between ages 20 and 40 years. A secondary peak of incidence in the elderly has also been described.

Etiology and Pathogenesis

The etiology has remained elusive. Several theories have been proposed including infection, dietary allergy, autoimmunity, immune reaction to bacteria, and psychosomatic causes. In addition, a genetic predisposition has been identified.

Genetics

About 10% to 20% of patients have one or more affected family members. A study in twins has shown that, of 20 dizygote twins, all 20 were affected, while only one of 16 monozygotic twins had the disease.[16] Nevertheless, the genetic influences are greater in CD than in CUC.

Infection

No specific infecting microorganism has been consistently isolated, so CUC is unlikely to be due to infection. *E. coli* isolated from CUC patients express higher amounts of adhesion molecules, suggesting they may adhere better to and damage the colonic mucosa.

Dietary Allergy

Sensitivity to milk has long been suspected as a trigger. Controlled clinical trials suggest that 20% of patients might benefit from a milk-free diet, and increased antibodies to milk proteins have been shown in these patients.[17] Despite these observations, there is little evidence that food allergy is the primary cause.

Autoimmune Response

Antibodies against polymorphonuclear neutrophils (PMNs) or perinuclear antineutrophil cytoplasmic antibodies (pANCAs) have been shown to be more prevalent in CUC, especially in the aggressive form. But the true relevance of these autoantibodies is unknown.

Immune Response

Both humoral and cell-mediated responses are probably involved in the pathogenesis of inflammation. In the inflamed tissue, cells that produce IgG are disproportionately increased, but this finding may be an epiphenomenon. In active disease, T cells and macrophages are activated and release an array of cytokines including IL-1β, TNF, and IL-6. Class II antigens are induced in the epithelial cell surface, making it capable of behaving as an antigen-presenting cell. In addition to cytokines, other substances released from activated mucosal cells include leukotrienes, thromboxane, platelet-activating factor, and reactive oxygen metabolites. This process contributes to the cause of diarrhea.

Role of Tachykinins

Neurogenic inflammation, mediated by substance P (SP) and the neurokinin-1 receptor (NK$_1$R), may be important in CUC. Both SP levels and SP-containing neurons are markedly increased in the colon in CUC.

Psychosomatic Causes

No convincing evidence exists to show that CUC is a psychosomatic disease. Many of the psychologic findings in patients with CUC are likely to be secondary to the chronic and anxiety-producing symptoms of the disease.

Pathology

Distribution of Disease

In 20% of patients, the disease involves the whole colon; in 30% to 40% the disease involves the rectum and sigmoid only, and in 40% to 50% disease is limited to the rectum. Disease is often more severe in the rectum.

Macroscopic Features

On sigmoidoscopy, the rectal mucosa is hyperemic, edematous, and granular, and it bleeds when touched with an instrument. More advanced disease is characterized by ulcers that look like they might penetrate into the lamina propria. In longstanding cases, pseudopolyps are present in the colon. At laparotomy, the involved bowel is not thickened as in CD and, since the disease is mucosal, bowel may appear nearly normal on the serosal surface. In advanced cases, however, the colon wall is thin and gray in appearance. The bowel is often foreshortened and haustral folds may be lost. Small abscesses may be present within the mesentery and the colon may dilate and perforate (Figure 8.21).

Microscopic Features

Inflammation is largely confined to the mucosa. The lamina propria is edematous and infiltrated with neutrophils, lymphocytes, plasma cells, and macrophages. Crypt abscesses may be present (Figure 8.22).

Complications of Ulcerative Colitis

Gastrointestinal Complications

HEMORRHAGE Hemorrhage occurs in 5% of cases. Emergency colectomy should be performed if 6 to 8U of blood for transfusion are required per 24h.

PERFORATION Perforation may occur with or without toxic megacolon. Perforation is associated with a high mortality rate.

TOXIC MEGACOLON The diagnosis of toxic megacolon is made when the diameter of the transverse colon is 6cm or more. The incidence is 5%. Factors that precipitate the development of toxic megacolon include the use of opiates (particularly in conjunction with anticholinergics), hypokalemia, and barium enema or colonoscopy during the course of severe acute colitis.

ACUTE TOXIC COLITIS Severe toxic colitis can occur without the development of megacolon. Patients with toxic colitis are septic and have peritoneal symptoms. Signs and symptoms of peritonitis may be partially masked by steroid therapy. An important symptom is frequent bloody diarrhea.

CARCINOMA OF THE COLON The incidence of colon cancer is 7.2% and 16.5% with 20- and 30-year history of disease, respectively.[18] Colon cancer is usually preceded with dysplasia. Performing colectomy if dysplasia is present prevents the development of carcinoma. There is the impression that colon cancer associated with CUC is more virulent than that occurring in an otherwise normal colon.

SCLEROSING CHOLANGITIS AND CHOLANGIOCARCINOMA Sclerosing cholangitis has a significant association with ulcerative colitis. It can antedate the development of the disease or develop in the course of the disease. There appears to be, however, no relationship between the severity of ulcerative colitis and the develement of sclerosing cholangitis. Sclerosing cholangitis is a significant risk factor for cholangiocarcinoma.

EXTRAGASTROINTESTINAL COMPLICATIONS These include:

1. Ocular: episcleritis and anterior uveitis.
2. Oral: Aphthus ulcers in the buccal mucosa.
3. Dermatologic: Pyoderma gangrenosa and erythema nodosum. Severe pyoderma gangrenosa is occasionally an indication for colectomy.
4. Musculoskeletal: sacroileitis, ankylosing spondilitis. The musculoskeletal complications of ulcerative colitis are rarely an indication for colectomy.

DIVERTICULAR DISEASE OF THE COLON

Diverticula, or outpouchings from the colon wall, may be true or false. True diverticula, which involve all layers of the colonic wall, are infrequent and occur singly or in multiples, mostly in the right colon. Pseudodiverticula, which lack muscular coat, are more common and are responsible for most diverticular diseases of the colon.

Epidemiology

Around the world, an inverse relationship exists between the prevalence of diverticular disease and colonic volvulus.[19] Diverticular disease is an affliction of Western civilization, most common in North America and Western Europe, where the incidence of volvulus of the colon is small. By contrast, volvulus is common in Eastern Europe, Asia, and Africa, where diverticular disease is rare. This epidemiologic contrast has been ascribed to dietary habits. In North America and Western Europe, the diet is low in fiber content. As a result, the stools are small, and the colon has a narrow caliber and is not fecally loaded. The opposite is true in areas where a high-fiber diet is consumed.

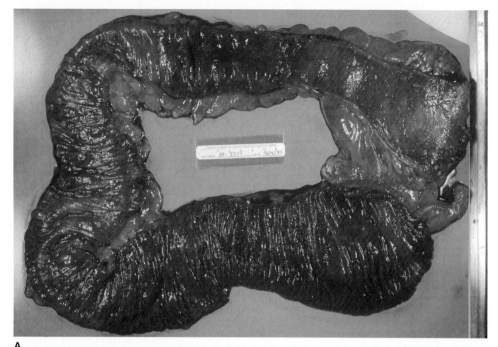

A

B

FIGURE 8.21. (A) Total colectomy specimens in severe ulcerative colitis show foreshortening of the bowel, loss of haustral markings, and (B) severe pseudopolyposis. (Courtesy of Theodore Schrock, MD, and Linda D. Ferrell, MD.)

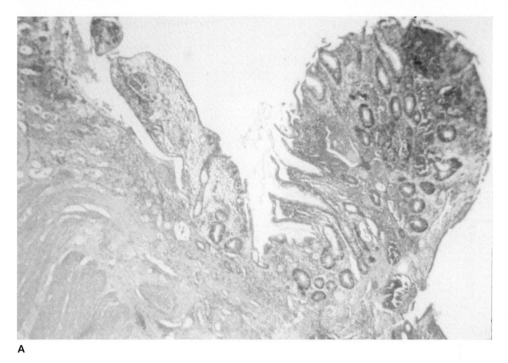

A

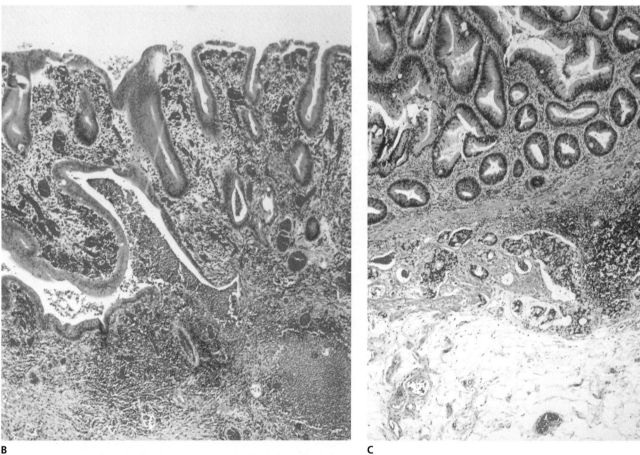

B   C

FIGURE 8.22. Ulcerative colitis. (A) Microscopically, pseudopolyps are formed as islands of inflamed mucosa by ulceration and denudation of surrounding mucosa. (B) Complications of ulcerative colitis include crypt abscess formation, in this case with a large collection of inflammatory cells and superficial inflammation, and (C) cancer, demonstrating high-grade dysplasia with overt carcinoma formation. (Courtesy of Linda D. Ferrell, MD.)

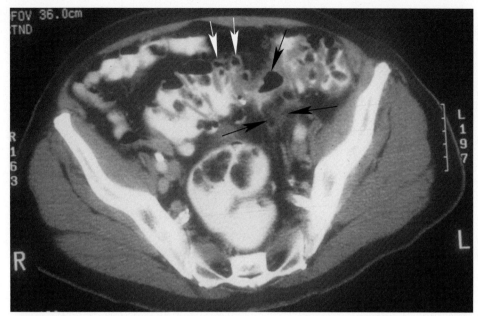

FIGURE 8.23. Diverticulitis. CT scan of the pelvis with contrast material in the sigmoid colon and small bowel shows sigmoid thickening, stranding of the pericolonic fat, and an air collection in the thickened wall (black arrows). These features are typical of diverticulitis with small intramural abscess. A few simple diverticula (white arrows) are also present. (Figure courtesy of Henry I. Goldman, MD.)

Distribution

Diverticulosis is a condition of the elderly. Its incidence is less than 10% under the age of 40 years and more than 40% after the age of 80 years. The sigmoid colon is involved in 95% of cases. Involvement decreases progressively as the disease moves proximally. In a small percentage of patients, the disease is distributed throughout the colon (Figure 8.23). Diverticula limited to the right colon are likely to be true diverticula and appear to be more frequent in Asian populations.

Pathogenesis

Diverticulosis

The presence of diverticula without inflammation is known as diverticulosis. Two etiologic factors have been proposed:

INCREASED INTRALUMINAL PRESSURE High intraluminal pressures due to colonic hypermotility occur in individuals whose diet has a low fiber content. The result is that the colonic musculature becomes thickened and shortened—a condition known as mychosis. The colon, particularly the sigmoid, has a small caliber, and contractions of its wall generate high luminal pressures. (This is in keeping with LaPlace's law, which states that the pressure within a tubular structure is inversely proportional to its radius.) The increased intraluminal pressure is believed to push out, through areas of weakness in the colon wall such as the sites of arterial entry, portions of mucosa surrounded by submucosa (Figure 8.24). Evidence for increased intraluminal pressure has been provided with manometric studies and demonstrations of occlusive contractions on cineradiography.

WEAKNESS OF COLONIC MUSCULATURE It is postulated that the high frequency of diverticulosis in the elderly is due to a weakness of the colonic musculature that develops with aging. Colonic diverticulosis is also associated with connective tissue diseases such as Ehlers–Danlos and Marfan's syndromes. When connective tissue weakness is present, pancolonic diverticulosis tends to develop.

Diverticulitis

When diverticula become inflamed, the precipitating event is thought to be microperforation of individual diverticuli due to increased intraluminal pressure. This causes infection and inflammation in the peridiverticular and pericolonic tissue. Obstruction of diverticular orifices with fecalith may also precipitate inflammation without initial perforation. At times, macroperforation of a diverticulum may occur with more acute septic complications. Patients who perforate a diverticulum because of steroids tend to develop free perforation and generalized peritonitis.

Uncomplicated diverticulitis is, in essence, peridiverticulitis, usually due to microperforations of diverticula. Macroperforation of diverticula may give rise to a pericolic abscess if the process is walled off or to general peritonitis if it is not (Figure 8.25). Also, a pericolic abscess can perforate secondarily to give rise to generalized peritonitis. Pericolic abscess or severe diverticulitis can lead to sigmoid obstruction.

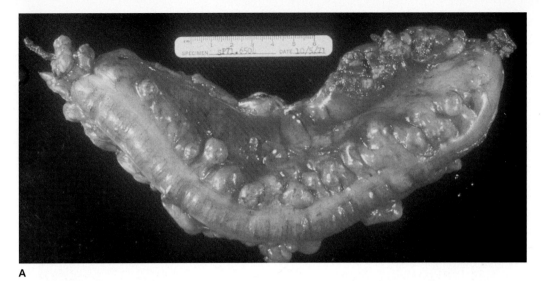

A

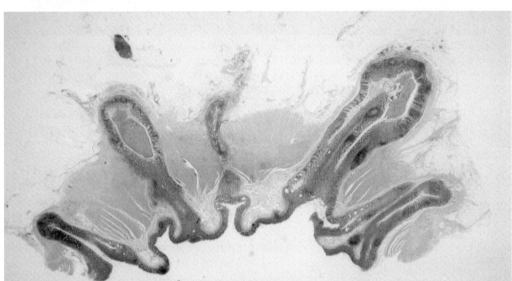

B

FIGURE 8.24. (A) Gross appearance of diverticulosis coli. (B) Microscopically, diverticula are manifest as outpouchings of the mucosa through the muscle wall and have no muscular coverings themselves (i.e., pseudodiverticula). (Courtesy of Linda D. Ferrell, MD.)

COMPLICATIONS Diverticulitis may be uncomplicated, although complications often occur (see Table 8.8). Colovesical fistula may manifest with recurrent polymicrobial urinary tract infections, pneumaturia, and fecaluria. Ureteric obstruction or colouretic fistula may be found in rare cases. Bleeding is a feature of diverticulosis and is less common in the presence of diverticulitis. Both right-sided and left-sided diverticula can bleed. At times, exsanguinating lower gastrointestinal hemorrhage can occur. Bleeding is usually from ruptured vas rectum arterioles at the dome of the diverticulum.

Diverticula of the Small Intestine

Small intestinal diverticula may be solitary or multiple. Solitary diverticula occur more commonly in the duodenum and in the ileum (Meckel's diverticulum). Diverticu-

losis of the small intestine may occur as an isolated condition or as part of a multiorgan syndrome.

DUODENAL DIVERTICULA All duodenal diverticula occur on the inner (medial) aspect of the duodenum.

Periampullary Diverticula Periampullary diverticula are common but most are asymptomatic. Nearly 70% are found near the insertion of the ampulla of Vater. On occasion, the ampulla enters the apex of the diverticulum. Periampullar diverticula become symptomatic if they develop diverticulitis or cause mechanical obstruction of the common bile duct or pancreatic duct. These diverticuli may lead to perforation. They may also make catheterization of the papilla more difficult during ERCP.

Diverticula of the Third and Fourth Portion of the Duodenum These diverticula are much less frequent than those found in the periampullary region. They are clinically

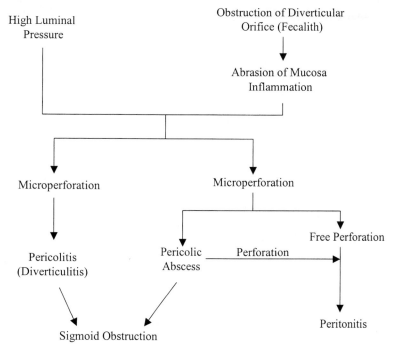

FIGURE 8.25. Pathogenesis of diverticulitis.

significant because they may cause upper GI bleeding that is difficult to localize. They are far less likely to cause diverticulitis.

MECKEL'S DIVERTICULUM This is a common true diverticulum that occurs on the antemesenteric aspect of the ileum, usually within 2 feet of the ileocecal valve. It is a remnant of the Vitelline duct. The Rule of 2 refers to the fact that Meckel's diverticulum occurs in 2% of the population, it is 2 feet proximal to the ileocecal valve, it is 2 inches long, and it is symptomatic in only 2% of adults (Figure 8.26). It is clinically important because it can cause three conditions; Meckel's diverticulitis, gastrointestinal hemorrhage, and small bowel obstruction.

Meckel's Diverticulitis Signs and symptoms are similar to those of acute appendicitis. Meckel's diverticulitis is thus an important item in the differential diagnosis.

Gastrointestinal Hemorrhage The mucosa of Meckel's diverticulum may contain heterotopic gastric mucosa that secretes acid. This produces a peptic ulcer in the adjacent normal ileal mucosa, which may sometimes lead to major hemorrhage and rarely to perforation. Techniques that help demonstrate the presence of Meckel's diverticulum

include enteroclysis and radionucleotide scan with ^{99m}Tc-pertechtinate, which is taken up by heterotopic gastric mucosa if present.

Small Bowel Obstruction In rare cases, the apex of a Meckel's diverticulum may be attached to the underside of the umbilicus through a persistent cord remnant of the Vitelline duct. Small bowel volvulus around this cord is a rare complication.

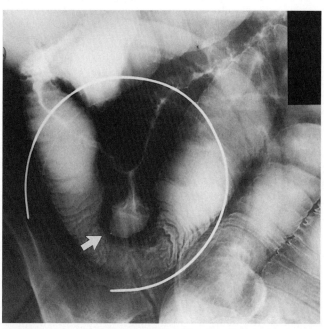

FIGURE 8.26. Meckel's diverticulum. The diverticulum (arrow) originates from a collapsed segment of ileum in the right lower quadrant. This barium small bowel examination was performed to look for metastatic melanoma, and the Meckel's diverticulum was incidentally found. (Courtesy of Henry Goldberg, MD.)

TABLE 8.8. Complications of Diverticular Disease

Localized pericolic abscess
Free perforation and generalized peritonitis
Sigmoid obstruction
Colovesical or colovaginal fistula and sequelae
Ureteric obstruction or colouretic fistula
Pylephlebitis and liver abscess
Lower gastrointestinal hemorrhage

DIVERTICULOSIS OF THE SMALL INTESTINE Diverticulosis of the small intestine is usually seen in conjunction with other underlying conditions such as abnormalities of the myenteric plexus and/or smooth muscle, and in the pseudo-obstruction syndrome. These are most common in the jejunum. Their clinical significance lies in their association with pseudo-obstruction and potential to cause malabsorption syndrome due to bacterial overgrowth within their lumen.

PATHOGENESIS AND GENETICS OF COLON POLYPS AND COLORECTAL CANCER

Although the exact cause of colorectal cancer is incompletely understood, significant advances in molecular genetics in the last 5 to 10 years have improved our understanding of the mechanism of carcinogenesis. Colorectal cancer is the second most common cause of cancer death in North America and in Western Europe after cancer of the lung. Approximately 55,000 deaths and 134,000 new cases of colon cancer are predicted each year.[20]

Etiology

It is now generally accepted that colorectal cancer develops as a multistep process. The epithelial cell receives multiple hits, first from environmental factors that damage the DNA, then with sequential genetic alterations within the cell involving oncogenes and tumor-suppressor genes. Four factors that have been found to have significance in the etiology of colorectal cancer are diet, genetic predisposition, premalignant conditions, and molecular genetics.

Dietary Factors

An association has been described between high fat intake and colorectal cancer. The likelihood is that cancer will develop more often when more than 5% of the diet is made up of fat. Not all fats are implicated in this equation, but the polyunsaturated and saturated fats are the primary culprits. Monounsaturated fats do not pose the same risk. Some theories have been advanced regarding the mechanism that makes a high-fat diet carcinogenic, including the carcinogenic effect of increased bile acids in the colon and the release of tumor-promoting prostaglandins. The exact mechanism is as yet unknown.

A second dietary risk factor may be a diet low in fiber. Countries with a high-fiber diet have a lower incidence of colon cancer, but how the high-fiber diet protects against cancer is unknown. One plausible theory is that a high-fiber diet increases transit time through the colon. As a corollary, a low-fiber diet prolongs transit time, increasing mucosal exposure to luminal carcinogens.

A number of substances are said to be protective. These include vitamins A, C, and E; β-carotenes; calcium; selenium; dithiothiones; thioethers; and terpenes. These substances are believed to act by reducing the generation of free-oxygen radicals at the mucosal surface.

Genetic Predisposition

About 15% of colorectal cancer is familial. The transmission is most obvious in familial adenomatous polyposis (see below). But other nonpolyposis hereditary conditions are also known. These include the cancer family syndrome (CFS), or Lynch syndrome II, and hereditary site-specific colon cancer (HSSCC), or Lynch syndrome I. In Lynch syndrome II, the cancers tend to be located in the proximal colon and are associated with noncolon cancers such as endometrial cancer. Lynch syndrome I is similar but not associated with extracolonic cancers. Even in the absence of these predisposing syndromes, first-degree relatives carry a risk that is two to three times higher than the general population.

Premalignant Conditions

Several hereditary and nonhereditary premalignant conditions of the colon are recognized.

ADENOMATOUS POLYPS Colon cancer often develops from polyps. The polyp to cancer sequence is depicted in Figure 8.27.

FAMILIAL ADENOMATOUS POLYPOSIS Familial adenomatous polyposis (FAP) is the best known premalignant condition (Figure 8.28). It is inherited as a dominant autosomal disorder with a genetic defect on chromosome 5, close to the q21 locus. The defective gene has been called the adenomatous polyposis coli or APC gene.

Colorectal cancer develops in all patients with FAP before age 40 years if untreated. Infants in affected families have congenital hypertrophy of the retinal pigment epithelium as early as 3 months of age.[21] This abnormality predicts FAP with an accuracy of 97%. Polyps begin to appear at puberty, but the average age of diagnosis of a new patient with FAP is 29 years.

FAP includes two other syndromes characterized by varying extracolonic manifestations.

Gardner's Syndrome Gardner's syndrome is characterized by colonic polyposis, sebaceous cysts, desmoid tumors, and osteomas of the mandible and skull.

Turcot's Syndrome Turcot's syndrome is characterized by colonic polyposis and brain tumors (medulloblastoma or glioma).

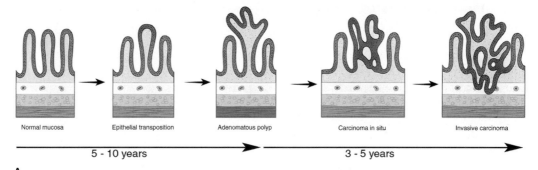

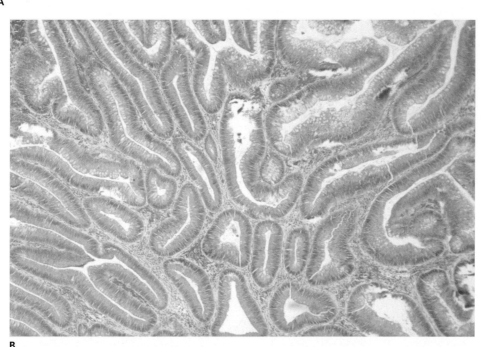

FIGURE 8.27. Polyp to cancer sequence. (A) Diagrammatic representation of the transition from normal colonic mucosa to adenomatous polyp, carcinoma in situ and invasive carcinoma. These stages of cancer development are shown in the photomicrographs demonstrating (B) benign adenomatous polyp, (C) high-grade dysplasia and carcinoma in situ, and (D) early invasive carcinoma. (Courtesy of Linda D. Ferrell, MD.)

Chronic Ulcerative Colitis In CUC involving the entire colon, the incidence of colon cancer is 1% per year after 10 years, that is, the cumulative incidence of cancer by 20 years is 10%.[22] The cancers are more advanced at the time of diagnosis, most being Duke C or D lesions. Dysplasia predates the development of colon cancer. Once dysplasia is diagnosed, colectomy is the best way to prevent the development of cancer.

Crohn's Disease The incidence of cancer in CD is lower than in CUC, estimated at 7% over 20 years of disease, including cancers in both the small and large intestine.[23] The incidence of cancer in the large bowel is much lower.

Molecular Genetics

The process of carcinogenesis involves: (1) alteration in proto-oncogene expression and (2) deletion of tumor suppressor genes.

Alteration in Proto-Oncogenes

Proto-oncogenes are human genes containing DNA sequences homologous to those of acute transforming retroviruses. They normally exist in inactive form. Their activation, it has been suggested, contributes to malignant transformation. The oncogenes of greatest interest are the *myc* and *ras* families. In colon cancer, c-myc levels are

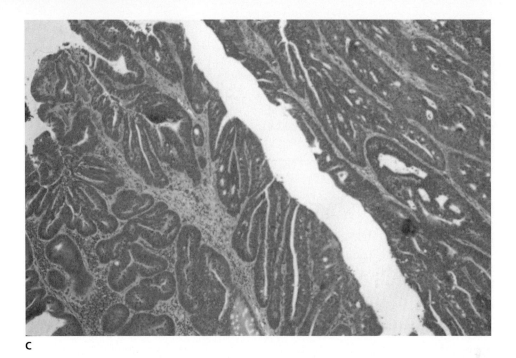

C

D

FIGURE 8.27. *Continued*

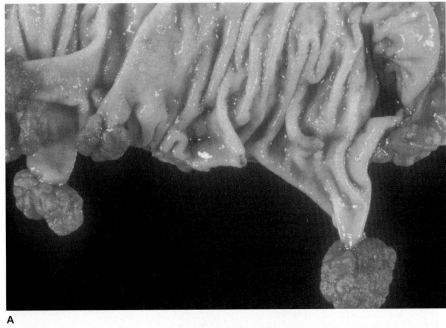

A

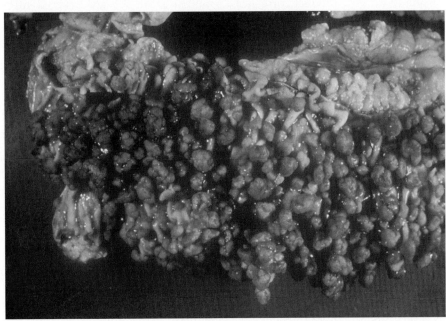

B

FIGURE 8.28. Familial multiple polyposis. (A) Discrete polyps occur separated by large surfaces of normal colonic mucosa. (B) In other cases, the entire surface of the colon may be covered with grape-like polyps. (Reprinted with permission from Fenoglio–Priese CM, et al., eds. Gastrointestinal Pathology: An Atlas and Text. Philadelphia: Raven Press, 1989.)

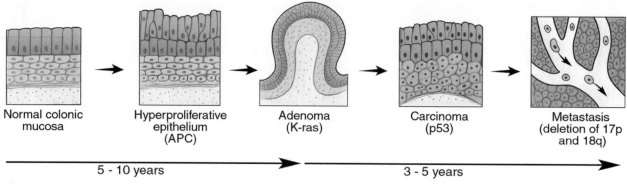

FIGURE 8.29. Proposed sequence of molecular genetic events in evolution of colon cancer. APC gene abnormalities lead to disruption of normal cell-to-cell adhesions and hyperproliferative epithelium. The K-ras gene is associated with adenoma formation, but loss of the p53 gene is required for conversion of an adenoma to adenocarcinoma. Distant metastases are associated with allelic loss of 17p and 18q. *Abbreviation*: APC, adenomatous polyposis coli.

elevated. In 40% to 50% of primary colon cancer cases, ras point mutations have been found. Ras gene mutations are an early event and occur in 58% of adenomas larger than 1 cm. Enhanced expression of ras gene product correlates with depth of tumor invasion.

Deletion of Tumor Suppressor Genes

Allelic losses occur at chromosome locations 5q, 17p, and 18q. Some 20%–36% of sporadic colon cancers have lost alleles at the 5q location. The familial polyposis gene is found at locus 5q21. The p53 gene is a major tumor suppressor gene located on chromosome 17p, and point mutations of p53 are believed to be implicated in the development of colon cancer. Another gene involved at locus 18q has been termed the DCC gene, that is, deleted in colon cancer.

Figure 8.29 illustrates the proposed sequence of molecular genetic events in the evolution of colon cancer.

CLINICAL DISORDERS AND MANAGEMENT

SMALL BOWEL OBSTRUCTION

Clinical Presentation

Simple Obstruction

The approximate site of a simple small bowel obstruction will be evident from the patient's presenting signs and symptoms. Vomiting and abdominal distension are present in all small bowel obstruction but differ considerably depending on whether the obstruction is in the high or low bowel (Table 8.9). Evidence from x-rays however, is apparent only in low small bowel obstruction.

TABLE 8.9. **Comparison of High and Low Small Bowel Obstruction**

	High	Low
Vomiting	Early, severe	Late, feculent
	Rapid dehydration	Slow dehydration
	Electrolyte imbalance	Little electrolyte imbalance
Distension	Absent or minimal	Significant, midabdominal
Abdominal x-ray	Little or no finding	Distended loops of bowel
		Air fluid levels
		Ladder formation

High Small Bowel Obstruction The presenting symptoms of high small bowel obstruction are colicky upper abdominal pain and profuse, bilious vomiting. The onset of vomiting is close to the onset of pain, and the vomitus is nonfeculent. On physical examination, vital signs are normal except late in the course, when dehydration is present. Distension, if present, is not prominent. The patient will be dehydrated if protracted vomiting has occurred. An abdominal scar from previous operation is usually present. Abdominal tenderness is absent, and bowel sounds are hyperactive, the crescendos of which coincide with attacks of colicky pain.

Low Small Bowel Obstruction Colicky, midabdominal pain, vomiting, and abdominal distension are the presenting symptoms of low small bowel obstruction. The interval between onset of pain and vomiting lengthens as the site of obstruction is more distal. Vomiting may be feculent. No gas or feces will have been passed through the rectum for variable periods of time. An abdominal scar may be present. Potential hernial sites in the abdominal wall and groin area should be carefully examined, especially the femoral hernia site beneath the midinguinal point. Abdominal tenderness is minimal or absent, and rectal examination is normal.

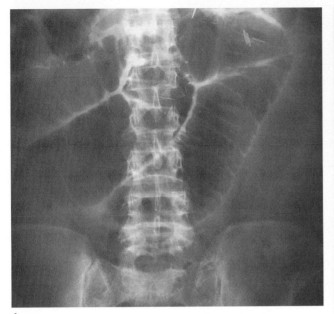

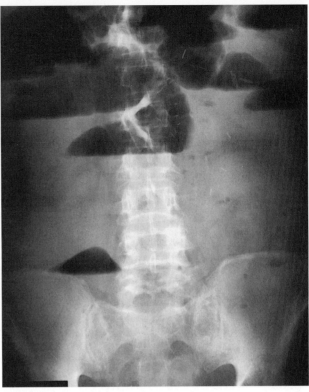

FIGURE 8.30. Simple bowel obstruction. (A) Supine radiographs are provided of a patient with a simple small bowel obstruction due to a postoperative adhesion. The bowel is identified as small bowel because of its central location, the presence of plicae circularis, which cross the entire air-filled lumen, and multiple sharp turns of small bowel segments. Notice that no air is seen in the colon. (B) Upright x-ray demonstrates multiple air-fluid levels in distended loops of bowel, a classic appearance of distal small bowel obstruction. (Courtesy of Henry I. Goldman, MD.)

Strangulated Obstruction

The presence of strangulation may be difficult to detect in complete small bowel obstruction, but historical and physical clues may be present. When recording the medical history, the most suggestive finding is the progression of colicky pain to constant and more intense pain. Fever and tachycardia may develop but are relatively late signs. The most significant physical finding is the presence of abdominal tenderness, which may or may not be associated with early rebound tenderness. Despite these distinctions, it should be noted that some 35% of strangulated obstructions are unsuspected before operation, underscoring the importance of early operation in all patients with complete small bowel obstruction. The old adage still holds true: "Never let the sun rise or set on complete bowel obstruction."

Investigations

Laboratory Studies

Laboratory findings are normal in the early stages. Later, hemoconcentration and some leukocytosis may develop. Electrolytes are usually normal in distal small bowel obstruction, but hypokalemia and hypochloremia may occur in high obstruction. Serum amylase levels are infre-

quently elevated and usually in the presence of strangulation. When strangulation is present, marked leukocytosis with a shift to the left occurs. Blood gases may show metabolic acidosis.

Abdominal X-Ray

Abdominal x-rays should include supine and upright views. The findings in simple obstruction (Figure 8.30) are:

1. Dilated loops of small intestine with air–fluid levels, a finding that may be absent when the level of obstruction is high in the small intestine.
2. No air in the colon if complete obstruction is present, although gas may be present in the rectum and sigmoid, especially if sigmoidoscopy was performed before x-rays.

The findings suggesting that strangulation has occurred are:

1. Thumbprinting and loss of mucosal pattern.
2. Air in the bowel wall or in the portal vein and its branches.
3. Free air in the peritoneum if perforation has occurred.

Management

All patients with complete mechanical small bowel obstruction need an emergent operation. Patients with incomplete obstruction can be treated expectantly with nasogastric suction and hydration. Long intestinal tubes (e.g., Miller–Abbot) are sometimes successful, but they are cumbersome and may not be well tolerated by the patient. Serial plain films of the abdomen should be obtained daily or more often and, if the obstruction becomes complete, an emergency operation is necessary.

In complete small bowel obstruction, rapid fluid and electrolyte resuscitation and early surgery are required. The management steps are described below.

Preoperative

A nasogastric tube is inserted and placed to suction early to prevent aspiration and reduce distension. Fluid and electrolyte resuscitation is commenced, as patients with small bowel obstruction have significant contraction of the extracellular volume. The fluid deficit should be corrected with either normal saline or lactated Ringer solution. A Foley catheter is inserted into the bladder to monitor urine output, which should be maintained at 50 cc/h or more, as an index of adequacy of hydration. When dehydration is severe or when the patient has serious cardiopulmonary disease, central venous or pulmonary artery pressure may need to be monitored. Most patients with low small bowel obstruction have normal electrolyte measurements. Despite this, potassium chloride should be administered as soon as adequate urine output is established, because hypokalemia develops with hydration. Patients with high small bowel obstruction may have severe hypokalemia, hypochloremia, and even metabolic alkalosis. Correction of these abnormalities is best accomplished with saline solution and potassium chloride.

Analgesia should be provided with either morphine or pethidine once a decision is made to operate. Broad-spectrum perioperative antibiotics should be administered.

Operation

The optimal time to operate is as soon as fluid and electrolyte resuscitation is complete. The type of incision depends on the cause of obstruction and on any preexisting abdominal scars. Wide exposure is necessary. A useful way to identify the site of obstruction is to locate the collapsed bowel and follow it proximally to the site of obstruction and proximal distension. Adhesion bands should be lysed, and if the obstruction is due to tumor or foreign body, these should be dealt with appropriately. If frank gangrene is present, the gangrenous bowel must be resected.

If there is any question about the viability of the obstructed bowel, it should be wrapped in warm towels after obstruction is relieved for 2 to 3 minutes and reinspected for color, peristaltic activity, and pulsation of vessels at the mesentery. Other helpful techniques are Doppler ultrasound to detect blood flow in the intestinal wall and the fluorescein test. Fluorescein (1000 mg) is injected intravenously over a period of 1 minute, and the bowel is then examined under ultraviolet light using Wood's lamp. Gangrenous parts of the intestine have no fluorescence. If the bowel is nonviable, or if there is serious doubt of its viability, it should be resected and end-to-end anastamosis performed.

If the cause of obstruction is a groin hernia, a standard groin incision is used. It is critical that the incarcerated bowel in a femoral or inguinal hernia be inspected for viability. This means that, if the hernia reduces spontaneously under anesthesia, laparotomy will be necessary through a midline incision. Otherwise, the entire procedure, including bowel resection if necessary, can be done through the groin incision. At times, it may be difficult to reduce a femoral hernia at operation. In such a case, incision of the lacunar ligament (the medial boundary of the femoral ring) or division of the inguinal ligament (the anterior boundary of the femoral ring) will be necessary.

Obstruction due to radiation enteritis presents a special problem. Dissection may be difficult, and the possibility of unintended enterotomy could be significant. The adhesions may be an important conduit of blood supply to the bowel. These and other considerations may indicate that the best course of action is to bypass the obstruction either by entero-enterostomy or enterocolostomy.

Some patients who have uncontrolled formation of adhesions may have several recurrences of bowel obstruction. In these special patients, the surgeon may wish to fix the bowel in a ladder fashion in the hope of preventing future obstruction. Fixing is best done by threading a long tube with an inflatable cuff at its end (e.g., the Baker tube) into the cecum through a gastrostomy or jejunostomy. The tube is left in place 14 to 21 days. The old technique of Nobel plication, in which antemesenteric portions of bowel were sutured in a ladder formation, is dangerous because of the associated high incidence of abdominal abscess and fistulas.

ACUTE MESENTERIC ISCHEMIA

Clinical Picture

Sudden mesenteric occlusion causes acute, severe and diffuse noncolicky abdominal pain. The patient may have a history of intestinal angina; recent abdominal angiography, cardiac catheterization, or cardiopulmonary bypass; or congestive heart failure and digoxin therapy. A history of atrial fibrillation may be an important clue. Nausea, vomiting, and diarrhea may or may not be present.

Abdominal examination shows diffuse tenderness, but frequently, the abdominal pain is out of proportion to the severity of abdominal finding. The abdomen is usually not rigid and rebound tenderness not very pronounced. Bowel sounds may be hypoactive or absent, but early in the course of the disease, they may be hyperactive. Often blood may be seen on the physician's finger after rectal examination. In later stages of the disease, generalized peritonitis and septic shock may develop, portending poor outcome.

Investigation

Laboratory Findings

Severe leukocytosis, with a white blood cell count of 20,000 to 30,000/cm^3, is a common finding. Metabolic acidosis and hemoconcentration are late findings. Other findings may include elevated serum amylase, serum inorganic phosphate levels, and coagulation abnormalities.

Radiological Studies

Plain abdominal film details the ileus, with diffuse distension of the small intestine and colon. Specific signs of intestinal necrosis (air in bowel wall or in portal vein radicals) are a late sign. CT scan helps to exclude acute pancreatitis as the cause. Specific diagnostic features of intestinal ischemia may be shown in 25% of patients. A CT scan is essential if the plain film does not provide definitive information for diagnosis.

The most specific diagnostic investigation is abdominal angiogram, which should include the celiac artery, the SMA, and the IMA. A lateral aortogram is useful and may show obstruction at the origin of the SMA if present (Figure 8.31). Angiography should be done early and is sometimes performed on the operating table. If angiography shows no vascular occlusion, nonocclusive mesenteric ischemia may be present, requiring continuous infusion of vasodilators (i.e., papaverin, nitroglycerin) directly into the SMA.

Operative Management

An algorithm for the management of acute visceral ischemia is given in Figure 8.32. The key is not to delay laparotomy unnecessarily. When abdominal findings suggest generalized peritonitis, immediate exploration should be performed, and if necessary, an on-table angiogram obtained. The entire bowel is examined and the area of ischemia noted (Figure 8.33). The relevant vessel, usually the SMA or its major branches, should be directly examined by reflecting the mesentery of the transverse colon superiorly and taking down the ligament of Treitz.

If an embolus or thrombus is encountered, catheter embolectomy should be performed through a transverse arteriotomy in the SMA, after anticoagulation and after obtaining proximal and distal control. The arteriotomy is closed when adequate back-bleeding is present. Once circulation is re-established, the bowel should be wrapped in warm saline sponges for several minutes and re-examined. All infarcted bowel or bowel of questionable viability

should be resected if this will not result in short bowel syndrome (i.e., resection of more than 50% of small intestine). Otherwise, bowel of questionable viability is not resected, primary anastomosis is completed, and a decision is made to re-explore within 24 h no matter how well the patient may look immediately postoperatively.

The most difficult decision is faced when all or most of the small intestine is infarcted. Patients can be kept alive with permanent total parenteral nutrition, but the most humane course of action in the elderly may be not to resect but close the abdomen and keep the patient comfortable until death.

Selected patients may benefit from revascularization procedures of the SMA, the celiac axis, or both. The best approach is medial visceral rotation, reflecting the spleen and pancreas medially. The procedure of choice is antegrade bypass from the supraceliac aorta using either saphenous vein or a prosthetic graft.

In contrast to the small intestine, acute vascular ischemia of the colon is treated with resection without significant attempt to restore circulation. It is usually not prudent to perform primary colo-colic anastomosis, whereas ileo-colic anastomoses seem to pose less risk of dehiscence.

Outcome

The mortality rate following acute mesenteric occlusion is very high, due primarily to delay in diagnosis and treatment. The mortality rate for mesenteric thrombosis and nonocclusive ischemia is over 50%, and that for mesenteric embolism 40%–50%.[24]

LARGE BOWEL OBSTRUCTION

As mentioned earlier, carcinoma and diverticulitis account for nearly 90% of all large bowel obstruction. Volvulus and inflammatory bowel disease are other important causes.

Clinical Presentation

Symptoms and signs include those of mechanical obstruction as well as those of underlying disease. The pain is crampy and suprapubic. Vomiting is a late symptom, and the vomitus is typically feculent. Constipation and obstipation are constant features. Abdominal distension can be prominent, especially in sigmoid volvulus. Bowel sounds are hyperactive and high pitched.

Superimposed on these symptoms and signs are those of the underlying disease producing the obstruction. Patients with colon cancer may complain of a change in bowel habits and rectal bleeding. Patients with diverticulitis may have a history of alternating diarrhea and constipation and usually have signs of the inflammatory process: fever, tachycardia, and tenderness or mass in the left lower quadrant. Patients with sigmoid volvulus are generally elderly and may reside in nursing homes.

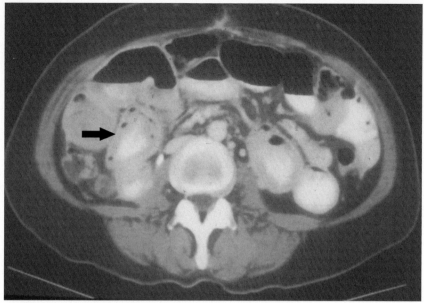

A

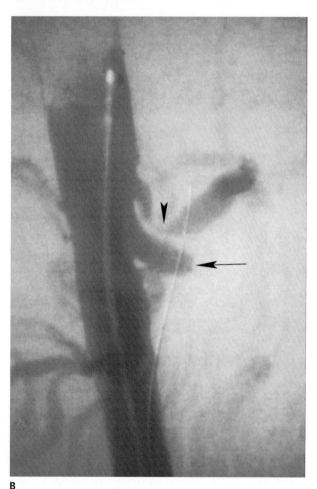

B

FIGURE 8.31. Acute mesenteric ischemia. (A) A CT scan of the midabdomen demonstrates thickened segments of small bowel containing air bubbles within the wall (arrow). In this patient with severe abdominal pain and distention, these findings, as well as metabolic acidosis, are diagnostic of acute mesenteric ischemia. (B) The aortogram of the same patient shows an occluded superior mesenteric artery (arrow), the cause of the ischemic small bowel. Compression of the celiac artery by an arcuate ligament (arrowhead) is also present. (Courtesy of Henry I. Goldman, MD.)

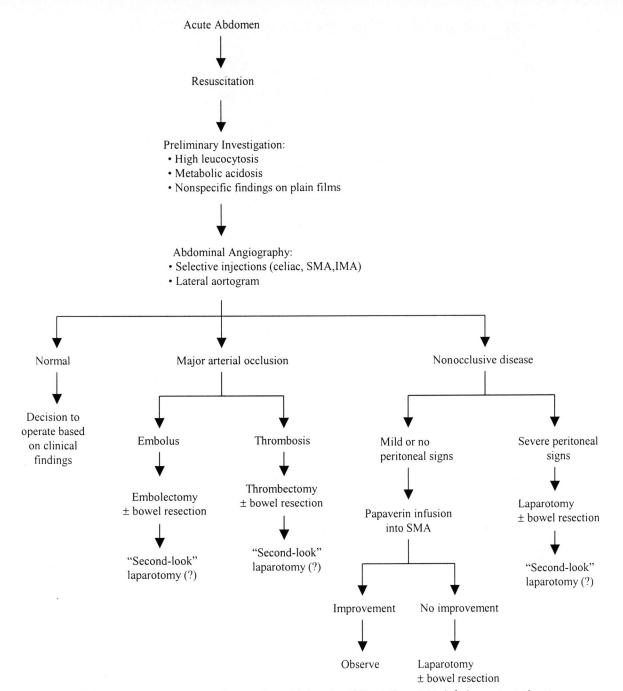

FIGURE 8.32. Management of acute visceral ischemia. *Abbreviations*: IMA, inferior mesenteric artery; SMA, superior mesenteric artery.

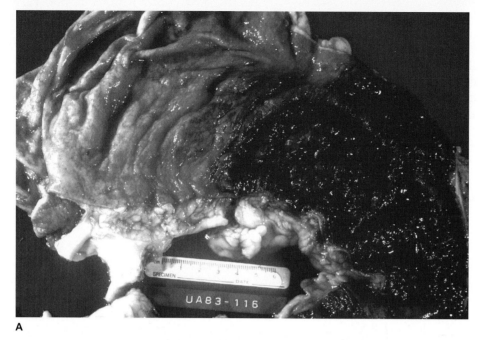

A

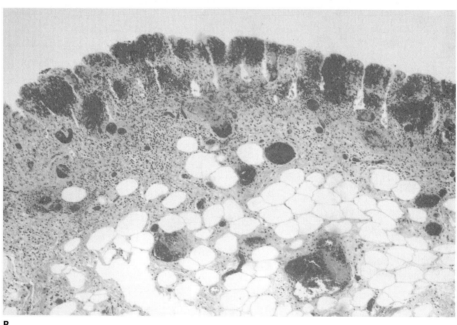

B

FIGURE 8.33. Acute ischemic colonic infarction. (A) Grossly, there is sloughing of the mucosa, and (B) microscopically, the vessels in the submucosa and serosa are filled with microthrombi. (Figures courtesy of Linda Ferrell, MD.)

Investigation

Endoscopy

Sigmoidoscopy may show a carcinoma in the upper rectum, sigmoid, or descending colon. In diverticulitis, the examination is painful and no tumor is seen. Colonoscopy may be indicated in some cases.

Radiological Studies

Plain films demonstrate distended colon with its typical haustral markings and absence of air in the rectum. CT scan with rectal contrast enema is usually a conclusive examination. In general, barium enema should not be performed in a patient with left lower quadrant tenderness and inflammatory mass. However, if abdominal tenderness is absent, a careful barium enema may yield useful information. If this is done, the radiologist should be instructed that a limited examination is needed to show only the site and nature of the obstruction and not a full study of the colon. If too much barium with significant head pressure is used, two catastrophic complications can follow:

1. Perforation of the cecum or at the site of diverticulitis, causing barium peritonitis.
2. Barium loading of the colon proximal to the obstruction, a problem that complicates surgical treatment.

Management

The goals of treatment are rapid decompression of the bowel, removal of the underlying lesion, and restoration of bowel continuity. Specific management details in obstruction due to diverticulitis and volvulus are discussed below.

When obstruction is due to cancer, the management decision depends on the condition of the patient, the condition of the bowel (e.g., distension, fecal loading), and the lesion site. Three questions must be asked:

1. Should decompressing ileostomy or colostomy precede resection?
2. Should resection be performed and an end-colostomy created with a plan for anastomosis in a second operation?
3. Could primary resection and anastomosis be accomplished in one operation?

In general, the safest operation should be chosen. Whenever the lesion can be removed without compromising the resection necessary to treat the cancer, primary resection without anastomosis is preferred. Some prefer to perform resection with intraoperative colonic lavage and primary anastomosis. Another option is to perform anatomosis with the use of a coloshield, a device that provides intraluminal bypass to divert the fecal stream from the anastomosis, thereby reducing anastomotic leak rate. When the obstructing lesion is proximal or in the splenic flexure, extended right hemicolectomy with ileocolostomy is the preferred operation.

SIGMOID VOLVULUS

Clinical Picture

Intermittent suprapubic colicky pain and striking abdominal distension are the usual presenting symptoms. The patients, usually elderly and from nursing homes, may have longstanding constipation and may, indeed, have had prior attacks of sigmoid volvulus that resolved spontaneously.

Radiologic Studies

Plain abdominal films show an extremely dilated single loop of bowel arising from the pelvis, typically with a coffee bean shape (see Figure 8.16). Barium enema, if necessary, must be performed with caution. It shows obstruction at the rectosigmoid with a characteristic bird's beak deformity and spiral narrowing of the bowel.

Management

Sigmoidoscopic Reduction

Sigmoidoscopic reduction should be attempted only when strangulation has not occurred. This is best assessed with flexible sigmoidoscopy. The presence of dusky or black mucosa is a contraindication to sigmoidoscopic decompression. Otherwise, the procedure is performed by advancing a rigid sigmoidoscope to a point a few centimeters below the obstruction, then passing a well-lubricated large rectal tube through the sigmoidoscope and gently pushing it through the obstruction. The resulting decompression may be somewhat explosive, and the surgeon and surgical assistants should place themselves appropriately to escape the deluge.

If successful decompression is possible, elective sigmoid resection should be planned after bowel preparation. In very elderly patients, expectant management may be appropriate after the first episode.

If sigmoidoscopic decompression is unsuccessful or if strangulation or perforation occurs, an emergency operation is needed. The goal is to resect the sigmoid and perform an end-descending colostomy. In selected patents with megacolon, total colectomy may be the best option.

CECAL VOLVULUS

Clinical Presentation

The presentation of cecal volvulus is distal small bowel obstruction. The patient may have a history of similar past attacks.

Investigation

Plain films of the abdomen show distal small bowel obstruction with a dilated cecum in the epigastrium or the left upper quadrant. Barium enema is usually diagnostic, showing the level of obstruction and the ileocecal junction to the right of the cecal bubble (see Figure 8.17).

Management

After fluid resuscitation, all patients should undergo an operation. The goals of surgery are to decompress the obstruction and fix the cecum in the right lower quadrant, either by creating a pocket in the parietal peritoneum and suturing the cecum to the peritoneum or by using tube cecostomy. If strangulation has occurred, right hemicolectomy is the definitive procedure.

FISTULAS OF THE SMALL INTESTINE

About 95% of external small bowel fistulas develop as a complication following surgery. In the remaining 5%, spontaneous fistulas may occur as a result of primary disease, such as Crohn's disease, actinomycosis, tuberculosis, or neoplasm. Postoperative small bowel fistulas occur as a result of either suture-line dehiscence, unrecognized intraoperative bowel injury, or because the small bowel is incorporated into a suture during closure of the abdominal wall. Suture-line dehiscence is apt to occur in previously irradiated bowel. The fistula may be a high-output fistula (producing more than 500 mL/24 h) or a low-output fistula.

Clinical Picture

The typical picture is a patient who, 2 or more days postabdominal surgery, develops sepsis with fever and leukocytosis. Abdominal pain and tenderness are present. The incision becomes red and, when opened, intestinal contents discharge through the wound. The discharge of succus entericus may excoriate the skin of the abdominal wall. After drainage of the wound, the sepsis subsides unless there is associated intra-abdominal abscess or abscesses. A high-output fistula from the duodenum or jejunum can lead to severe fluid and electrolyte abnormalities.

Investigation

Laboratory Studies

Leukocytosis is common and, in high-output fistula, hemoconcentration and electrolyte abnormalities may occur. Low serum albumin levels may indicate preexisting malnutrition.

Radiological Studies

Plain abdominal films are likely to be less helpful than CT scan and ultrasound, which are the best way to look for an intra-abdominal abscess. The location of the fistula and whether or not distal obstruction is present may be detected by oral or rectal administration of contrast medium. In regard to the fistulous tract, information about the number of fistulas and whether or not there is associated abscess is best obtained with a fistulogram by injecting hypaque into the fistula tract.

Treatment

A well-planned management approach is indicated, including:

1. Replacement of fluids and electrolytes. Restoration of lost fluids requires estimating the existing deficit and measuring continuing losses. An ileostomy bag or a suction system is used to collect fistula output. Careful daily input-output charting and daily weighing of the patient are essential.

2. Reduction of fistula output. This is done through institution of nasogastric suction, use of H_2-receptor antagonists, or, in the case of a high-output fistula, use of subcutaneous injection of the longacting somatostatin analogue octreotide.

3. Control of fistula and wound care. As much as possible, fistula output should be drained directly into a bag or by a suction catheter to limit skin damage. Various pastes may be applied to the surrounding skin to prevent excoriation.

4. Drainage of any associated abscess. Drainage is best handled by interventional radiology using CT-guided insertion of a catheter into the abscess cavity through the fistulous tract. If the fistula cannot be drained successfully in this way, operative drainage is necessary.

5. Supplemental nutrition. Total parenteral nutrition may need to be instituted, providing 2500 to 3000 kcals/day.

6. Operative treatment. Operative treatment is indicated when a fistula fails to heal, usually due to the presence of:
   a. Undrained pus.
   b. Foreign body.
   c. Distal obstruction.
   d. Short fistulous tract.
   e. Active disease (e.g., Crohn's disease, malignancy) at the site of perforation.

The key decision is choosing the timing of surgery. If sepsis is controlled and adequate nutrition established, the operation should be delayed 8 to 12 weeks. During that time, about a third of patients spontaneously heal their fistula. If the fistula persists, reoperation is necessary to resect the fistulous segment. If this is technically difficult, the fistula may be bypassed. The latter procedure is rarely needed if the second operation is delayed 8 to 12 weeks after the onset of the fistula.

DIVERTICULITIS OF THE COLON

Diverticulitis is the second most common disease of the colon and the second most common cause of colonic obstruction following colon cancer.

Clinical Presentation

Uncomplicated Diverticulitis

Uncomplicated diverticulitis typically presents with acute onset of nausea, vomiting, fever, and left lower quadrant (LLQ) pain similar to the pain of acute appendicitis but on the wrong side. Diarrhea alternating with constipation is a typical antecedent complaint. Physical examination reveals LLQ tenderness and mass. The mass is best appreciated with bimanual examination with one finger in the rectum and the other hand palpating the abdomen. Leukocytosis with a shift to the left will be present. Sometimes, patients may complain of dysuria.

Complicated Diverticulitis

Diverticulitits may cause complications, which include obstruction of the sigmoid, localized perforation with pericolic abscess, free perforation with generalized peritonitis, and colovesical fistula.

1. Colonic obstruction due to diverticulitis. Colonic obstruction is always associated with acute flare-up of diverticulitis and the signs and symptoms of sigmoid inflammation, as well as left-sided colon obstruction with distension and late-onset vomiting.

2. Pericolic abscess. The patient is more ill, and impressive signs of localized peritonitis and tender mass may be present in the LLQ of the abdomen. High fever and leukocytosis with bandemia are common. Nausea and vomiting, including signs of large bowel obstruction, may be present.

3. Generalized peritonitis. Free perforation of colonic diverticula with fecal peritonitis is a serious, life-threatening illness. Generalized peritonitis could also be secondary to perforation of a previously localized pericolic abscess, in which case the peritonitis is purulent. The findings in both are those of generalized peritonitis with severe sepsis with or without accompanying septic shock.

4. Colovesical fistula. This is rarely an acute problem and manifests itself with recurrent attacks of polymicrobial urinary infection and history of pneumoturia.

Investigations

Laboratory Studies

Leukocytosis with a shift to the left occurs. In severely septic patients, gram-negative bacteria may be grown in blood culture. Mild dehydration may be present. Anemia and severe electrolyte imbalance are not characteristically seen.

RADIOLOGICAL STUDIES

Plain Films of the Abdomen Obstruction associated with diverticulitis involves the left colon. When pericolic abscess is present, the picture is that of ileus. When perforation has occurred, free air may be present in the peritoneum.

CT Scan CT scan is the most useful study to investigate septic process in the lower abdomen. Sigmoid thickening and effacement of pericolic fat are seen in diverticulitis. Pericolic abscesses are readily visualized and their accessibility for percutaneous drainage determined.

Rectal Contrast Studies Barium enema is contraindicated in acute diverticulitis. The use of water-soluble enema has now been largely replaced by CT scan. Barium enema is a useful study 2 or 3 weeks following resolution of acute diverticulitis and may show multiple diverticula and a sinus tract with or without communication to an abscess cavity outside the colon.

ENDOSCOPY The role of sigmoidoscopy is limited, and colonoscopy should be avoided. If rigid sigmoidoscopy is performed, the scope cannot be passed beyond the rectosigmoid, where erythema and edema may be visible. The examination is painful.

Surgical Management

Uncomplicated Diverticulitis

Patients with mild attacks can be treated on an outpatient basis with clear fluid diet and broad-spectrum oral antibiotics or triple antibiotics (i.e., ampicillin, an aminoglycoside, and metronidazole). Patients with more severe symptoms should be admitted to hospital and treated with intravenous fluids and intravenous antibiotics. Resolution of symptoms occurs within 5 to 10 days. Rarely is operation required unless the condition has recurred three or more times. Full colon investigation is done 2 to 3 weeks after discharge from hospital.

Colonic Obstruction due to Diverticulitis

Patients with colonic obstruction should be admitted to a hospital. They are given intravenous fluids and nasogastric suction is instituted. Broad-spectrum antibiotic or triple antibiotic therapy is administered intravenously. Adequate analgesia is provided with meperidine or pentazocin. Morphine should be avoided because it increases colonic pressure. Typically, symptoms resolve in 5 to 10 days. Surgery is not indicated if this is the first, and perhaps even the second, attack. If it is the third attack, or if obstruction fails to resolve in 12 to 14 days, sigmoid resection is necessary. The safest operation is the Hartmann procedure

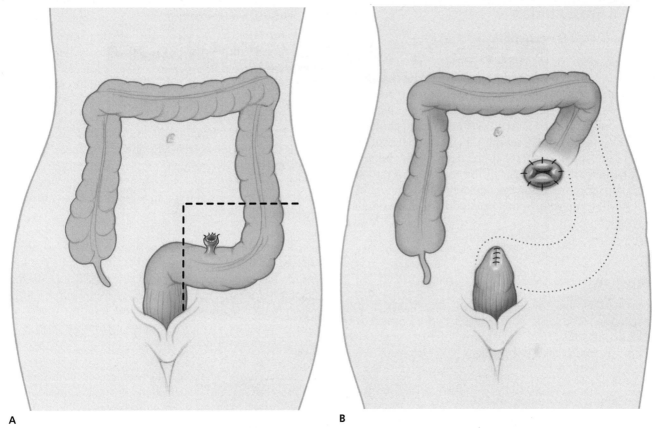

FIGURE 8.34. Hartmann procedure. (A) The affected sigmoid colon is resected, (B) the descending colostomy is then constructed, and the rectal stump closed in layers. (Adapted from Schwartz SI, ed: Principles of Surgery, 6th ed. New York: McGraw Hill, 1994:1282.)

(Figure 8.34), in which the sigmoid is resected; the rectal stump closed, and end-descending colon colostomy constructed. The colostomy would then be taken down and colorectal anastomosis performed in a second operation 2 to 6 months later. Some surgeons advocate colonic lavage performed on the operating table and resection with primary colorectal anastomosis to avoid a second operation.

Pericolic Abscess

Pericolic abscesses can be drained with a CT-guided percutaneous catheter if they are 4 cm or larger and readily accessible (Figure 8.35). The drainage procedure, done in conjunction with antibiotic therapy, resolves symptoms in most patients. The catheter is removed when drainage is 10 mL or less per day, and the patient is discharged to await definitive colectomy in about 6 weeks time. At any time during the treatment, if sepsis worsens or fails to resolve, an emergency Hartmann procedure is performed and the abscess is drained. During operation on patients like these, it may be wise to insert a ureteric catheter in place in the left or both ureters to aid in identification of the ureters and thus help prevent inadvertent injury.

Generalized Peritonitis

Generalized peritonitis is a complication that requires rapid resuscitation, institution of nasogastric and intravenous antibiotic therapy, and emergency laparotomy. The diseased segment with perforation is resected; the abdomen is washed with multiple liters of saline; the rectal stump is closed or, if long enough, brought out as a mucous fistula; and end-colostomy is constructed. During operation for severe diverticulitis complicated with pericolic abscess or perforation—where the pelvis is frozen and safe dissection of the diseased sigmoid is difficult—the descending colon should be divided just above the diseased bowel and end-colostomy and mucous fistula constructed. Closed-suction drainage of the pelvis is also instituted.

Treatment of colonic perforation is associated with a high incidence of intra-abdominal abscesses postoperatively. These patients require vigilant abdominal examination and CT scan if a septic picture develops. They are, of course, kept on broad-spectrum antibiotics postoperatively. Any intra-abdominal abscess that develops might be amenable to percutaneous drainage. Otherwise, surgical drainage will be necessary.

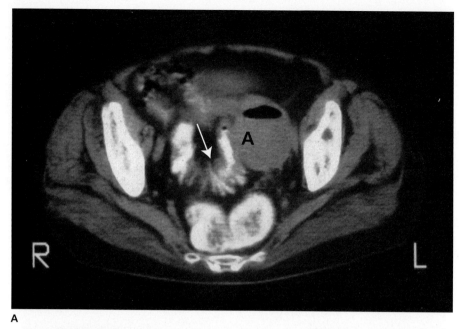

A

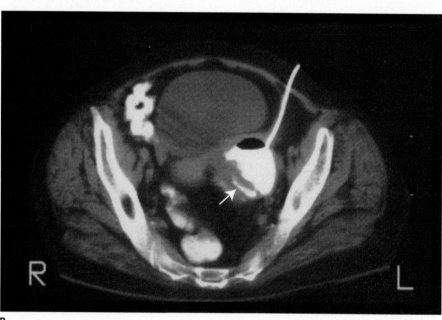

B

FIGURE 8.35. Drainage of pericolic abscess in diverticulitis. (A) The pelvic CT scan, performed with water-soluble contrast material in the rectum and sigmoid, demonstrates a 6–cm mass (letter A) with an air-fluid level adjacent to a thickened sigmoid segment (arrow). This mass represents an extramural pericolic abscess. (B) After a drainage catheter was placed percutaneously in the abscess cavity using CT guidance, contrast injected into the abscess demonstrated a connection with the sigmoid colon (arrow). (Courtesy of Henry I. Goldman, MD.)

Colovesical Fistula

Patients who develop colovesical fistula are treated with elective resection after mechanical and antibiotic bowel preparation. The colovesical fistula is taken down. Usually, the fistula is exceedingly small but may be large enough to require closure of the bladder with nonabsorbable sutures. Sigmoid resection with primary colorectal anastomosis is then performed.

CROHN'S DISEASE

Crohn's disease may present as a chronic disease or as an acute abdomen simulating acute appendicitis. The distinction between Crohn's disease and chronic ulcerative colitis is generally evident, based on the different manifestations and treatment responses of the two diseases (Table 8.10), but occasionally the distinction may be difficult.

TABLE 8.10. Comparison of Crohn's Disease and Chronic Ulcerative Colitis

	Crohn's disease	Chronic ulcerative colitis
Distribution	Small intestine in 90% Ileocolitis in 40%–60% Large bowel alone in 25%–30% Rectum infrequently involved	Small intestine involved only in backwash ileitis Rectum usually involved

Pathology	Transmural granulomatous
	  inflammation
	Extensive superficial ulceration
	Bowel wall and mesentery
	  thickened
	Pseudopolyps uncommon
		Inflammation limited to mucosa
		
		Longitudinal ulcers, transverse fissures
		No thickening of bowel wall or
		  mesentery
		Pseudopolyps common

Clinical features	Diarrhea less severe, less bloody Gross bleeding uncommon Bowel obstruction common Severe perianal disease common Toxic megacolon uncommon Fistula formation common Perforation rare	Severe diarrhea, usually bloody Gross bleeding characteristic Bowel obstruction rare Perianal disease uncommon Toxic megacolon more common Fistula formation rare Perforation common
Radiology	Skip areas Cobblestone mucosa Fistulas and strictures common	Continuous involvement Finely granular mucosa with ulcers Fistulas and strictures uncommon

Endoscopy	Rectal sparing common
	Cobblestone mucosa with
	  linear ulcers and skip lesions
		Rectum usually involved
		Erythematous mucosa with contact
		  bleeding and discreet ulcers

Treatment response	Less responsive to medical
	  treatment
	High recurrence rate after
	  surgical resection
		Good response to medical treatment
		  in 85%
		Cured by colectomy and mucosal
		  proctectomy

Malignancy	<10% after 20 years	20%–25% after 20 years

Acute Presentation

Acute ileitis may present as an acute abdomen, mimicking acute appendicitis in abdominal findings and leukocytosis. Some patients, however, have, in addition, anemia that is not usually seen in acute appendicitis.

Treatment

An emergent operation, usually through a right lower quadrant incision, is performed for presumed acute appendicitis. The appendix is normal, but the terminal ileum is grossly inflamed with thickening of the bowel wall and mesentery. Mesenteric lymph nodes may also be enlarged. The condition could be Crohn's disease or ileitis due to other causes, particularly *Yersinia enterocolitica*. About 15% of cases initially presumed to be due to *Yersinia* are determined to be chronic Crohn's disease.

Appendectomy should be performed to remove acute appendicitis as a possible diagnosis during future attacks. However, it may be unwise to perform appendectomy if granulomatous inflammation is present at the base of the appendix in the cecum because of the risk of postoperative fistula formation. Resection of the diseased ileum may be necessary if obstruction is present.

Chronic Crohn's Disease

Clinical Presentation

Onset of disease is usually insidious. Chronic diarrhea and abdominal pain are the presenting symptoms in 90% of cases. Patients may describe a course characterized by exacerbations and remissions. Diarrhea is frequent, with loose bowel movements occurring sometimes 10 to 15 times/day. The stool usually contains no blood unless Crohn's colitis is present. Fatigue, weight loss, malaise, and fever are frequent symptoms. Other presenting symptoms include fever of unknown origin, recurrent anorectal lesions, or iron-deficiency anemia. Patients may also present with obstruction, abdominal abscess, or occasionally, with one or more of the extra-intestinal manifestations described earlier.

Investigation

LABORATORY FINDINGS Anemia is a frequent finding, and leukocytosis is present if sepsis has developed. An elevated sedimentation rate is a feature of active disease. Hypoalbuminemia is common. Steatorrhea is present when the ileum is extensively involved. A number of malabsorption tests may be abnormal, including the D-xylose absorption test, and hydrogen and $^{14}CO_2$ breath tests. Both ^{111}indium and ^{99m}technitium have been used semiquantitatively to measure tracer activity in fecal leukocytes and to perform scintigraphy to establish disease location and extent.

RADIOLOGICAL STUDIES

Plain Films of the Abdomen Plain films often are negative or show nonspecific gas patterns within the small intestine unless an obstruction is present.

BARIUM CONTRAST STUDIES Barium studies often establish the diagnosis. Barium enema should be the initial examination because, not only will it detect the presence of Crohn's colitis, but it also provides the best image of the terminal ileum (Figure 8.36). Following barium enema, the small bowel should be investigated with barium swallow and small bowel follow-through or enterocylosis. Positive findings include edema of the mucosa; edema of the entire wall, which manifests as a separation between adjacent loops of bowel; and aphthous ulcers, which progress to create denuded areas that give the characteristic cobblestone appearance. A characteristic radiological finding is the string sign, due to thickening of the bowel wall and luminal narrowing (Figure 8.37). Signs of more advanced disease include strictures, fistulas, and abscesses. Also characteristic in Crohn's disease are skip lesions, where affected segments of bowel are separated by segments of normal bowel. When extramural complications are suspected, CT scan provides the most information.

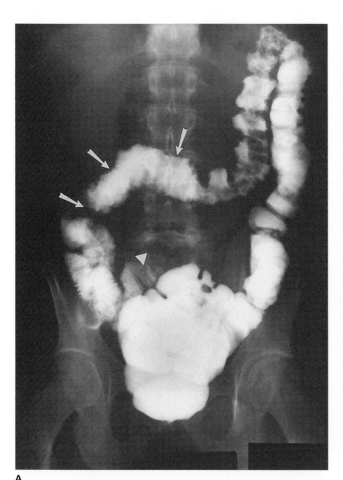

A

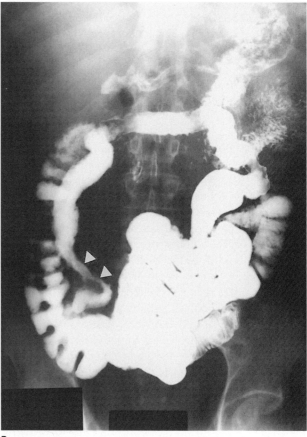

B

FIGURE 8.36. Diagnosis of chronic Crohn's colitis. (A) A barium enema in a patient with ileocolic Crohn's disease demonstrates a normal appearance of the rectosigmoic and extensive ulceration and nodularity of the transverse and ascending colon (arrows), typical of Crohn's disease. The terminal ileum appears normal (arrowhead). (B) The small bowel barium examination illustrates the presence of Crohn's disease in the terminal ileum (arrowheads), while the cecum in this patient appears normal. (Courtesy of Henry I. Goldman, MD.)

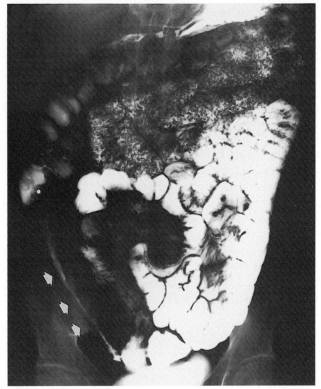

FIGURE 8.37. String sign in Crohn's colitis. This small bowel barium examination illustrates the string sign, due to extensive transmural ileal Crohn's disease (arrows). The ileum is extremely narrowed and widely separated from adjacent bowel segments because of both transmural thickening and reactive mesenteric fat. (Courtesy of Henry I. Goldman, MD.)

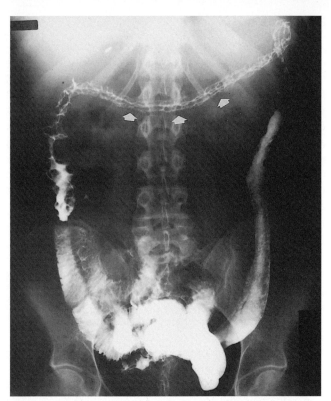

FIGURE 8.38. Cobblestoning in Crohn's disease. In Crohn's disease of the colon, the presence of linear and transverse ulcers characteristically produces a cobblestone pattern (arrows). In this patient, the pattern is manifest primarily in the transverse colon. (Courtesy of Henry I. Goldman, MD.)

Endoscopy Both colonoscopy and upper GI endoscopy may be necessary. Colonoscopy should attempt to examine the terminal ileum by intubation of the ileocecal valve. Pancolonoscopy is generally contraindicated during severe bouts of colitis for fear of precipitating toxic megacolon, a complication that is sometimes seen in CD but is more common in CUC. Colonoscopy should be preceded by careful evaluation of the perianal region. The presence of perianal fissures, fistulas, or abscess is most suggestive of CD. The rectum is relatively spared. Colonic involvement, if present, is segmental, with cobblestoning from intersections of longitudinal and transverse ulcers (Figure 8.38). The terminal ileum is involved in some 80% of cases of CD. Multiple biopsies of affected areas should be obtained, particularly areas of stenosis or stricture formation. The diagnostic role of capsule video endoscopy is now under evaluation.

Clinical Management

MEDICAL THERAPY

Nutritional Therapy CD is treated medically; surgery is reserved for complicated cases (see below). Nutritional therapy is important as a supplement to other medical therapy and to help induce growth in children. Both elemental diet and total parenteral nutrition are useful. Medical and surgical approaches are summarized in Table 8.11.

Aminosalicylates These include sulfasalazine and a growing number of 5-aminosalicylic acid (mesolamine) derivatives. Sulfasalazine has been shown by several controlled prospective trials to provide effective therapy, particularly in patients with Crohn's colitis and ileocolitis.

TABLE 8.11. Essentials: Treatment of Crohn's Disease
Medical
▪ Sulfasalazine
▪ Mesalamine (5-ASA) 500–1000 mg tid
▪ Corticosteroid 0.25–0.75 mg/kg
▪ Clarithromycin 250 mg bid
▪ Growth hormone
▪ 6-mercaptopurine 15 mg/wk
▪ Azathioprine
Surgical
▪ Ileal obstruction: right hemicolectomy
▪ Acute refractory disease: conservative resection
▪ Chronic stricutre: stricturoplasty

These drugs can be used orally or topically. A combination of oral and rectal administration may be required.

Steroids While steroids are the mainstay of acute therapy, they are associated with severe toxicity. Less toxic, newly developed drugs (e.g., budesonide) may prove useful. Steroids should be used at the lowest possible dose and for the shortest period necessary. Steroids block the production and effects of cytokines and other inflammatory mediators. The use of steroids, particularly in the presence of abdominal masses and fistulas, may mask abdominal signs of severe sepsis. Steroids may be administered orally or rectally.

Immunomodulatory Agents Four immunomodulatory drugs are in use: azathioprine (AZA), 6-mercaptopurine (6-MP), methotrexate (MTX), and cyclosporine. The beneficial effect of AZA and 6-MP is slow, developing in 3 to 4 months. Hence, these agents are useful only as maintenance therapy to reduce recurrence rates. MTX is particularly useful in patients who are refractory to AZA. Cyclosporine is the most controversial choice because it is associated with serious systemic toxicity (i.e., renal failure, upper GI bleeding, bowel infarction). Cyclosporine may be a useful drug to treat pyoderma gangrenosum.

Antibiotics Clarithromycin, ciprofloxacin, and metronidazole are currently used in inflammatory bowel disease therapy. Metronidazole has been shown to prolong postresection remission.

INDICATIONS FOR SURGICAL THERAPY Surgery is reserved for complications of Crohn's disease or for failure of medical treatment. Possible complications of CD include: acute abdomen due to acute ileitis, obstruction, fistula, perforation, hemorrhage, growth retardation, ureteral obstruction, or anorectal disease. Acute abdomen due to acute ileitis was discussed earlier (see Acute Presentation, under Crohn's Disease, earlier in this chapter).

Obstruction Intestinal obstruction is the most common indication for surgery in CD. The indication for operation may be complete obstruction or, more frequently, nonresolving incomplete obstruction. The guiding principle of surgical treatment in bowel obstruction due to CD is to conserve as much intestine as possible. There is no advantage to extending resection beyond macroscopic disease. The practice of performing frozen sections to determine microscopically free margins has been abandoned. Any segment of normal intestine measuring 10 cm or longer between skip lesions should be preserved. Narrowings due to burnt-out Crohn's can be treated with stricturoplasty. This procedure is used primarily in patients with multiple short fibrotic strictures, particularly those vulnerable to short bowel syndrome. Strictures as long as 15 to 20 cm can be treated with stricturoplasty. Operated

sites should be biopsied to exclude lymphoma or carcinoma.

Fistula Enteroenteral fistulas that are asymptomatic require no surgical correction. Often, however, fistulas are either associated with sepsis or involve other organs (e.g., bladder, vagina, uterus). Sometimes enterocutaneous fistulas may develop and cause severe abdominal wall excoriation. Surgical management of fistulas requires excision of the bowel from which the fistula arises and drainage of any associated abscess.

Perforation Perforation is a rare complication of CD and requires emergency operation, appropriate resection, and drainage.

Hemorrhage Massive, life-threatening hemorrhage is a rare but important complication of CD, especially Crohn's colitis. Selective angiography is useful to localize areas of bleeding. Operative treatment requires resection of the involved segment of bowel.

Growth Retardation Approximately 25% of children with CD have growth retardation. If aggressive medical and nutritional therapy fails to reverse growth retardation, resection of the diseased bowel is indicated.

Ureteral Obstruction The ureter may become obstructed either because of a retroperitoneal abscess or retroperitoneal fibrosis. The treatment for abscess is drainage with or without bowel resection. In the case of fibrosis, extensive ureterolysis may be necessary.

Anorectal Disease Perineal abscesses and fistulas are treated with conservative surgery without performing large excisions.

FAILURE OF MEDICAL THERAPY Failure to achieve remission in severe CD involving the small or large bowel is an indication for surgery, particularly when patients cannot tolerate medication or develop complications from drug therapy. Severe perianal disease that recurs frequently or fails to respond to local surgery is an indication for surgery. While bowel conservation is a top priority in small intestinal resection, the same is not true for colonic resection. Stricturoplasty, for example, is not indicated in colonic stricture. Pancolonic disease requires total proctocolectomy with Brook's ileostomy. Continent ileostomy, either the Kock's type or pelvic, is contraindicated.

PROGNOSIS It is estimated that 70% of patients with CD require surgical treatment. Postresection recurrence rates are high and endoscopically 70% recur within 1 year. If defined by the need for reoperation, however, some 25% to 30% have recurrent disease within 5 years, and 40% to 45% develop recurrent disease within 20 years.[25] Neither medical nor surgical therapy can cure CD. A partnership between patient, physician, gastroenterologist, and surgeon is required to provide optimum care.

CHRONIC ULCERATIVE COLITIS

Clinical Presentation

The predominant clinical picture in a patient with chronic ulcerative colitis (CUC) is one of rectal bleeding and diarrhea. The stools are watery, containing blood, mucous, and pus, and may be frequent. Tenesmus and rectal urgency are frequent symptoms. Most patients complain of abdominal pain. The onset may be either mild, characterized by bloody diarrhea, or fulminant with fever, abdominal pain, and tenderness. Abdominal examination in severe cases shows tenderness with or without rebound tenderness. Rectal examination may show superficial anal fissures from severe diarrhea, and blood may be present on the examining finger. Sigmoidoscopy should be performed as part of the physical examination. The rectal mucosa is usually erythematous and bleeds on contact; in severe cases, it has been aptly described as "bleeding velvet." Paradoxically, rectal ulcers are not frequently seen in CUC, whereas rectal involvement in Crohn's disease is often associated with longitudinal ulcers in the rectal mucosa.

Investigations

Laboratory Findings

Anemia, leukocytosis, and elevated sedimentation rates are usually present. In fulminant disease, severe leukocytosis, and bandemia are present. Severe diarrhea may lead to hypokalemia, hypoproteinemia, and significant contraction of the extracellular fluid volume. Stool studies may be necessary to exclude salmonellosis and shigellosis. *Campylobacter* and *C. difficile* infections must also be excluded.

Colonoscopy

If sigmoidoscopy suggests the presence of CUC, colonoscopy will be needed to show the extent of colon involvement, the presence of pseudopolypi (Figure 8.39), and to facilitate biopsy. Following colonoscopy, barium enema may or may not be necessary to obtain additional information. Colonoscopy must be performed with great care in severe disease because of the danger of perforation. Colonoscopy should not be performed in the presence of toxic megacolon or toxic colitis.

Radiology

PLAIN FILMS In patients with severe disease, plain films of the abdomen may show edematous, thickened

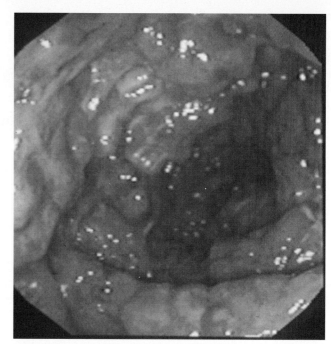

FIGURE 8.39. Colonoscopy in a patient with chronic ulcerative colitis shows extensive polyposis. (Courtesy of John Cello, MD.)

colon with irregular interface between luminal gas and the edematous mucosa. Dilatation of the colon and small bowel may be present.

BARIUM ENEMA Barium enema should be performed carefully to avoid overinflation and should be avoided if toxic colitis or toxic megacolon is present. The mucosa is granular, thickened, with superficial ulcers. Haustral folds are lost, and the colon is foreshortened if disease has been longstanding. Pseudopolyps may be present (Figure 8.40).

SPIRAL CT Spiral CT with 3-D reconstruction may be useful when barium enema is too risky to perform.

Clinical Management

CUC is treated medically, with surgery reserved for medical failure or complications.

Medical Therapy

The medical therapy for CUC is the same as that described above for Crohn's disease. When only the rectum is involved, steroid retention enemas are used first in combination with oral preparation of 5-ASA. Systemic corticosteroid therapy is reserved for cases in which local therapy fails. Disease beyond the rectum is treated with oral prednisone in mild cases or intravenous prednisone in severe cases. Once remission is achieved, maintenance therapy is usually instituted, using 5-ASA preparations (e.g., mesalazine, olsalazine).

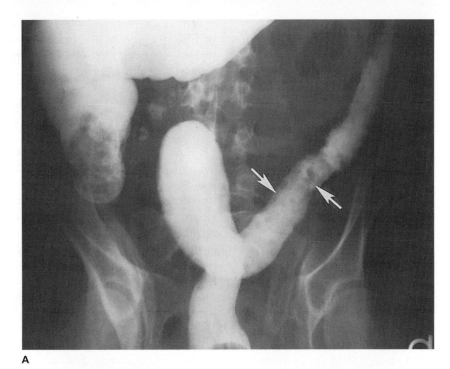

FIGURE 8.40. Manifestations of CUC. (A) Pseudopolyps (arrows) produce multiple filling defects in this barium-filled descending colon. These are seen in chronic ulcerative colitis in the acute phase and as part of the healing spectrum. (B) The entire colon is foreshortened and has lost its normal haustral pattern, a condition known as "lead pipe colon," due to long-standing chronic ulcerative colitis. (Courtesy of Henry I. Goldman, MD.)

TABLE 8.12. Chronic Ulcerative Colitis: Indications for Surgery

Emergent
- Perforation
- Hemorrhage (6–8 U of blood/24 h)
- Toxic colitis that is nonresponsive to 72–84 h of maximal medical therapy
- Toxic megacolon that is nonresponsive to 24–48 h of maximal medical therapy

Elective
- Failure of or intolerance to medical therapy
- Dysplasia
- Carcinoma

Surveillance for Cancer

Colonoscopic surveillence for cancer is recommended after 7 years of pancolitis or 10 years of left-sided colitis. Colonoscopy and multiple random biopsies, as well as biopsies of any suspicious lesions are performed every 1 to 2 years. If dysplasia is found, colonoscopy and biopsy are repeated in 2 months. If dysplasia persists, colectomy is recommended.

Surgical Treatment

The indications for surgery are complications and failure of medical therapy (Table 8.12).

PREOPERATIVE MANAGEMENT Preoperative management requires correction of any fluid deficit, hypokalemia, and anemia. Preoperative total parenteral nutrition is indicated in elective settings where the patient has evidence of malnutrition. Because most patients have been on steroids, a perioperative steroid regimen is administered, with 100 mg of cortisol intramuscularly or intravenously just before the operation, followed by 50 to 100 mg every 6 h during surgery. Postoperatively, the steroid dose can be decreased by half each day from postoperative day 1 until maintenance doses are reached. Thereafter, a steroid tapering program is started until the patient is completely off the drug. Preoperatively, intraoperatively and postoperatively, careful monitoring of the volume status, serum potassium, and blood pressure should be performed.

OPERATIVE MANAGEMENT Elective surgery is indicated when the patient's condition is refractory to treatment, when severe extraintestinal manifestations develop, or when risk for cancer is identified. The current operation of choice is total colectomy, mucosal protectomy, and ileo-anal anastomosis using a reservoir ileal pouch (Figure 8.41). The preferred pouch is a 30-cm duplicated J (15 cm per limb). Other pouch constrictions are the Sand W-types. The operation removes all mucosa susceptible to CUC and cancer development, avoids permanent ileostomy, and maintains anal continence. Successful outcome can be expected in at least 95% of patients.

Other alternatives—including total procolocolectomy with continent (Kock) ileostomy or abdominal colectomy with ileoproctostomy—are less appealing. The latter, of course, does not eliminate the risk of cancer in the rectal mucosa.

Emergency surgery may be indicated for toxic colitis, toxic megacolon, perforation, or hemorrhage.

Toxic Colitis Toxic colitis, or fulminant colitis, affects 5% to 15% of patients with CUC. Toxic colitis may represent the initial presentation of disease in approximately one-third of patients with CUC. It carries a mortality rate of 8% to 10%, which rises more than 25% if the colitis is accompanied by perforation.[26] Clinical features include fever, abdominal pain and tenderness with signs of peritonitis, absent bowel sounds, distension, and leukocytosis with bandemia. Steroid therapy inhibits the full clinical expression of peritonitis, and this fact must always be borne in mind. Other causes of acute colitis should be excluded, especially *Clostridium difficile* enterocolitis. Plain films of the abdomen show ileus of the small intestine but no megacolon. Free peritoneal fluid may be present. The presence of free air, of course, indicates that perforation has occurred, In which case barium enema and colonoscopy must be avoided.

This complication, like toxic megacolon, is best managed by a team approach between the surgeon and gastroenterologist. A decision is made how to administer

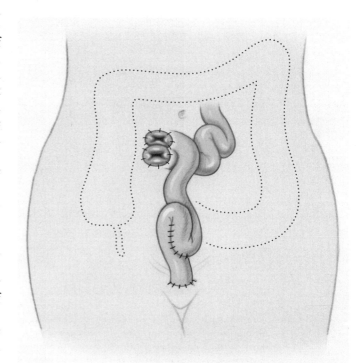

FIGURE 8.41. Elective surgery for ulcerative colitis includes total colectomy with mucosal protectomy and ileo-anal anastomosis using an ileal pouch and protective divided ileostomy. (Adapted from Schwartz SI, ed: Principles of Surgery, 6th ed. New York: McGraw Hill, 1994:1247.)

maximum medical therapy, to follow the patient with frequent abdominal examinations, and to operate if no improvement is seen in 48 to 72 h. Treatment consists of:

1. Nasogastric suction.
2. Fluid administration monitored by urine output and central venous pressure or pulmonary artery pressure measurements.
3. Maximum doses of intravenous steroids (hydrocortisone 100 to 300 mg/24 h, or, if the patient does not respond to steroids, ACTH by intravenous drip at 120 U/24 h).
4. Intravenous antibiotics, usually triple antibiotics consisting of ampicillin, aminoglycoside, and metronidazole.

On this regimen, approximately 60% to 75% of patients improve. The 25% to 40% who do not improve require an emergency proctocolectomy with concurrent or subsequent mucosal protectomy and ileo-anal anastomosis with pelvic reservoir. A temporary diverting loop ileostomy is often necessary. If perforation has occurred, the procedure must be staged by first performing total abdominal colectomy (Figure 8.42), followed by the pelvic operation several weeks later.

Toxic Megacolon This complication consists of fulminant colitis associated with persistent dilatation of the

TABLE 8.13. Essentials: Toxic Megacolon in Chronic Ulcerative Colitis

Incidence: 5%

Precipitating factors
- Hypokalemia
- Opiates or anticholinergics
- Barium enema, colonoscopy

Clinical picture
- Frequent bloody diarrhea
- Fever, tachycardia
- Abdominal distention
- Abdominal tenderness (may be masked by steroid therapy)

X-ray findings
- Dilated transverse colon (>6 cm)
- Ileus

Management
- Initial conservative treatment
  - ➤ Nasogastric tube
  - ➤ Intravenous fluids
  - ➤ Intravenous steroids (hydrocortisone 100 mg q 6 h)
  - ➤ Broad-spectrum antibiotics
- If no improvement in 24–48 h, total abdominal colectomy with ileostomy
- Definitive treatment is delayed mucosal proctectomy, ileo-anal anastomosis with ileal pouch

Prognosis
- 50% respond to medical therapy; 50% of these will ultimately require surgery
- Postoperative mortality rate of 10%–15%

colon. The essentials are summarized in Table 8.13. Colonic dilatation is assessed by measuring the diameter of the transverse colon in a supine abdominal x-ray film (Figure 8.43). Transverse colon diameter in excess of 6 cm represents dilatation. On the same film, the size of the cecum should also be noticed. The clinical picture and management is the same as for toxic colitis, except that there is more urgency in toxic megacolon because of potential complications. Thus, if the patient fails to improve clinically, and dilatation does not subside within 24 to 48 h, emergency operation is indicated. The principles of operative management are similar to those for toxic colitis.

Factors that precipitate toxic megacolon include the use of opiates or anticholinergic drugs, hypokalemia, and recent colonoscopy or barium enema.

Perforation Perforation is a dreaded and potentially lethal complication of CUC. It can complicate both toxic colitis and toxic megacolon. The incidence of perforation in toxic megacolon has been reported to be as high as 33%.[27] Physical findings may be masked by steroid therapy, but free peritoneal air is present on plain abdominal films. Immediate abdominal colectomy and Brook's ileostomy are indicated. Rectal mucosectomy, construction of a pelvic pouch, and ileo-anal anastomosis are postponed to a second operation weeks or months after colectomy.

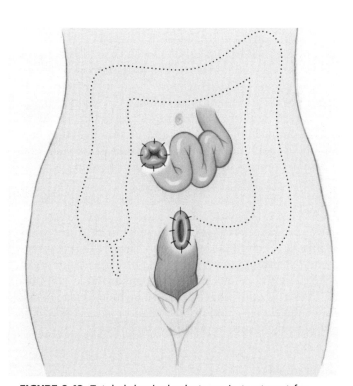

FIGURE 8.42. Total abdominal colectomy. In treatment for emergent complications of ulcerative colitis, a total abdominal colectomy with ileostomy is performed and the divided rectum is brought out as a stoma. (Adapted from Schwartz SI, ed: Principles of Surgery, 6th ed. New York: McGraw Hill, 1994:1247.)

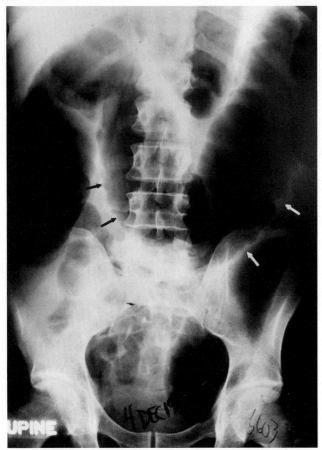

FIGURE 8.43. Colonic dilatation in toxic megacolon. This supine abdominal x-ray, taken because the patient had abdominal pain and distention and known acute ulcerative colitis, shows a greatly dilated colon. The colon contour lacks the usual haustral pattern and, in the transverse colon (arrows), an irregular contour is present, suggesting ulceration. This patient had systemic signs and symptoms as well as laboratory values consistent with the term toxic megacolon. (Courtesy of Henry I. Goldberg, MD.)

Hemorrhage Massive hemorrhage is an indication for surgery in fewer than 5% of cases. Hemorrhage requiring 6 to 8 U of blood transfusion per 24 h should be treated with emergency colectomy or proctocolectomy.

OTHER INFLAMMATORY DISEASES OF THE SMALL AND LARGE BOWEL

Specific infections of the small and large intestine are very common in developing countries but less so in North America and Europe. They must be differentiated from Crohn's disease or chronic ulcerative colitis. Causes include bacteria, viruses, parasitic infestations, or fungal infections.

Bacterial Enterocolitis

Bacteria may infect either the small bowel, the colon, or both.

Yersenia Enteritis

The pathogen *Yersenia enterocolitica* typically causes terminal ileitis and mesenteric adenitis that simulate acute appendicitis. But it can also cause gastroenteritis and colitis and even liver and spleen abscesses. Diagnosis can be made by culturing the pathogen from stool and/or by measuring blood antibody titer, which rises and falls with the course of the disease. Effective antibiotic therapy is provided by trimethoprim-sulfamethoxazole or doxycycline.

Campylobacter Enteritis

The pathogen is *Campylobacter jejuni.* This common infection is transmitted by contaminated water, milk, or undercooked poultry. The usual picture is similar to that of viral gastroenteritis, although severe enterocolitis with bloody diarrhea—resembling CD or CUC—can develop. Diagnosis is made by microscopic (darkfield or phase-contrast) examination of stool, or by culturing the Gram-negative rod from stool or blood. The treatment of choice is oral erythromycin.

Typhoid

Typhoid, caused by *Salmonella typhi,* is endemic in regions with poor public health services. The disease is an acute systemic infection with high fever. In the GI tract, the infection concentrates on Peyer's patches, causing severe enteritis and colitis with ulcerations. Gross hemorrhage or perforation can occur. Diagnosis is established by demonstrating high titer of agglutinins for the O and H antigens in samples of blood or feces. The drug therapy of choice is chloramphenicol or trimethoprim-sulfamethoxazole (TMP-SMX). Parenteral amoxicillin is a second choice. Perforation requires immediate surgery, but in severe disease limited to the ileum and cecum that does not rapidly respond to antibiotic therapy, early operation before perforation develops may prove lifesaving.

Shigella

Shigella organisms cause bacillary dysentery. Four groups of shigella are the major pathogens. They include *S. dysenteriae, S. flexneri, S. boydii,* and *S. sonnei.* The major organ affected is the colon. The stool contain large amounts of PNMs and blood. Treatment includes rehydration, ampicillin therapy, and avoidance of opiates. Ampicillin-resistant organisms are treated with TMP-SMX.

Tuberculosis

Primary tuberculosis of the intestine is rare and is caused by *Mycobacterium tuberculosis.* The cecum and terminal ileum are most commonly involved, but the ascending colon, jejunum, duodenum, stomach, esophagus, and sigmoid colon may also be involved. Complications include hemorrhage, perforation, fistula formation, and malabsorption. If an operation is carried out, the findings are similar to those in CD, and resection should be conservative. The mainstay of therapy is, of course, the use of antituberculosis drugs.

Clostridium Difficile Enterocolitis

Clostridium difficile elaborates a toxin that causes pseudomembranous enterocolitis. The most common precipitating cause is antibiotic therapy, particularly with oral clindamycin, ampicillin, cephalosporins, and several others. Antibiotic therapy leads to unopposed proliferation of *C. difficile* and invasion of the colonic mucosa. The clinical findings are severe watery diarrhea (15–30 stools per day), associated with abdominal pain and high fever. Sigmoidoscopy shows a confluent pseudomembrane covering an erythematous and swollen mucosa. Diagnosis is further established by showing *C. difficile* cytotoxin in the stool and culturing the organism from stool. Occasionally, pseudomembranous colitis may cause toxic megacolon or perforation, requiring colectomy.

Viral Diseases

Several viruses cause gastroenteritis, which is rarely of surgical interest. Rotavirus, Norwalk virus, enteric adenovirus, and others are involved.

Parasitic Infestations

Intestinal Amebiasis

The pathogen *Entamoeba histolytica*, transmitted by oral-fecal contact, can cause three forms of disease: amebic dysentery, amebic colitis, and intestinal ameboma. Amebic colitis may be severe; it causes severe bloody and mucousy diarrhea, abdominal pain, high fever, toxicity, and high leukocytosis. Sigmoidoscopy shows typical amebic ulcers, which are small with white caps. Ameba may be recovered from their exudate. Colonic dilatation may develop, resulting in a picture similar to that of toxic megacolon in CUC. The distinction is critical, however, because steroid therapy for amebic colitis leads to perforation. Amebic colitis is treated with metronidazole and tetracycline. Other antiamebic drugs include paromomycin (Humatin®), dehydroemetin, and iodoquinol. Very rarely colectomy may be necessary. Intestinal ameboma may rarely cause intestinal obstruction requiring resection.

Fungal Infection

Actinomycosis

The infection is due to *actinomycetes*, Gram-positive, nonacid-fast filamentous organisms. Typically, the ileum, cecum, and ascending colon are involved. Multiple sinuses may form within the abdomen and into the skin. The characteristic and diagnostic finding is the presence of sulfur granules in the discharging pus. The disease is treated with high doses of penicillin. Right hemicolectomy may be necessary to remove the diseased bowel for cure.

Nocardiosis

The pathogen is *Nocardiae*, Gram-positive branching filamentous organisms. Abdominal nocardiosis resembles actinomycosis and is characterized by abscess, granuloma, and sinus formation. The treatment of choice is sulfonamides. Surgical intervention may be necessary to drain abscesses and excise fistulas.

NEOPLASMS OF THE SMALL INTESTINE

Neoplasms of the small intestine comprise about 3% of all gastrointestinal tumors. They tend to be associated with neoplasms elsewhere. Benign lesions are the most common, but they are rarely symptomatic unless they cause intussusception or bleeding. Lymphomas and adenocarcinomas are the most common tumors. In general, lymphomas are more common distally and their incidence declines more proximally in the small intestine. Adenocarcinomas have the opposite distribution.

Benign Neoplasms

Solitary Polyps

Both villous and adenomatous polyps occur but very rarely. The most common site is the duodenum. Large periampullary villous adenomas nearly always have a malignant component, which is often difficult to detect on biopsy. Solitary polyps are asymptomatic unless they cause intussusception or bleeding. They are then treated by limited resection.

Leiomyomas

These benign tumors are usually asymptomatic. Bleeding is rare unless malignant degeneration is present.

Multiple Polyps

Peutz–Jeghers Syndrome An inherited disorder of multiple polyposis, Peutz–Jeghers syndrome is associated with skin pigmentation. Patients often have café-au-lait pigmentation in the circumoral area and in the buccal mucosa. The lesions rarely become malignant, but they can cause bleeding or obstruction when they are treated with resection.

MULTIPLE HAMARTOMATOUS POLYPS These polyps are usually asymptomatic.

FAMILIAL ADENOMATOUS POLYPOSIS These polyps occur as part of Gardner's syndrome (see section on familial adenomatous polyps of the colon).

JUVENILE POLYPS Also known as retention polyps, juvenile polyps are benign and are probably hamartomas. They may cause bleeding or intussusception in childhood.

Malignant Tumors

Primary Tumors

LYMPHOMA Primary lymphoma is probably the most common malignant lesion of the small intestine. It is most common in the ileum but may occur in the jejunum in association with celiac disease. These tumors present clinically with colicky abdominal pain, anorexia, weight loss, and sometimes anemia. They may also present with small bowel obstruction and intussusception. Rarely, lymphomas may cause perforation. Treatment includes limited small bowel resection followed by whole abdominal radiation and/or chemotherapy.

Several histologic subtypes of lymphoma exist, including:

1. Diffuse large- or small-cell lymphoma.
2. Immunoproliferative intestinal disease (IPSID lymphoma).
3. Mucosa-associated lymphoid tumors (MALT).
4. Multiple lymphoid polyposis.
5. Enteropathy-associated T cell lymphoma.

ADENOCARCINOMA Adenocarcinoma is more common in the jejunum. It remains asymptomatic for a long period and, by the time surgery is performed, the tumor is invasive and 80% has metastasized (Figure 8.44). Treatment is resection of the involved bowel and its mesentery. The 5-year survival rate is 15% to 35%.[28] Adenocarcinoma may occur in the bypassed segment of bowel when bypass is used to treat Crohn's disease.

CARCINOID TUMOR See Chapter 5 for a full discussion of carcinoid tumors of the small intestine. A characteristic small intestinal carcinoid tumor is shown in Figure 8.45.

LEIOMYOSARCOMA Leiomyosarcoma can occur anywhere in the small intestine and tends to cause bleeding from central ulceration of the mucosa overlying it. Less commonly, leiomyosarcoma may cause obstruction. The major mode of spread is hematogenous. Treatment is segmental resection. Recently, imatinib mesylate has been shown to be effective in the treatment of stromal tumors of the gastrointestinal tract.[29] Other types of sarcoma can also occur. In HIV/AIDS, Kaposi sarcoma may develop in the small intestine.

Metastatic Disease

The most common metastatic tumor in the small intestine is malignant melanoma. Approximately 50% of patients dying from melanoma have secondary tumors in the submucosa of the small intestine. Other neoplasms that may metastasize to the small intestine include breast, lung, kidney, and cervix. Useful palliation can be achieved by resection if bleeding or obstruction occurs.

COLORECTAL CANCER

Colon cancer has a doubling time of 130 days and may remain asymptomatic for 5 to 10 years. When it becomes symptomatic, the clinical picture varies depending on whether the tumor is located in the right colon, the left colon, or the rectum. Colon cancer may be of the polypoid, ulcerating, or napkin-ring type (Figure 8.46).

Clinical Presentation

Carcinoma of the Right Colon

Because of the large caliber of the right colon and the fluid nature of the intestinal contents, carcinoma of the right colon does not frequently produce obstruction, and the tumor can become large in size. The clinical presentation may include:

1. Iron-deficiency anemia causing fatigue and weakness.
2. Right-sided abdominal pain.
3. Abdominal mass discovered by the patient or by the physician in routine physical examination.
4. Obstruction of the ileocecal valve causing low small bowel obstruction.
5. Obstruction of the base of the appendix causing acute appendicitis (rare presentation).

When a patient over 40 years of age, particularly a man, presents with unexplained iron-deficiency anemia, carcinoma of the right colon must be excluded. Bleeding is usually occult, but when it is gross, the stools become melanotic, and the patient may not suspect bleeding. Occasionally, patients present with advanced disease including liver metastasis and ascites.

Carcinoma of the Left Colon

Because the left colon has a smaller diameter, the stools in it are more solid, and the lesion is more distal, carcinoma of the left colon causes symptoms earlier than cancer of the right colon. The clinical presentation may include the following symptoms:

1. A change in bowel habits develops, usually constipation.

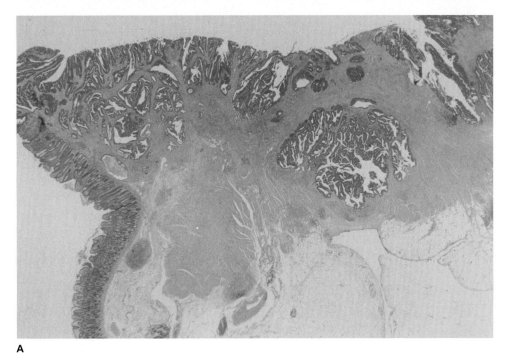

A

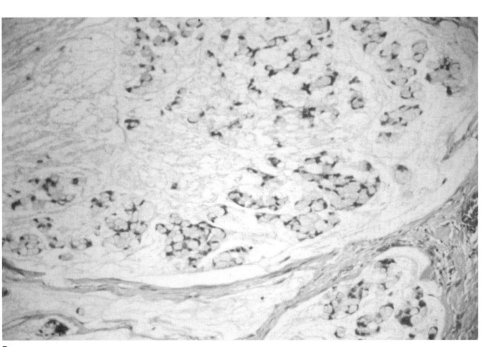

B

FIGURE 8.44. (A) Adenocarcinoma of the colon with invasion of the muscularis propria. (B) Some colon cancers are mucin-producing, in which case the prognosis is worse. (Courtesy of Linda D. Ferrell, MD.)

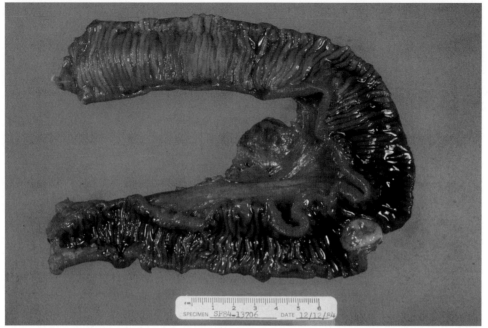

A

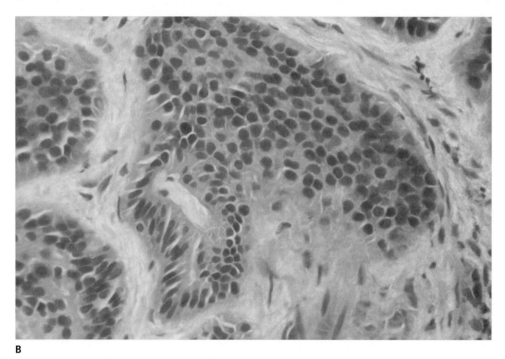

B

FIGURE 8.45. (A) Carcinoid tumor of the small intestine causes a characteristic knuckling, due to fibrosis. (B) Carcinoid tumors are formed from nests of uniform cells with small round nuclei. (Courtesy of Linda D. Ferrell, MD.)

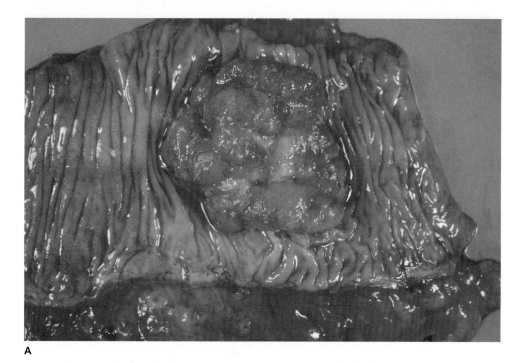

A

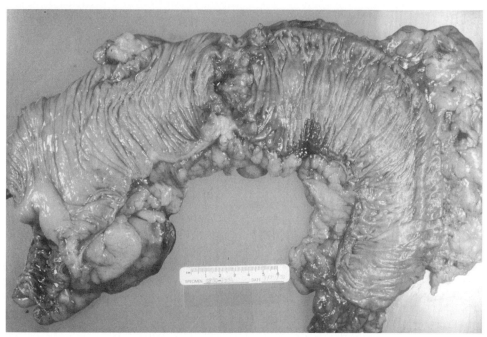

B

FIGURE 8.46. Differing patterns of growth in colon cancer. Colectomy specimens demonstrate (A) polypoid carcinoma, more commonly found in the right colon; and (B) napkin-ring carcinoma, more commonly found in the left colon. (Courtesy of Linda D. Ferrell, MD.)

2. Rectal bleeding usually presents as blood mixed with or streaking the stool, which often also contains mucous. More severe bleeding is possible, but profuse bleeding is rare.
3. Left colon obstruction causes partial obstructive symptoms (i.e., suprapubic colicky pain and constipation) before complete obstruction develops.

Carcinoma of the Rectum

Presenting symptoms and signs include the following:

1. Rectal bleeding is the most significant symptom.
2. Red blood is passed with stools (hematochezia) and, at times, bleeding may be severe.
3. A rectal mass is found on digital examination, with or without blood on the examining finger.
4. Rectal examination can determine the size and fixation of the tumor.

Investigations

Laboratory Studies

Anemia is a very frequent finding. Liver function tests should be obtained. Elevated alkaline phosphatase might suggest the presence of hepatic metastasis. Carcinoembryonic antigen (CEA), a glycoprotein expressed in the embryo and in cell membranes of many adult tissues, is elevated in approximately 70% of patients, particularly those with Duke C or D lesions. CEA levels not only provide diagnostic guidance but serve to determine whether all tumor has been extirpated by colonic resection. If CEA levels return to normal postoperatively after complete resection, an elevation of these levels during follow-up usually indicates a recurrence of tumor. Measurement of susceptibility genes and telomerase activity in biopsy specimens and other genetic markers hold promise for earlier and improved diagnosis and treatments in the future.

Radiologic Studies

Barium enema is the best radiological technique to diagnose colon cancer. Cancers in the right colon appear as intraluminal masses, while those in the descending colon typically show as apple core lesions due to annular tumor growth. All diagnosed or suspected lesions require colonoscopic examination and biopsy. Chest x-ray should always be obtained. CT scan or MRI are useful, not only in detecting liver metastasis, but also in evaluating extramural extension of tumor and pericolonic lymph node involvement.

Endoscopy

Flexible sigmoidoscopy and biopsy are often the initial steps. Endoscopic evaluation of the entire colon requires colonoscopy in every patient. When a distal lesion is seen on sigmoidoscopy, colonoscopy evaluates for synchronous lesions. Fully 60% to 70% of colon cancers are beyond the reach of sigmoidoscopy. Colonoscopy and barium enema complement one another in examination of the entire colon.

Endorectal Ultrasonography

This examination is an accurate way to determine depth of tumor invasion and presence of enlarged pararectal lymph nodes. In both evaluations, endorectal ultrasound is more accurate than CT scan.

Surgical Treatment

Surgery provides the only definitive treatment for colorectal cancer. Colectomy is usually contraindicated in patients with advanced tumor who have bilobar multiple metastases and peritoneal seeding. Even in these patients, however, it may be best to perform surgical decompression of the colon to treat obstruction and palliative colectomy to control hemorrhage. The type of curative surgical resection required depends on tumor location. An attempt must be made to minimize intraoperative spread by:

1. Ligating the tumor-bearing bowel at both ends to prevent transluminal spread.
2. Ligating the mesenteric vein early to minimize hematogenous spread during manipulation.
3. Limiting the amount of manipulation of the tumor.

Preoperative Bowel Preparation

Mechanical and bacteriologic preoperative bowel preparation reduces the incidence of anastomotic dehiscence, intra-abdominal abscesses, and wound infection. Even after the recommended bacteriological preparation, the colon is not sterilized, and elective colectomy is considered a clean-contaminated operation. Mechanical cleansing is achieved either by mono and dibasic sodium phosphate purgatives or, more commonly, by whole-gut lavage using 4L of isotonic solution containing polyethylene glycol (Golytely®). The solution can be taken orally or instilled by nasogastric tube over a period of 4h. Bacteriologic preparation may be accomplished by using a combination of poorly absorbed oral antibiotics, typically 1g of neomycin and 1g of erythromycin given in three doses the preceding day, at 19, 18, and 9h prior to operation. Intravenous, broad-spectrum antibiotic is administered just before the procedure.

Operative Treatment

Figure 8.47 depicts the various types of resections required for tumors at different locations.

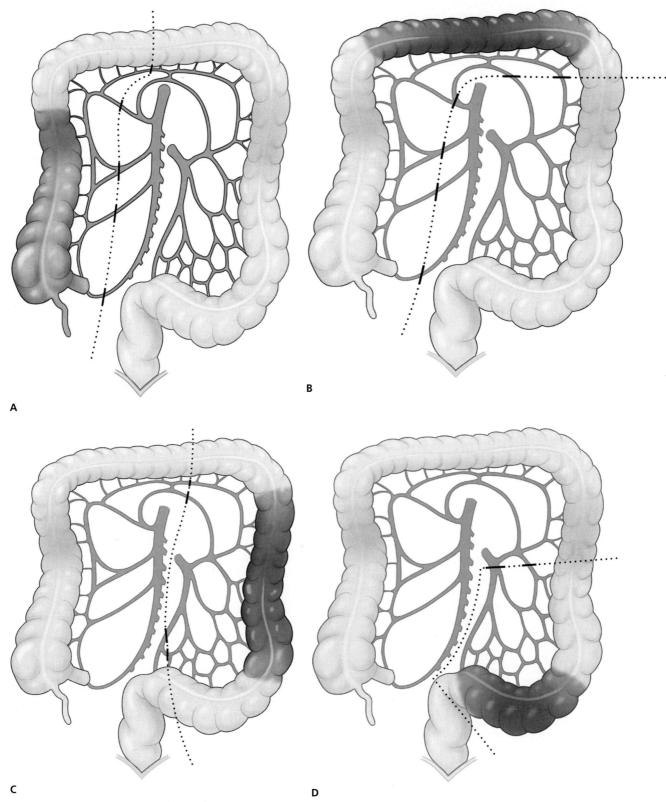

FIGURE 8.47. (A–D) Extent of colon resection depends on the location of the primary carcinoma.

CARCINOMA OF THE RIGHT COLON Cecal cancer is treated by right hemicolectomy and ileotransverse colectomy. Resection lines are 6 to 8 inches proximal or distal to the ileocecal valve and the hepatic flexure of the colon, respectively. This requires division of both the ileocolic and right colic arteries and resection of the mesentery to the origin of these vessels.

Carcinoma of the ascending colon requires extending the resection distally to the left of the midtransverse colon and sacrificing the right branch of the middle colic.

Transverse colon cancer is treated by transverse colectomy and colocolic anastomosis in which the entire middle colic is sacrificed. In some cases, it may be technically preferable to remove the entire right colon and perform ileodescending colostomy.

CARCINOMA OF THE LEFT COLON Carcinoma of the splenic flexure is treated by resection of most of the descending colon and the left half of the transverse colon and their mesentery. Descending colon carcinoma requires resection of most of the sigmoid, the entire ascending colon and splenic flexure. Sigmoid carcinoma requires removal of the upper rectum, the sigmoid, and half of the descending colon. The splenic flexure has to be mobilized completely so that colorectal anastomosis can be performed without tension.

CARCINOMA OF THE RECTUM The advent of intraluminal surgical stapling instruments has allowed the performance of lower and safer anastomosis deep in the pelvis after rectal resection. Low anterior resection of the rectum requires: (1) adequate blood supply and absence of tension at the anastomosis, and (2) preservation of adequate anal sphincter function. Resection of the rectum for cancer requires division of the inferior mesenteric artery at its origin and removal of the mesorectum and most of the pararectal tissue. Resection margins should be at least 10 cm proximally and 2 cm distally. Low anastomoses are often protected with temporary diverting loop ileostomy.

When a sphincter-saving resection is not feasible, the treatment of choice is abdominoperineal resection of the rectum (Mile's procedure). In this operation, the rectum is mobilized through the abdomen and perineum and the entire rectum and anus are removed. An end-sigmoid colostomy is then constructed in the left lower quadrant of the abdomen.

Colostomy and ileostomy sites should be marked preoperatively with ink. This practice is an important consideration in the surgical management of rectal cancer.

SURGICAL RESECTION OF LOW-LYING RECTAL CANCER The definitive surgical treatment of low-lying rectal cancer is abdominoperineal resection (Mile's procedure). If the anal sphincter can be preserved without compromising surgical cure, however, more limited resection is desirable. Sometimes this can be accomplished by performing a low anterior resection if a distal surgical margin of 2 to 3 cm can be achieved. Such anastomoses are usually covered with temporary diverting ileostomy.

Low-lying rectal cancer can also be locally resected either transacrally (Kraske procedure) or transanally.

Sacral Resection Sacral resection, or the Kraske procedure, is rarely performed today. Using the sacral approach, the rectum containing the lesion can be resected and intestinal continuity restored by anastomosis. The procedure is associated with a high rate of anastomotic leakage and recurrence and has now been supplanted by transanal excision.

Transanal Excision Lesions less than 4 cm in size, located within 8 cm of the anal verge, and unassociated with lymph node metastases may be treated by local excision. The procedure is performed after dilating the rectum widely. The goal is to accomplish full-thickness excision with 1 cm normal margins and closure of the defect preferably in two layers.

A preoperative transanal ultrasonography is important to assess depth of invasion and whether lymph node metastases are present. When transanal resection is preferred to abdominoperineal resection in patients who are fit and have small lesions, the following principles must be observed:

1. The excised specimen must be regarded as total biopsy and the patient informed that further decision as to whether abdominoperineal resection should be done will await the results of pathologic examination.
2. Abdominoperineal excision should be considered if:
   a. Tumor is present at excision margins.
   b. Histology shows poorly differentiated, high-grade carcinoma.
   c. Tumor is transmural.

In patients who are poor candidates for abdominoperineal resection because of concurrent illness, transanal excision or transanal destruction of the tumor by electrocautery or radiation therapy may be used.

Transanal Endoscopic Microsurgery Using instruments similar to those used in laparoscopic surgery and with appropriate rectal insufflation with carbon dioxide, excision is performed with electrocautery. Full-thickness resection should be undertaken only for lesions that are extraperitoneal (i.e., 8 cm anteriorly or 12 cm posteriorly or lower).

Endocavitory Radiation This form of primary therapy is indicated in frail patients considered not suitable for surgery. It can also be used as postexcision therapy.

Staging and Prognosis

The TNM classification for colorectal cancer is given in Table 8.14. Although Dukes' classification is most widely used, the TNM classification provides more pathological detail. Table 8.15 compares Dukes' classification to TNM stages and provides 5-year survival rates. These figures make it clear that earlier diagnosis is the most important strategy to improve survival. Surveillance for colorectal cancer in individuals over the age of 50 has improved survival in the past 25 years. Important tests include periodic fecal occult blood evaluation, sigmoidoscopy and colonoscopy, and more careful follow-up in high-risk individuals (e.g., polyps, CUC, CD). The exploding knowledge of the genetics of colorectal cancer is providing additional tools, which will become more precise and in the future help us to detect colorectal cancer early.

The prognosis is adversely affected by the following circumstances:

1. Poor histological differentiation and vascular and perineural invasion.
2. Presence of obstruction or perforation.
3. Aneuploid tumor cells.
4. Mucin-producing and signet cell tumors (intracytoplasmic mucin).
5. Elevated CEA levels.

TABLE 8.15. Staging of Colorectal Cancer and Survival Rates According to Dukes' Classification and TNM Stage

Dukes' Classification	Stage	TNM Classification	5-Year Survival
A	I	T1 or T2, N0, M0	90%
B	II	T3 or T4, N0, M0	60%–80%
C	III	Any T, N1, N2, or N3, M0	20%–50%
D	IV	Any T, Any N, M1	5%

Furthermore, younger patients appear to have a worse prognosis than older ones, and preoperative blood transfusion may have an adverse effect.

Adjuvant Chemotherapy

Colorectal cancer is relatively resistant to chemotherapy. Nevertheless, it appears to be more effective when the burden of carcinoma is lowest and when cell division is maximal.

Large clinical trials have now shown that the combination of levamisole and 5-fluorouracil (5-FU), given after curative resection, improves disease-free survival rate and overall survival rates after surgery in Stage III (Dukes' C) cancer.[30] Recurrence rate was reduced by 39%, cancer-related deaths by 32%, and overall death rate by 31% in patients receiving the combination therapy postoperatively compared with those who underwent resection but received no chemotherapy. No survival advantage was seen in Stage II cancer.

Adjuvant chemotherapy does not appear as effective in rectal cancer as it does in colon cancer. Even then, some randomized prospective trials have shown that there may be modest gain in the use of levamisole and 5-FU in Stage II and Stage III rectal cancer in combination with radiation.[31]

ANORECTAL DISORDERS

Anorectal disorders are a common human affliction. They include hemorrhoids, anorectal abscesses and fistulae, fissure-in-ano, pruritus ani, condylomata, and malignant neoplasms of the anus. In this section, we also consider rectal prolapse and pilonidal disease.

Hemorrhoid

Hemorrhoidal plexus of veins occur above and below the dentate line. Those above the dentate are internal and are covered by rectal mucosa. Those below are external and are covered by the anoderm of the anal canal. Engorgement and enlargement of the internal hemorrhoids can be symptomatic. The main clinical significance of external hemorrhoids is that they may produce painful thrombosis (Figure 8.48).

TABLE 8.14. TNM Staging of Colorectal Cancer

Designation	Involvement
Primary Tumor (T)	
TX	Primary tumor cannot be assessed
T0	No evidence of primary tumor
Tis	Carcinoma in situ: intraepithelial or invasion of lamina propria
T1	Tumor invades submucosa
T2	Tumor invades muscularis propria
T3	Tumor invades through muscularis propria into subserosa or into non-peritonealized pericolic or perirectal tissues
T4	Tumor directly invades other organs or structures, and/or perforates visceral peritoneum
Regional lymph nodes (N)	
NX	Regional lymph nodes cannot be assessed
N0	No regional lymph node metastasis
N1	Metastasis in 1 to 3 regional lymph nodes
N2	Metastasis in 4 or more regional lymph nodes
Distant metastasis	
MX	Distant metastasis cannot be assessed
M0	No distant metastasis
M1	Distant metastasis

Source: Reprinted with permission from the American Joint Committee on Cancer (AJCC), Chicago, Illinois. The original source for this material is the *AJCC Cancer Staging Manual*, 6th ed. (2002) published by Springer-Verlag New York, www.springer-ny.com.

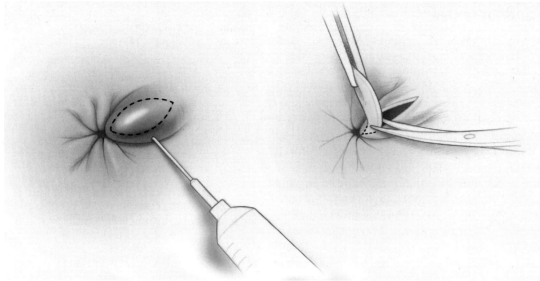

FIGURE 8.48. Surgical drainage of thrombosed hemorrhoid. Thrombosed hemorrhoids are treated with excision of the thrombosed hemorrhoid and the clot. (Adapted from Sabiston DC, ed: Textbook of Surgery: The Biological Basis of Modern Surgical Practice, 15th ed. Philadelphia: WB Saunders, 1997:1038.)

Internal Hemorrhoid

Internal hemorrhoids are caused by increased abdominal pressure during straining or lifting, from chronic constipation, portal hypertension, or obstruction of the superior hemorrhoidal vein by tumor. They occur at three primary positions as seen in Figure 8.49.

CLINICAL PRESENTATION Bleeding is the earliest and most common symptom of internal hemorrhoids. Rectal bleeding should never be ascribed to hemorrhoids until carcinoma is ruled out. Typically, the bleeding is seen in the surface of the stool or on toilet tissue. As the hemorrhoids enlarge, they begin to prolapse. At the outset, prolapse occurs with defecation and is followed by spontaneous reduction (first-degree hemorrhoid). At a later stage, spontaneous reduction does not occur and the patient must manually replace the hemorrhoid (second-degree). Eventually, the hemorrhoids may remain permanently prolapsed, causing mucoid discharge and soiling (third-degree). In the latter stage, acute thrombosis may occur, causing edematous enlargement of the hemorrhoids (fourth degree), which may be very acute and painful.

INVESTIGATION Physical examination and anoscopy suffice to establish the diagnosis. Bleeding, when present, requires sigmoidoscopic or colonoscopic examination to

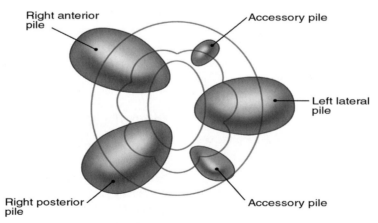

FIGURE 8.49. Common location of internal hemorrhoids. The three primary sites of internal hemorrhoids are 3, 7, and 11 o'clock. (Adapted from Goligher JC. Surgery of the Anus, Rectum, and Colon, 3rd ed. London: Balliere Tindall, 1975:117.)

rule out neoplasm and chronic inflammatory bowel disease. Examination of the perineum during straining may lead to prolapse of the hemorrhoids. Anoscopy allows visualization of enlarged and protruding hemorrhoid(s).

TREATMENT

Conservative Treatment First- and second-degree hemorrhoids can be treated successfully with local measures (e.g., suppositories, ointment) and with diet. The goal is to prevent constipation by increased daily fluid intake, high-fiber diet, and bulk-forming laxatives. When edema and prolapse are present, bed rest, local astringent compresses (witch hazel), and warm sitz baths may help.

Rubber-band Ligation Rubber-band ligation can be an effective way of treating second- and third-degree hemorrhoids. One hemorrhoid is banded at a time. The tissue over the hemorrhoid is grasped and pulled into the barrel of the rubber-band applicator, and the rubber band is placed at the base of the hemorrhoid. Placement must be well above the mucocutaneous junction or the patient will experience severe pain, and the band will have to be replaced. The ligated hemorrhoid undergoes ischemic necrosis and sloughs off in several days. Ligation of hemorrhoidal complexes is performed 2 to 3 weeks apart.

Injection Sclerosis of the hemorrhoid may be achieved by injecting 5% phenol in almond oil into the submucosa at the base of each hemorrhoid. The procedure must be performed in a manner that does not cause sloughing of the mucosa.

Cryosurgery A cryoprobe using carbon dioxide or nitrous oxide can be applied to generate necrosis of the hemorrhoid. However, it is difficult to control the depth of necrosis, and mucosal sloughing tends to occur.

Direct Current Coagulation Each hemorrhoid cushion is coagulated for 10 minutes.

Hemorrhoidectomy Large and refractive third- or fourth-degree hemorrhoids are treated surgically. The procedure requires conservative excision of normal anoderm and skin, dissection of the hemorrhoid cushion off the internal sphincter, high suture ligation of the hemorrhoid pedicle, and amputation of the hemorrhoid distal to the ligature (Figure 8.50). The skin defects are packed open. Several techniques have been described for hemorrhoidectomy. The Whitehead technique, which involves circumferential excision of the anoderm and dentate line, is prone to cause anal stricture.

Thrombosed External Hemorrhoid

This is an acute, painful thrombosis of a subcutaneous vein just outside the anal verge. The thrombosed vein pro-duces a very tender and tense bluish tumor. A common problem, few patients are as grateful as those with this lesion, when, under local anesthesia, the tumor is incised and the clot evacuated. Relief is instantaneous. Some surgeons prefer excision of the hemorrhoid to avoid recurrence.

Anorectal Abscesses

Anorectal abscesses are common and can occur in one of several potential spaces shown in Figure 8.51. Most probably they begin as an infection of an anal crypt, from which the infection spreads into one of the potential spaces. The infection is due to mixed flora consisting of *E. coli*, bacteroides, streptococci, *Proteus vulgaris*, and staphylococci.

Anorectal abscesses include:

1. Perianal abscess, which occurs under the skin of the anus within the anal canal.
2. Submucosal abscess, in the submucosa just superior to the anal canal.
3. Intermuscular abscess, lying between layers of the sphincter muscle.
4. Ischiorectal abscess, which develops in the ischiorectal fossae.
5. Supralevator or pelvirectal abscess, which lies above the levator but below the peritoneum and is often associated with supralevator rectal disease.
6. Retrorectal abscess, lying behind the rectum.

Treatment

Prompt incision and adequate drainage is the proper treatment. Except for superficial abscesses, which may be drained under local anesthesia, drainage under general anesthesia is required in most patients. The abscesses are larger than they appear, and all loculations must be broken. The wound is left open. A fistular tract from the primary site of origin may be found. This should be excised without significantly damaging the internal sphincter. Ischiorectal abscesses are drained through the perineum and may require the placement of a catheter drain. Supralevator abscesses are drained transrectally.

A high percentage of operated anorectal abscesses may develop an anal fistula following surgery. Patients should be informed of this possibility preoperatively. Inadequate or delayed drainage can result in major necrotizing anorectal infection. At times, this type of infection may involve the entire perineum and the scrotum (Fournier's disease). This complication requires major debridement, diverting colostomy, and skin grafting after infection has been eradicated.

When anorectal abscesses recur, the possibility of underlying inflammatory bowel disease should be investigated with colonoscopy and barium enema. The anorectal abscess wall should be biopsied whenever possible to

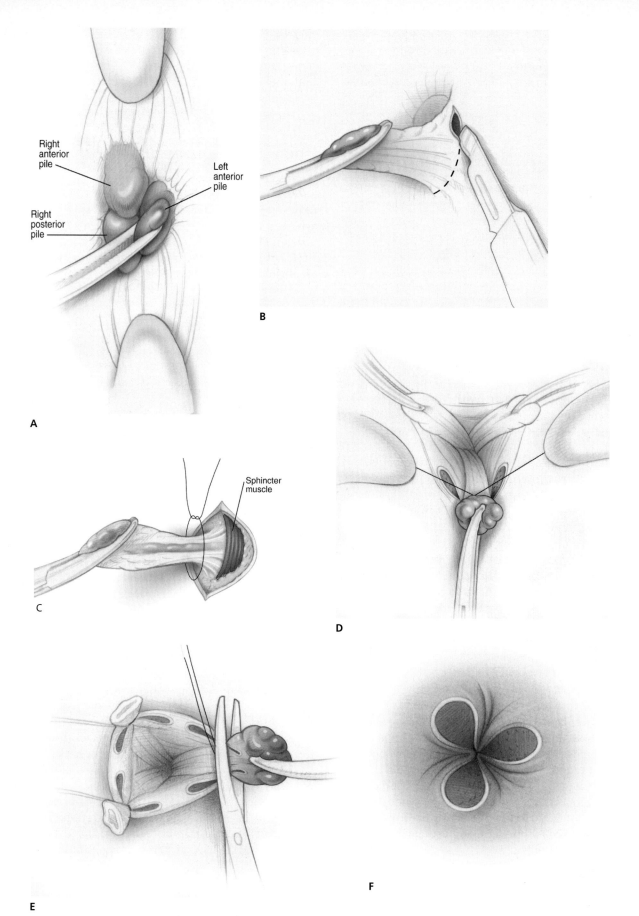

FIGURE 8.50. (A–F) Internal hemorrhoidectomy. Open internal hemorrhoidectomy involves dissection of the hemorrhoid cushion off the internal sphincter, high-suture ligation, and amputation of the hemorrhoid. (Adapted from Goligher JC. Surgery of the Anus, Rectum, and Colon. London: Baillière Tindall, 1975;155–156.)

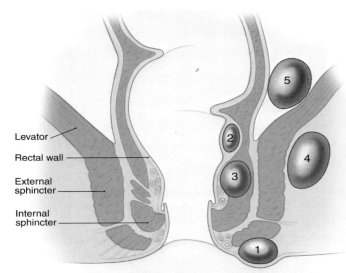

FIGURE 8.51. Anorectal abscess. The sites where anorectal abscesses occur include: (1) perianal, (2) submucus, (3) intrasphincteric, (4) ischerorectal, and (5) supralevator (pelvirectal). Anorectal abscesses can also occur retrorectally (not shown).

determine any possible unusual cause (e.g., tuberculosis, Crohn's disease, malignancy).

Anorectal Fistulas

Most anorectal fistulas originate as crypt infection at the anorectal junction. The internal opening may not correspond to the external opening. The second opening in skin can be in one of several sites in the perianal perineum. Fistulas are usually due to bacterial infection that starts in the crypts. Approximately 40% to 50% of patients in whom a perianal abscess has been drained have a residual fistula. Crohn's disease and tuberculosis can also cause anorectal fistulas.

The Salmon–Goodsall rule predicts the location of the secondary opening in the skin, depending on the location of the primary opening in the crypt (Figure 8.52). A fistula that has its external opening anterior to an imaginary transverse line drawn through the center of the anal orifice opens internally in a crypt radially opposite. When the external opening is posterior to this transverse line, however, the internal opening is always in a crypt in the midline posteriorly. While this rule holds most of the time, exceptions do exist.

Clinical Picture

The presenting complaint in patients with anorectal fistulas is drainage, usually pus, issuing from the perianal perineum. Inspection of the perineum reveals the site of the external fistula, and a cord-like tract towards the anal canal may be palpable. A lacrimal probe inserted into the fistula may reveal its relation to the anal sphincter, and the site of the internal opening may be determined with a con-

comitant digital exam. Recurrent fistulas should raise the possibility of Crohn's disease or tuberculosis.

Investigation

Digital rectal examination may reveal the site of the internal opening with or without a probe in the fistula. Proctoscopic examination is essential to rule out inflammatory bowel disease. If rectal inflammation is present or if the fistula is recurrent, colonoscopy with or without barium enema will be necessary.

Treatment

The most successful treatment is fistulotomy, in which the fistulous tract is laid open without damage to the sphincter. Curettage or cautery of the fistula is performed and the wound allowed to heal by secondary intention.

Trans-sphincteric fistulas result from drained ischiorectal abscess and cross both the internal and external sphincters. Fistulotomy divides the internal sphincter and part of the external. The procedure may produce incontinence in some patients. When the trans-sphincteric fistula is high, a seton suture may be inserted through it and the sphincter divided slowly over many days by progressively tightening the knot. This procedure is rarely used now, and the use of the seton suture is no guarantee against incontinence.

Fissure-in-ano

Fissure-in-ano, or anal fissure, is a painful crack or longitudinal ulcer in the anal canal overlying the internal sphincter. The base of the fissure is the internal sphincter,

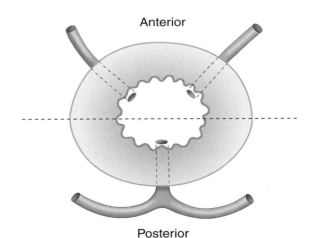

FIGURE 8.52. Salmon–Goodsall rule. When the secondary opening in the skin is located anterior to the transverse line drawn through the center of the anal orifice, the internal opening is radially opposite. When the external opening is posterior to this transverse line, however, the internal opening is in the midline.

which may go into spasm and aggravate the pain. Acute fissures are common in conditions producing constipation or following bouts of diarrhea. Most heal spontaneously without treatment. It is the chronic fissure that requires specific treatment.

Clinical Presentation

Severe anal pain on defecation is the primary symptom. A small amount of bright red bleeding may be noted on the toilet tissue. Fear of painful defecation leads to constipation. The patient often will not allow digital rectal examination because of pain, but a prominent localized swelling of the skin at the distal end of the fissure—the sentinel pile—may be observed externally. Digital rectal and anoscopic examination may be possible after liberal use of topical anesthetic.

Treatment

A dietary regimen to soften the stools, use of topical anesthetic and hydrocortisone, and sitz bath are the mainstay of medical therapy. If conservative treatment fails to heal the fissure in 4 to 6 weeks or less and pain is severe, lateral internal sphincterotomy should be performed. The sentinel pile is also excised. The fissure heals quickly after this procedure.

Forceful anal dilatation under anesthesia, known as the Lord maneuver, is not recommended because of the associated high incidence of incontinence.

Pilonidal Disease

Pilonidal disease consists of either a draining sinus or an abscess in the intergluteal region. Controversy exists as to its origin. Some believe it is congenital, while others believe it is acquired and results from ingrown hair. Indeed, deep in the sinus or abscess a tuft of hair is usually found. It is common in soldiers who ride in Jeep®-type vehicles.

Clinical Presentation

Patients usually present with acute pain due to an abscess. Some patients present with a draining sinus, the abscess having drained spontaneously. On examination, a midline abscess or one or more draining sinuses in the sacrococcygeal region is noted.

Treatment

The simplest surgical treatment is incision and drainage, with curettage to remove all hair follicles. The wound is then allowed to heal by secondary intention. Alternatively, the entire pilonidal complex can be excised and the wound allowed to heal secondarily. This procedure leaves a large wound, which requires a long time to heal. The third alternative is excision and primary closure, suitable only when pilonidal sinus is present without abscess. The procedure is best reserved for recurrent disease after prior incision and drainage.

Pruritis Ani

Severe perineal itching may be caused by a multitude of conditions. In children, a common cause is pinworm infestations (*Enterobius vermicularis*). The diagnosis can be made by applying a piece of cellophane tape to the anus at night to recover eggs, which are then examined under the microscope. In adults the causes range from dermatological diseases, to fungal or bacterial infections, to systemic diseases such as diabetes. Some causes are psychogenic, but most often no cause can be identified and the condition is idiopathic.

Treatment

The treatment is that of the underlying cause. The patient is advised to keep the perianal region dry and to avoid foods that exacerbate itching (e.g., coffee, tea, chocolate, tomatoes, etc.). Water-soluble corticosteroid cream with an acid pH applied three or four times a day may be helpful.

Rectal Prolapse

Rectal prolapse (procidentia) is a protrusion of the full thickness of the rectum through the anus. The proposed causes are colonic intussusception or a sliding hernia. Essential defects may be poor rectal support and increased intra-abdominal pressure. The condition is seen more commonly in the elderly, particularly those from nursing homes or on psychotropic drugs. Anatomically, patients with rectal prolapse have deep rectovesical space (Douglas pouch); lax levator muscles; a weak puborectalis, with loss of the acute angle it produces between the rectum and anus by pulling anteriorly; poor fixation of the rectum to the sacrum posteriorly; and poor support from the lateral ligaments.

Clinical Presentation

The patient complains of the prolapse, rectal bleeding, or discharge. Prolapse occurs on straining and, early in the course of the disease, it reduces spontaneously. With time, the patient has to reduce it manually. As the prolapse increases, anal sphincter incompetence and incontinence develop. A situation of full procidentia, where the prolapse cannot be reduced, may occur.

Investigation

It is essential that the prolapse be demonstrated. Full evaluation of the colon is necessary with colonoscopy and barium enema.

Treatment

Surgical treatment combines elements of bowel resection and rectal fixation. The procedures have a success rate of approximately 85% and include:

1. Anterior resection and suture fixation of the fully mobilized rectum to the sacrum is appropriate for low-risk patients who have normal anal sphincter function.

2. The Ripstein procedure, in which the rectum is fully mobilized and anchored to the presacral fascia with a Teflon or Mersilene mesh, may be useful for low-risk patients with incompetent anal sphincter.

3. The Thiersch loop, used in high-risk elderly patients, is a loop of stainless steel wire placed subcutaneously around the circumference of the anus. This procedure can provide effective palliation but may be complicated by fecal compaction, infection, or erosion of the wire into the rectum.

REFERENCES

1. Richards WO, Williams LF Jr. Obstruction of the large and small intestine. *Surg Clin North Am* 1988;68:355–376.
2. Nakashima H, Ueo H, Shibuta K, et al. Surgical management of patients with radiation enteritis. *Int Surg* 1996;81:415–418.
3. Crohn BB, Ginzburg L, Oppenheimer GD. Regional ileitis: a pathologic and clinical entity. *JAMA* 1932;99:1232–1329.
4. Rose JD, Roberts GM, Williams G, et al. Cardiff Crohn's disease jubilee: the incidence over 50 years. *Gut* 1988;29:346–351.
5. Elton E, Hanauer SB. Review article: the medical management of Crohn's disease. *Aliment Pharmacol Ther* 1996;10: 1–22.
6. Townsend CM, Thompson JC. Small intestine. In: Schwartz SI, Shires GT, Spencer FC, eds. *Principles of Surgery*. 6th ed. New York: McGraw Hill; 1994.
7. Taoka Y. Ecological approach to the patients with digestive diseases in Kitakyushu City and its suburbs. *J UOEH* 1986; 8(Suppl):381–399.
8. Mousen. Kough Carolinska Medico Chirurgiska Institute [thesis], VI, 1990:18.
9. Hugot JP, Chamaillard M, Zouali H, et al. Association of NOD2 leucine-rich repeat variants with susceptibility to Crohn's disease. *Nature* 2001;411:599–603.
10. Fielding JF. Clinical features of Crohn's disease in Ireland. *Am J Gastroenterol* 1986;81:524–528.
11. Sachar DB. Cancer in Crohn's disease: dispelling the myths. *Gut* 1994;35:1507–1508.
12. Wilks S. Morbid appearances in the intestine of Miss Bankes. *Med Times Gazette* 1859;19:264.
13. Hawkins HP. An address on the natural history of ulcerative colitis and its bearing on treatment. *BMJ* 1909;1:765.
14. Hurst AF. Ulcerative colitis. *Guy's Hosp Rep* 1909;71:26.
15. Jewell DP. Ulcerative colitis. In: Feldman M, Sleisenger MH, Scharschmidt BF, et al., eds. *Gastrointestinal and Liver Disease: Pathophysiology, Diagnosis, Management*. 6th ed. Philadelphia: Saunders; 1998:1735–1761.
16. Satsangi J, Jewell DP, Rosenberg WM, Bell JI. Genetics of inflammatory bowel disease. *Gut* 1994;35:696–700.
17. Wright R, Truelove SC. A controlled therapeutic trial of various diets in ulcerative colitis. *BMJ* 1965;2:138.
18. Gyde SN, Prior P, Allan RN, et al. Colorectal cancer in ulcerative colitis: a cohort study of primary referrals from three centres. *Gut* 1988;29:206–217.
19. Madiba TE, Mokoena T. Pattern of diverticular disease among Africans. *East Afr Med J* 1994;71:644–646.
20. Welton ML, Madhulika GV, Amerhause A. Colon, rectum, and anus. In: Norton JA, Bollinger RR, Chang AE, et al., eds. *Surgery: Basic Science and Clinical Evidence*. New York: Springer; 2001: 667–762.
21. Winawer SJ, Zauber AG, Gerdes H, et al. Risk of colorectal cancer in the families of patients with adenomatous polyps. National Polyp Study Workgroup. *N Engl J Med* 1996;334:82–87.
22. Devroede GJ, Taylor WF, Sauer WG, et al. Cancer risk and life expectancy of children with ulcerative colitis. *N Engl J Med* 1971;285:17–21.
23. Greenstein AJ, Sachar DB, Smith H, et al. A comparison of cancer risk in Crohn's disease and ulcerative colitis. *Cancer* 1981;48:2742–2745.
24. Guttormson NL, Bubrick MP. Mortality from ischemic colitis. *Dis Colon Rectum* 1989;32:469–472.
25. Wolff BG. Factors determining recurrence following surgery for Crohn's disease. *World J Surg* 1998;22:364–369.
26. Turnbull RB Jr, Hawk WA, Weakley FL. Surgical treatment of toxic megacolon. Ileostomy and colostomy to prepare patients for colectomy. *Am J Surg* 1971;122:325–331.
27. Kodner IJ, Fry RD. Inflammatory bowel disease. *Clin Symp* 1982;34:3–32.
28. Ouriel K, Adams JT. Adenocarcinoma of the small intestine. *Am J Surg* 1984;147:66–71.
29. Savage DG, Antman KH. Imatinib mesylate—a new oral targeted therapy. *N Engl J Med* 2002;346:683–693.
30. Moertel CG, Fleming TR, Macdonald JS, et al. Levamisole and fluorouracil for adjuvant therapy of resected colon carcinoma. *N Engl J Med* 1990;322:352–358.
31. Gastrointestinal Tumor Study Group. Prolongation of the disease-free interval in surgically treated rectal carcinoma. *N Engl J Med* 1985;312:1465–1472.

SELECTED READINGS

Small Bowel Obstruction

Bass KN, Jones B, Bulkley GB. Current management of small-bowel obstruction. *Adv Surg* 1997;31:1–34.

Maglinte DD, Balthazar EJ, Kelvin FM, et al. The role of radiology in the diagnosis of small-bowel obstruction. *AJR Am J Roentgenol* 1997;168:1171–1180.

Vanderhoof JA, Langnas AN. Short-bowel syndrome in children and adults. *Gastroenterology* 1997;113:1767–1778.

Small Bowel Tumors

Arnold R. Medical treatment of metastasizing carcinoid tumors. *World J Surg* 1996;20:203–207.

Ashley SW, Wells SA Jr. Tumors of the small intestine. *Semin Oncol* 1988;15:116–128.

Cheek RC, Wilson H. Carcinoid tumors. *Curr Probl Surg* 1970;Nov: 4–31.

Cunningham JD, Aleali R, Aleali M, et al. Malignant small bowel neoplasms: histopathologic determinants of recurrence and survival. *Ann Surg* 1997;225:300–306.

Kulke MH, Mayer RJ. Carcinoid tumors. *N Engl J Med* 1999;340: 858–868.

Loehr WJ, Mujahed Z, Zahn FD, et al. Primary lymphoma of the gastrointestinal tract: a review of 100 cases. *Ann Surg* 1969;170: 232–328.

Moertel CG, Sauer WG, Dockerty MB, et al. Life history of the carcinoid tumor of the small intestine. *Cancer* 1961;14:901–912.

Neugut AI, Marvin MR, Rella VA, et al. An overview of adeno-carcinoma of the small intestine. *Oncology (Huntingt)* 1997;11:529–536.

North JH, Pack MS. Malignant tumors of the small intestine: a review of 144 cases. *Am Surg* 2000;66:46–51.

Crohn's Disease

Fazio VW, Marchetti F. Recurrent Crohn's disease and resection margins: bigger is not better. *Adv Surg* 1999;32:135–168.

Fazio VW, Wu JS. Surgical therapy for Crohn's disease of the colon and rectum. *Surg Clin North Am* 1997;77:197–210.

Herfarth H, Scholmerich J. IL-10 therapy in Crohn's disease: at the crossroads. Treatment of Crohn's disease with the anti-inflammatory cytokine interleukin 10. *Gut* 2002;50:146–147.

Hodgson HJ. Pathogenesis of Crohn's disease. *Baillieres Clin Gastroenterol* 1998;12:1–17.

Jess T, Winther KV, Munkholm P, et al. Mortality and causes of death in Crohn's disease: follow-up of a population-based cohort in Copenhagen County, Denmark. *Gastroenterology* 2002;122:1808–1814.

Yang YX, Lichtenstein GR. Corticosteroids in Crohn's disease. *Am J Gastroenterol* 2002;97:803–823.

Colon and Rectum

Anatomy and Physiology

Bassotti G, Germani U, Morelli A. Human colonic motility: physio-logical aspects. *Int J Colorectal Dis* 1995;10:173–180.

Hajivassiliou CA, Carter KB, Finlay IG. Anorectal angle enhances faecal continence. *Br J Surg* 1996;83:53–56.

Nano M, Levi AC, Borghi F, et al. Observations on surgical anatomy for rectal cancer surgery. *Hepatogastroenterology* 1998;45: 717–726.

Diverticulitis

Cullen JJ, Kelly KA, Moir CR, et al. Surgical management of Meckel's diverticulum. An epidemiologic, population-based study. *Ann Surg* 1994;220:564–569.

Eggesbo HB, Jacobsen T, Kolmannskog F, et al. Diagnosis of acute left-sided colonic diverticulitis by three radiological modalities. *Acta Radiol* 1998;39:315–321.

Khan AL, Ah-See AK, Crofts TJ, et al. Surgical management of the septic complications of diverticular disease. *Ann R Coll Surg Engl* 1995;77:16–20.

Nirula R, Greaney G. Right-sided diverticulitis: a difficult diagnosis. *Am Surg* 1997;63:871–873.

Spivak H, Weinrauch S, Harvey JC, et al. Acute colonic diverticuli-tis in the young. *Dis Colon Rectum* 1997;40:570–574.

Wedell J, Banzhaf G, Chaoui R, et al. Surgical management of complicated colonic diverticulitis. *Br J Surg* 1997;84:380–383.

Colonic Polyps

Bazzoli F, Fossi S, Sottili S, et al. The risk of adenomatous polyps in asymptomatic first-degree relatives of persons with colon cancer. *Gastroenterology* 1995;109:783–788.

Debinski HS, Love S, Spigelman AD, et al. Colorectal polyp counts and cancer risk in familial adenomatous polyposis. *Gastroen-terology* 1996;110:1028–1030.

Kronborg O. Colon polyps and cancer. *Endoscopy* 2002;34:69–72.

Moisio AL, Jarvinen H, Peltomaki P. Genetic and clinical character-isation of familial adenomatous polyposis: a population based study. *Gut* 2002;50:845–850.

Vasen HF, van der Luijt RB, Slors JF, et al. Molecular genetic tests as a guide to surgical management of familial adenomatous polyposis. *Lancet* 1996;348:433–435.

Colon Cancer

Beart RW, Melton LJ 3rd, Maruta M, et al. Trends in right and left-sided colon cancer. *Dis Colon Rectum* 1983;26:393–398.

Beart RW, Steele GD Jr, Menck HR, et al. Management and survival of patients with adenocarcinoma of the colon and rectum: a national survey of the Commission on Cancer. *J Am Coll Surg* 1995;181:225–236.

Chau I, Cunningham D. Cyclooxygenase inhibition in cancer—a blind alley or a new therapeutic reality? *N Engl J Med* 2002;346: 1058–1087.

Dukes CE. The classification of cancer of the rectum. *J Pathol Bacteriol* 1932;35:323.

Easson AM, Cotterchio M, Crosby JA, et al. A population-based study of the extent of surgical resection of potentially curable colon cancer. *Ann Surg Oncol* 2002;9:380–387.

Harrison LE, Guillem JG, Paty P, et al. Preoperative carcinoembry-onic antigen predicts outcomes in node-negative colon cancer patients: a multivariate analysis of 572 patients. *J Am Coll Surg* 1997;185:55–59.

Mandava N, Kumar S, Pizzi WF, et al. Perforated colorectal carcino-mas. *Am J Surg* 1996;172:236–238.

Marohn M. Endorectal ultrasound. Postgraduate Course Syllabus. *SAGES* 1997;126–153.

Varma MG, Rogers SJ, Schrock TR, et al. Local excision of rectal carcinoma. *Arch Surg* 1999;134:863–868.

Fistulas

Orringer JS, Mendeloff EN, Eckhauser FE. Management of wounds in patients with complex enterocutaneous fistulas. *Surg Gynecol Obstet* 1987;165:79–80.

Present DH, Rutgeerts P, Targan S, et al. Infliximab for the treatment of fistulas in patients with Crohn's disease. *N Engl J Med* 1999;340:1398–405.

Reber HA, Roberts C, Way LW, et al. Management of external gastrointestinal fistulas. *Ann Surg* 1978;188:460–467.

9

Appendix

ANATOMY

The appendix is a 5–8 cm diverticulum arising from the cecum at the convergence of the teniae coli. It is typically 2–3 cm below the ileocecal valve. The appendix most commonly lies in the ileocecal location but may also be retrocecal (16%), retroileal, or pelvic (Figure 9.1). The position of the appendix may affect the clinical presentation of acute appendicitis.

Inflammation of the appendix, appendicitis, is the most important condition of this vestigial organ. Diagnosing appendicitis may be simple or difficult. Hence, it is wise to include acute appendicitis in the top two or three items in the differential diagnosis of the acute abdomen.

The lumen of the appendix communicates with the cecum. The appendiceal wall has mucosal, submucosal, muscular, and serosal layers. The mucosa is colonic in appearance with goblet cells. The submucosa is rich with lymphoid tissue that aggregates as numerous lymphoid follicles. The muscle wall and serosa are similar to those of the cecum. The appendix, like the small intestine and right colon, originates from the midgut of the embryo and, as such, is supplied by the ileocolic branch of the superior mesenteric artery (Figure 9.2) and is innervated by T-10, the same somatic innervation as the skin surrounding the umbilicus. Thus, in early appendicitis, when only the visceral wall of the appendix is involved, the pain is initially referred to the region of the umbilicus. Parenthetically, it must also be pointed out that when the jejunum, ileum or right colon are obstructed, the colicky abdominal pain initially felt by the patient is periumbilical.

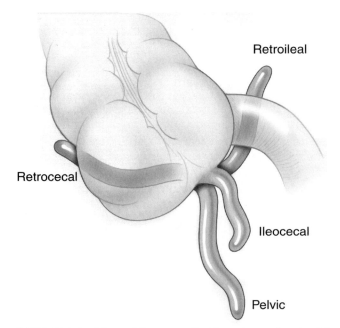

FIGURE 9.1. Positions of the appendix. The retrocecal and pelvic positions are likely to result in atypical presentation of acute appendicitis.

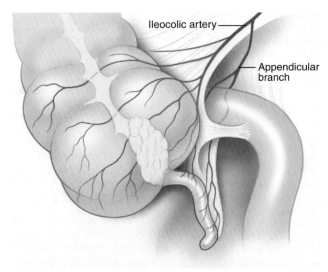

FIGURE 9.2. Blood supply of the appendix. The appendiceal artery is a branch of the ileocolic, which is a branch of the superior mesenteric artery.

PHYSIOLOGY

The function of the appendix in the adult human is unknown but is likely to be related to the role of the lymphoid tissue in immunologic processes. Early studies suggested an increased incidence of colon cancer following appendectomy, but larger reviews subsequently found no support for that observation.

PATHOPHYSIOLOGY

ACUTE APPENDICITIS

A primary event in the initiation of acute appendicitis is luminal obstruction, which in over 70% of cases is caused by fecalith, foreign body, tumor of the appendix or cecum, parasites, or fibrous bands. When such definitive obstruction is present, appendicitis is likely to progress rapidly and result in gangrene and perforation, known as acute obstructive appendicitis. In approximately 25% to 30% of patients with acute appendicitis, no luminal cause for obstruction is found. Instead, hyperplasia of the submucosal lymphoid follicles appears to compromise the appendiceal lumen. Such lymphoid hyperplasia has been related to recent or concurrent incidences of upper respiratory tract or other viral infections, particularly in children.

Acute obstructive appendicitis can progress within 12 to 24 h to gangrene of the wall of the appendix and perforation. Perforation may become rapidly confined by the omentum and/or small bowel and develop into an appendiceal abscess. When the perforation is not localized, general peritonitis develops. Unless quickly treated, pelvic, intramesenteric and/or subphrenic abscesses ensue. Acute appendicitis may lead to hematogenous spread of bacteria and infection of the portal vein (pylephlebitis) or liver abscesses.

The diagnosis of acute appendicitis can be difficult in the very young, the very old, and in individuals on steroid therapy, in whom the classic signs and symptoms may not be evident.

CARCINOID TUMOR OF THE APPENDIX

The most common tumor of the appendix is carcinoid. Usually, these tumors are benign and found either incidentally at laparotomy or because they cause obstructive appendicitis. A small proportion of carcinoid tumors of the appendix are malignant and may metastasize. Liver metastases may cause the carcinoid syndrome. Metastases to mesenteric lymph nodes may cause small bowel obstruction due to intense local fibrosis.

CLINICAL MANAGEMENT

ACUTE APPENDICITIS

Clinical Presentation

Classic Presentation

Acute appendicitis may start with vague periumbilical pain, nausea, and vomiting. Several hours later (4–8 h), the pain moves to the right lower quadrant (RLQ) as the parietal peritoneum becomes involved with the inflammation. At this point, tenderness develops at McBurney's point (Figure 9.3), and rebound tenderness is present in the RLQ. The presence of generalized peritonitis is indicative of development of gangrene or perforation. In uncomplicated appendicitis, tachycardia and fever are low grade.

Retrocecal Appendicitis

Abdominal pain, which starts in the periumbilical region, remains poorly localized without migration to the RLQ. Abdominal tenderness may be difficult to elicit until late, although some patients have point tenderness in the right flank. Diarrhea and urinary symptoms may develop because of the proximity of the inflamed appendix to the cecum and the right ureter, respectively.

Pelvic Appendicitis

Early symptoms are similar to those in classic presentation. Nausea and vomiting are significant and diarrhea develops from irritation of the pelvic colon. RLQ tender-

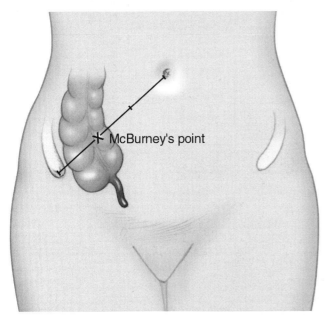

FIGURE 9.3. McBurney's point lies at the junction of the medial two-thirds and lateral third of a line drawn between the umbilicus and the superior anterior iliac spine. Typically, maximal tenderness is elicited at this point during abdominal palpation in acute appendicitis.

ness does not develop, but point tenderness is elicited on the right side of the rectum on digital examination.

Two clinical tests that may sometimes be helpful are the Rovsing and psoas signs. The Rovsing sign is elicited by abdominal compression over the descending colon, which tends to cause distension of the cecum and to elicit RLQ pain in the presence of acute appendicitis. The psoas sign is elicited by placing the patient supine, with his or her right side up, then extending the right hip while the knee is in full extension. The maneuver stretches the psoas muscle and, if retrocecal appendicitis is present, elicits abdominal pain due to the location of the inflamed retrocecal appendix over the right psoas.

Appendicitis during Pregnancy

Acute appendicitis occurs during pregnancy with the same frequency as in nonpregnant women of similar age. The condition is a true emergency requiring rapid diagnosis and surgical treatment. The cecum and appendix are displaced upwards to the right upper quadrant by the pregnant uterus. The initial symptoms of midabdominal pain, nausea, vomiting, and mild leukocytosis are common in pregnancy, even in the absence of appendicitis. The most important finding is tenderness and rebound in the right abdomen, above McBurney's point.

Investigation

Diagnosis of acute appendicitis is made largely on clinical grounds. When the diagnosis is not immediately evident, the patient should have repeated abdominal examination, preferably by the same examiner, every 2 to 3 h. Labora-

tory tests and radiologic examination are also useful, particularly when the diagnosis is uncertain.

Laboratory Tests

Mild leukocytosis with some shift to the left is the most common finding. Absence of any leukocytosis suggests—but by no means proves—the absence of acute appendicitis. Urinalysis is usually normal, although a preexisting urinary tract infection may be present. In retrocecal appendicitis, the urine may contain red cells and leukocytes, but gross hematuria should suggest renal calculus.

Radiological Studies

Plain abdominal x-rays are useful in ruling out perforation of another viscus. Free air in the peritoneum is rarely, if ever, seen in perforated appendicitis. In acute appendicitis, the findings are frequently nonspecific, showing either no abnormal findings or a mild ileus. In well-established acute appendicitis, soft tissue density may be apparent in the region of the cecum. Barium enema is not indicated except in the rare patient. If the appendix fills with dye, acute appendicitis can be excluded. In the presence of acute appendicitis, the appendix fails to fill, and an impression on the barium-filled cecum from an adjacent inflammatory mass may be appreciated. CT examination is indicated in the evaluation of RLQ mass when this is present.

Ultrasound examination is indicated when the diagnosis is uncertain (Figure 9.4), particularly during pregnancy and in children. It is helpful in ruling out tubo-ovarian pathology and, in acute appendicitis, it may show an abscess-filled appendix with thickened wall.

Laparoscopy

Laparoscopy provides the opportunity not only to establish the diagnosis but also to perform appendectomy. Hence, its value and the frequency with which it is used have risen sharply in the past 10 years.

Differential Diagnosis

Several conditions must be considered in the differential diagnosis of acute appendicitis (Table 9.1). The diagnosis is most often difficult in women of childbearing age who are susceptible to pelvic inflammatory disease, tubal pregnancy, and ovarian pathology. It is particularly in these patients that ultrasound examination and early laparoscopy are indicated.

Urinary tract disease, particularly right ureteral calculus and acute pyelonephritis, are important conditions that must be excluded. The pain in pyelonephritis is usually in the right flank with tenderness in the right costophrenic angle. The pain from a calculus in the right ureter is more severe, colicky, and tends to spread from the loin to the groin. Tenderness and guarding in the RLQ is uncommon. Urinalysis is often diagnostic, but ultrasonography and/or an intravenous pyelogram (IVP) may be necessary.

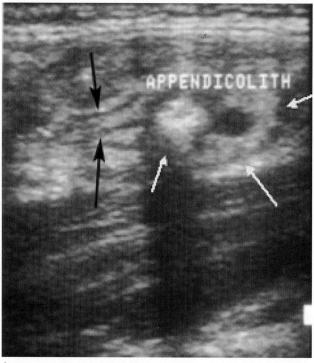

A

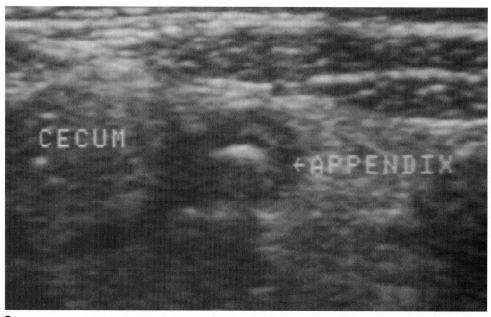

B

FIGURE 9.4. Ultrasound in acute appendix. (A) Ultrasonogram in a patient with RLQ pain illustrates normal proximal appendix (black arrows) and an inflamed portion of distal appendix containing an appendicolith (white arrows). (B) Ultrasonogram in early nonruptured appendicitis demonstrates the cecum and a thick-walled appendix containing fluid (arrow). *Abbreviation*: RLQ, right lower quadrant.

In perforated duodenal ulcer, gastric juice may sometimes track to the RLQ, where it incites acute inflammation simulating acute appendicitis. When generalized peritonitis is present, the conditions to consider include perforated viscus, acute cholecystitis, acute pancreatitis, and acute vascular compromise of the bowel. Free air in the peritoneum is not a feature of perforated appendicitis or perforated small intestine. Approximately 70% of patients with perforated peptic ulcer and most patients with free right or left colonic perforation have free intraperitoneal air.

Patients with inflammatory bowel disease tend to have antecedent symptoms of diarrhea or abdominal pain. No such medical history may accompany acute regional ileitis, although the patient often exhibits anemia.

TABLE 9.1. Differential Diagnosis of Acute Appendicitis

Gastrointestinal
  Perforated peptic ulcer
  Intestinal perforation
  Intestinal ischemia
  Meckel's diverticulitis
  Colonic diverticulitis
  Terminal ileitis
  Gastroenteritis

Biliary tract/pancreas
  Acute cholecystitis
  Acute pancreatitis

Urinary tract
  Ureteral calculus
  Acute pyelonephritis

Gynecologic
  Ruptured ovarian cyst or follicle
  Torsion of ovary
  Tubal (ectopic) pregnancy
  Acute salpingitis

Abdominal wall
  Rectus muscle hematoma

Supradiaphragmatic
  Right lower lobe pneumonia

Endocrine/metabolic
  Diabetic ketoacidosis
  Acute porphyria

Nervous system
  Tabes dorsalis
  Herpes zoster

Surgical Treatment

Uncomplicated Appendicitis

Once diagnosis is established, an operation should be performed as early as possible, before perforation occurs. Appendectomy can be done either laparoscopically or with an open technique. When appendectomy is performed laparoscopically, the position of the ports is as indicated in Figure 9.5. When performed with an open technique, a small oblique or transverse incision centered on McBurney's point is sufficient. If the diagnosis is uncertain, either a vertical (midline or right paramedian) or transverse incisions are used (Figure 9.6). These incisions may be extended to address other conditions should the diagnosis of acute appendicitis prove wrong. If an oblique incision has been used but the problem proves to be located in the upper or left abdomen, the prudent thing to do is to close the incision and perform a midline incision. During pregnancy, the incision must be higher in the right abdomen, preferably guided by the point of maximal tenderness.

SURGICAL TECHNIQUE The technique of open appendectomy is depicted in Figure 9.7. After the abdomen is entered, the cecum is identified and the teniae followed to their convergence to locate the appendix. Often small bowel and/or omentum covers the inflamed appendix. These are gently moved aside to free the appendix. The apex of the inflamed organ is grasped to expose the mesoappendix. The appendiceal vessels in the mesoappendix are then divided and ligated. The appendix is freed to its base, which

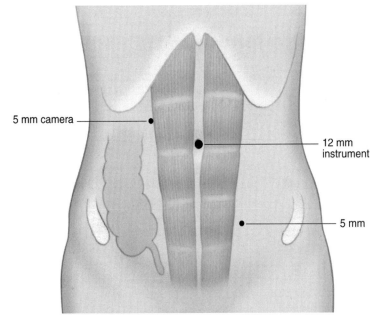

5 mm camera

12 mm
instrument

5 mm

FIGURE 9.5. Ports for laparoscopic appendectomy.

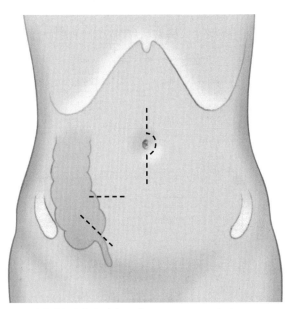

FIGURE 9.6. Incisions for open appendectomy.

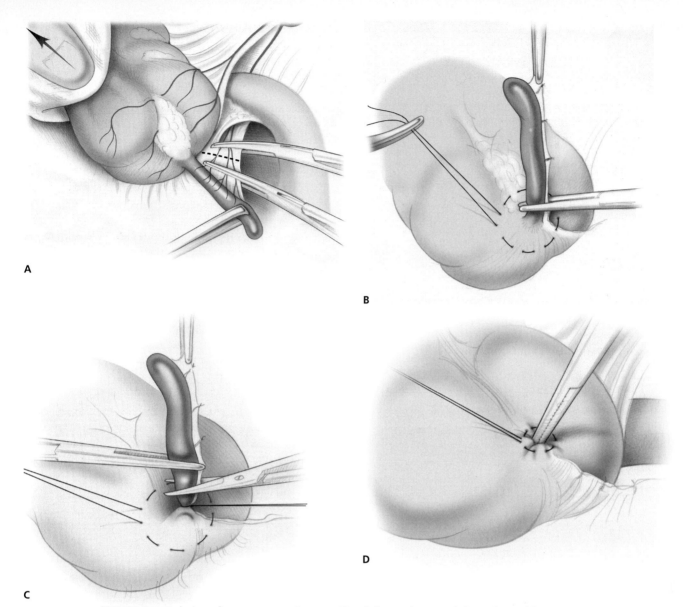

FIGURE 9.7. Technique for open appendectomy. The abdomen is opened through an oblique or transverse incision centered on McBurney's point. (A) The appendix is grasped and retracted, and the appendiceal artery is divided between ligatures. (B) The appendix is dissected to its base, (C) where it is ligated, divided distal to the ligature, and removed. (D) The appendiceal stump is inverted into the cecum using a pursestring suture. (Adapted from Sabiston DC, Jr, ed. Atlas of General Surgery. Philadelphia: WB Saunders, 1994:967.)

is often remarkably free of acute inflammation. The base is gently crushed with a hemostat and the hemostat reapplied a few millimeters distally. The crushed portion of the appendix is ligated with 2-0 silk. The appendix is amputated distal to the ligature and removed. Some surgeons cauterize the mucosa of the stump of the appendix with phenol or electric cautery. More importantly, the appendiceal stump is inverted using a pursestring suture in the surrounding cecum.

If the appendix is perforated, a search for a fecalith is undertaken in the surrounding area, in the pelvis and between loops of small intestine. These areas are liberally irrigated, and a drain is usually placed in the right lower quadrant of the abdomen.

When the procedure is performed laparoscopically, the appendix is identified and its tip is grasped and retracted to display the mesoappendix. The appendiceal artery is then dissected off the wall of the organ, and the mesoappendix containing the artery is divided by a linear-cutting stapling device. The appendix is amputated at its base, also done with a stapling device, and retrieved. No inversion is attempted. Most uncomplicated appendectomies can be performed laparoscopically. However, if the procedure proves difficult because of either access problems, presence of abscess, or large inflammatory mass, the operation should be converted to open appendectomy.

Complicated Appendicitis

PERFORATION Most patients with perforated appendicitis can be treated with routine appendectomy. The base of the appendix proximal to the obstruction is often reasonably normal, and secure closure is possible. An attempt should be made to find and remove the fecalith. Rarely is the perforation right at the cecum. The cecal edges may be so indurated that the perforation cannot be closed. The surgeon has two alternatives: Either place a cecostomy tube and drain the RLQ or perform a limited right hemicolectomy. This book's author prefers the latter.

APPENDICEAL ABSCESS A patient may present with a medical history of several days' duration of a well-developed mass in the RLQ. Ultrasound and/or CT scan confirms the diagnosis. If the patient has generalized abdominal signs, immediate surgery is indicated to drain the abscess and perform appendectomy. If, on the other hand, tenderness is localized to the RLQ with no evidence of generalized peritonitis, the abscess may be drained with a catheter placed percutaneously under ultrasound guidance. The patient is placed under broad-spectrum antibiotics and carefully followed clinically. If the patient fails to improve or deteriorates, surgical intervention is indicated. Often the patient improves, and the purulent catheter drainage subsides slowly. Such a patient may be discharged from hospital and readmitted for interval appendectomy 6 to 8 weeks later.

CARCINOID TUMOR OF THE APPENDIX

Clinical Presentation

Carcinoid tumors of the appendix are discovered either incidentally or because they have caused obstructive appendicitis. Rarely do they present with the carcinoid syndrome if they have metastasized to the liver or with small bowel obstruction from cicatrization associated with mesenteric lymph node metastasis.

Surgical Treatment

Appendectomy is performed when the carcinoid tumor is encountered incidentally during exploratory laparotomy or during treatment of acute appendicitis. Right hemicolectomy is indicated when the tumor is:

1. Too close to the base at the cecum.
2. Two centimeters in diameter or larger.
3. Malignant as evidenced by metastasis to lymph nodes or liver; isolated liver metastasis may be locally resected.

SELECTED READINGS

Appendicitis

Al-Mulhim AA. Acute appendicitis in pregnancy. A review of 52 cases. *Int Surg* 1996;81:295–297.

Baron EJ, Bennion R, Thompson J, et al. A microbiological comparison between acute and complicated appendicitis. *Clin Infect Dis* 1992;14:227–231.

Birnbaum BA, Balthazar EJ. CT of appendicitis and diverticulitis. *Radiol Clin North Am* 1994;32:885–898.

Bohnen MA, Solomkin JS, Dellinger EP, et al. Guidelines for clinical care: anti-infective agents for intra-abdominal infection: a Surgical Infection Society policy statement. *Arch Surg* 1992;127: 83–89.

Chen SC, Chen KM, Wang SM, et al. Abdominal sonography screening of clinically diagnosed or suspected appendicitis before surgery. *World J Surg* 1998;22:449–452.

Fisher KS, Ross DS. Guidelines for therapeutic decision in incidental appendectomy. *Surg Gynecol Obstet* 1990;171:95–98.

Gahukamble DB, Gahukamble LD. Surgical and pathological basis for interval appendicectomy after resolution of appendicular mass in children. *J Pediatr Surg* 2000;35:424–427.

Garbutt JM, Soper NJ, Shannon WD, et al. Meta-analysis of randomized controlled trials comparing laparoscopic and open appendectomy. *Surg Laparosc Endosc* 1999;9:17–26.

Hale DA, Molloy M, Pearl RH, et al. Appendectomy: a contemporary appraisal. *Ann Surg* 1997;225:252–261.

Halvorsen AC, Brandt B, Andreasen JJ. Acute appendicitis in pregnancy: complications and subsequent management. *Eur J Surg* 1992;158:603–606.

Jeffrey RB Jr, Laing FC, Lewis FR. Acute appendicitis: high-resolution real-time US findings. *Radiology* 1987;163:11–14.

Keller MS, McBride WJ, Vane DW. Management of complicated appendicitis. A rational approach based on clinical course. *Arch Surg* 1996;131:261–264.

McBurney C. Experience with early operative interference in cases of disease of the vermiform appendix. *N Y Med J* 1889;50:676–684.

McCahill LE, Pellegrini CA, Wiggins T, et al. A clinical outcome and cost analysis of laparoscopic versus open appendectomy. *Am J Surg* 1996;171:533–537.

Nitecki S, Assalia A, Schien M. Contemporary management of the appendiceal mass. *Br J Surg* 1993;80:18–20.

Rao PM, Rhea JT, Novelline RA, et al. Effect of computed tomography of the appendix on treatment of patients and use of hospital resources. *N Engl J Med* 1998;338:141–146.

Neoplasms of the Appendix

Deans GT, Spence RA. Neoplastic lesions of the appendix. *Br J Surg* 1995;82:299–306.

Kulke MH, Mayer RJ. Carcinoid tumors. *N Engl J Med* 1999;340:858–868.

Nitecki SS, Wolff BG, Schlinkert R, et al. The natural history of surgically treated primary adenocarcinoma of the appendix. *Ann Surg* 1994;219:51–57.

Parkes SE, Muir KR, al Sheyyab M, et al. Carcinoid tumours of the appendix in children 1957–1986: incidence, treatment and outcome. *Br J Surg* 1993;80:502–504.

Sandor A, Modlin IM. A retrospective analysis of 1570 appendiceal carcinoids. *Am J Gastroenterol* 1998;93:422–428.

10

Spleen

The spleen, an organ of the reticuloendothelial system, plays a valuable role in the body's immune response and in the removal of effete red cells and cellular debris from circulation. Its principal importance to the surgeon is that it is the organ most frequently ruptured in blunt abdominal trauma, and it is susceptible to inadvertent operative trauma. Furthermore, splenectomy is a significant therapeutic option in several hematologic disorders and is also used to stage lymphomas.

ANATOMIC RELATIONSHIP

The spleen, normally 80 to 100g in weight, is located in the left upper quadrant of the abdomen and has several important anatomic relationships (Figure 10.1). It lies along the ninth rib and is protected by the left rib cage. It is attached to the left diaphragm by the lienophrenic ligament. Other suspensory ligaments include the gastrosplenic, splenocolic, and splenorenal. Short gastric vessels travel in the gastrosplenic ligament, and the relationship of the spleen to the gastric fundus—which is anterior and medial—is also important. The hilum of the spleen is related to the tail of the pancreas and, during splenectomy, the tail of the pancreas must be carefully dissected before clamping the splenic vessels at the hilum to avoid pancreatic injury and pancreatic fistula formation. Laterally and inferiorly, the spleen is related to the splenic flexure of the colon. Posteriorly and inferiorly lie the left kidney and left adrenal gland.

The structure of the spleen is depicted in Figure 10.2. The spleen has an outer capsule that encloses the pulp. The splenic capsule is relatively better defined in children than in adults. The splenic pulp consists of three zones: (1) the white pulp, which is structurally similar to lymph nodes and contains lymphocytes, macrophages, and plasma cells in a reticular network of supporting structure; (2) the red pulp, consisting of cords of reticular cells and parallel sinuses; and (3) the marginal zone, consisting of vascular spaces between the pulps. It is here that foreign material, cell fragments, and plasma are sequestered.

BLOOD SUPPLY

The main arterial blood supply occurs through the splenic artery, a branch of the celiac axis. The main venous drainage is through the splenic vein, which joins the superior mesenteric vein behind the neck of the pancreas to form the portal vein. Within the spleen, the splenic artery branches into trabecular arteries that course through the trabeculae to reach the white pulp, where they become central arteries. Central arteries terminate in the red pulp. From the red pulp, blood collects in splenic sinuses, which drain into the central veins, then into the trabecular veins, and finally into the splenic vein. Splenic pulp pressure, which can be measured through a percutaneously inserted needle, is 8mmHg and approximates portal venous pressure.

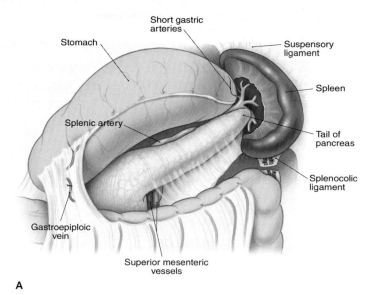

A

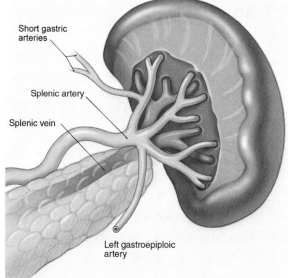

B

FIGURE 10.1. Surgical anatomy of the spleen. (A) The spleen has key anatomic relationships to the gastric fundus, pancreatic tail, and splenic flexure of the colon, including the suspensory (lienorenal and splenocolic) ligaments. (B) The terminal branching of the splenic artery and vein at the splenic hilum and relation to the tail of the pancreas are shown. (Adapted from Warren KW, Jenkins RL, Steele GD Jr. Atlas of Surgery of the Liver, Pancreas, and Biliary Tract. Norwalk, CT: Appleton & Lange, 1991:319.)

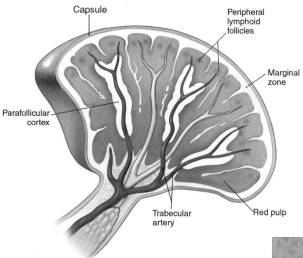

A

FIGURE 10.2. Structure of the spleen. (A) The cross-section of the spleen shows peripheral lymphoid follicles with T cell zone forming the parafollicular cortex and the splenic medulla with its medullary cords and sinuses. (B) Distribution of the blood supply to the spleen shows the relationship of splenic arterioles to the periarteriolar lymphoid sheath (PALS) and attached lymphoid follicles. (Figure A adapted from Atlas of Human Anatomy, with illustrations by Frank H. Netter, MD. Teterboro, NJ: Icon Learning Systems, 1989. All rights reserved; Figure B adapted from Abbas AK. Basic Immunology: Functions and Disorders of the Immune System. Philadelphia: WB Saunders, 2001.)

B

In human fetal life, the spleen is a site of production of both red and white cells. This function is lost in the adult human, in whom the spleen serves mainly to filter blood and to mediate immune function.

FILTERING FUNCTION

The spleen removes old, effete red cells, cellular elements, and bacterial debris from circulation. Every day, the spleen removes about 20 mL of aged red cells. Cells that have immunoglobulin G (IgG) on their surfaces are removed by monocytes. The spleen also removes abnormal white cells, platelets, and cell debris.

IMMUNOLOGIC PROCESSES

The spleen, a necessary portion of the peripheral lymphoid system, is populated by mature T and B lymphocytes. The T lymphocytes are responsible for cell-mediated immune functions, and the B lymphocytes produce a humoral (immunoglobulin) or antibody response to antigen. The immunologic functions of the spleen may be summarized as follows:

1. Opsonin production. The spleen produces tuftsin and properdin. Tuftsin coats granulocytes, promoting their phagocytosis. Properdin initiates complement activation to produce destruction of bacteria and foreign bodies trapped within the spleen.
2. Antibody synthesis. Immunoglobulin M (IgM) is produced by the white pulp in response to soluble antigens.
3. Protection from infection. Splenectomy leaves some patients prone to infection, sometimes to fulminant sepsis. While the known immunologic functions of the spleen are undoubtedly important in protection from infection, the mechanism is not fully understood.
4. Storage function. About one-third of the body's platelets are stored in the spleen at any time.

The spleen is enlarged in a number of pathologic conditions. Some forms of splenomegaly are associated with hypersplenism, which causes an increase in destruction of red cells, white cells, and/or platelets. The increased destruction is a result of either abnormally shaped blood elements getting entrapped in and destroyed by the spleen or splenic enlargement leading to entrapment and destruction of normal blood cells.

PRIMARY HYPERSPLENISM

A rare condition that primarily affects women, primary hypersplenism is a diagnosis of exclusion of all possible causes of secondary hypersplenism (see below). The cause is unknown. It is characterized by splenomegaly and exaggerated destruction or sequestration of circulating blood elements. Anemia, leukopenia, and/or thrombocytopenia may occur. Recurrent fever and infections are common.

SECONDARY HYPERSPLENISM

Congestive Splenomegaly

Portal Hypertension

Portal hypertension causes splenomegaly in approximately 60% of cases. Of these, only 25% develop hypersplenism with mild anemia and thrombocytopenia. Splenomegaly is more common when portal hypertension is due to presinusoidal block. Nearly always, portal hypertension that causes splenomegaly also causes esophageal and sometimes gastric varices (Figure 10.3).

Splenic Vein Thrombosis

Splenic vein thrombosis may occur secondary to acute or chronic pancreatitis and pancreatic neoplasm. It can occur spontaneously in women taking birth control pills. It may also complicate polycythemia vera. Splenomegaly caused

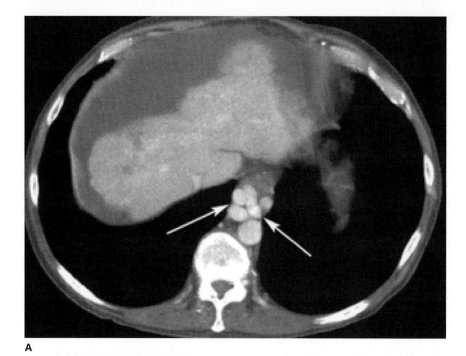

A

B

FIGURE 10.3. Varices in splenomegaly and portal hypertension. (A) A CT scan of the upper abdomen in a patient with end-stage cirrhosis demonstrates large esophageal varices (arrows) as well as a nodular liver. (B) Portal venogram obtained during a transjugular, intrahepatic, portosystemic shunt (TIPS) procedure demonstrates gastric varices and portal hypertension. (Courtesy of Henry I. Goldberg, MD.)

by splenic vein thrombosis is rarely associated with hypersplenism. When it causes varices, these are nearly always gastric rather than esophageal.

Sequestrative Splenomegaly

The most common causes of sequestrative splenomegaly are congenital diseases of the red cells and hemoglobinopathies. The red cells are abnormal either because they are too large or misshapen. In either case, the cells become trapped in the splenic pulp because of their inability to undergo the necessary deformation to pass through the capillary microcirculation.

Diseases of Red Blood Cells

HEREDITARY SPHEROCYTOSIS Hereditary spherocytosis, the most commonly diagnosed of the congenital hemolytic anemias, is transmitted through autosomal dominant inheritance. It is a disease of the red cell, in which the membrane lacks the necessary structural protein assembly. The cell becomes small, dense, and lacking in deformability. Clinically, the disease is manifested by hemolytic anemia, splenomegaly, and nonconjugated hyperbilirubinemia with negative Coombs' test. Special staining of peripheral blood shows the spherocytes, and reticulocyte count in the blood is elevated. Intravenous injection of the patient's own red cells labeled with ^{51}Cr shows greatly shortened half-life. The enlarged spleen may cause left upper quadrant discomfort and is more susceptible to traumatic rupture. As a result of the large hemoglobin load secondary to hemolysis, pigment stones form in approximately 85% of patients.

HEREDITARY ELLIPTOCYTOSIS As the name implies, hereditary elliptocytosis is a congenital disease in which over 25% of red cells in the peripheral blood are elliptic in shape. Again, the abnormality is in the red cell membrane, and the abnormally shaped red cells are destroyed by the spleen. Splenomegaly, mild anemia, and jaundice result as clinical manifestations in 10% to 15% of affected individuals.

Hemoglobinopathies

SICKLE-CELL ANEMIA Another hereditary disease, sickle-cell anemia, occurs predominantly in blacks and is due to the replacement of the normal hemoglobin-A (Hb-A) by sickle hemoglobin (Hb-S). Under conditions of reduced oxygen tension, Hb-S molecules crystallize within the red cell, causing it to elongate and become sickle-shaped. Conditions of reduced pH and circulatory stasis aggravate sickling. The sickle cells contribute to increased blood viscosity and increased incidence of vascular thrombosis. The condition is associated with splenomegaly in the early stages, but as the spleen undergoes repeated infarctions, its size may decrease in later stages.

Approximately 9% of the African American population in the United States have the sickle trait, but only approximately 1% are clinically symptomatic.[1] Symptoms include anemia, jaundice with intermittent acute attacks, or sickle-cell crises related to vascular occlusion. The acute attacks can cause an acute abdomen, acute bone or joint pain, and acute neurological deficits. The symptoms manifest in childhood in the first decade of life. Most affected individuals die before the age of 60 years.

Evaluation of anemia shows the presence of characteristic sickle cells in peripheral blood. On hemoglobin electrophoresis, more than 80% of the hemoglobin is Hb-S. Mild, nonconjugated hyperbilirubinemia and increased incidence of pigment stone formation may also occur.

THALASSEMIA (MEDITERRANEAN ANEMIA) Thalassemia is also transmitted by a dominant genetic trait characterized by a deficit in the synthesis of the peptide chain. Three forms are recognized: alpha, beta, and gamma. The most common form in the United States and Southern Europe is beta-thalassemia, characterized by quantitative reduction in the synthesis of the beta chain, which results in decreased Hb-A. Intracellular deposition of hemoglobin creates Heinz bodies that contribute to the fragility of the red cell.

Clinically, the disease occurs in two forms of severity: major and minor. Thalassemia major usually presents in the first year of life and is manifested by failure to thrive, a large head, splenomegaly, leg ulcers, and anemia. Increased susceptibility to infection and pigment stone formation occur. Most patients with thalassemia minor are asymptomatic. A peripheral blood smear shows hypochromic, microcytic anemia with target cells, and other misshapen red cells. Alkaline denaturation studies show reduction in Hb-A levels and persistence of fetal hemoglobin (Hb-F).

Autoimmune Hemolytic Anemia

The disease develops when an individual generates hemagglutinin-type antibodies to antigens in his or her red blood cells. The spleen is the likely source of the antibodies. As a result of immune reaction, red cells undergo hemolysis, and their lifespan is shortened as the cells are destroyed in the spleen. Splenomegaly and mild jaundice develop. Autoimmune hemolytic anemia is twice as common in women as in men, and peak age of incidence is the fifth decade. A severe form of the disease associated with severe anemia, hemoglobinuria, and renal tubular necrosis has a mortality rate of up to 50%.[2] A diagnostic feature of this hemolytic anemia is a positive Coombs' test done with peripheral blood.

Diseases of Platelets

IDIOPATHIC THROMBOCYTOPENIC PURPURA (ITP) This acquired disease results from destruction of platelets by circulating IgG antiplatelet factors originating from the spleen. Idiopathic thrombocytopenic purpura (ITP) is three times more prevalent in women than in men. The platelet count is reduced below 50,000 mm^3. Bleeding time is prolonged, while clotting time is normal.

Clinically, the most common presentation pertains to petechiae, easy bruisability, bleeding gums, or bleeding from the gastrointestinal or genitourinary tracts. Cerebrovascular accidents occur in 1% to 2% of these patients. The spleen is not enlarged and there is no abnormality in red cell or white cell counts. Bone marrow examination shows normal or an elevated megakaryocyte count.

ITP is the most common hematologic indication for splenectomy, usually performed following failure of medical therapy (e.g., steroids, IgG, plasmapheresis).

THROMBOTIC THROMBOCYTOPENIC PURPURA (TTP) Abnormalities of capillaries and arterioles, which are irregularly narrowed by subendothelial deposition of collagen, cause thrombotic thrombocytopenic purpura (TTP). This vascular abnormality leads to diffuse platelet trapping, leading further to thrombocytopenia. In these patients, thrombocytopenia is associated with hemolytic anemia, the symptoms of which include fever and neurological and renal abnormalities. The disease is so effectively treated with plasmapheresis that splenectomy is only occasionally required.

MYELOPROLIFERATIVE DISORDERS Replacement of the bone marrow in myeloproliferative disorders leads to anemia, splenomegaly, and thrombocytopenia (two-thirds of cases) or thrombocytosis (one-third of cases). Splenectomy is required when splenomegaly becomes symptomatic (multiple splenic infarcts) or medical therapy (chemotherapy, transfusions) fail. In those patients with thrombocytosis, splenectomy may be complicated with splenic and portal vein thrombosis. This complication may be avoided by perioperative treatment with anticoagulants or with drugs that prevent platelet aggregation.

SPLENIC CYSTS AND NEOPLASMS

Splenic Cysts

Splenic cysts are rare and may be true or false depending on whether or not they have epithelial lining. True cysts may be parasitic or nonparasitic. Approximately 10% of all splenic cysts are congenital, nonparasitic cysts. By far, the most common cysts are false, and most (75%) of them are secondary to post-traumatic hematoma.[3] Splenic cysts may be asymptomatic or may cause vague left upper quadrant abdominal discomfort. Diagnosis is readily established by ultrasonography; CT examination is usually not necessary. The cysts may be treated with splenectomy, cyst excision, or marsupialization.

Splenic Neoplasms

Primary splenic neoplasms are rare and may be lymphoid or nonlymphoid.

Lymphoid Tumors

Lymphoid tumors include Hodgkin's lymphoma and non-Hodgkin's lymphoma. Hodgkin's lymphoma of the spleen is usually a manifestation of disseminated Hodgkin's disease. NonHodgkin's lymphoma may be lymphocytic (small cell) or histiocytic, with the latter carrying a poorer prognosis. The spleen may also be involved in chronic myelocytic leukemia (CML) and chronic lymphocytic leukemia (CLL).

Nonlymphoid Tumors

The most common nonlymphoid tumors are vascular and include hemangiomas, lymphangiomas, and hemangioendotheliomas.

Tumors Metastatic to the Spleen

The spleen is an infrequent site of metastatic tumor. The neoplasms that metastasize to the spleen include breast, lung, and melanoma.

Splenic Abscess

Splenic abscess is rare and may be due to fungal or bacterial infection.

Fungal Abscess

Fungal abscesses occur mainly in patients undergoing prolonged antibiotic or steroid therapy, in those undergoing chemotherapy, and in immunocompromised patients. Approximately 75% of these abscesses are due to candida infection.

Bacterial (Pyogenic) Abscess

Predisposing conditions for bacterial splenic abscess include diabetes, bacterial endocarditis, conditions causing splenic infarcts, intravenous drug use, and steroid therapy. Splenic abscesses may also occur following colectomy or gastrectomy by contiguous spread. The most common bacteria involved are *Escherichia coli*, *Streptococcus viridans*, *Staphylococcus aureus*, and *Bacteroides fragilis*. Splenic abscesses may be treated with percutaneous drainage when unilocular or with splenectomy. Splenic abscess is one of the causes of fever of unknown origin.

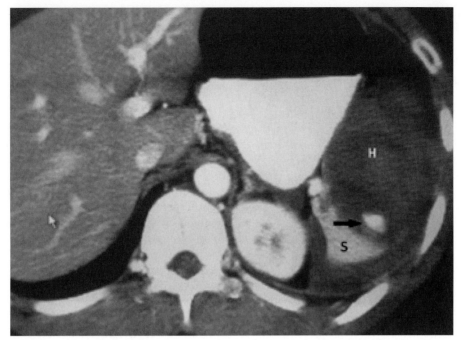

FIGURE 10.4. Ruptured spleen. The CT scan of a patient following a motor vehicle accident shows a macerated spleen (S) with a large perisplenic hematoma (H) and some active bleeding (black arrow). (Courtesy of Vincent McCormick, MD.)

SPLENIC TRAUMA

The spleen is the intraabdominal solid organ most commonly injured by blunt trauma (Figure 10.4). The spleen may also be damaged by penetrating injury or as a result of operative trauma during abdominal surgery. Operative trauma is responsible for approximately 20% of splenectomies and is most common during left colectomy, gastric surgery, and hiatal hernia repair. In reoperative surgery, a typical mechanism of injury is avulsion of adhesions to the spleen by traction. The enlarged spleen is more susceptible to rupture from abdominal trauma and may also undergo spontaneous rupture, although it is rare. Approximately 5% of blunt injuries to the spleen may cause delayed rupture of a contained hematoma occurring days to weeks after trauma. Grading systems for splenic trauma, such as the one shown in Table 10.1, provide a useful guide to management.

TABLE 10.1. Grading of Traumatic Splenic Injuries

Grade*	Type of injury	Injury description
I	Hematoma	Subcapsular, <10% surface
	Laceration	Capsular tear, <1 cm parenchymal depth
II	Hematoma	Subcapsular, 10%–50% surface area; intraparenchymal hematoma, <5 cm in diameter
	Laceration	1–3 cm parenchymal depth that does not involve a trabecular vessel
III	Hematoma	Subcapsular, >50% surface area or expanding; ruptured subcapsular or parenchymal hematoma; intraparenchymal hematoma >5 cm or expanding
	Laceration	>3 cm parenchymal depth or involving trabecular vessels
IV	Laceration	Laceration involving segmental or hilar vessels producing major devascularization (>25% of spleen)
V	Laceration	Completely shattered spleen
	Vascular	Hilar vascular injury that devascularizes spleen

* Advance one grade for multiple injuries, up to grade III.
Adapted with permission from Moore EE, Cogbill TH, Jurkovich GJ, et al. Organ injury scaling: spleen and liver (1994 revision). J Trauma 1995;38:323.

NONOPERATIVE MANAGEMENT OF SPLENIC INJURY

Not all patients with traumatic injury require splenectomy. It is particularly important to avoid surgery whenever possible in infants and children because they have a higher susceptibility to postoperative sepsis. Nonoperative management of splenic injury is possible in some 25% of patients where the cause is blunt abdominal trauma. The decision to manage nonoperatively should be made judiciously and be accompanied by implementation of a strict clinical monitoring protocol in the intensive care unit. Once imaging studies establish the presence of splenic injury, the conditions that permit nonoperative approach include: (1) hemodynamic stability, (2) absence of peritonitis, (3) absence of associated injuries that require operative treatment, and (4) total transfusion requirements not exceeding 2 U.

SPLENECTOMY

Indications

The indications for splenectomy are summarized in Table 10.2. The conditions listed as absolute indications represent only those conditions in which splenectomy is always indicated and is either lifesaving or associated with predictable response.

Over the past 25 years, management of splenic trauma has undergone significant change as the complications of postsplenectomy sepsis became more appreciated, as successful techniques of splenorrhaphy have been developed, and as the role of conservative management of splenic trauma—particularly in children—has become established. As sophisticated imaging techniques have developed, the incidence of using laparotomy for staging Hodgkin's disease has decreased, although the procedure continues to be useful in determining therapy.

Idiopathic thrombocytopenic purpura (ITP) continues to be the most common condition for which splenectomy is indicated. When steroid therapy, intravenous immunoglobulins, and plasmapheresis fail to aid the patient with ITP, splenectomy has a positive response rate in 85%. Platelet counts rise to $100,000/mm^3$ or higher in approximately 70% of patients. A patient's failure to respond initially or relapse of thrombocytopenia after successful response to splenectomy may be associated with the presence of an accessory spleen.

Preoperative Preparation for Splenectomy

To minimize postsplenectomy sepsis, patients should undergo immunization against pneumococcus, *Hemophilus Influenza B*, and meningococcus at least 2 to 3 weeks before surgery. Antibiotics (cephalosporins) are used perioperatively to reduce wound infection. In patients with massive splenomegaly, preoperative splenic artery embolization with coils is a useful technique to reduce the size of the spleen and minimize risk of major intraoperative bleeding. In patients undergoing splenectomy for ITP, platelets are administered only after the splenic artery is ligated. The essential features of postsplenectomy sepsis are summarized in Table 10.3.

TABLE 10.2. Indications for Splenectomy

Absolute indications
  Bleeding varices due to splenic vein thrombosis
  Hereditary spherocytosis
  Massive splenic trauma
  Primary splenic malignancy

Relative indications
  Autoimmune hemolytic anemia
  Hypersplenism due to portal hypertension
  Idiopathic thrombocytopenic purpura
  Leukemia (esp. CML)
  Lymphoma
  Myelofibrosis
  Primary hypersplenism
  Sickle-cell disease
  Splenic abscess
  Staging for Hodgkin's lymphoma
  Thalassemia
  Thrombotic thrombocytopenic purpura

Abbreviation: CML, chronic myleogenous leukemia.

TABLE 10.3. Essential Features: Postsplenectomy Sepsis

Scope of problem
  Increase in mortality rate 200-fold
  Frequency of pneumonia, septicemia, and meningitis increased
    166 times
  Incidence of overwhelming sepsis: 4%

Pathophysiology
  Decreased clearance of bacteria
  Reduced phagocytosis
  Reduced opsonin production
  Reduced IgM production

Prophylaxis
  Postpone splenectomy until age 6 years
  Presplenectomy vaccination for
  ■ Pneumococcus
  ■ *Hemophilus Influenza B*
  ■ Meningococcus
  Use of penicillin
  ■ Perioperative
  ■ Continuous use in children under 2 years
  ■ Prescription for all adults

Abbreviation: IgM, immunoglobulin M.

Surgical Technique

Splenectomy can be performed with the open technique or laparoscopically. Laparoscopic splenectomy is rapidly gaining popularity but should be performed only by surgeons with advanced laparoscopic training.

Open Splenectomy

The type of incision selected depends not only on the surgeon's choice but also on whether the splenectomy is part of a larger procedure, e.g., staging laparotomy, in which case a midline incision is preferred. Otherwise, a midline or a subcostal incision can be used. In patients with massive splenomegaly, a double subcostal incision probably affords the best exposure, allowing early control of the splenic artery in the lesser sac. Early control of the splenic artery is not routinely required.

The first step in splenectomy is to mobilize the spleen by retracting it medially and inferiorly to expose the suspensory ligaments (Figure 10.5A). The splenorenal, lienorenal, and splenocolic ligaments are divided with scissors or electrocautery. Using gentle blunt dissection with the fingers behind the spleen, the organ can then be delivered onto the abdomen. Next, the short gastric arteries can be individually divided and ligated. (Figure 10.5B). The hilum of the spleen is then approached, and the distal extent of the pancreatic tail is carefully examined. The splenic artery and vein are readily identified at the hilum. The splenic artery is first divided between large clamps. The proximal end is ligated with 0-silk and then ligated with sutures distal to the ligature. The distal end is ligated singly and the artery divided between ligatures. The splenic vein is then handled similarly, taking care not to avulse smaller tributary veins. Any residual attachments of the spleen to surrounding strictures are divided and the spleen removed. The splenic bed is now thoroughly irrigated with saline and examined for any bleeding. The abdomen is closed in the usual fashion, leaving a closed sump drain in the left upper quadrant. The drain is brought out through a separate stab wound.

Removal of the massively enlarged spleen requires special precautions that have already been discussed. The two techniques include preoperative obliteration of the splenic artery using coils inserted by interventional radiology or intraoperative ligation of the splenic artery in the lesser sac before mobilizing the spleen. Another circumstance that requires special precaution is the performance of splenectomy for ITP. In this case, care must be taken not to breach the splenic capsule and spill out splenic tissue. This unfortunate occurrence might lead to splenosis and recurrence of ITP postoperatively. Another useful precaution in ITP is to carefully search for accessory spleen in the region of the splenic flexure, at the tail of the pancreas, and in the greater omentum attached to the transverse colon.

Placing a nasogastric tube in the patient postoperatively is prudent, although not all surgeons use it. If used, it is inserted after induction of anesthesia and usually removed within 24 h. In the older surgical literature, the complication of acute gastric dilatation, causing hemodynamic collapse, was seen not infrequently following splenectomy.

Laparoscopic Splenectomy

Removing the enlarged spleen laparoscopically is a challenge that should probably be avoided. Laparoscopic splenectomy is, however, rapidly becoming the preferred procedure in conditions such as ITP, where the spleen is normal in size. The patient is positioned on the operating table with the left side elevated 45°, using a bean bag. The lateral position provides excellent exposure of the splenic hilum, although some surgeons routinely use the supine approach.

Five trocars are placed as shown in Figure 10.6. After institution of pneumoperitoneum, the camera trocar is first inserted in the subumbilical area. To accommodate instruments, which the surgeon uses with his or her left hand, two (10–11 mm) trocars are placed in the midline, one in the subxiphoid area and another midway between this trocar and the xiphoid. A lateral trocar (10–11 mm) is placed in the left axillary line, midway between the costal margin and the iliac crest. Finally, a 12-mm trocar, which will be used to introduce the endovascular cutter, is inserted to the left of the rectus sheath and slightly above the umbilicus.

Following a general inspection of the abdomen, the splenic artery is identified and ligated with a clip in the lesser sac. This step is performed first to avoid hemorrhage during dissection of the spleen. Not all surgeons do this, nor is it always necessary. Next, the spleen is mobilized by dividing the splenocolic ligament after retracting the spleen superiorly and the splenic flexure inferiorly. This brings into complete view the inferior pole of the spleen and makes the splenic hilum accessible. The lienophrenic and splenorenal ligaments are then divided to mobilize the spleen. The hilar vessels are dissected with right-angled instruments and divided between clips and/or ligatures. The short gastric vessels are then ligated and divided individually.

Once the spleen is completely freed, it is placed in a specimen bag, a procedure that needs to be learned. The opening of the specimen bag is triangulated and held by three graspers introduced through the two upper midline trocars and the left lateral trocar. The specimen is extracted within the bag either intact through a small incision in the abdominal wall or after breaking up the tissue within the bag by morcellation and then removing it through the 12-mm trocar.

Conversion into open splenectomy occurs in less than 5%. Laparoscopic splenectomy takes an average of 30 to 60 minutes longer, but it is at least as safe as open splenectomy in terms of morbidity. It is likely, but as yet unproven, that laparoscopy will prove to be the best

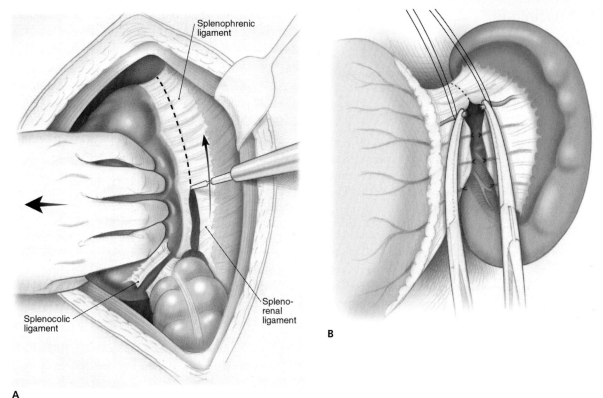

A

B

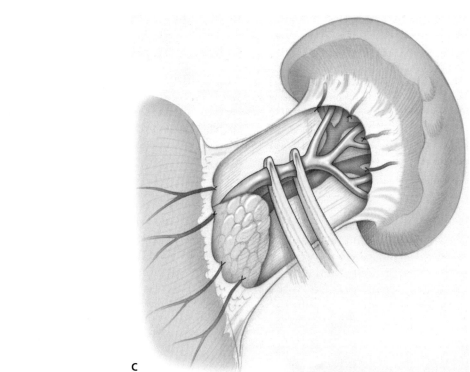

C

FIGURE 10.5. Technique of open splenectomy. (A) The spleen is mobilized by dividing the splenophrenic and splenorenal ligaments and brought forward onto the wound using blunt dissection. (B) The short gastric vessels are then divided between clamps and ligated, making sure not to incorporate gastric wall in the ligature. (C) The splenic artery and vein are then isolated at the splenic hilum, divided between clamps, and ligated with sutures, while avoiding damage to the tail of the pancreas. (Adapted from Norton JA, ed. Surgery: Basic Science and Clinical Evidence. New York: Springer, 2001:772.)

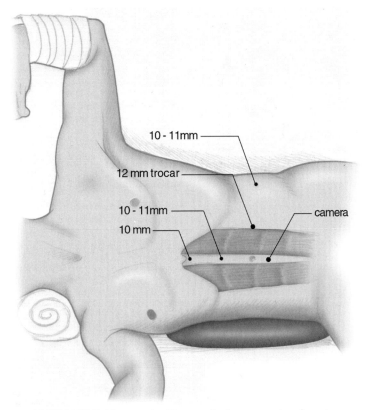

FIGURE 10.6. Placement of trocars for laparoscopic splenectomy.

technique in identifying accessory spleens. Approximately 10% of patients are said to have accessory spleens, but the figure is probably higher in patients who have previously sustained splenic injury.

Partial Splenectomy

Subtotal splenectomy has been used in recent years in order to salvage at least some splenic function. The main indications are hypersplenism or traumatic injury in children that requires splenectomy. In hypersplenism, approximately 80% of the spleen is resected. All patients undergoing a partial splenectomy should receive the same immunization as patients undergoing total splenectomy.

The technique of partial splenectomy requires excellent exposure and full mobilization of the spleen. Arrangement of the splenic vessels at the hilum is inspected. The splenic artery usually divides into three main branches before entering the spleen: a superior branch supplying 20% to 25% of the spleen, a large central branch supplying 60% to 70%, and a small inferior branch supplying 10% to 20%. In elective partial splenectomy, the inferior portion of the spleen is usually easier to preserve. Next, the splenic veins are carefully dissected. The vessels to that portion of the spleen to be resected are ligated and divided. The devascularized region then turns dark purple. The spleen is transected either with electrocautery or a carefully performed finger-fracture technique. The cut edge of spleen is sutured with overlapping horizontal mattress

sutures of 1-0 absorbable material over Teflon® pledgets (Du Pont,™ Wilmington, DE), using long straight needles (Figure 10.7).

Incidental Intraoperative Injury of the Spleen

The spleen may be inadvertently injured in a number of upper abdominal operations, especially gastric, hiatal hernia, and left colon operations. Inadvertent injury to the spleen is more common in patients who have had previous abdominal surgery because of adhesions to the splenic capsule. In these circumstances, splenic injury may be avoided by early division of adhesions to the spleen before retraction is applied. Another cause of operative trauma to the spleen is the use of deep and unprotected retractors and vigorous application of retraction. The most common injury is a linear capsular tear or avulsion of a small piece of spleen. Massive injury or injury extending to the hilum is infrequent. Bleeding from capsular tears can frequently be managed without splenectomy, provided the bleeding can be controlled. Successful techniques include:

1. Temporary firm packing.
2. Application of hemostatic agents in combination with packing, including thrombin-impregnated Gelfoam® (Pharmacia Upjohn, Peapack, NJ) and Avitene®-microfibrillar collagen (Davol Inc., Cranston, RI).

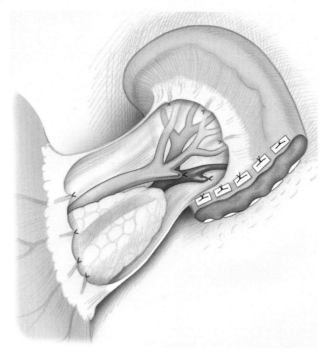

FIGURE 10.7. Technique for partial splenectomy.

3. Splenorrhaphy, which requires ligation of individual vessels and approximation of the splenic capsule with 1-0 absorbable sutures tied over Teflon® pledgets (Figure 10.8).

Postsplenectomy Course and Complications

Complications that may occur following splenectomy are summarized in Table 10.4.

Hematologic Changes

Leukocytosis and increased platelet counts are seen in most patients following splenectomy. The changes develop within 24 to 48h and may last for weeks or months. Peripheral blood shows typical Howell–Jolly bodies.

TABLE 10.4. Complications of Splenectomy
Hematologic changes
Thrombocytosis
Leukocytosis
Atelectasis
Injury to surrounding structures
Gastric perforation
Colonic injury
Pancreatic fistula
Postoperative hemorrhage
Subphrenic abscess
Postsplenectomy sepsis
Increased incidence of pneumonia, septicemia, meningitis
Overwhelming postsplenectomy sepsis of
■ 0.8% in adults
■ Higher in children

Pulmonary Complications

Left lower lobe atelectasis may sometimes develop postsplenectomy.

Subphrenic Hematoma

Subphrenic hematoma presents with left upper quadrant pain, nausea, and sometimes fever. Abdominal ultrasound or CT scan establishes the diagnosis. Treatment with percutaneous catheter drainage is effective.

Subphrenic Abscess

Although subphrenic abscess is frequently due to secondary infection of blood or fluid collection, it is important to rule out injury to either the stomach or the splenic flexure of the colon as an underlying cause. Gastric and colonic injury are ruled out with upper and lower gastrointestinal studies with barium or Gastrografin (Figure 10.9). The abscess is usually readily drained percutaneously.

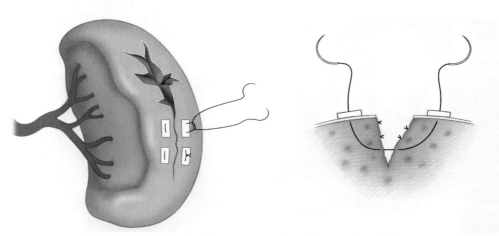

FIGURE 10.8. Repair of spleen rupture using splenorraphy and pledgets.

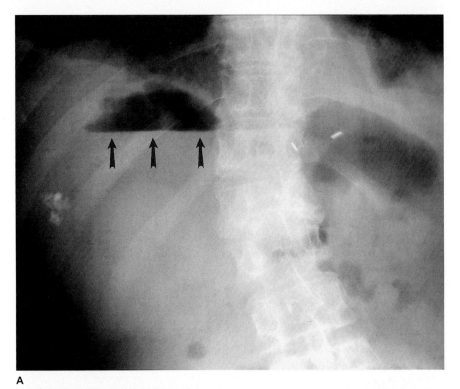

A

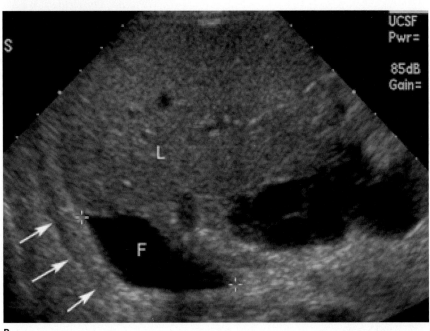

B

FIGURE 10.9. Subphrenic abscess can be demonstrated with contrast and ultrasound studies. (A) Upright radiograph of the abdomen in a patient with previous liver trauma due to a bullet wound demonstrates an air–fluid level typical of a subphrenic abscess (arrows). (B) Ultrasonography demonstrates the subphrenic fluid collection (F), bordered by the diaphragm (arrows) and by the liver (L). (Courtesy of Henry I. Goldberg, MD.)

Gastric Perforation

Gastric perforation is a rare complication probably occurring from inadvertent inclusion of the gastric wall in a ligature, although direct inadvertent injury is also possible. The clinical course is sepsis, often accompanied by respiratory failure. A Gastrografin study can show the leak from the gastric fundus. Reoperation is nearly always necessary to close the gastric perforation and adequately drain the left subphrenic space.

Colonic Injury

Injury to the splenic flexure usually presents as subphrenic abscess. Percutaneous drainage results in evacuation of purulent and fecal material. If sepsis is rapidly controlled and peritonitis is not present, conservative management may be possible so that a controlled fecal fistula develops. The fistula closes with time. On the other hand, if sepsis is not controlled, and particularly if signs of peritoneal irritation are present, reoperation will be necessary. The options then are to resect the splenic flexure and perform primary anastomosis or to create a diverting colostomy. Adequate antibiotic coverage is essential.

Injury to the Pancreas

The proximity of the tail of the pancreas to the splenic hilum has been emphasized. Typically, injury to the pancreas occurs during ligation and division of the splenic artery and vein at the hilum. The usual presentation is persistent fluid from the drainage tube. The fluid tends to be slightly cloudy but clear. The amylase content of the fluid should be measured and will be found to be high, indicating that a pancreatic fistula has developed.

Pancreatic fistulas are typically self-limited and close within 1 to 3 weeks on a regimen of no oral intake and administration of the longacting somatostatin analog octreotide (50–100 mg q8h subcutaneously). Rarely will pancreatic fistula fail to heal. Operative management may be necessary to accomplish distal pancreatectomy or a Roux-en-Y pancreaticojejunostomy.

Postsplenectomy Sepsis

Singer reported that deaths from sepsis in splenectomized patients are 200 times as frequent as in the general population.[4] Furthermore, the incidence of pneumonia, septicemia, and meningitis is 166 times greater in patients who have undergone splenectomy for trauma.[4] This finding is the basis for vaccination for pneumococcus, *H. influenza*, and meningococcus presplenectomy or immediately after surgery. Overwhelming postsplenectomy infection occurs in 0.3% of children and 0.1% of adults with a mortality rate of 1% to 7%.[5] This complication occurs within 2 years of splenectomy in two-thirds of cases.[6]

The increased susceptibility to infection following splenectomy is probably due to: (1) decreased clearance of bacteria from the blood; (2) reduced phagocytosis; (3) reduced formation of IgM; and (4) decreased production of opsonins, which contributes to reduced phagocytosis. Children, especially those less than 2 years old, are particularly susceptible. Preventive measures include: (1) vaccination as described above, (2) prophylactic penicillin administration in all children under 2 years of age, (3) a prescription to all adults for penicillin or other antibiotic, and (4) education about the symptoms of sepsis, so that they can start treatment if necessary before they go to the hospital.

REFERENCES

1. Schwartz SI, Shires GT, Spencer FC, eds. *Principles of Surgery*. 6th ed. New York: McGraw Hill; 1994:1440.
2. Schwartz SI. Splenectomy for hemorrhagic disorders. In: Hiatt JR, Phillips EH, Morgenstern L, eds. *Surgical Diseases of the Spleen*. New York: Springer-Verlag; 1996.
3. Sheldon GF, Croom RD III, Meyer AA. The spleen. In: Sabiston DC Jr, ed. *Textbook of Surgery: The Biological Basis of Modern Surgical Practice*. Philadelphia: WB Saunders; 1997:1207–1208.
4. Singer DB. Postsplenectomy sepsis. In: *Perspectives in Pediatric Pathology*. Vol 1. Chicago: Year Book Medical; 1973:285–331.
5. Styrt B. Infection associated with asplenia: risks, mechanisms, and prevention. *Am J Med* 1990;88:33N–42N.
6. Cullingford GL, Watkins DN, Watts AD, et al. Severe late postsplenectomy infection. *Br J Surg* 1991;78:716–721.

SELECTED READINGS

Adekile AD, Owunwanne A, Al-Za'abi K, et al. Temporal sequence of splenic dysfunction in sickle cell disease. *Am J Hematol* 2002;69:23–27.

Alonso Cohen MA, Galera MJ, Ruiz M, et al. Splenic abscess. *World J Surg* 1990;14:513–517.

Badura RA, Oliveira O, Palhano MJ, et al. Spontaneous rupture of the spleen as presenting event in infectious mononucleosis. *Scand J Infect Dis* 2001;33:872–874.

Bohnsack JF, Brown EJ. The role of the spleen in resistance to infection. *Annu Rev Med* 1986;37:49–59.

Brodsky J, Abcar A, Styler M. Splenectomy for non-Hodgkin's lymphoma. *Am J Clin Oncol* 1996;19:558–561.

Bynum B. The spleen. *Lancet* 2002;359:1624.

Cusack JC Jr, Seymour JF, Lerner S, et al. Role of splenectomy in chronic lymphocytic leukemia. *J Am Coll Surg* 1997;185:237–243.

Delaitre B, Pitre J. Laparoscopic splenectomy versus open splenectomy: a comparative study. *Hepatogastroenterology* 1997;44:45–49.

George JN, Woolf SH, Raskob GE, et al. Idiopathic thrombocytopenic purpura: a practice guideline developed by explicit methods for the American Society of Hematology. *Blood* 1996;88:3–40.

Glasgow RE, Yee LF, Mulvihill SJ. Laparoscopic splenectomy. The emerging standard. *Surg Endosc* 1997;11:108–112.

Herneth AM, Pokieser P, Philipp MO, et al. Role of Doppler sonography in the evaluation of accessory spleens after splenectomy. *J Ultrasound Med* 2001;20:1347–1351.

Horowitz J, Smith JL, Weber TK, et al. Postoperative complications after splenectomy for hematologic malignancies. *Ann Surg* 1996;223:290–296.

Katkhouda N, Hurwitz MB, Rivera RT, et al. Laparoscopic splenectomy: outcome and efficacy in 103 consecutive patients. *Ann Surg* 1998;228:568–578.

Lipshy KA, Shaffer DJ, Denning DA. An institutional review of the management of splenic trauma. *Contemp Surg* 1996;48:330.

Moore EE, Cogbill TH, Jurkovich GH, et al. Organ injury scaling: spleen and liver (1994 revision). *J Trauma* 1995;38:323–324.

Morgenstern, L. A History of splenectomy. In: Hiatt JR, Phillips EH, Morgenstern L, eds. *Surgical Diseases of the Spleen.* New York: Springer-Verlag, 1996.

Prevention of pneumococcal disease: recommendations of the Advisory Committee on Immunization Practices (ACIP). *MMWR* 1997 Apr 4;46(RR-8):1–24.

Schwab CW. Selection of nonoperative management candidates. *World J Surg* 2001;25:1389–1392.

Schwartz SI. Role of splenectomy in hematologic disorders. *World J Surg* 1996;20:1156–1159.

Taylor MA, Kaplan HS, Nelsen TS. Staging laparotomy with splenectomy for Hodgkin's disease: the Stanford experience. *World J Surg* 1985;9:449–460.

Tsiotos G, Schlinkert RT. Laparoscopic splenectomy for immune thrombocytopenic purpura. *Arch Surg* 1997;132:642–646.

Uranus S, Pfeifer J. Nonoperative treatment of blunt splenic injury. *World J Surg* 2001;25:1405–1407.

Abdominal Trauma

Abdominal trauma is a major cause of death. Nearly 40% of deaths from abdominal trauma are due to blunt trauma caused primarily by motor vehicle accidents. In these circumstances, abdominal trauma is often associated with head, chest, and extremity injury. Delay in diagnosis and treatment is a major contributing factor to mortality, which is often due to hemorrhage, sepsis, and multiple organ failure. Penetrating abdominal trauma, whether due to handguns or knives, is a significant problem associated with the use of alcohol and drugs. These injuries affect individuals in the most productive part of their lives. Organized trauma systems, including prehospital care, transport, and trauma centers, have improved the care of the injured patient. But much remains to be done to prevent trauma and improve legislation and the socioeconomic factors that contribute to the trauma environment.

This chapter focuses primarily on injuries of the gastrointestinal tract and only mentions injuries of the genitourinary system and the great vessels in the retroperitoneum.

MECHANISMS OF INJURY

Abdominal trauma occurs as a result of either acceleration–deceleration injuries or missile injuries.

ACCELERATION–DECELERATION INJURY

Most blunt abdominal trauma, whether caused by motor vehicle accidents, falls, or direct blow to the abdomen, is due to acceleration–deceleration injury. When the body is suddenly accelerated or halted, intra-abdominal organs, which are either filled with fluids or tethered, can undergo shearing or avulsion. Such injuries can cause tearing of the mesentery and hemorrhage, as well as fracture of the spleen and avulsion of the renal pedicle.

MISSILE INJURY

Several types of missile injury are possible: low velocity, high velocity, and bullet wounds.

Most civilian bullet wounds are low velocity. Missiles fired from handguns have a velocity in the range of 600 to 1100 ft/sec.[1] Typically, wounds from low-velocity missiles are restricted to the path of the bullet. It must be remembered, however, that the bullet may be deflected within the abdomen, and the path may not be direct from the entry to the exit wound. High-velocity missiles typically have a small entrance wound and a large exit wound, and they cause extensive damage to the tissue in their path. The damage caused by shotguns depends on whether they are fired at short or long range.

Short-range injuries cause massive soft tissue destruction. Long-range shotgun injuries are multiple, low-velocity pellet injuries. They cause widespread penetration but do not generally cause severe injury unless the missile directly hits an organ or blood vessel.

The reader is referred for full discussion to the excellent literature that exists on trauma. This chapter only briefly recapitulates the principles. The ABCDE mnemonic recommended by the American College of Surgeons Advanced Trauma Life Support (ATLS) is indispensable to prioritize the initial management of the traumatized patient. It recommends investigating the extent of injury in this sequence: airway, breathing, circulation, disability, and environment (Table 11.1).

Rapid control of the airway by early intubation is indicated if the patient: (1) is comatose or semicomatose; (2) is apneic or cyanosed; (3) has sustained major injury of the head, face, or neck; (4) has sustained chest trauma; or (5) is profoundly hypotensive. Abdominal trauma is often associated with thoracic injury, and tension pneumothorax should be ruled out. Signs of tension pneumothorax are: (1) hypotension; (2) distended neck veins; (3) inadequate ventilation, cyanosis, absence of breath sounds in one chest cavity; and (4) shift of the mediastinum and trachea to the opposite side. A chest tube must be inserted immediately.

Two large-bore intravenous lines are required when the patient is hemodynamically unstable. Volume resuscitation begins with the rapid administration of crystalloids. A urinary catheter is needed to monitor urine output, and

TABLE 11.1. Initial Management of Trauma: ATLS* Recommendations

A: Airway (establish patent airway)
B: Breathing (ensure both lungs are ventilated)
C: Circulation (restore circulating blood volume; control external bleeding by compression)
D: Disability (assess neurologic deficit; look for C-spine fracture)
E: Environment (expose patient completely to assess entire body)

* Advanced Trauma Life Support System recommended by American College of Surgeons.

a decision must be made whether monitoring of central venous or pulmonary artery pressure is required. Colloid resuscitation with albumin, plasma, or blood will be needed if hypotension is not reversed with the rapid infusion of 1 to 2 L of crystalloids. The goal of volume resuscitation is to restore tissue perfusion as judged by adequate urine output (50 ml/h), systolic pressure (>100 mm Hg), pulse rate (<100/min), central venous pressure (>6 mm Hg), and pulmonary artery pressure (>8 mm Hg). Inability to restore hemodynamic stability with rapid fluid administration usually indicates serious internal bleeding in the chest, the abdomen, or the soft tissues of the extremity.

EVALUATION OF ABDOMINAL TRAUMA

THE UNCONSCIOUS PATIENT

If the patient with multiple trauma is unconscious, it should be assumed that intraabdominal injury is present until specifically excluded. The quickest way to determine this is with diagnostic peritoneal lavage (DPL) after emptying the patient's bladder with a catheter. The open technique is preferred. A small infraumbilical incision is made and carried down to the peritoneum, which is then grasped with forceps and opened under direct vision. A lavage catheter is inserted. If no blood is immediately encountered, 1 L of saline is instilled into the peritoneal cavity and then withdrawn. The peritoneal tap is positive if: (1) gross blood is present; (2) more than 100,000 red blood cells/mL are present; and/or (3) bile, fecal matter, or bacteria are present.

If the unconscious patient with multiple trauma is hemodynamically stable, particularly if injury to a solid abdominal organ is suspected, abdominal CT examination may be preferable because liver or splenic fractures can be visualized.

THE CONSCIOUS PATIENT

The clinician is aided by the knowledge of symptoms and signs when the patient is lucid. The patient may complain of abdominal pain and/or may clearly demonstrate peritoneal irritation. A rapid increase in abdominal girth usually indicates severe intraabdominal bleeding. The absence of peritoneal signs, however, does not exclude the possibility of intraabdominal injury. Such patients, if hemodynamically stable, can be followed by repeated abdominal examination. If, however, the patient requires operative treatment for injury of other systems (head, extremity), peritoneal dialysis should be performed before surgery.

Abdominal injury may be associated with the use of motor vehicle seat belts. The most specific abdominal injury associated with seat belts is Chance's fracture: fracture of an upper lumbar vertebra, usually L-1, associated with rupture of the small intestine, usually the jejunum (Figure 11.1). But abdominal seat belt injuries may include lacerations of the colon, small bowel, liver, and spleen.

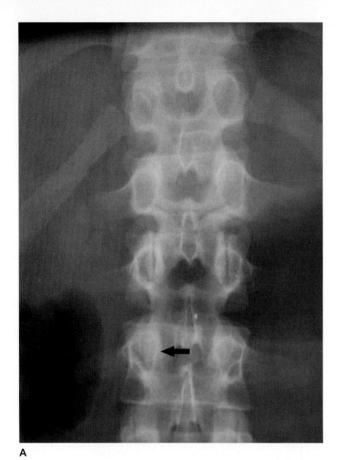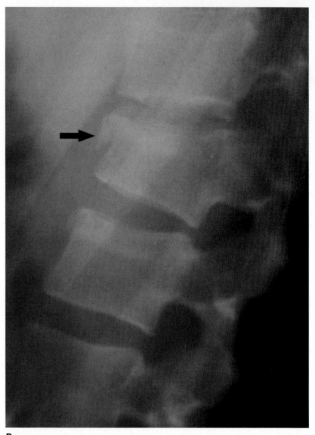

A   B

FIGURE 11.1. Chance's fracture. (A) Frontal view of the lumbar vertebrae in a patient with a seat belt injury shows lateral displacement of the pedicles (arrow), indicating fracture. (B) Lateral view of the lumbar spine in the same patient shows the compression fracture of the L-3 vertebral body (arrow). (Courtesy of Vincent McCormick, MD.)

MANAGEMENT OF SPECIFIC INTRAABDOMINAL ORGAN INJURIES

GASTRIC INJURY

Gastric injuries may be caused by blunt trauma but are more often due to penetrating injury, either by bullet or knife wounds. Penetrating wounds are often associated with injury to the diaphragm or colon. Gastric perforations are easily treated by debridement and two-layer closure. Both the anterior and posterior walls of the stomach must be inspected. Associated diaphragmatic injuries significantly raise the likelihood of postoperative empyema of the left chest.

DUODENAL INJURY

Duodenal injuries may result from either blunt or penetrating trauma and may vary in their severity. Table 11.2 provides a useful scale of duodenal trauma. Generally, severe injury (Grades IV and V) is seen in bullet wound trauma. Two important types of duodenal injury seen in blunt trauma are intramural hematoma and retroperitoneal rupture.

TABLE 11.2. Management of Duodenal Injury

Injury	Surgical treatment
Duodenal hematoma (Grade I)	Conservative (NG suction and TPN) Duodenojejunostomy if no resolution of obstruction in 2–3 weeks
Retroperitoneal rupture	
Grade II	Primary repair and closed drainage
Grade III	Primary repair, pylorus exclusion, tube decompression of duodenum
Major disruption (Grade IV)	Primary repair, pyloric exclusion, or pancreatico-duodenectomy
Massive disruption (Grade V)	Pancreaticoduodenectomy

Abbreviations: NG suction, nasogastric suction; TPN, total parenteral nutrition.

Duodenal Hematoma (Grade I)

Duodenal hematoma is an uncommon injury caused by blunt trauma. It occurs more frequently in children than in adults; the mechanism is often blunt injury to the upper abdomen caused by a fall on the handlebar of a bicycle. The trauma may be trivial and symptoms may not occur for 8 to 12 h.

Clinical Presentation

The presenting symptom is persistent vomiting and inability to eat or drink. Abdominal pain is uncommon. Duodenal hematoma typically occurs distal to the entrance of the common bile duct, and the vomitus is typically bilious. Abdominal examination may show bruising in the upper abdomen but is otherwise negative. A nasogastric tube should be inserted.

Diagnosis

Diagnosis can be established either by upper gastrointestinal examination with a water-soluble contrast medium or abdominal CT scan (Figure 11.2). If an upper GI examination is done, complete obstruction is seen, usually between the second and third parts of the duodenum. Characteristically, the contrast medium ends in obstruction that has a "spring-coil" appearance. No contrast medium, however, leaks out of the duodenum. The hematocrit and white blood count are usually normal. Rarely, associated trauma to the head of the pancreas may cause elevation of the serum amylase.

Management

In the past, acute obstruction of the duodenum from intramural hematoma was an indication for urgent surgery. Most patients now, however, are given time to resolve their obstruction.

Initial conservative management is instituted with nasogastric suction, correction of fluid and electrolytes, and total parenteral nutrition. Institution of acid reduction therapy with an H_2-receptor antagonist or proton-pump inhibitor significantly decreases nasogastric suction. Gastrografin swallow is repeated within 10 to 15 days. If obstruction has resolved, nasogastric suction is discontinued; oral fluids are then started slowly and advanced to a solid food diet as tolerated. If obstruction has not resolved completely, further conservative management for another week is appropriate.

Surgical treatment is indicated if the obstruction fails to resolve within approximately 3 weeks. No attempt should be made to evacuate the intramural hematoma. Instead, the site of obstruction should be bypassed. The bypass procedure of choice is side-to-side duodenojejunostomy (Figure 11.3). Gastrojejunostomy should be avoided whenever possible because: (1) it bypasses the pylorus and can lead to the dumping syndrome, and (2) late occurrence of anastomotic ulcer is a possible complication.

Retroperitoneal Rupture of the Duodenum (Grades II and III)

Retroperitoneal rupture of the duodenum most commonly results from steering wheel injury in motor vehicle

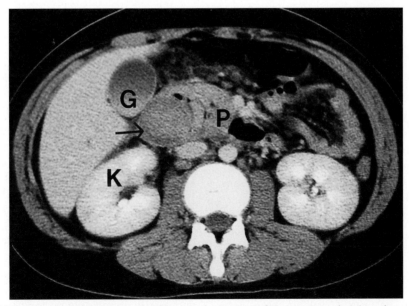

FIGURE 11.2. Duodenal hematoma. The CT scan of a patient after a motorcycle injury demonstrates a large duodenal hematoma (arrow) occupying the space between the head of the pancreas (P), the gallbladder (G), and the kidney (K). (Courtesy of Henry I. Goldberg, MD.)

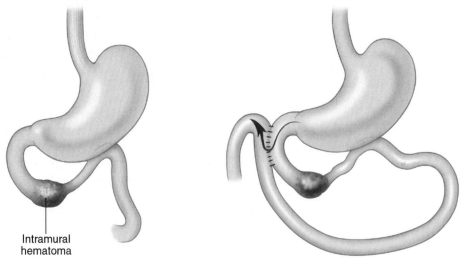

Intramural
hematoma

FIGURE 11.3. Side-to-side duodenojejunostomy.

accidents. The mechanism of injury is violent compression of the duodenum against the vertebra—particularly when the duodenum is closed at both ends—by the contracted pylorus proximally and by closure of the duodenojejunal flexure distally by the ligament of Treitz. The site of rupture is typically between the second and third portions of the duodenum, with extravasation of intestinal contents into the retroperitoneum.

Clinical Presentation

Because the duodenal rupture is retroperitoneal, peritoneal signs take time to develop. As a result, diagnosis is often delayed for 24 to 48h, increasing morbidity and mortality. Hence, in any severe injury of the upper abdomen, the possibility of retroperitoneal duodenal rupture must be considered. The symptoms are upper abdominal and thoracolumbar back pain. Fever and tachycardia are present and, with time, signs of peritonitis. If not treated emergently, full-blown peritonitis and septic shock ensue.

Diagnosis

Diagnosis is confirmed with radiologic studies. Plain films of the abdomen may show free retroperitoneal air, either alveolar in appearance or outlining retroperitoneal organs such as the kidney (Figure 11.4). Free air in the abdominal cavity is very rare. A picture of ileus may be present. Gastrografin upper GI studies or abdominal CT scan shows duodenal rupture and extravasation of dye into the retroperitoneum. CT scan is preferable because it facilitates diagnosis of any associated pancreatic injury.

Management

Fluid resuscitation and nasogastric suction should be instituted. Broad-spectrum antibiotics should be given intravenously and laparotomy performed as soon as the diagnosis is established. A midline incision is used to open and carefully explore the abdomen for associated injuries. The duodenum is best exposed by the Cattell maneuver, which consists of incising the lateral peritoneum and reflecting the right and transverse colon to the left (Figure 11.5). The Kocher maneuver can then be performed and the rupture will become apparent, usually between the second and third portions of the duodenum. The required surgical treatment depends on duration of injury and extent of damage to the duodenal wall. When treatment is undertaken early and the tear is simple, the edges of the perforation can be debrided and the duodenum closed in two layers. The peritoneum is then thoroughly irrigated with saline, and the abdomen is closed after instituting closed-suction drainage of the periduodenal area using a large-bore sump drain.

When duodenal injury is more complex (Grade III) or treatment delayed, postoperative complications must be anticipated. Usually, the edges of the defect can be debrided and duodenal closure accomplished without compromising the duodenal lumen. Jejunal serosal patch may be used for further protection. If this is not possible, the duodenal defect may be managed by creating a side-to-side duodenojejunostomy. In either case, not only must adequate closed-drainage of the retroperitoneum be established, but tube gastrostomy and feeding jejunostomy should also be constructed in anticipation of protracted postoperative course and/or duodenal leak. On occasion, intraluminal decompression of the duodenum may be advisable and is accomplished by threading a catheter into the duodenum through a jejunostomy and bringing the catheter out through a stab wound in the left upper quadrant. If the duodenal repair is such that the surgeon has serious concern about dehiscence, the judicious procedure is pyloric exclusion, in which the pylorus is stapled closed and gastrojejunostomy performed (Figure 11.6). In addition, tube decompression of the duodenum should be performed.

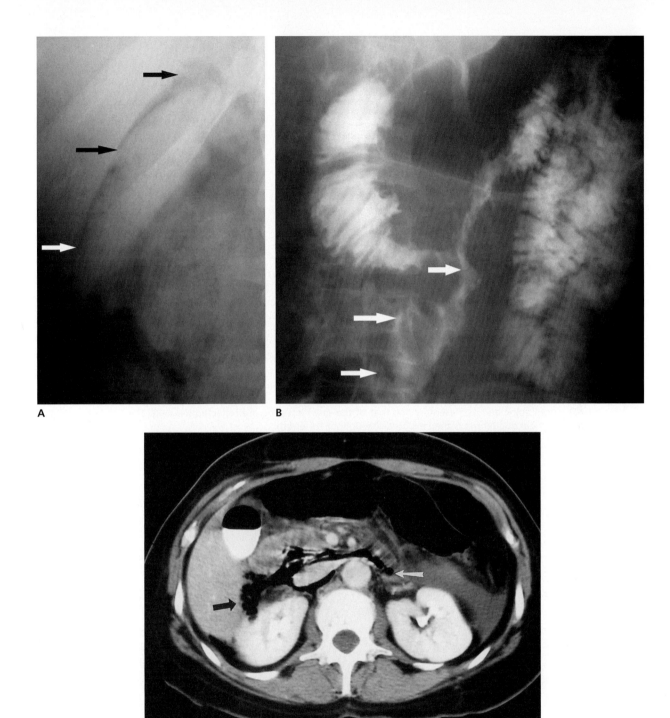

FIGURE 11.4. Duodenal retroperitoneal rupture. (A) The plain abdominal radiograph after blunt trauma shows streaks of retroperitoneal air around the right kidney (arrows), indicating duodenal rupture. (B) Water-soluble contrast material given orally shows the site of rupture in the transverse duodenum (arrows). (C) This CT scan demonstrates the extent of the retroperitoneal air from the duodenal rupture. The air dissects around the kidney, inferior vena cava, and aorta (arrows). (Courtesy of Vincent McCormick, MD, and Henry I. Goldberg, MD.)

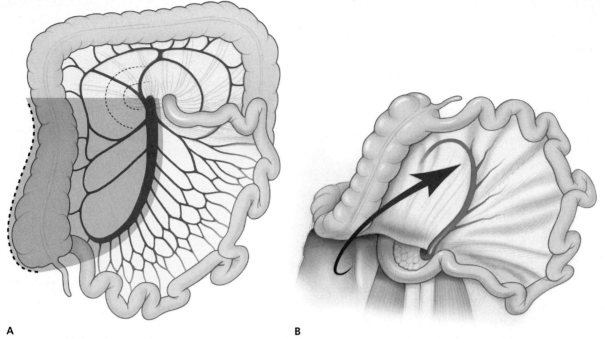

FIGURE 11.5. Cattel maneuver. The best exposure of the retroperitoneal duodenum is obtained using the Cattel maneuver. (A) The peritoneal reflection lateral to the ascending colon is incised sharply. (B) The right colon and its mesentery and that of the small intestine are reflected medially. The retroperitoneal duodenum is then exposed throughout its length.

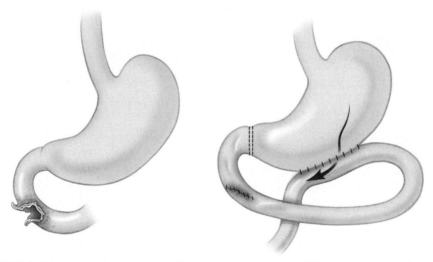

FIGURE 11.6. Pyloric exclusion procedure. The retroperitoneum should be adequately drained with a soft closed-drainage system.

The most important complications of this type of rupture are: duodenal leak, retroperitoneal abscess, delayed gastric emptying, and pancreatitis. The ancillary procedures described above anticipate all of these complications. The morbidity and mortality rates of this injury are significant and increase with delay in treatment and presence of other associated injuries.

Major Duodenal Disruption Involving Ampulla or Distal Common Bile Duct (Grade IV Injury)

Grade IV injury of the duodenum is fortunately rare and usually the result of a bullet wound. In this injury, major disruption of the duodenum occurs involving the ampulla or distal common bile duct (CBD). The diagnosis is usually made on abdominal exploration. When the injury is amenable to repair, surgical treatment consists of repair of the duodenal tear followed by pyloric exclusion. Otherwise, pancreaticoduodenectomy is required.

Massive Disruption of Duodenopancreatic Complex; Devascularized Duodenum (Grade V Injury)

This type of injury is serious and associated with a high mortality rate. The only treatment option is pancreaticoduodenectomy.

PANCREATIC INJURY

The pancreas may be injured in blunt or penetrating trauma. In either case, associated injury of the duodenum may be present. A simple classification of pancreatic injury is given in Table 11.3 and serves to guide treatment. Penetrating pancreatic trauma is often associated with vascular injury.

Diagnosis

Penetrating pancreatic injury is diagnosed and evaluated in the operating room. Pancreatic injury due to blunt trauma, on the other hand, can be difficult to diagnose. The mechanism of injury is usually a blow to the upper abdomen, often caused from being slammed against the steering wheel in car accidents. The patient may complain of upper abdominal pain radiating to the region of L-1. Ecchymosis may be present in the epigastrium. Signs of peritoneal irritation may or may not be present. Serum amylase is elevated in approximately 70% of cases; hence, normal levels of serum amylase do not exclude the presence of pancreatic injury. When the possibility of pancreatic injury is seriously entertained, or when the serum amylase level is elevated, a CT scan should be obtained. The CT scan may show swelling of the pancreas, mass

effect, or rarely, fracture of the pancreas at its neck (Figure 11.7). Pancreatic duct injury may sometimes be detected.

Management

All patients with penetrating trauma require prompt abdominal exploration. The indication for surgery in blunt trauma is not clear. A patient who is hemodynamically stable and without peritoneal signs, but who has evidence of pancreatic injury because of CT findings or elevated serum amylase, may be observed with repeated abdominal examinations. Such a patient usually has a Class I injury. Patients with severe disruption of the pancreas, however, require operative treatment.

A midline incision is performed and careful exploration of the abdomen undertaken. Thorough examination of the pancreas requires complete mobilization of the head by the Kocher maneuver. An associated duodenal injury will be evident if present. The lesser sac is entered through the gastrocolic omentum, and the anterior surface of the pancreas is carefully examined. Complete examination of the body and tail of the pancreas requires reflecting the spleen and the pancreas medially after division of the lateral attachments of the spleen. Further management depends on extent of the injury.

Class I Injury

Simple contusions (Class I injury) of the pancreas should be treated nonoperatively. If an operation must be performed for other indications, however, it is judicious to establish closed-suction drainage of the lesser sac.

Class II Injury

Class II injury involves laceration of the body or tail of the pancreas. One such injury is fracture of the pancreas at its neck as a result of blunt trauma (Figure 11.7). In these injuries, the surgeon encounters a hematoma of the body or tail of the pancreas. The key question at that point—whether there is disruption of the pancreatic duct—is

TABLE 11.3. Classification and Surgical Management of Pancreatic Injury

Class	Type of injury	Treatment
I	Simple contusions	Observation ± lesser sac drainage
II	Lacerations of the parenchyma in the body or tail	No ductal injury: Drainage of lesser sac
III	Severe disruption of the head or body	■ Involving head: Drainage ± gastrostomy and jejunostomy ■ If severe: Pancreaticoduodenectomy ■ If involving body: Distal pancreatectomy
IV	Associated with duodenal injury	■ Simple duodenal injury: Primary repair and drainage ■ Complex duodenal injury: Primary repair and pylorus exclusion ■ Severe disruption: Pancreaticoduodenectomy

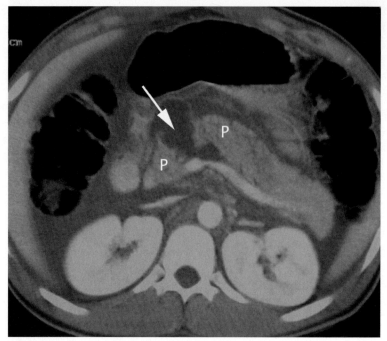

FIGURE 11.7. Pancreatic fracture. This CT scan shows a fracture (arrow) of the neck of the pancreas due to blunt abdominal trauma. The pancreas (P) is surrounded by fluid but otherwise appears normal. (Courtesy of Vincent McCormick, MD.)

often difficult to answer. Operative pancreatogram can be obtained but requires opening the duodenum. This procedure is used rarely and only if ductal injury is seriously suspected. If available, on-table endoscopic retrograde cholangiopancreatography (ERCP) should be done. Otherwise, the hematoma should be opened to facilitate operative evaluation for ductal injury. If no ductal injury is present, only drainage of the lesser sac is necessary. If ductal disruption is present, however, distal pancreatectomy should be performed.

Class III Injury

Class III injury involves severe disruption of the head or body of the pancreas. When the body of the pancreas is involved, the injury is treated with distal pancreatectomy. When the head is disrupted, however, the options are simple drainage or pancreaticoduodenectomy. The latter procedure is associated with a high mortality rate, and the surgeon may opt instead for drainage. If drainage is elected, a pancreatic fistula and protracted postoperative course should be anticipated. Hence, gastrostomy and feeding jejunostomy are advisable. Opening the gastrointestinal tract, however, increases the risk of infection; therefore, some surgeons prefer only total parenteral nutrition (TPN) and nasogastric drainage.

Class IV Injury

In Class IV trauma, both the pancreas and the duodenum are injured. Typically, the injury is to the pancreatic head. Surgical treatment depends on the severity of injury.

Simple duodenal injuries are primarily repaired, and the pancreatic injury is managed by drainage. If this is possible, the addition of tube gastrostomy and feeding jejunostomy is wise. More complicated injury of the duodenum requires the pylorus exclusion procedure. Massive injuries of the duodenum and pancreas require pancreaticoduodenectomy.

HEPATIC INJURY

The liver, the largest solid organ in the abdomen, is frequently injured in both blunt and penetrating trauma. Blunt trauma is more common, accounting for 85% of all cases of liver injury. In the urban setting, however, the incidence of penetrating trauma may be higher. The most common cause of blunt hepatic trauma is motor vehicle accident. The force required to injure the liver causes associated injuries of other organs in approximately 65% of cases of penetrating trauma and approximately 10% of blunt trauma. The single most important recent change in management of blunt trauma to the liver is the application of nonoperative treatment. Perhaps the single most important recent development that has made nonoperative management possible is accurate imaging of the liver and abdomen by CT, ultrasound, and MRI. The incidence of missed injury when nonoperative treatment is applied to blunt liver trauma is now less than 1%; most of these associated injuries are enteric.

Table 11.4 gives the organ injury scale of the American Association for the Surgery of Trauma. With each increase in injury grade, there is an associated increase in the sever-

TABLE 11.4. Liver Injury Scale: American Association for the Surgery of Trauma

Grade		Injury
I	Hematoma	Subcapsular, <10% surface area
	Laceration	Capsular tear, <1 cm depth
II	Hematoma	Subcapsular, 10%–50% surface area
		Intraparenchymal, <10 cm diameter
	Laceration	1–3 cm depth, <10 cm in length
III	Hematoma	Subcapsular, >50% surface area or expanding
		Intraparenchymal, >10 cm or expanding
	Laceration	>3 cm depth
IV	Laceration	Parenchymal disruption of 25%–75% hepatic lobe or 1–3 segments within single lobe
V	Laceration	Parenchymal disruption of >75% hepatic lobe or >3 segments within single lobe
	Vascular	Juxtahepatic venous injuries, i.e., retrohepatic vena cava/central major hepatic veins
VI	Vascular	Hepatic avulsion

Source: Reprinted with permission from Moore EE, et al. Organ injury scaling: spleen and liver. *J Trauma* 1995;38:323–324.

ity of the injury. Most liver injuries are Grades I through III and most can be treated nonoperatively.

Diagnosis

Physical examination alone is not reliable because it can miss 50% of hepatic injuries. Diagnostic peritoneal lavage (DPL) was once the mainstay of diagnosis and remains so wherever modern imaging techniques are unavailable. DPL, however, does not enable a physician to assess the severity of liver injury itself and, when a positive tap is the basis for laparotomy, 3% to 25% of patients undergo unnecessary exploration. Indeed, more than 50% of patients with liver injuries are not bleeding when laparotomy is performed on the basis of positive DPL.

Ultrasound scanning, often done by the surgeon, is an expeditious way to determine whether or not liver injury is present. Major limitations of the technique are that its accuracy is operator-dependent and, unless the injury is appreciated during the examination, the test lacks specificity when free fluid within the abdomen is the only sign. Hence, CT scan and, increasingly, MRI are necessary to assess liver trauma, even after DPL has indicated the presence of injury. CT scan may show a fracture of the liver or large parenchymal injury (Figure 11.8). CT scan or MRI, however, can be done safely only if the patient is hemodynamically stable. A patient with positive DPL who is hemodynamically unstable requires prompt surgical exploration of the abdomen. CT scan facilitates accurate assessment of the severity of liver injury, but even then, the decision to operate depends not on the CT findings, but on the patient's hemodynamic stability.

Blunt Liver Trauma

ATLS guidelines are used for resuscitation. The response to resuscitation is a key determinant of whether operative treatment is necessary.

Nonoperative Treatment of Hepatic Trauma

Patients can almost always be treated nonoperatively. Many are adequately resuscitated with crystalloids. Patients who require blood transfusions and never become stable during resuscitation require surgery. Another group of patients comprises those who are resuscitated to hemodynamic stability but require continuous administration of large amounts of fluids and blood transfusions to maintain blood pressure. Surgical decision-making is most difficult in this group. The issue is whether to undertake early surgical exploration or better evaluate vascular trauma by performing angiography, which may also enable transcatheter embolization to control bleeding (Figure 11.9). The latter choice depends on available physical resources and technical expertise. Table 11.5 outlines the criteria for nonoperative management of patients with blunt liver injuries. When these criteria are used, nonoperative management is usually successful, but failure necessitates immediate operation.

COMPLICATIONS OF NONOPERATIVE TREATMENT

1. Hemobilia. This condition results from the formation of an intrahepatic vascular fistula and is seen in 0.2% to 0.3% of blunt liver injuries. Symptoms include: (a) upper gastrointestinal bleeding, manifested usually as melena and infrequently as hematemesis; (b) jaundice; and (c) right upper quadrant colicky pain. CT scan shows intrahepatic artery pseudoaneurysm and hepatic angiography confirms this. Nearly all patients can be successfully treated with angiographic embolization.

2. Delayed hemorrhage. This occurs in fewer than 3% of patients with blunt trauma treated nonoperatively. Hepatic angiography can identify the site of bleeding. Control of bleeding is usually accomplished with transcatheter embolization.

3. Liver abscess and biloma. These occur with an incidence of less than 0.5%. Liver abscess and a persistent biloma are successfully treated with percutaneous catheter drainage. When abscess is present, broad-spectrum antibiotic treatment is also required.

4. Extrahepatic bile duct injury. This infrequent complication is probably a result of increased survival of patients with serious liver injury. Jaundice and subhepatic fluid accumulation seen on ultrasonographic examination suggest the diagnosis. Definite confirmation is obtained by ERCP. The injury may be amenable to treatment by endoscopic stenting but in most cases requires operative intervention and, ultimately, hepaticojejunostomy.

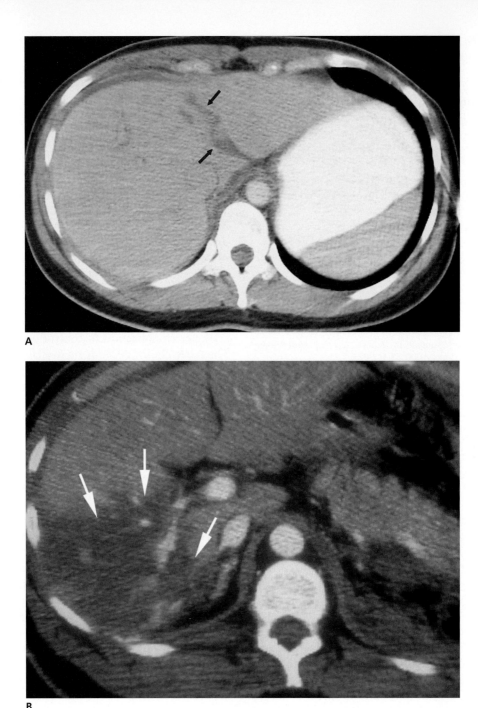

FIGURE 11.8. Major hepatic trauma. (A) This CT scan of the liver demonstrates a well-defined fracture of the left lobe due to a steering wheel injury (arrows). (B) CT scan in another patient following a motor vehicle accident demonstrates a large intrahepatic parenchymal injury (arrows) in the right lobe of the liver. (Courtesy of Henry I. Goldberg, MD, and Vincent McCormick, MD.)

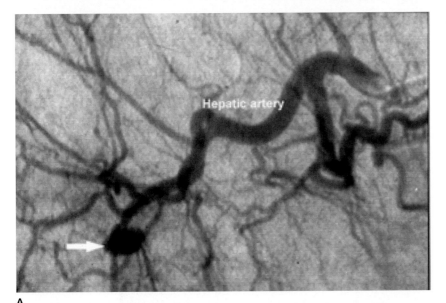

A

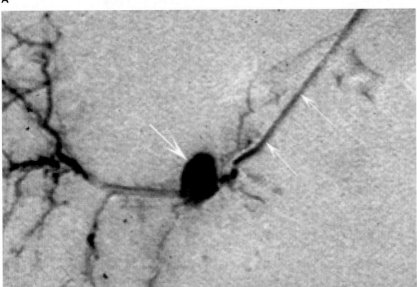

B

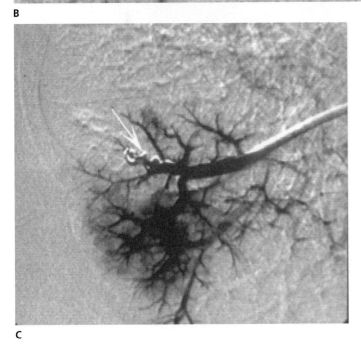

C

FIGURE 11.9. Selective hepatic angiogram in trauma. (A) Arteriogram performed after a CT scan demonstrates hepatic laceration with extravasation of contrast material. The arterial supply of the bleeding site (arrow) is a branch of the hepatic artery. (B) A catheter is placed selectively (small arrows) into the hepatic artery branch feeding the bleeding site (large arrow). (C) The bleeding site (arrow) is embolized by instilling coils through the selectively placed catheter to control bleeding. (Courtesy of Henry I. Goldberg, MD.)

1. Hemodynamic stability on admission or after initial resuscitation
2. CT-scan evidence of liver injury and little free intraperitoneal blood
3. Absence of CT evidence of enteric or retroperitoneal injury
4. Liver-related blood transfusion of 4 U or less
5. CT-documented improvement or stabilization of liver injury, when indicated

Source: Reprinted with permission from Carrillo EH, Wohltmann C, Richardson JD, et al. Evolution in the treatment of complex blunt liver injuries. *Curr Probl Surg* 2001;38:1–60.
Abbreviation: CT, computerized tomography.

5. Posttraumatic liver cyst. This rare complication causes right upper quadrant pain, mild jaundice, increased abdominal girth, and anorexia. Diagnosis is established by ultrasound or CT scan. Treatment with percutaneous drainage may be attempted, but the scant available experience with this complication suggests that operative drainage with decortication is often required.

Operative Treatment of Hepatic Trauma

All patients with penetrating injuries and those who fail nonoperative management of blunt liver trauma require operative treatment. A midline incision is used and can be extended into median sternotomy or a right anterior thoracotomy incision if necessary. Subcapsular

hematomas due to blunt injury (Figure 11.10) require surgical treatment if they undergo progressive expansion as detected by CT scan or if ongoing bleeding is documented by angiography.

The required procedure depends on type and extent of injury, but the principles of surgical treatment are always the same. They include: (1) control of bleeding, (2) removal of devitalized tissue, and (3) establishment of adequate drainage. Any associated diaphragmatic injury must be located and repaired.

Specific Approaches to Hepatic Injuries

Specific approaches to specific types of hepatic injuries are as follows:

1. Subcapsular hematoma. The hematoma is opened and evacuated. Control of bleeding is accomplished by exploration of the underlying liver fracture and ligation of bleeders. If control cannot be accomplished by ligation of bleeders within the liver parenchyma, the Pringle maneuver should be attempted. The Pringle maneuver is accomplished by compressing the portal triad manually or using noncrushing vascular clamps. If the Pringle maneuver controls bleeding, it may be necessary to ligate the hepatic artery as close to the liver as possible.

2. Major parenchymal disruption. Parenchymal disruption requires removal of all dead tissue and control of bleeding. When the injury is unilobar and extensive, the treatment of choice is formal lobectomy. When the parenchymal disruption is central or massive, if bleeding cannot be controlled and coagulopathy develops, the injury should be packed and the abdomen closed. Subse-

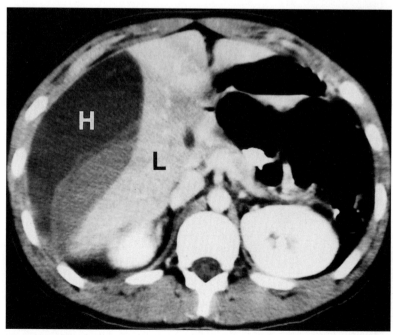

FIGURE 11.10. Subcapsular liver hematoma. The CT scan in a patient hit by a tractor shows a large subcapsular hematoma (H) deforming the liver (L). (Courtesy of Henry I. Goldberg, MD.)

quent operation to remove the packing is undertaken in 24 to 72 h, by which time bleeding may have stopped. If not, suture control or hepatic resection is performed (see Figure 6.20). Adequate sump drainage must also be instituted.

3. Retrohepatic caval injury. This Grade IV injury is associated with a high rate of mortality. Survival depends on promptness of operation and speed with which bleeding is controlled. The diagnosis is usually made intraoperatively when the Pringle maneuver fails to control bleeding. The midline abdominal incision is extended into a median sternotomy. Control of the infrahepatic inferior vena cava above the renal veins and the suprahepatic vena cava is obtained. A large shunt is then inserted through a pursestring suture in the right atrium, advanced into the inferior vena cava to below the renal arteries, and secured in place by occlusion at the previously dissected infra- and suprahepatic sites. Although repair of retrohepatic caval injury may be attempted with total venous occlusion, intracaval shunt is preferred due to the significant incidence of severe hypotension associated with the former approach.

Complications of Operative Treatment of Liver Injury

COMPLICATIONS DUE TO MASSIVE BLOOD TRANSFUSION In severe liver injury, where bleeding is excessive and massive blood transfusion is needed, hypothermia and coagulopathy commonly occur. Prevention of these complications requires warming of all fluids and blood administered intravenously. To prevent dilutional coagulopathy, coagulation studies including platelet count should be measured after 8 to 10 U of blood are transfused; based on these measurements, fresh-frozen plasma and/or platelets should be given as necessary.

COMPLICATIONS DUE TO HEPATIC RESECTION When a significant portion of liver is resected, complications may develop including hypoglycemia, coagulopathy, hyperbilirubinemia, and hypoalbuminemia. Hypoglycemia is caused by a loss of glycogenolysis and can be prevented by continuous administration of 10% glucose in water. Coagulopathy is treated with administration of fresh-frozen plasma or specific coagulation factors. Hyperbilirubinemia is transitory and requires no specific therapy. Hypoalbuminemia may require albumin administration, but patients with mild symptoms can be treated with TPN. These four complications are transient and improve with rapid liver regeneration.

COMPLICATIONS DUE TO BILE DUCT INJURY Intrahepatic injuries can lead to hemobilia or biloma (see discussion above under "Management of Blunt Liver Trauma"). Extrahepatic bile duct injury can lead to biliary fistula or stricture. Some of these injuries may be amenable to endoscopic stenting with ERCP but many require hepaticoje-

junostomy at a later date. Fortunately, these complications are uncommon.

SEPTIC COMPLICATIONS Intraabdominal or intrahepatic abscess can occur and cause fever and leukocytosis. Diagnosis is confirmed with ultrasound or CT scan. The abscess may be successfully treated with percutaneous catheter drainage and broad-spectrum antibiotics.

INJURY OF THE SMALL INTESTINE

Although uncommon in blunt abdominal trauma, injury of the small intestine is the most commonly encountered injury after penetrating abdominal trauma. Injuries can vary from simple bruising to small perforation, massive disruption, and devascularization.

Diagnosis

All patients with penetrating trauma are promptly explored, looking for small intestinal injury by carefully examining the small bowel from the ligament of Treitz to the ileocecal valve. Diagnosis of small bowel injury in blunt trauma is readily made in the conscious patient who develops symptoms of peritoneal irritation. It is considerably more difficult in the unconscious patient, in whom intestinal injury is best diagnosed with DPL. DPL is positive if gross blood is present in free aspiration or if, after peritoneal irrigation with 1 L of saline, there are $\geq$100,000 RBC/μL; $\geq$500 WBC/μL; $\geq$175 U amylase/dL; bacteria on Gram stain; bile; or food particles. The presence of amylase, bacteria, bile, and food particles is particularly suggestive of small bowel injury. Plain films of the abdomen may show an ileus but rarely, if ever, free air in the peritoneal cavity.

Treatment

An operation should be performed promptly. A midline incision is used and complete exploration undertaken. Two types of injury are seen in blunt abdominal trauma: mesenteric tear and intestinal perforation. Tears of the mesentery may be small and bleeding readily controlled without compromising the blood supply of the small bowel. At times, however, rents in the mesentery are large, and blood supply of a segment of the small intestine is compromised. In this case, bowel resection and primary anastomosis are necessary.

Perforation of the jejunum or ileum usually occurs in association with other injuries. In Chance's fracture, caused by a seat belt injury in motor vehicle accidents, a proximal jejunal or distal ileal perforation, usually single, is found in association with vertebral fracture. This injury can usually be repaired in two layers transversely without compromising bowel lumen.

As mentioned earlier, penetrating injuries are more common. Wounds from sharp objects may be single or multiple and may involve other organs in the abdomen.

They are amenable to debridement of the edges and closure in two layers. It is critical to examine the whole length of the small intestine and colon before beginning repair. Bullet wounds of the abdomen cause more severe and more complex injuries.

Whether trauma is blunt or penetrating, the surgical decision to be made is whether to close individual perforations or to resect a segment of small intestine. Resection is indicated when: (1) half the circumference of the bowel is missing after debridement; (2) several holes are present within a short segment of intestine (e.g., 2–3 feet); and (3) perforation of the terminal ileum is associated with injury of the right colon, in which case right hemicolectomy may be the appropriate treatment.

COLONIC INJURY

Ninety-five percent of colon injuries are due to penetrating trauma, caused most often by bullet wounds. The diagnosis and evaluation, therefore, is relatively simple. Colon perforation nearly always results in signs and symptoms of peritonitis. Should plain abdominal films be obtained, free air is usually seen in the peritoneal cavity (Figure 11.11). The key to minimizing morbidity and mortality is early surgical treatment.

Treatment

All patients with suspected colon injury should be given broad-spectrum antibiotics intravenously. Selective use of tetanus toxoid is indicated, depending on the vaccination history. Controversy has raged for years over whether or not to perform primary closure of perforation and, if resection is required, whether or not to perform primary anastomosis. The surgeon should use common sense. Simple perforations of the colon not associated with much contamination can be treated with debridements and primary closure, especially when treated early. When treatment is delayed or when there is significant fecal peritonitis, exteriorization of the perforated colon or diversion of the fecal stream may ultimately be safer.

When resection is necessary, primary anastomosis can be performed safely in low-risk patients; these include those with early injury, absence of preoperative hypotension, fewer than three organs injured, and less than 1 L of blood in the peritoneal cavity. Some surgeons advocate on-table colon irrigation to achieve mechanical preparation; others have used intracolonic bypass tube (Coloshield) to protect the anastomosis. Several contraindications to primary anastomosis must be cited when:

1. Colon injury is associated with multiple organ trauma.
2. The patient is in shock.
3. The colon is fecally loaded or significant fecal contamination of the peritoneal cavity is present.
4. Treatment is delayed more than 6 h and peritonitis has developed.

RECTAL INJURY

Most rectal injuries are due to bullet wounds. The rectum can also be perforated by displaced pelvic fracture as a result of a motor vehicle accident or sexual misadventure.

Diagnosis

When rectal perforation is above the peritoneal reflection, signs and symptoms are similar to those of colonic perforation. Rectal perforation below the peritoneal reflection may be difficult to diagnose unless suspected. Most rectal injuries are diagnosed preoperatively. Blood on digital examination is seen in approximately 80% of cases. Proctosigmoid examination establishes the diagnosis in fewer than 75% of cases. If the diagnosis is still in question, a low-pressure x-ray examination with water-soluble contrast medium should be performed.

Treatment

Perforation of the intraperitoneal rectum is treated with debridement and closure in two layers, then protection by sigmoid loop colostomy. If the injury is severe, however, Hartman's procedure is more appropriate.

Rectal injury below the peritoneal reflection is more difficult to treat. The main principles are:

1. Closure of perforation whenever possible.
2. Construction of diverting sigmoid loop colostomy.
3. Closed sump drainage of the pelvis.
4. Presacral drainage via the perineum posterior to the anus.
5. Irrigation of distal rectal stump.

Retroperitoneal Hematoma

Retroperitoneal hematoma is diagnosed with imaging techniques or at the time of laparotomy. For decision-making purposes, retroperitoneal hematoma is classified by three zones (Figure 11.12).

SURGICAL MANAGEMENT

1. Zone 1 retroperitoneal hematoma must *always* be explored. This is best done by reflecting the ascending colon and small intestine to the left after incising the peritoneal reflection laterally (Cattell maneuver). The most common injuries associated with this type of hematoma are: (a) retroperitoneal duodenal rupture, (b) injury to the head of the pancreas, and (c) vascular injury.

2. Zone 2 retroperitoneal hematomas need not be explored provided: (a) they are not expanding, (b) colon injury is not suspected, and (c) CT or angiographic studies have shown a functioning kidney on that side. Expanding hematomas must be explored and may be due to avulsion of the renal pedicle. Hence, before opening the hematoma,

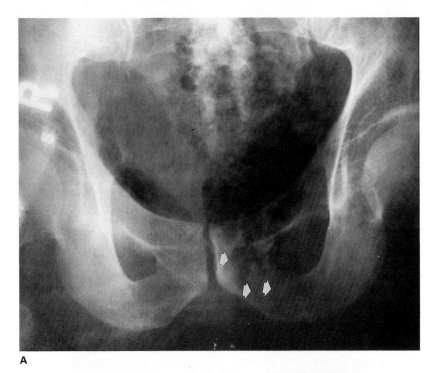

A

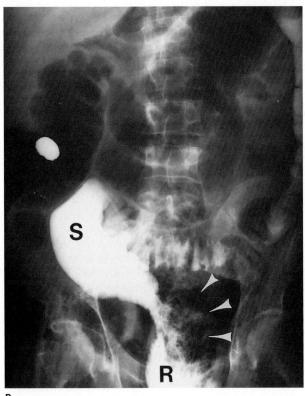

B

FIGURE 11.11. Rectal traumatic injury. (A) Plain film of the pelvis of an elderly patient in a nursing home after traumatic insertion of a rectal thermometer shows the unusual location of multiple air collections (arrows) suggestive of rectal perforation. (B) Water-soluble contrast material is instilled through a soft rubber catheter to define the site of rupture. The radiograph shows contrast material in the rectum (R) and sigmoid (S), and extravasation into the perirectal area (arrowheads). (Courtesy of Henry I. Goldberg, MD.)

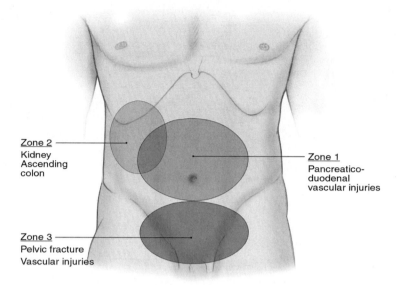

FIGURE 11.12. Classification of retroperitoneal hematoma. Zone 1 hematoma is associated with pancreaticoduodenal and vascular trauma and must always be explored. Zone 2 hematoma is associated with injury to the kidney and ascending colon and is explored selectively when either colon injury is suspected or the hematoma is expanding. Zone 3 hematoma is usually associated with pelvic fracture and is generally not opened. When low abdominal hematoma is not associated with pelvic fracture, the hematoma must be explored.

vascular control should be obtained by controlling the renal artery, or, if this is not possible, by obtaining aortic control below the diaphragm.

3. Zone 3 retroperitoneal hematomas are often associated with pelvic fracture and, as a general rule, are not explored. If they are expanding, angiogram is performed to identify the site of bleeding and to obtain angiographic control of bleeding. Retroperitoneal hematomas not associated with pelvic fracture, as seen in penetrating trauma, however, are explored to exclude and, if present, repair major retroperitoneal vessel injury.

REFERENCE

1. Nance FC, Wennar MH, Johnson LW, et al. Surgical judgment in the management of penetrating wounds of the abdomen: experience with 2212 patients. *Ann Surg* 1974;179:639–646.

SELECTED READINGS

Stomach and Duodenum

Harrison CR, Debas HT. Injuries of the stomach and duodenum. *Surg Clin North Am* 1972;52:635–648.

Levison MA, Peterson SR, Sheldon GF, et al. Duodenal trauma: experience of a trauma center. *J Trauma* 1984;24:475–480.

Pancreas

Cogbill TH, Moore EE, Morris JA Jr, et al. Distal pancreatectomy for trauma: a multicenter experience. *J Trauma* 1991;31:1600–1606.

Feliciano DV, Martin T, Cruse PA, et al. Management of combined pancreaticoduodenal injuries. *Ann Surg* 1987;205:673–680.

Lucas CE. Diagnosis and treatment of pancreatic and duodenal injury. *Surg Clin North Am* 1977;57:49–65.

Wisner DH, Wold RL, Frey CF. Diagnosis and treatment of pancreatic injuries. An analysis of management principles. *Arch Surg* 1990;125:1109–1113.

Liver

Carrillo EH, Wohltmann C, Richardson JD, et al. Evolution of the treatment of complex blunt liver injuries. *Curr Probl Surg* 2001;38:1–60.

Knudson MM, Lim RC Jr, Oakes DD, et al. Nonoperative management of blunt liver injuries in adults: the need for continued surveillance. *J Trauma* 1990;30:1494–1500.

Pachter HL, Spencer FC, Hofstetter SR, et al. Significant trends in the treatment of hepatic trauma: an experience with 411 injuries. *Ann Surg* 1992;215:492–502.

Yellin AE, Chaffee CB, Donovan AJ. Vascular isolation in treatment of juxtahepatic venous injuries. *Arch Surg* 1971;102:566–573.

Colon and Rectum

Burch JM, Martin RR, Richardson RJ, et al. Evolution of the treatment of injured colon in the 1980s. *Arch Surg* 1991;126: 979–984.

Chappuis CW, Frey DJ, Dietzen CD, et al. Management of colon injuries: a prospective randomized trial. *Ann Surg* 1991; 213:492–498.

Ivatury RR, Licata J, Gunduz Y, et al. Management options in penetrating rectal injuries. *Am Surg* 1991;57:50–55.

Thomas DD, Levison MA, Dykstra BJ, et al. Management of rectal injuries: dogma versus practice. *Am Surg* 1990;56:507–510.

Abdominal Wall, Peritoneum, and Retroperitoneum

The primary clinical significance of the abdominal wall is herniation, which constitutes a typical surgical problem. Peritonitis and intraabdominal abscesses also require surgical intervention. While secondary malignancies are common, primary tumors of the peritoneum are rare. Disorders of the retroperitoneum are far less common.

ANATOMY AND EMBRYOLOGY

The abdominal wall consists of skin, subcutaneous fascia, and Scarpa's fascia overlying the musculature. From superficial to deep, the muscular wall layers include the external oblique, the internal oblique, and the transversus. The muscles are fleshy laterally and become aponeurotic medially, where the aponeurosis fuses before separating to the anterior and posterior fascia that invest the rectus muscles. The anterior and posterior rectus fascia fuse in the midline to form the linea alba (Figure 12.1). The transversus muscle ends at the semilunar line, where the transversalis fascia begins. The transversalis fascia extends down to the groin.

The innermost layer of the abdomen, the peritoneum, invests continuously all the abdominal viscera. In the male embryo, peritoneum may project as a sac through the processus vaginalis at the internal inguinal ring if, following testicular descent, the processus vaginalis fails to obliterate completely. An oval defect exists in the external oblique aponeurosis just above and lateral to the pubic tubercle—the external inguinal ring. The internal ring is a defect in the transversalis fascia about 1 inch above the midinguinal point, midway between the anterior superior iliac crest and the public tubercle. The oblique space extending from the internal ring superiorly and laterally, and to the external ring inferiorly and medially, constitutes the inguinal canal. The spermatic cord in men and the round ligament in women course through the inguinal canal, which is bounded anteriorly by the external oblique aponeurosis, superiorly by the internal oblique and trans-

versus abdominis aponeurosis, and inferiorly by the inguinal and lacunar ligaments. The transversalis fascia forms the floor (posterior wall) of the inguinal canal. Hernias commonly form because of weaknesses in the inguinal canal floor or in the femoral ring. The boundaries of the femoral ring are, anteriorly, the inguinal ligament; laterally, the femoral vein; posteriorly, the pectinius fascia, which condenses to create Cooper's ligament; and medially, the lacunar ligament, also known as Gimbernat's ligament. The anatomy of inguinal hernia is summarized in Table 12.1.

INGUINAL OR GROIN HERNIAS

Three types of inguinal or groin hernia are common: the indirect inguinal hernia, the direct inguinal hernia and the femoral hernia. An indirect inguinal hernia is associated with a peritoneal sac that protrudes through the internal ring into the inguinal canal and lies anteromedial to the spermatic cord or round ligament. The sac and its contents, which may include omentum or small intestine, may protrude so extensively in men that they reach the scrotum (scrotal hernia). Direct inguinal hernias do not often have well-developed sacs. They are protrusions through Hesselbach's triangle as a result of weakness of the posterior wall of the inguinal canal. Femoral hernias occur when a segment of the peritoneum protrudes through the femoral ring. The sac is usually small and has a narrow neck, allowing only a small piece of omentum or part of the wall of the small intestine to herniate. The sites of the three main groin hernias are shown in Figure 12.2.

Pathogenesis

The development of a hernia requires an abdominal wall defect and an increase in abdominal pressure.

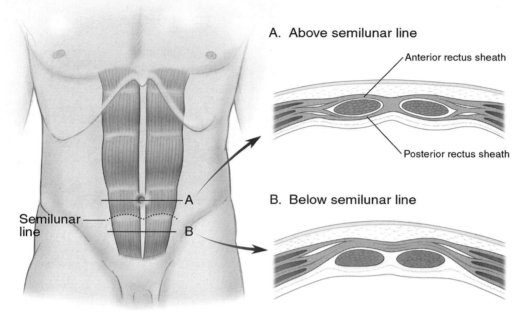

A. Above semilunar line

Anterior rectus sheath

Posterior rectus sheath

B. Below semilunar line

Semilunar line

A

B

FIGURE 12.1. (A and B) Muscles and fascia of the abdominal wall showing fusion of anterior and posterior rectus fascia in midline to form the linea alba. (Adapted from Norton, JA, ed. Basic Science and Clinical Evidence. New York: Springer, 2001:788.)

Defect in the Abdominal Wall

A key anomaly in indirect inguinal hernia is the presence of a hernial sac in the inguinal canal. The sac is a vestige of the processus vaginalis, a structure important in boys for descent of the testes from the retroperitoneum to the scrotum. It is likely, however, that an indirect hernial sac may develop *de novo* in the adult. With time, enlargement of an indirect inguinal hernia is associated with weakness of the posterior wall of the inguinal canal and thinning and bulging of the transversalis fascia.

In direct inguinal hernia, the primary abnormality is weakness of the posterior wall of the inguinal canal, leading to a bulge through Hesselbach's triangle. Direct inguinal hernias typically occur in elderly men. The sac may not be prominent, although a well-developed sac may sometimes be encountered. Such sacs are rarely large enough to merit excision and may be managed by pushing them into the abdomen and applying a few sutures to hold them in place.

Femoral hernia involves not only weakness of the posterior inguinal wall but also widening of the femoral ring. A hernial sac is formed as part of the peritoneum descends through the ring.

Increased Abdominal Pressure

Increased abdominal pressure is sometimes an acute precipitating event. The construction worker who attempts to lift a heavy object and suddenly experiences tearing pain in the groin is an example. More commonly, however, increased abdominal pressure is caused by chronic cough, constipation, or straining to urinate as a result of prostatic hypertrophy. Occasionally, constipation may be associated with development of colonic cancer.

Whenever possible, the condition of increased abdominal pressure should be improved or eliminated before herniorrhaphy. The correction of abdominal pressure is particularly important in prostatic hypertrophy, where prostatectomy (transurethral or otherwise) should be performed before hernia repair.

Progression of Disease

In the early stages, the hernia bulge develops intermittently, often associated with activities that generate sudden elevation in intraabdominal pressure. The patient experiences a dull pain in the groin and can feel the bulge. The bulge may either reduce spontaneously or can easily be pushed back by the patient—the stage of reducible inguinal hernia. As

---

TABLE 12.1. Essentials: Inguinal Hernia Anatomy

External inguinal ring: Defect in external oblique aponeurosis

Internal ring: Defect in transversalis fascia

Hesselbach's triangle: Site of direct hernia

Boundaries
- Medially: Rectus fascia
- Superiorly: Inferior epigastric vessels
- Inferiorly: Inguinal ligament

Relation of neck of hernia sac
- Direct hernia: Medial to inferior epigastric vessels
- Indirect hernia: Lateral to inferior epigastric vessels

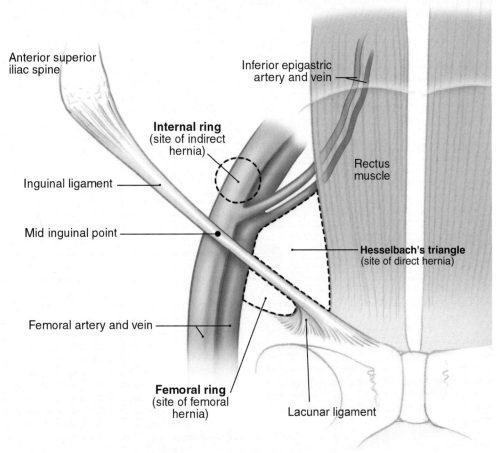

FIGURE 12.2. Anatomical sites of groin hernias.

time passes, the herniation may become permanent, and the patient may be unable to reduce it—the stage of incarcerated (irreducible) inguinal hernia. An irreducible inguinal hernia may exist as a chronic abnormality without serious symptoms or complications. At times, an incarcerated inguinal hernia is associated with small bowel obstruction within the hernia. In some cases, the blood supply of the herniated structures (omentum or bowel) may become compromised, causing an acute clinical problem—the stage of irreducible, strangulated hernia. The wall of a viscus may descend to form part of the hernial sac. This type of hernia is known as sliding hernia.

Bowel obstruction or strangulation is uncommon in direct inguinal hernia but much more common in indirect inguinal and femoral hernias, which have a narrow neck. The swelling in an irreducible femoral hernia is in the groin below the inguinal ligament, just lateral to the pubis and medial to the femoral vessels. When strangulation develops, the swelling becomes tender. Because the femoral ring is narrow, only a portion (usually the antimesenteric aspect) of the small intestine may become incarcerated and, when strangulated, only part of the small intestine may become gangrenous. This type of hernia, called Richter's hernia, presents with a tender groin lump below the inguinal ligament and is associated with small

bowel obstruction. The essentials of femoral hernia are summarized in Table 12.2.

Management

Techniques Common to All Types of Inguinal Hernia Repair

ANESTHESIA Most inguinal hernia repair is performed on an outpatient basis, admission to hospital being

TABLE 12.2. Essentials: Femoral Hernia
Boundaries of femoral ring
■ Anteriorly: Inguinal ligament
■ Laterally: Femoral vein
■ Posteriorly: Pectineus fascia
■ Medially: Lacunar ligament
Femoral hernia
■ More common in women
■ Causes small bowel obstruction in 20%
■ Richter's hernia: Strangulated femoral hernia involving infarction of part of the small intestine wall
Treatment: McVay repair

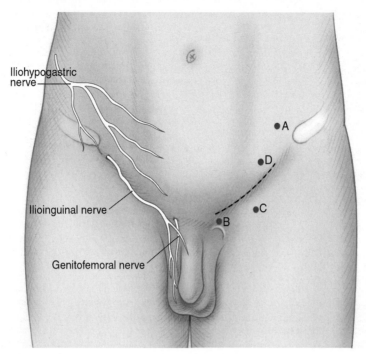

FIGURE 12.3. Technique for administering local anesthesia in preparation for hernia repair. Effective local anesthesia can be provided by directing the local anesthetic to points A, B, C, and D to desensitize the iliohypogastric, the genitofemoral, the ilioinguinal, and hypogastric branches of the iliohypogastric nerves, respectively. (Adapted from Flanagan L, Bascom JU. Repair of the groin hernia: outpatient approach with local anesthesia. Surg Clin North Am, 1984;64:257–267.)

reserved only for patients who have other confounding medical problems. Anesthesia may be general, epidural (spinal), or local. Increasingly, hernia repair is being done either under epidural or local anesthesia with parenteral sedation (Figure 12.3).

INCISION The midpoint of the incision should be over the internal ring, the surface marking for which is 0.5 inch above the midinguinal point. An oblique or transverse skin incision (6–8 cm) is made and deepened to the external oblique aponeurosis after dividing Scarpa's fascia and superficial veins.

OPENING THE INGUINAL CANAL The external ring, a defect superior and lateral to the pubic tubercle, is first identified. The genitofemoral nerve is seen issuing from it. The anterior wall of the inguinal canal is opened along the fibers of the external oblique aponeurosis, taking care to preserve the nerve. The spermatic cord is mobilized at the pubic tubercle, encircled, and then retracted using a .25-inch Penrose drain.

IDENTIFYING THE HERNIA SAC An indirect hernia sac is found on the anteromedial aspect of the spermatic cord. Its apex is picked with clamps and the sac is dissected proximally to the internal ring. Its neck lies lateral to the inferior epigastric vessels. A direct hernia sac, on the other hand, is found in Hesselbach's triangle. The direct hernia

sac is usually not prominent but can be at times. When dissected proximally, its neck is found medial to the inferior epigastric vessels.

EXCISION OR INVERSION OF THE HERNIAL SAC All indirect hernia sacs are opened at their apex; any omental or bowel content is reduced into the abdomen. The neck of the sac is closed using suture ligature flush with the peritoneum. The sac is then excised distal to the ligature. Most direct hernia sacs are inverted, but large sacs are excised.

Open Surgical Approaches to Hernia Repair

The major surgical approaches to inquinal hernia repair are summarized in Table 12.3.

BASSINI REPAIR The Bassini repair, introduced in 1890, is a simple and effective repair. The essential element is approximation of transversalis fascia and the internal oblique muscle to the inguinal ligament using interrupted sutures (Figure 12.4). Some believe that this procedure predisposes to future development of femoral hernia, although the evidence is anecdotal.

MCVAY (COOPER LIGAMENT) REPAIR The McVay repair has two important components: the repair itself and a relaxing incision. The repair is accomplished by approx-

| TABLE 12.3. | Essentials: Surgical Approaches to Inguinal Hernia Repair |

Bassini
Approximation of internal oblique, transversus abdominus and transversalis fascia to inguinal ligament

Shouldice (modified Bassini)
- Division of posterior inguinal canal and imbrication of lateral and medial edges
- Suturing of free edge of medial flap to shelving edge of inguinal ligament
- Approximation of internal oblique to inguinal ligament

McVay
Approximation of transversalis fascia to Cooper's ligament

Lichtenstein
Tension-free repair suturing synthetic mesh to transversalis fascia superiorly and inguinal ligament inferiorly

Preperitoneal
Approximation of transversalis fascia to inguinal ligament

is formed when the spermatic cord is reached. The new ring should be snug but should permit introduction of the small finger next to the cord to avoid compression of the spermatic veins and subsequent scrotal swelling.

The second step in the McVay repair is to perform a relaxing incision by vertical division of the anterior rectus sheath (Figure 12.5B).

SHOULDICE REPAIR The Shouldice herniorrhaphy, popularized in Canada, is a modified Bassini repair (Figure 12.6) and is typically performed under local anesthesia.

TENSION-FREE HERNIORRHAPHY OF LICHTENSTEIN The major concept of this repair, performed under local anesthesia is to avoid tension at the suture line by the use of prosthetic mesh (Figure 12.7).

PREPERITONEAL (CHEATLE–HENRY) REPAIR The preperitoneal approach was not frequently used until the advent of laparoscopic herniorrhaphy. The preperitoneal repair, most often indicated in bilateral hernias in which bilateral herniorrhaphy is accomplished through a single incision, is also an excellent technique for repair of recurrent inguinal hernia. A transverse skin incision is made about 3 cm above the inguinal ligament, and transverse incisions are made in the rectus sheath, the external and internal obliques, and the transversus abdominus aponeurosis. The rectus muscle is retracted medially, the transversalis fascia is incised, and the preperitoneal space is entered. With blunt dissection, the pelvic peritoneum is separated from the pelvic floor. Femoral and direct hernial sacs are easily visualized and reduced. An indirect hernia sac can also be dissected and excised using this approach. A McVay-type repair can then be performed from the back of the transversalis fascia.

imating the transversalis fascia to Cooper's ligament (Figure 12.5). Interrupted nonabsorbable sutures, either 2.0 or 0, are used, beginning at the public tubercle and moving laterally. The first suture to the pubic tubercle is important because this is a frequent site of recurrence. A sturdy needle is used so that the fascial insertion and the periosteum of the pubis can be incorporated.

As approximation of the transversalis fascia to Cooper's ligament proceeds laterally, the femoral vein is reached. At this point, a transition stitch is required incorporating Cooper's ligament, the femoral sheath covering the vein and the inguinal ligament. Lateral to this point, the transversalis fascia is approximated to the inguinal ligament. As the repair proceeds laterally, a new internal ring

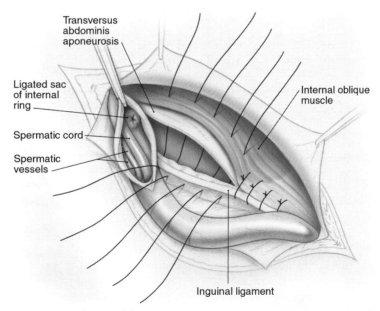

FIGURE 12.4. Bassini repair. (Adapted from Wartz GE. The operation of Bassini as described by Attilo Catterina. Surg Gynecol Obstet 1989;168:67–80.)

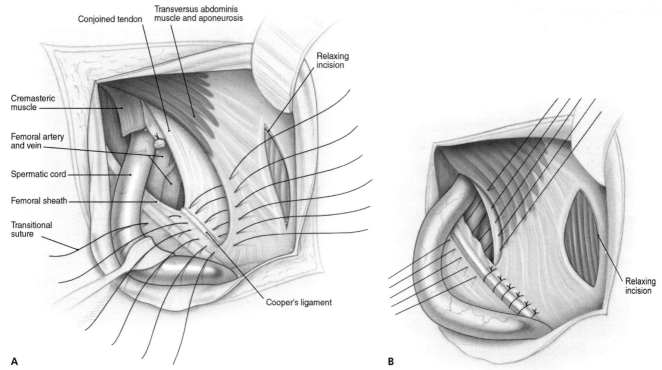

FIGURE 12.5. McVay or Cooper repair. (A) After dissection and excision of the hernial sac, the transversalis fascia is approximated to Cooper's ligament, beginning at the pubic tubercle and extending laterally to the femoral vein, beyond which the transversalis fascia is approximated to the inguinal ligament. (B) Tension at the repair is avoided by making a relaxing incision, 3 to 4 inches long, in the fusion of the external oblique and rectus fascia starting just above the pubic tubercle. (Adapted from Wartz GE. Atlas of Hernia Surgery. Philadelphia: Lippincott Williams & Wilkins, 1991:76.)

COMPLICATIONS OF INGUINAL HERNIA REPAIR Complications specific to inguinal herniorrhaphy may occur early or late following the operation. Early local complications include wound infection or hematoma (1% to 2%), scrotal and testicular swelling (7%), compression of the femoral vein (1%), and urinary retention (up to 30%). Scrotal swelling usually occurs when the internal ring is too tightly closed. Acute ischemic orchitis occurs when the spermatic cord or spermatic vessels are severed. Compression of the femoral vein is most likely to occur after McVay (Cooper ligament) repair. The resulting complications may include femoral thrombophlebitis or even pulmonary embolism.

Late complications include hydrocele formation, testicular atrophy, neuroma formation, nerve entrapment of the genitofemoral or ilioinguinal nerves, and recurrence. A late-developing hydrocele is usually due to incomplete excisions of the distal extension of the sac. Testicular atrophy occurs in fewer than 2% of cases and may represent partial interruption of the blood supply during surgery or may follow early acute testicular swelling. Neural complications are most distressing and are not always successfully treated. Local anesthetic blocks directly in the region of the neuroma or nerve entrapment or blocks of L1 and L2 (genitofemoral nerve) are sometimes used. Some surgeons have reported success after excising the entrapped nerve or after separating the genitofemoral nerve proximal to the entrapment.

Laparoscopic Hernia Repair Techniques

Several randomized clinical trials have shown that laparoscopic hernia repairs are safe and effective. The cost is higher than for open repair, but laparoscopic procedures are associated with less postoperative pain and shorter recovery time for the patient. Definitive statements comparing laparoscopic to open hernia repair await the conclusion of a large ongoing randomized U.S. Department of Veterans Affairs Medical Center trial. Most surgeons agree, however, that the laparoscopic approach is preferred only in bilateral and recurrent hernias.

Three techniques have emerged as the most popular laparoscopic procedures for inguinal hernia repair: transabdominal preperitoneal (TAPP), intraperitoneal onlay mesh (IPOM), and totally extraperitoneal (TEP). Laparoscopic hernia repair techniques that violate the peritoneum pose risks of trocar injury to viscera and an increased risk of adhesion formation. In the TAPP

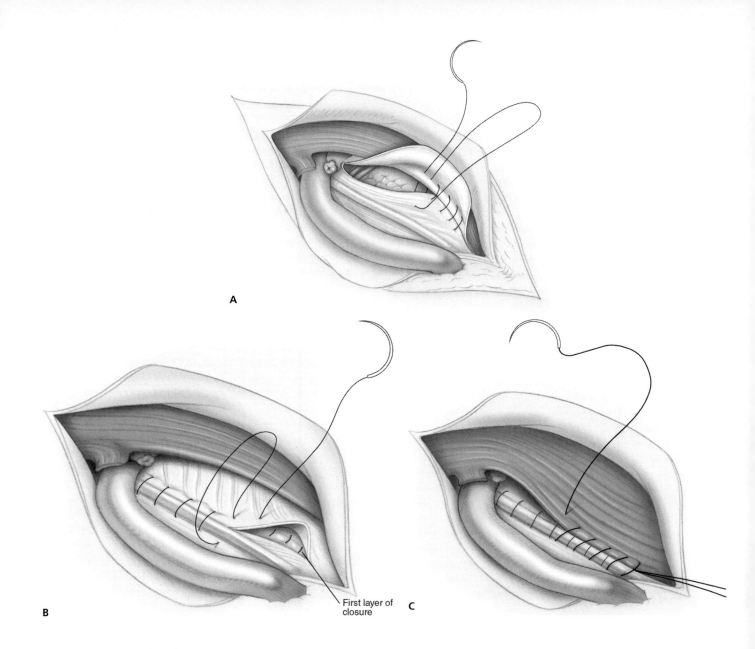

A

B

First layer of closure

C

FIGURE 12.6. Shouldice repair. (A) The procedure begins with complete division of the cremaster muscle, the external spermatic artery and vein, and the inguinal branch of the genitofemoral nerve. Then the posterior wall of the inguinal canal, including the transversalis fascia, is divided about 1 cm above the inguinal ligament. The internal ring is destroyed, leaving the spermatic cord mobile. The medial edge of the flap is elevated to the rectus sheath. (B) Repair is accomplished by imbricating the lateral and medial edges in a "vest-over-pants" fashion using continuous sutures (usually 34-gauge stainless steel), and the free edge of the medial flap is sutured to the shelving edge of the inguinal ligament. (C) With a second suture, the aponeurosis of the internal oblique muscle is approximated to the inguinal ligament. (Adapted from Wartz GE. Atlas of Hernia Surgery. Philadelphia: Lippincott Williams & Wilkins, 1991:67.)

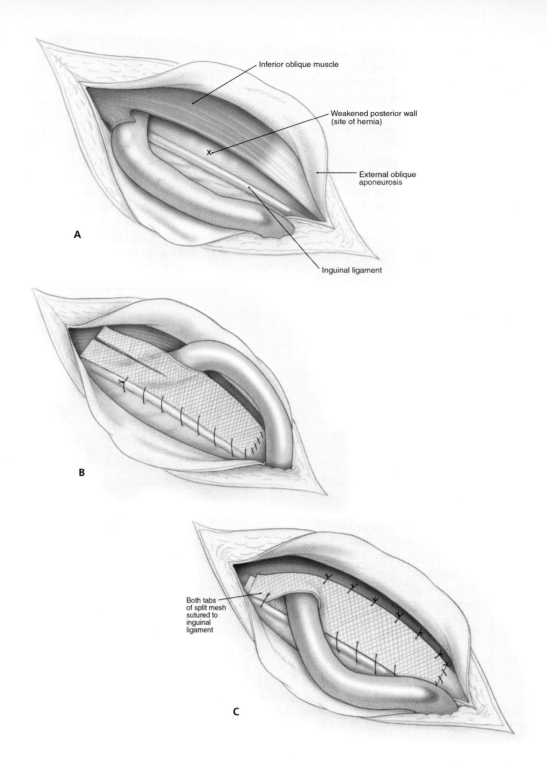

Inferior oblique muscle

Weakened posterior wall
(site of hernia)

External oblique
aponeurosis

Inguinal ligament

A

B

Both tabs
of split mesh
sutured to
inguinal
ligament

C

FIGURE 12.7. Lichtenstein repair. (A and B) Under local anesthesia, an appropriate patch of prosthetic mesh is sutured to the inguinal ligament from the pubic tubercle to the internal ring, using continuous 3.0 Prolene® and Novafil® (U.S. Surgical, Norwalk, CT) sutures. A slot is made in the mesh at the internal ring to allow emergence of the spermatic cord. (C) The superior edge of mesh is then sutured to the rectus sheath and conjoined tendon. (Adapted from Arregui ME, Nagan RD, eds. Inguinal Hernia: Advances or Controversies. Oxford, England: Radcliffe Medical, 1994.)

procedure, the mesh is embedded in peritoneal flaps, but the IPOM repair leaves the prosthetic mesh in direct contact with the bowel and has led to bowel erosion and obstruction according to published reports.[1]

TAPP Procedure In the transabdominal preperitoneal procedure (TAPP), three trocars are inserted into the peritoneal cavity after inducing pneumoperitoneum. One trocar is situated in the midline just below the umbilicus. The other two are situated laterally at the edge of the rectus muscles. The hernia site is approached by transversely incising the peritoneum cephalad to the groin, extending laterally to the internal ring. The hernia is reduced. Large indirect sacs are excised. Blunt preperitoneal dissection exposes Cooper's ligament below and the transversalis fascia above; it facilitates clear definition of Hesselbach's triangle and the femoral canal and vessels. A large polypropylene mesh (12 × 15 cm) is placed over the entire myopectineal orifice with generous overlap. The mesh is secured in place by applying fasteners medially to the rectus muscle, superiorly to the transversus abdominus, inferiorly to Cooper's ligament, and laterally to the iliopubic tract.

IPOM Procedure In the intraperitoneal onlay mesh (IPOM) approach, performed transabdominally and laparoscopically, hernial contents are reduced, and the defect is closed with a large piece of mesh, which is secured in place by staples.

TEP Procedure The totally extraperitoneal procedure (TEP) necessitates a preperitoneal approach and creates a working space by dissection with the laparoscope or a balloon. Three trocars are used to perform the procedure, as in the TAPP procedure. The key is not to enter the peritoneal cavity; otherwise, the dissection and repair with mesh is identical to the TAPP procedure.

Special Considerations

Hernia Repair in Women Herniorrhaphy in women is identical to the technique used in men. The significant difference in anatomy is that the spermatic cord is replaced by the round ligament, which may be divided if it facilitates the repair. The incidence of femoral hernia is higher in women than in men.

Combined Direct and Indirect Inguinal Hernias Combined hernias, also known as "pantaloon" hernias, are uncommon. The technique of choice is to divide the inferior epigastric vessels and make a single sac of the two hernial sacs. The sac is then resected and herniorrhaphy accomplished.

Sliding Hernia In sliding inguinal hernia, a viscus forms part of the wall of the hernia sac, either the cecum on the right (Figure 12.8) or sigmoid colon on the left. On either side, the bladder may also be involved. A sliding hernia must be diagnosed by opening the hernia at its apex so that the viscus can be protected and reduced. Otherwise, colon or bladder perforation occurs. Once the condition is recognized, the sac is carefully trimmed without injuring the viscus and closed. The viscus is then reduced into the abdomen, and surrounding tissue is carefully approximated to maintain reduction while adequate hernia repair is accomplished in the classic way.

Bilateral Hernia Most bilateral hernias can be repaired at the same time either through separate incisions or using the preperitoneal approach. The latter approach is ideally suited to laparoscopic repair of bilateral hernias. Some surgeons advocate repairing only one side, deferring the second side for 2 to 3 months in order to reduce recurrence. No convincing evidence exists to support this contention, however, and the surgeon is left to make his or her

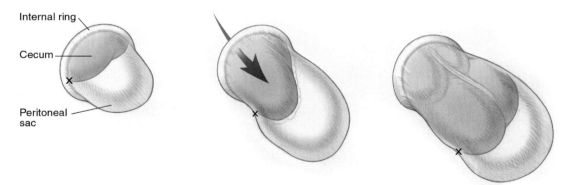

FIGURE 12.8. Genesis of a sliding inguinal right hernia. The attachment of the cecum, which is normally within the peritoneal cavity, progressively gets pulled into the lining of the hernia sac; eventually, the cecum forms the posterior portion of the hernia sac itself. The sliding organ can be the bladder on either side and the sigmoid colon on the left.

own decision. In a retrospective study, Miller and colleagues compared the results of unilateral hernia repair in 333 patients with simultaneous bilateral repair in 329 other patients.[2] Recurrence rates at 5 years were 4% to 8% in the unilateral group and 5% in the bilateral group.

Orchiectomy In older men with large scrotal hernias, particularly if the hernia is recurrent, preoperative consent to perform orchiectomy to facilitate repair should be obtained. The usual incidence of planned orchiectomies is fewer than 5% in primary hernia cases and 15% to 20% in recurrent hernia repair cases. Unplanned orchiectomy may be necessary if the spermatic cord is inadvertently divided. Under these circumstances, the surgeon should inform the patient of the complication.

Use of Pneumoperitoneum in Repair of Massive Hernias Patients with massive hernias containing large amounts of small bowel and omentum may experience respiratory difficulty if the contents of the hernia are reduced into the abdomen. Such patients can be prepared effectively with progressive pneumoperitoneum before repair. Progressive pneumoperitoneum is accomplished with an injection of 500 to 1500 ml of air into the peritoneal cavity every 1 to 3 days over a period of 2 to 3 weeks.

Recurrent Inguinal Hernia The incidence of recurrent hernia after primary repair is reported to be 2% to 10%.[3] The best results have been achieved with the Shouldice repair. Glasgow reported recurrence rates of 0.6% in 13,108 patients with primary repair and 1% in 1874 patients with repair of recurrent hernias.[4] No other type of repair has matched these results. Once a recurrent hernia is repaired, re-recurrence rates of over 20% have been reported.[3] Thus, the preferred approach to recurrent hernia is the Shouldice technique or the use of prosthetic mesh, either laparoscopically or with the open technique.

VENTRAL HERNIA

Ventral hernias include incisional, epigastric, and umbilical hernias. Incisional hernias are by far the most common of the three.

Incisional Hernia

Reported incidence of incisional hernia is approximately 4% (0.5%–10%).[5] Predisposing factors include wound infection, severe malnutrition (rapid weight loss greater than 10%, albumin <2g/dL), obesity, increased intra-abdominal pressure (e.g., chronic cough, urinary tract obstruction), development of bowel obstruction, chronic steroid therapy, age, and an inexperienced surgeon. Type of incision may also be important. Incisional hernias are less commonly associated with transverse than with the vertical incisions. Wound infection is strongly associated with the development of incisional hernia. Bucknall et al. reported that incisional hernias develop four times more often with wound infection.[6] Technical factors associated with the development of incisional hernia include use of inappropriate suture (e.g., catgut suture) and improper placement of sutures (e.g., <1 cm from fascial edges).

The incidence of incisional hernia in susceptible patients can be reduced by appropriate preoperative, intraoperative, and postoperative measures. Preoperative measures include correction of nutritional deficit, improvement of respiratory function, and correction of urinary tract obstruction. Vitamin A administration has been used to counteract the negative effect of steroids on wound healing. Intraoperative measures include meticulous tissue handling and procedures that reduce wound infection, including use of perioperative antibiotics. In patients with significant risk factors, retention sutures may reduce wound dehiscence, but there is no evidence that they reduce the incidence of incisional hernia. Postoperatively, abdominal distension should be minimized with appropriate use of nasogastric decompression and, in patients with urinary obstruction, catheter drainage should be maintained for 10 to 14 days. The wound should be closely examined postoperatively and any wound infection treated promptly by opening the skin incision.

Repair

Whenever possible, incisional hernias should be repaired without prosthetic mesh. The principles are to accomplish closure without tension, using strong sutures placed in healthy tissue at least 1 cm from fascial edges. Nearly two-thirds of incisional hernias can be repaired with this simple approximation of the musculofascial edges.

In one-third of patients, however, simple repair is not possible because either the defect is too large or the musculofascial layer at the edges of the hernia defect is not robust enough. In these circumstances, the weakened fascial edges should be excised and the defect closed using a prosthetic mesh. Various types of mesh have been used; Marlex® (Chevron Phillips Chemical Company LP, The Woodlands, TX) or Prolene® (Ethicon Inc., Cornelia, GA) mesh or Gortex are usually preferred. Whenever possible, the omentum should be mobilized to cover the intestines so that the mesh is not in direct contact with them. The mesh is sewn to strong fascia with interrupted, nonabsorbable sutures. When large incisional hernias are repaired in this fashion, closed subcutaneous sump drainage is used to prevent accumulation of serum. Some surgeons, fearing infection of the foreign material, have used the patient's own fascia lata to cover the defect. Patients with large, full-thickness loss of abdominal wall, may require major wound reconstruction. Such repairs will require rotation of pedicle flaps.

Epigastric Hernia

Epigastric hernia occurs through a defect in the linea alba above the umbilicus. The defects are often small but may be multiple. Epigastric hernias in children are best managed expectantly because most disappear by the age of 6 years. In adults, surgical repair is recommended in symptomatic hernias. The simplest technique is excision of the sac, closure of the peritoneum and approximation of the fascia with nonabsorbable, interrupted sutures. Some hernias require a two-layered repair using the posterior and anterior rectus sheaths.

Umbilical Hernia

Umbilical hernia is present in 10% to 20% of infants. Most of these hernias close spontaneously in the first 4 or 5 years of life. In older children, the incidence of incarceration and/or strangulation of bowel is 5%. Incarcerated hernias and hernias larger than 1.5 cm in diameter should be repaired. In adults, most umbilical hernias should be repaired because they tend to enlarge and cause bowel obstruction. Two types of repair are available. The most popular is the Mayo repair in which a transverse incision is used and a "vest-over-pants" repair performed. The second method is a simple, transverse approximation of the fascia.

OTHER HERNIAS

Parastomal Hernias

A parastomal hernia is an incisional hernia that develops in the vicinity of an ileostomy or colostomy. It is among the more common complications of stoma formation and is usually located adjacent to the mesentery of the bowel. The hernia may achieve a large size and interfere with the positioning and functioning of stomal appliances. It may cause pain and, rarely, small bowel obstruction within the hernia sac. It is caused by technical error and may be prevented by proper sitting of the stoma, particularly by avoiding placing the stoma lateral to the rectus or through a previous incision. The stoma is best brought out through the rectus muscle.

Small parastomal hernias can be managed expectantly. Larger hernias, particularly if they interfere with stomal function, require surgical treatment. Two approaches are possible: The stoma may be relocated to another site and the abdominal wall defect repaired, or the hernia may be repaired locally with or without reinforcing prosthetic mesh. Stoma relocation yields better results.

Spigelian Hernia

The semilunar (Spigelian) line represents the end of the transversus abdominis and the beginning of the aponeurosis or transversalis fascia that extends into the pelvis. A Spigelian hernia occurs through a defect in the abdominal wall at the juncture of the semilunar line and the lateral edge of the rectus abdominus muscle. The hernia is rare and occurs with equal frequency on both sides of the abdomen. Although some are congenital, it is believed that most are acquired. The most common symptom is localized pain. Although a swelling may be absent on physical examination, the patient may have previously observed a local swelling. Physical examination may reveal a hernia, but most often a hernial impulse or swelling is detected only on straining or Valsalva maneuver. The diagnosis may be difficult. The treatment is simple herniorrhaphy performed either through a midline or paramedian incision. The sac is excised and the defect closed with nonabsorbable simple sutures.

Lumbar Hernia

The lumbar area of the abdominal wall is bounded superiorly by the 12th rib, inferiorly by the iliac crest, medially by the sacrospinal muscles, and laterally by the posterior border of the external oblique muscle. This area is divided into a superior and inferior space. The inferior space, the triangle of Petit, is bound inferiorly by the iliac crest, medially by the lateral border of the latissimus dorsi muscle, and laterally by the external oblique muscle. Rarely, hernias may occur either in the superior or inferior lumbar space. The clinical presentation is usually back pain associated with a tender mass. When symptomatic, the treatment is surgical through a transverse incision over the mass. The defect is usually small, and the fascial defect readily approximated with nonabsorbable interrupted sutures.

Pelvic Floor Hernias

Pelvic floor hernias are rare and often present diagnostic dilemmas. They include obturator hernia, sciatic hernia, and perineal hernia.

Obturator Hernia

Fewer than 1,000 cases of obturator hernia have been reported in the literature.[7] Approximately 80% occur in thin, elderly women in the seventh or eight decade of life. They are also seen in women of childbearing age, especially in multiparity, which leads to relaxation of pelvic tissues. Approximately 60% occur on the right side.

The hernia occurs through the obturator foramen and may thus compress the obturator nerve, causing pain in the medial thigh (Howship–Romberg sign). When pain in the medial thigh is associated with intestinal obstruction, the diagnosis of an obturator hernia should be seriously entertained. Intestinal obstruction in an obturator hernia often leads to strangulation and high risk of death because the diagnosis is not made promptly. Spiral CT has recently proven to be an excellent diagnostic study.

All symptomatic obturator hernias should be treated surgically. If the diagnosis is certain, a preperitoneal approach may be used. Most often, however, the approach is transabdominal. The sac is usually medial to the neurovascular bundle. The hernia should be reduced and any herniated small intestine carefully examined for nonviability. Occasionally, the appendix or a Meckel's diverticulum may be found in the hernia. If the hernia cannot be reduced easily, the ring should be incised medially or posteriorly to avoid the neurovascular bundle. The sac is closed with a pursestring suture, and the defect is also closed using either fascia lata or a synthetic mesh. The contralateral side should always be inspected because bilateral hernias occur in 5% to 10% of these cases.

Sciatic Hernia

Sciatic hernia is exceedingly rare, with fewer than 100 cases reported in the literature. It occurs through the greater or lesser sciatic notch.[7] The greater sciatic notch is divided into superior and inferior portions by the piriformis muscle. Most hernias occur through the suprapiriformis part, along the course of the superior gluteal artery and nerve. The first symptom of the hernia may be bowel obstruction and pain in the gluteal region, suggesting compression of the sciatic nerve. Sciatic nerve compression may lead to pain that radiates down the posterior thigh and is aggravated by dorsiflexion of the foot. A palpable and sometimes reducible hernia may be present.

Treatment is surgical by the transabdominal route. The sac is found behind the broad ligament and superior to the uterosacral ligament in women and between the rectum and bladder in the posterolateral pelvis in men. After reduction of the hernia and excision of the sac, the defect is closed with a patch of either Marlex® or fascia lata.

Perineal Hernia

This rare hernia may be congenital or acquired following abdominoperineal resection. The hernia may be anterior or posterior to the transverse perineal muscle. Anterior hernias occur almost exclusively in women and represent a defect of the urogenital diaphragm. Posterior hernias occur between the bladder and rectum and appear in the ischiorectal fossa. Symptoms are unimpressive; the presentation is usually a soft, reducible mass. The treatment is surgical, and a transabdominal approach is recommended. A prosthetic mesh may be required to close the defect.

PERITONEUM

ANATOMY

The peritoneal cavity is the abdominal space bounded by the diaphragm superiorly, the pelvic floor inferiorly, the retroperitoneum posteriorly, and the anterior abdominal wall anteriorly. It contains all the abdominal viscera except those that lie in the retroperitoneum, which include the second, third, and fourth portion of the duodenum, the distal rectum, the pancreas, the kidneys and ureters, the adrenal glands, and the aorta and inferior vena cava. The peritoneal cavity is lined with the parietal peritoneum, made of mesothelium. The peritoneal lining reflects to cover partially or completely the intraabdominal viscera, thus creating the visceral peritoneum.

The parietal peritoneum is supplied by segmental nerves that also supply the abdominal wall directly in contact. The nerve supply of the visceral peritoneum, however, is the nerve supply of the viscus it covers. The entire small intestine, the appendix, ascending and right colon, and the visceral peritoneum covering these structures are supplied by thoracic C-10, which also supplies the skin in the preumbilical region. Hence, pain due to distension, ischemia, or inflammation in these structures is first referred to the periumbilical region (Figure 8.8). Only when the parietal peritoneum overlying the diseased bowel is involved does the pain localize to the region where the diseased bowel is actually located.

A number of potential spaces in the peritoneal cavity can be the site of intraabdominal abscesses. Figure 12.9 shows a simplified classification of the peritoneal spaces. The colon divides the abdomen into the supra- and infracolic spaces and into the right and left paracolic gutters. The supracolic space contains the left and right subphrenic spaces and the subhepatic space, which is continuous with the hepatorenal space. When a patient is lying supine, the hepatorenal space is the most dependent part of the peritoneal cavity. The supracolic space also contains the lesser sac behind the lesser omentum. The infracolic space is divided by the mesentery of the small intestine, whose oblique attachment to the retroperitoneum extends from the right side of L-4 to the left side of L-1, into a right and left infracolic space. The pelvic cavity begins at the promontory of the sacrum. The rectum divides the pelvic cavity into a prerectal space anteriorly—rectovesical in men and rectovaginal (pouch of Douglas) in women—and posteriorly into a retrorectal or presacral space.

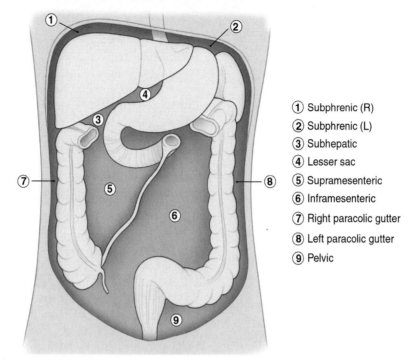

FIGURE 12.9. Simplified classification of the various spaces within the peritoneal cavity in which abscesses can form or fluid can accumulate.

① Subphrenic (R)
② Subphrenic (L)
③ Subhepatic
④ Lesser sac
⑤ Supramesenteric
⑥ Inframesenteric
⑦ Right paracolic gutter
⑧ Left paracolic gutter
⑨ Pelvic

All of these spaces are potential sites of intraabdominal abscesses. Abdominal abscesses may also develop between loops of small intestine, where they are referred to as interloop abscesses.

PHYSIOLOGY

The peritoneum and omentum play several roles of physiologic significance:

1. Provision of a surface that allows smooth gliding of the small intestine within the peritoneal cavity. This function is aided by the presence of free fluid (50 mL of transudate) within the peritoneal cavity.

2. Fluid exchange. Approximately 500 mL of fluid or more per hour may be exchanged between the peritoneal cavity and the circulation across the peritoneum. This remarkable property is exploited in the performance of peritoneal dialysis in renal failure. In infants, circulating blood volume may be replenished by the administration of fluid intraperitoneally.

3. Response to tissue damage or infection. The mesothelial and mast cells secrete histamine and other vasodilators in response to injury or infection. This leads to vascular permeability and the exudation of fibrinogen-rich plasma, complement, and opsonins. Together with the arrival of neutrophils and macrophages, this process contributes to bacterial destruction.

4. Omental migration. The omentum migrates to areas of inflammation, perforation, or ischemia. This well-vascularized tissue attempts to isolate the pathology and also exerts bacteriophagic function.

5. Elimination of bacteria and toxic products. Bacteria that are not destroyed and other toxic products of infection are circulated to the subdiaphragmatic surfaces, particularly on the right, and absorbed into lymphatic channels and delivered into the right thoracic duct. Undoubtedly, the circulation of fluid from the lower abdomen to the subdiaphragmatic space is due to negative pressure generated in the subdiaphragmatic space with respiration.

PATHOPHYSIOLOGY

Peritonitis

The peritoneum mounts rapid response to infection, injury, and leakage into the peritoneal cavity of digestive fluid, bile, pancreatic juice, urine, or blood. The result is vascular permeability, fluid exudation, and both neutrophil and cytokine response. Pain fibers within both the visceral and parietal peritoneum are activated. These fibers are believed to be C-fibers containing substance P and calcitonin gene-related peptide (CGRP). Reflex pathways cause muscular contraction in the abdominal wall to limit movement (guarding and rigidity). Similarly, peristaltic movement of the intestine is arrested (hypoactive or absent bowel sounds).

Earlier, it was indicated that vascular permeability, as a result of tissue damage or infection, causes fibrin-rich plasma to flow into the peritoneal cavity. This leads to the formation of fibrin, which later organizes into collagen and causes adhesion formation. Untreated, generalized peritonitis most commonly cause death secondary to gram-negative septicemia, septic shock, and disseminated intravascular coagulation. On other occasions, generalized peritonitis leads to intraabdominal abscesses, which tend to be multiple.

Ascites Formation

Ascites formation as a result of portal hypertension is discussed in detail in Chapter 6. Ascites can also occur secondary to hypoproteinemia caused by the nephrotic syndrome. Another important cause of ascites is malignancy. Patients with peritoneal metastases, especially secondary to ovarian cancer, may have extensive malignant ascites.

Chylous ascites can result from disruption of the main lymphatic channels as a result of external trauma or operative damage. The most common cause of chylous ascites, however, is malignancy—either lymphoma or metastatic adenocarcinoma—obstructing lymphatic channels.

CLINICAL DISORDERS

Primary Peritonitis

Primary (spontaneous) peritonitis is most commonly seen in cirrhotic patients with ascites. It may also be seen as the nephrotic syndrome in postsplenectomy patients and in systemic lupus erythematosus (SLE). The essentials of primary peritonitis are summarized in Table 12.4.

The diagnosis is confirmed by paracentesis, which shows monomicrobial infection (*Escherichia coli*, Klebsiella, or streptococcus). By contrast, secondary peritonitis is always polymicrobial. Fluid obtained by paracentesis is examined microscopically with Gram stain and is cultured. The fluid is mildly acidic (pH 7.3 or less) and will contain more than 500 WBC/μl, of which greater than 25% are polymorphonuclear cells.

Treatment is nonsurgical, using appropriate antibiotics intravenously. The mortality rate is greater than 50% and most often is due to liver or renal failure.[8]

TABLE 12.4. Essentials: Primary (Spontaneous) Peritonitis

Uncommon condition seen in
- Cirrhosis with ascites
- Nephrotic syndrome
- Following splenectomy
- Systemic lupus erythematosus

Pathogen: Monomicrobial infection (*Escherichia coli*, Klebsiella organisms, or streptococcus)

Treatment: Intravenous antibiotics

Prognosis: High mortality rate, usually from associated liver or kidney failure

---

Secondary Peritonitis

Secondary peritonitis occurs from septic invasion of the peritoneal cavity either from the gastrointestinal tract (perforation, anastomotic failure, or gangrene) or due to penetrating trauma, especially when a foreign body is introduced into the peritoneal cavity. The clinical presentation, diagnosis, and treatment of secondary peritonitis are discussed fully elsewhere under several headings in this book.

Intraabdominal Abscess

Both the incidence and management of intraabdominal abscess have changed significantly in the last three decades. Advances in management—including antibiotic prophylaxis, availability of potent antibiotics to treat abdominal infection, and better surgical technique—have reduced their incidence, but an even more significant revolution has occurred in their management. Abdominal imaging techniques (ultrasound, computed tomography, and magnetic resonance) have enabled early and accurate localization as well as percutaneous drainage of these abscesses.

Surgical treatment is indicated when abscesses are: (1) not readily accessible for percutaneous drainage, (2) multiloculated or intermesentery, or (3) fail to resolve following percutaneous drainage. Often, laparotomy and extensive debridement and drainage will be necessary. External drainage is accomplished through closed suction catheters, which can, if indicated, be used for irrigation.

Drainage of Subphrenic Abscess through the Bed of the Twelfth Rib

Occasionally, the need arises to provide dependent surgical drainage for resistant subphrenic abscess. This is best accomplished extraperitoneally through the bed of the twelfth rib. The tip of the rib is palpated, a transverse incision (8–10 cm) is placed over it, then deepened by splitting the abdominal wall muscles. Again, the tip of the twelfth rib is palpated, dissected, and resected. The abscess can be localized by needle aspiration. The peritoneum is opened, carefully avoiding entrance into the pleural space. On the left side, the surgeon should avoid damage to the spleen. By blunt dissection, the abscess cavity is entered and drained. Two large sump drains are left in place, and the wound is closed in layers.

Transrectal Drainage of Pelvic Abscess

A deep pelvic abscess that is palpable rectally but inaccessible for percutaneous catheter drainage may be readily drained through the rectum. With the patient in the lithotomy position, the anus is dilated. The soft bulge of the abscess is palpated with a finger and a long hemostat is inserted along the finger and pushed into the abscess cavity and spread. A soft rubber catheter is left in place and, if possible, sutured with catgut to the adjacent rectal wall. Before undertaking such drainage, careful radiological examination should be obtained to ascertain that the small intestine is out of harm's way. In women, an abscess in the pouch of Douglas may be drained transvaginally.

Ascites

Management of ascites in the cirrhotic patient is detailed in Chapter 6. Selected patients with serious malignant ascites who are resistant to medical therapy may be treated with peritoneovenous catheter. Malignant cells entering the circulation do not appear to cause a significant problem. Patients with chylous ascites resistant to supportive therapy are treated by TPN, chemotherapy, and/or radiotherapy.

Disorders of the Omentum

Torsion or infarction of the omentum may present with acute abdominal pain, nausea, and vomiting. The diagnosis is difficult, but localized tenderness and a mobile tender mass may be present in one-third of patients. Definitive diagnosis is only possible at laparotomy. The infarcted or torqued omentum is excised. Primary tumors and cysts of the omentum are rare, although they frequently occur at

the site of metastatic tumors from the gastrointestinal tract and ovaries.

Internal Abdominal Hernia

Internal abdominal hernias may occur in various locations (Figure 12.10). The main types are foramen of Winslow (lesser sac), paraduodenal, and pericecal. Other rare internal hernias are intersigmoid and transmesenteric.

Foramen of Winslow (Lesser Sac) Hernia

In rare instances, the small intestine herniates through the foramen of Winslow into the lesser sac. The symptoms are those of upper abdominal pain and small bowel obstruction. Typically, the pain is relieved by bending forward or by assuming the knee-chest position. Plain films of the abdomen show gas-containing loops of small intestine in the lesser sac. Barium examination of the upper gastrointestinal tract is diagnostic, showing anterior displacement of the stomach and displacement of the duodenum to the left.

Paraduodenal Hernia

These hernias represent more than 50% of all internal abdominal hernias. Approximately 75% occur on the left

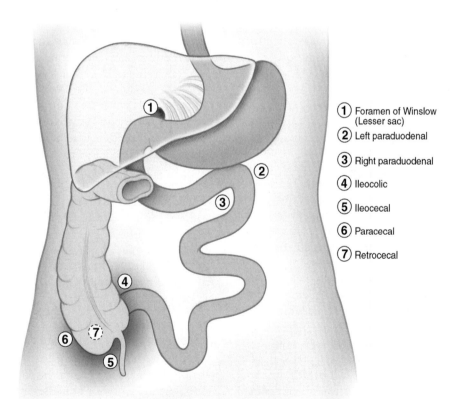

1 Foramen of Winslow (Lesser sac)
2 Left paraduodenal
3 Right paraduodenal
4 Ileocolic
5 Ileocecal
6 Paracecal
7 Retrocecal

FIGURE 12.10. Locations of internal abdominal hernias include the foramen of Winslow (1); around the duodenojejunal junction (2, 3); and around the cecum (4, 5, 6 and 7).

at the paraduodenal fossa of Landzert. Right paraduodenal hernias occur through an abnormal pocket of jejunal mesentery next to the duodenum and immediately behind the superior mesenteric artery. The clinical manifestation is variable and ranges from intermittent and mild digestive complaints to intestinal obstruction. A left paraduodenal hernia results in a characteristic sign in barium studies: an ovoid mass of several loops of small intestine immediately lateral to the ascending duodenum. Treatment is surgical reduction and obliteration of the abnormal paraduodenal spaces.

Pericecal Hernia

There are four peritoneal fossae in the ileocecal region—ileocolic, retrocecal, ileocecal, and paracecal—and herniation can occur into any of these sites. Symptoms are those of intermittent low small bowel obstruction. Chronic obstruction may simulate periappendiceal abscess or regional enteritis. The treatment is surgical.

Malignancy of the Peritoneum

While metastatic tumors to the peritoneum are common, primary malignancies in the peritoneum are rare and include peritoneal mesothelioma and pseudomyxoma peritonei.

Peritoneal mesothelioma is most common in men exposed to asbestos. The latent period may be 40 years. Peritoneal mesothelioma is not as frequently diagnosed as pleural mesothelioma. Computed tomography may show free peritoneal fluid, soft tissue mass, and mesenteric and peritoneal thickening. The diagnosis is best made by laparoscopy and biopsy. Treatment is with chemotherapy (cisplatinum and doxorubicin) or with radiation. Surgery is indicated if bowel obstruction develops, and debulking can also be accomplished simultaneously.

Pseudomyxoma peritonei is a rare tumor due to mucinous cystadenoma of the ovary or appendix. Symptoms occur late and consist of intermittent abdominal distension and pain accompanied by weight loss. Abdominal ultrasound or CT scan may show a mass, fluid, and calcified plaque. The treatment is surgical. If the tumor originates in the appendix, a right hemicolectomy is performed. Ovarian tumors are treated by oophorectomy and, if complete excision is not possible, tumor debulking may be helpful. Postoperative treatment includes chemotherapy (systemic and/or intraperitoneal) or radiotherapy. The 5-year survival rate of 50% is cited.[9]

RETROPERITONEUM

Retroperitoneal conditions requiring surgical attention are rare and include hematoma, abscesses, fibrosis, and tumors.

HEMATOMA

Retroperitoneal hematoma is most often seen in motor vehicle accidents and may be high in the region of the kidneys and duodenum or low as an extension of a pelvic hematoma. Retroperitoneal hematoma is best evaluated by CT scan if the patient is stable. In the unstable patient, associated intraabdominal injury is common, and diagnostic peritoneal lavage (DPL) is an appropriate diagnostic test. Lower retroperitoneal hematomas are usually not explored and, because they are nearly always associated with pelvic fracture, they are best managed with transcatheter angiographic control of bleeding with embolization.

Upper retroperitoneal hematomas represent a different and potentially serious injury. On either side, renal injury must be suspected, sometimes even renal pedicle disruption. On the right, injury of the retroperitoneal duodenum must be excluded. In either case, the principles of management are the same and include:

1. Examination of renal injury and status of the contralateral kidney with either flush aortogram or IVP.

2. Achievement of vascular control before opening the hematoma. Vascular control may be accomplished by controlling the renal vessels outside the hematoma, but supraceliac aortic and IVC control will usually be required.

3. Exploration of the hematoma and evaluation of the kidney, renal pedicle ureters and, on the right, duodenum. Renal injury may be amenable to repair, to partial nephrectomy or may require total nephrectomy if a normal contralateral kidney is present. Management of duodenal trauma was discussed in Chapter 11.

Retroperitoneal hematoma can occur spontaneously in patients who are on anticoagulants. Abdominal distension may develop as a result of ileus. The management is conservative with proper control of anticoagulation.

RETROPERITONEAL ABSCESS

Retroperitoneal abscesses may be anterior (medial) or posterior (lateral). Anterior abscesses are related to pathology in the pancreas, duodenum, colon, and kidneys. Posterior retroperitoneal abscess is usually sepsis that tracks down on the anterior surface of the psoas, either from infection in the vertebral column or other pathology, such as ruptured retrocecal appendicitis. The clinical picture is characterized by hip pain, flexion of the hip joint, and pain on hip extension.

Retroperitoneal abscess is best evaluated by CT scan and may be amenable to percutaneous drainage. If percutaneous drainage is impossible or fails, surgical drainage and debridement will be necessary. Posterior abscesses are best drained extraperitoneally, but anterior abscesses often require a transabdominal approach. The infection is usually due to mixed flora (i.e., *E. coli*, Klebsiella, bacteroides, and *Streptococcus fecalis*). Appropriate antibiotic coverage should be instituted. When a psoas abscess is encountered, the possibility of tuberculosis must be excluded. Tuberculous psoas abscess is often associated with spinal tuberculosis (Pott's disease).

RETROPERITONEAL FIBROSIS

Two-thirds of cases of retroperitoneal fibrosis are idiopathic. The other third are due to drugs, particularly methysergide and beta-adrenergic blocking agents. Occasionally, retroperitoneal fibrosis is seen in association with abdominal carcinoid tumor, Crohn's disease, and even post-trauma if urine has been extravasated in the retroperitoneum. Most cases are seen in men over the age of 50 years.

The clinical picture is usually due to obstruction of the urinary tract and includes bilateral hydroureter, hydronephrosis, and median deviation of the ureter, seen on IVP studies. Bowel obstruction may occur as a secondary complication. Diagnosis is best established by CT scan or MRI. The offending drug, if present, must be discontinued. Treatment may require urinary decompression by ureteric stenting or nephrostomy. Occasionally, surgical ureterolysis with omental wrap of the ureters may be necessary.

RETROPERITONEAL TUMORS

Retroperitoneal tumors are rare and include: (1) lymphatic: lymphomas; (2) mesenchymal: liposarcoma, leiomyosarcoma, or fibrosarcoma; (3) neural: neuroblastoma or schwannoma; or (4) embryonic: malignant teratoma, chondroma.

The most common symptoms are abdominal pain, weight loss, or fever. Large retroperitoneal liposarcomas may produce symptoms of intermittent hypoglycemia. Investigation may include IVP, contrast-enhanced CT, MRI, or angiography. Definitive diagnosis may be possible with FNA but frequently requires open laparotomy. Treatment is en bloc resection with postoperative radiation and/or chemotherapy.

REFERENCES

1. Toy FK, Moskowitz M, Smoot RT Jr, et al. Results of a prospective multicenter trial evaluating the ePTFE peritoneal onlay laparoscopic inguinal hernioplasty. *J Laparoendosc Surg* 1996;6: 375–386.
2. Miller AR, van Heerden JA, Naessens JM, et al. Simultaneous bilateral hernia repair. A case against conventional wisdom. *Ann Surg* 1991;213:272–276.
3. Ijzermans JN, deWilt H, Hop WC, et al. Recurrent inguinal hernia treated by classical hernioplasty. *Arch Surg* 1991;126: 1097–1100.
4. Glassow F. The Shouldice Hospital technique. *Int Surg* 1986; 71:148–153.
5. Read RC, Yoder G. Recent trends in the management of incisional herniation. *Arch Surg* 1989;124:485–488.
6. Bucknall TE, Cox PJ, Ellis H. Burst abdomen and incisional hernia: a prospective study of 1129 major laparotomies. *BMJ* 1982;284:931–933.
7. Marchal F, Parent S, Tortuyaux JM, et al. Obturator hernias—report of seven cases. *Hernia* 1997;1:23–26.
8. Conn HO. Spontaneous bacterial peritonitis: variant syndromes. *South Med J* 1987;80:1343–1346.
9. Carr NJ, McCarthy WF, Sobin LH. Epithelial noncarcinoid tumors and tumor-like lesions of the appendix. A clinicopathologic study of 184 patients with a multivariate analysis of prognostic factors. *Cancer* 1995;75:757–768.

SELECTED READINGS

Hernias

Cali RL, Pitsch RM, Blatchford GJ, et al. Rare pelvic floor hernias. Report of a case and review of literature. *Dis Colon Rectum* 1992;35:604–612.

Champault GG, Rizk N, Catheline JM, et al. Inguinal hernia repair: totally preperitoneal laparoscopic approach versus Stoppa operation, randomized trial of 100 cases. *Surg Laparosc Endosc* 1997; 7:445–450.

Flanagan L, Bascom JU. Repair of the groin hernia: outpatient approach with local anesthesia. *Surg Clin North Am* 1984;64:257–267.

Ghahremani GG. Internal abdominal hernia. *Surg Clin North Am* 1984;64:393–406.

Glassow F. Inguinal hernia repair. A comparison of the Shouldice and Cooper ligament repair of the posterior inguinal wall. *Am J Surg* 1976;131:306–311.

Lichtenstein IL, Shulman AG, Amid PK, et al. The tension-free hernioplasty. *Am J Surg* 1989;157:188–193.

Nyhus LM, Condon RE, Harkins HN. Clinical experiences with preperitoneal hernia repair for all types of hernia of the groin: with particular reference to the importance of transversalis fascia analogues. *Am J Surg* 1960;100:234–244.

Payne JH Jr, Grininger LM, Izawa MT, et al. Laparoscopic or open inguinal herniorrhaphy? A randomized prospective trial. *Arch Surg* 1994;129:973–981.

Rutledge RH. Cooper's ligament repair: a 25-year experience with a single technique for all groin hernias in adults. *Surgery* 1988;103:1–10.

Skandalakis JE, Gray SW, Skandalakis LJ, et al. Surgical anatomy of the inguinal area. *World J Surg* 1989;13:490–498.

Wantz GE. Complications of inguinal hernia repair. *Surg Clin North Am* 1984;64:287–298.

Wantz GE. Suture tension in Shouldice's hernioplasty. *Arch Surg* 1981;116:1238–1239.

Zieren J, Zieren HU, Jacobi CA, et al. Prospective randomized study comparing laparoscopic and open tension-free inguinal hernia repair with Shouldice's operation. *Am J Surg* 1998;175:330–333.

Peritoneum and Retroperitoneum

Ablan CJ, Littooy FN, Freeark RJ. Postoperative chylous ascites: diagnosis and treatment. A series report and literature review. *Arch Surg* 1990;125:270–273.

Bullock N. Idiopathic retroperitoneal fibrosis. *BMJ* 1988;297:240–241.

Crepps JT, Welch JP, Orlando R 3rd. Management and outcome of retroperitoneal abscesses. *Ann Surg* 1987;205:276–281.

Deveney CW, Lurie, Deveney KE. Improved treatment of intraabdominal abscess. *Arch Surg* 1988;123:1126–1130.

Edney JA, Hill A, Armstrong D. Peritoneovenous shunts palliate malignant ascites. *Am J Surg* 1989;158:598–601.

Haaga JR. Imaging intraabdominal abscesses and nonoperative drainage procedures. *World J Surg* 1990;14:204–209.

Hallak A. Spontaneous bacterial peritonitis. *Am J Gastroenterol* 1989;84:345–350.

Hau T, Haaga JR, Aeder MI. Pathophysiology, diagnosis and treatment of abdominal abscesses. *Curr Probl Surg* 1984;21:1–82.

Mann WJ Jr, Wagner J, Chumas J, et al. The management of pseudomyxoma peritonei. *Cancer* 1990;66:1636–1640.

Plaus WJ. Peritoneal mesothelioma. *Arch Surg* 1988;123:763–766.

Storm FK, Mahvi DM. Diagnosis and management of retroperitoneal soft-tissue sarcoma. *Ann Surg* 1991;214:2–10.

Perioperative Care

Major gastrointestinal surgery imposes significant insult on the patient's metabolic, endocrine, and immunologic equilibrium. Some operations, particularly if followed by postoperative complications, can result in prolonged inability to use the gastrointestinal tract to sustain nutrition. Operations in the upper abdomen can also compromise a patient's ability to breathe well and to cough. Finally, whenever the gastrointestinal tract is opened, the risk of developing intraabdominal or wound infection is markedly increased. Hence, it is critically important to perform careful preoperative general assessment; correct any fluid, electrolyte, and nutritional deficits; and institute prophylaxis for infection and/or thromboembolism. Patients with specific preexisting cardiopulmonary, metabolic, renal, endocrine, and hematologic disorders require special assessment and preoperative preparation.

GENERAL PATIENT EVALUATION

CLINICAL EVALUATION

A careful medical history must determine several factors: whether the patient has any allergies or coexisting disease, whether he or she is taking any medications, and whether problems were encountered with prior anesthesia or surgery. A history of a tendency to bruise or bleed should be sought. A family medical history should also be obtained to rule out bleeding disorders and anesthetic complications.

Physical examination should assess the presence or absence of anemia, contraction of the extracellular fluid volume, and nutritional deficit. Subclinical hypovolemia is best assessed at the bedside by looking for orthostatic changes in blood pressure. Patients who have lost 10% or more of their body weight have lost all their body fat and exhibit hollowed cheeks. They require preoperative correction of their nutritional deficit. Nutritional deficit is more difficult to assess in the obese patient.

LABORATORY EVALUATION

In all patients undergoing major abdominal surgery, the following tests are required: hemogram, urinalysis, blood urea nitrogen (BUN), creatinine, serum electrolytes, prothrombin time (PT), and partial prothrombin time (PTT). Those patients with hepatobiliary disease require liver function tests (total and direct bilirubin, alkaline phosphatase, and liver enzymes).

ROUTINE CARDIOPULMONARY EVALUATION

Patients without underlying cardiopulmonary disease who are undergoing major abdominal injury should have a chest x-ray and electrocardiogram. The evaluation of patients with preexisting cardiopulmonary disease is discussed below.

Patients with preexisting conditions require specific evaluation directed at assessing the degree of physiological impairment so that their condition can be optimized preoperatively.

PREEXISTING CARDIAC DISEASE

Elective surgery in a patient with a history of recent myocardial infarction (MI) carries a significantly increased risk of reinfarction. The risk of reinfarction if elective surgery is done within 3 months of MI is 30%, but this risk falls to less than 5% just 6 months after MI. Hence, elective surgery should be postponed at least 6 months after MI.

A useful method of assessing cardiac risk is to compute the cardiac risk index (CRI) with the method described by Goldman et al.[1] (Table 13.1). Zeldin has used the CRI to classify into four groups patients who undergo noncardiac surgical procedures.[2] The incidence of life-threatening complication and mortality rate in each of these classes is summarized in Table 13.2.

Patients with a history of coronary artery disease or angina should undergo evaluation with a thalium perfusion scan at rest and during exercise or after administra-

TABLE 13.2. Correlation of Cardiac Index and Life-Threatening Operative Complications*

Class	Points	Complication (%)	Mortality (%)
I	0–5	0.7	0.2
II	6–12	5	2
III	13–25	11	2
IV	>25	22	56

*Life-threatening complications include myocardial infarction, pulmonary edema, and ventricular tachycardia.
Source: Reprinted with permission from Zeldin R. Assessing cardiac risk in patients who undergo noncardiac surgical procedures. Can J Surg 1984; 27:402–404. Canadian Medical Association.

tion of dipyridamole. Perfusion defects indicate ischemic regions. Another method of evaluation is the use of stress echocardiography with infusion of dobutamine. Echocardiography is not only cheaper but is better at assessing valve function, quantifying wall motion abnormalities, and estimating left ventricular ejection fraction. Patients who have serious cardiac disease as demonstrated by one or both of these tests should undergo coronary angiography and have the coronary artery disease treated surgically or by angioplasty and stenting before major elective abdominal surgery is undertaken. Preoperative coronary angiography is also indicated in patients with symptoms or a history of poorly controlled congestive heart failure. Individuals with underlying cardiac disease require intraoperative monitoring of systemic arterial and pulmonary artery pressure.

RESPIRATORY DISEASE

The presence of lung disease significantly increases the risk of postoperative pulmonary complications, particularly in patients undergoing upper abdominal operations. A history of cigarette smoking (20 pack-years or smoking more than 20 cigarettes per day) also significantly increases the risk of postoperative pulmonary complications including atelectasis and pneumonia. Preoperative assessment of pulmonary function using spirometry and arterial blood gasses is indicated in patients with chronic obstructive lung disease (COPD), those with productive cough and dyspnea, and those with a history of heavy smoking of 20 pack-years or greater. Table 13.3 summarizes abnormal pulmonary function tests that predict increased operative risk as described by Pett and Wernly.[3]

The forced expiratory volume in 1 second (FEV_1) and the functional volume capacity (FVC) provide adequate evaluation of lung function. FEV_1 of less than 1.2 L (<70% of predicted) or FVC of less than 1.7 L (<70%) is associated with an increased risk of pulmonary complication (e.g., atelectasis, pneumonia). On arterial blood gas analy-

TABLE 13.1. Calculation of Cardiac Risk Index

Factor	Points
History	
Age >70 years	5
MI in previous 6 mo	10
Physical Examination	
S_3 heart sound or JVD	11
Significant valvular aortic stenosis	3
Electrocardiogram	
Nonsinus rhythm or PACs	7
>5 PVCs/min preoperatively	7
General Medical Status	3
PO_2 <60 or Pco_2 >50 mm Hg	
K^+ <3.0 or HCO_3 <20 mEq/dl	
BUN >50 or creatinine >3.0 mg/dL	
Chronic liver disease, abnormal SGOT	
Bedridden for noncardiac cause	
Surgical Procedure	
Intraperitoneal, intrathoracic, aortic	3
Emergency surgery	4
Total	53

Abbreviations: BUN, blood urea nitrogen; JVD, jugular venous distention; MI, myocardial infarction; PAC, premature atrial contraction; PVC, premature ventricular contraction; S_3, third heart sound; SGOT, serum glutamic-oxaloacetic transaminase.
Source: Reprinted with permission from Goldman L, Caldera D, Nussbaum E, et al. Multifactorial index of cardiac risk in noncardiac surgical procedures. N Engl J Med 1977;297:845–850. Copyright© 1977 Massachusetts Medical Society. All rights reserved.

TABLE 13.3. Pulmonary Function Test Results that Suggest Increased Operative Risk

FVC	<50%–70% predicted
FEV₁	<35%–70% predicted
FEF	<50% predicted
MVV	<35%–55% predicted
MEFR	<200 L/min
RV	<47%
DCO	<50%
PaCO₂	>45 mm Hg
PAP	>22–35 mm Hg
PVP	>190 dynes/cm/sec
VO₂	<15 ml/kg/min

Abbreviations: DCO, diffusion capacity of carbon monoxide; FEF, forced expiratory flow; FEV₁, forced expiratory volume in 1 sec; FVC, forced vital capacity; MEFR, maximum expiratory flow rate; MVV, maximum voluntary ventilation; PaCO₂, arterial partial pressure of carbon dioxide; PAP, pulmonary artery pressure; PVR, pulmonary vascular resistance; RV, residual volume; VO₂, oxygen uptake.
Source: Reprinted with permission from Pett SB Jr, Wernly JA. Respiratory function in surgical patients. Perioperative evaluation and management. Surg Annu 1988;20:311–329.

sis, arterial oxygen tension in room air of 60 mm Hg or less and pCO₂ of 45 mm Hg or greater are associated with increased postoperative complications. Cigarette smoking should be discontinued at least 8 weeks preoperatively, but discontinuation of smoking even for far shorter periods is beneficial. Patients with COPD may benefit from preoperative treatment with bronchodilators (e.g., aminophylline), mucolytic drugs (e.g., acetylcysteine) and aerosol β₂ agonists. Patients with COPD who have purulent sputum may benefit from a short course of antibiotic therapy preoperatively. Patients with asthma require bronchodilator therapy to eliminate wheezing preoperatively, and some may require steroid therapy.

RENAL DISEASE

Renal failure can cause hyperkalemia, metabolic acidosis, and coagulopathy, all of which must be corrected preoperatively. Patients with established renal failure should undergo dialysis about 24 h before elective surgery. The 24-h period facilitates the reestablishment of fluid and electrolyte equilibrium postdialysis and allows the effects of heparin given at the time of dialysis to subside before operation.

The presence of renal disease may be discovered de novo during preoperative assessment. If serum creatinine is below 6 mg/dL or glomerular filtration rate (GFR) greater than 15 mL/min, the patient must be adequately hydrated and the hematocrit kept above 32%. In such patients, adequate blood volume should be strictly monitored and maintained during operation and postoperatively to avoid acute renal failure.

Patients with renal failure are more prone to infection and are susceptible to drug toxicity, particularly to nephro-

toxic antibiotics such as gentamycin, amphotericin B, and methicillin. Gentamycin administration should be based on measurement of plasma levels of the antibiotic. The dose and frequency of administration of hypnotics and digitalis must be titrated to renal function. Patients with renal failure are susceptible to coagulopathy. This complication is prevented by preoperative dialysis. Coagulopathy that develops intra- or postoperatively may be treated by administration of fresh-frozen plasma or diamino-8-D-argenine vasopressin (DDAVP).

ENDOCRINE COMPLICATIONS

Diabetes Mellitus

Patients with mild diabetes maintained on oral hypoglycemic agents may require no specific perioperative management. Oral hypoglycemic agents should be discontinued the day of surgery, and longer acting sulfonylurea drugs should be discontinued at least 1 day preoperatively. Intravenous 5% glucose-in-water should be administered at 100 ml/h. If blood glucose rises over 250 mg/dL, 5 U of insulin should be added to each liter of 5% glucose solution.

Patients with insulin-dependent diabetes require insulin during surgery and monitoring of blood glucose levels. One method of managing insulin requirement during surgery is to administer one-half to two-thirds of the daily insulin dose as neutral protamine Hagedorn (NPH) insulin. Alternatively, regular insulin may be infused intravenously in glucose solution (5% or 10%). The amount of insulin infused depends on the initial blood glucose concentration and may vary from 0.5 to 1.5 U/h. Whatever method is used, hypoglycemia must be avoided with frequent determination of blood glucose. Diabetic ketoacidosis is another complication to be avoided. Except in the patient with brittle diabetes or severe sepsis, ketoacidosis is rare when modern techniques of perioperative care are used.

Adrenal Insufficiency

Patients with adrenal insufficiency or those on long-term steroid therapy may develop Addisonian crises if adequate corticosteroid therapy is not maintained during and after surgery. Any preexisting hypokalemia should be corrected and serum potassium monitored intra- and postoperatively.

Patients on chronic corticosteroid therapy should receive stress doses of cortisol (approximately 300 mg/day). If adrenal insufficiency is established, adequate blood volume and electrolyte balance must be achieved preoperatively. Saline solution containing potassium chloride should be administered and adequacy of circulating volume assessed with central venous pressure monitoring. Adequate preparation of the patient may require 2 to 3 days of daily cortisol administration, 20 mg in the morning and 10 mg in the afternoon, for a total daily dosage of 30 mg. Just before the operation, the patient is given another 100 mg intravenously, followed by 50 to 100 mg every 6 h. Postoperatively, the cortisol dosage is reduced by half each day until the maintenance dose is reached, usually in 3 to 4 days.

Thyroid Disease

The hyperthyroid patient is susceptible to developing cardiac arrhythmias, hypertension, and hyperthermia. Surgery can also precipitate thyroid storm. Thus, the hyperthyroid patient should be rendered euthyroid before elective surgery by the administration of propylthiouracil, 800 to 1000 mg daily for about 1 week, followed by a maintenance dose of 200 to 400 mg daily. If emergency surgery is to be undertaken in a hyperthyroid patient, β-adrenergic blockade with propranolol and prevention of thyroid hormone release by the administration of potassium iodide (Lugol's solution) is required. This regimen is also used in treatment of thyroid storm, which may in addition require sedation, hydration, oxygen administration, and corticosteroid therapy.

Hypothyroidism, if present, should be corrected preoperatively to avoid acute hypotension and hypothermia during surgery. Hypothyroidism is corrected with the administration of levothyroxine. Hypothyroid patients may develop severe CO_2-retention immediately postoperatively and may fail to awaken from general anesthesia. In the severe case, myxedema coma may result with CO_2 narcosis and hypothermia. This condition is treated by intravenous administration of levothyroxine sodium.

PREEXISTING HEMATOLOGIC DISORDERS

The Anticoagulated Patient

If major surgery is to be performed in a patient chronically anticoagulated with coumadin, conversion to heparin anticoagulation preoperatively is advisable. Conversion can be done by restoring the prothrombin time through parenteral administration of vitamin K, which takes 24 to 48 h. Concomitantly, the patient is started on heparin therapy. The coagulation time returns to normal about 4 h after administration of 5000 U of heparin intravenously. The effect of heparin is rapidly reversed by administration of protamine sulfate. If emergent operation is required in a patient anticoagulated with coumadin, the prothrombin time can be corrected in a few hours by administering 500 to 1000 mL of plasma. Plasma provides the normal levels of coagulation Factors II, VII, IX, and X that are lowered by coumadin therapy.

Thrombocytopenia

Surgery can be performed safely in the patient with thrombocytopenia if the platelet count is 50,000/mL or more. In patients undergoing splenectomy for idiopathic thromocytopenic purpura (ITP), platelets are given only after the splenic artery has been occluded.

A number of situations may cause qualitative platelet abnormality, including the presence in the patient's blood of aspirin and nonsteroidal anti-inflammatory drugs (NSAIDs) as well as renal failure. Patients are advised to discontinue taking aspirin or NSAIDs for 10 to 14 days before operation. The best way to treat the platelet abnormality of renal failure is by performing hemodialysis 24 h before surgery.

Hemophilia

Patients with hemophilia who require surgery need to receive enough antihemophilic factor (AHF) concentrate to restore factor VIII levels to at least 75% of normal preoperatively.

NUTRITIONAL DEFICIT

Accurate assessment of risk due to nutritional deficit is not available. Table 13.4 lists the available predictors of risk. Of these predictors, rapid weight loss and low serum levels of albumin are the two most important. Mild-to-moderate malnutrition is not associated with significant increase in major postoperative complications. Severe malnutrition, however, is associated with increased risk of noninfectious complications, which can be significantly prevented with 7 to 15 days of preoperative TPN. An increase in rate of postoperative complication is seen in patients who have lost 10% to 20% of their body weight. If weight loss is rapid and occurs within 1 month, 5% to 10% weight loss increases the complication rate. Poor wound healing with abdominal wound dehiscence is more commonly seen in the severely malnourished patient.

Enteral Feeding

General agreement exists that the enteral route should be used, whenever possible, to improve the nutritional status

---

TABLE 13.4. Predictors of Surgical Risk in Patients with Nutritional Deficit

Recent weight loss of >10%
Undernutrition <85% of ideal body weight
Serum albumin <3 g/100 ml
Transferrin <200 mg/100 ml
Skin anergy to recall antigens
Triceps skin fold

---

of the poorly nourished patient. Enteral therapy can be given via a nasogastric or nasoenteral tube if oral intake is inadequate or impossible. A feeding gastrostomy or feeding jejunostomy tube can also be inserted in the patient percutaneously prior to surgery. Feeding jejunostomy can be placed during abdominal surgery in patients with preexisting poor nutrition, in those who might be anticipated to develop delayed gastric emptying, and in those with a precarious anastomosis in the esophagus, stomach, or duodenum.

Enteral feeding avoids the infectious complications seen with TPN. Evidence also exists from studies of patients with trauma that enteral feeding is superior to parenteral nutrition with respect to outcome. Suggested explanations for the superiority of enteral feeding include that it prevents bacterial dislocation from the gut into the circulation; it preserves gut-based immune mechanisms (e.g., IgA production) and results in improved liver function, including synthesis of hepatic acute phase protein; and it avoids the risk of catheter sepsis. Another factor that should be considered is cost, which is significantly lower with enteral feeding. Recent advances in enteral feeding incorporate the use of enterocyte-specific nutritional substitutes such as glutamine and short-chain amino acids. Both blenderized and defined formula diets are available. In frequent clinical use at present are such commercial products as Ensure®, Isocal®, Osmolite® and Vivonex®.

Parenteral Nutrition

In many patients, either because the gastrointestinal tract is unavailable for use or for the sake of convenience and timeliness, parenteral nutrition is necessary. Although peripheral administration for short periods is possible, parenteral hyperalimentation should be given by a central catheter, usually into the superior vena cava. Several complications attend parenteral nutrition, from technical complications of catheter placement to late complications such as catheter sepsis, subclavian vein thrombosis, or even life-threatening septic thrombosis. Also possible are metabolic complications including hyperglycemia, liver dysfunction, diabetes mellitus and deficiencies of essential fatty acids and trace metals. A standard formula consists of 150 g of 15% dextrose, 50 g of 5% amino acids and 40 g of 4% fat emulsion. To this are added trace elements, vitamin K (5 mg weekly), and electrolyte sodium (30 mEq/L), potassium (18 mEq/L), calcium (4–5 mEq/L), magnesium (5 mEq/L), phosphate (10 mM), chlorides (37 mEq/L), and acetate. Adjustments are made to an individual patient's needs and conditions.

In nutritionally at-risk patients whose surgery cannot be postponed until optimal status is achieved, the common surgical practice is to provide parenteral nutrition for at least 6 to 10 days prior to surgery. In many such cases, a positive nitrogen balance can be achieved preoperatively.

PERIOPERATIVE PROPHYLAXIS

ANTIBIOTIC PROPHYLAXIS

Prophylactic Systemic Antibiotic Therapy

Prophylactic antibiotic therapy is not indicated in patients undergoing clean, uncontaminated operations. In all gastrointestinal operations where the viscus may be entered, however, perioperative antibiotic prophylaxis is indicated. The only possible exception might be in patients undergoing elective surgery for peptic ulcer disease. Antibiotic prophylaxis is indicated, however, when the operation is for bleeding or obstruction. Perioperative antibiotic therapy is indicated in all esophageal and small and large intestinal procedures, most biliary tract and pancreatic surgeries, and in all operations for penetrating abdominal trauma.

Prophylactic antibiotic therapy is more effective when given before the incision is made. The aim is to maintain a therapeutic level of antibiotics throughout the operation and also perhaps for 12 h following surgery but not beyond. The antibiotic selected in gastrointestinal surgery must be effective against anaerobes, especially against *Bacteroides* species. Cefotetan or cefoxitin is an appropriate choice. A combination of an aminoglycoside and clindamycin may also be used. Vancomycin is selected only for patients who are allergic to cephalosporins and clindamycin or in whom potential exists for methicillin-resistant *Staphylococcus aureus* infection.

Bowel Preparation for Colon Surgery

Prospective controlled clinical trials have established the effectiveness of preoperative suppression of both aerobic and anaerobic colonic flora in preventing infection after operations on the colon. Nonabsorbable antibiotics are used. A combination of neomycin and erythromycin are given orally 19, 18, and 9 h before the scheduled start of surgery. Another effective combination is that of neomycin and metronidazole. Effective antibiotic preparation of the colon cannot be achieved without thorough mechanical preparation. All patients undergoing colon surgery must also receive prophylactic intravenous antibiotics perioperatively.

Topical Antibiotics

Surgeons commonly instill topical antibiotics in the peritoneal cavity and in the wound as prophylaxis against infection. Topical antibiotics are inferior to systemic antibiotics, and there is no clear evidence that the combination is more effective than intravenous antibiotics alone.

PROPHYLAXIS AGAINST THROMBOEMBOLISM

All patients undergoing major abdominal surgery are at risk for developing venous thrombosis and pulmonary embolism. The risk is increased in cases involving obesity, cancer, cigarette smoking, previous history of thromboembolism, and several hematologic conditions that result in hypercoagulability. The type and duration of surgery itself may also increase the risk. Pelvic operations and those in which packing or retraction interferes with blood flow through the inferior vena cava or pelvic veins increase the risk of thromboembolism postoperatively. Patients undergoing lengthy laparoscopic surgery while intraperitoneal pressures of 15 mm Hg or more are maintained may also be at greater risk.

Prophylaxis involves both mechanical and chemical approaches:

1. Mechanical. An intermittent pneumatic compression device or graded-compression elastic stockings should be used on all patients.

2. Anticoagulation. During surgery, obstruction of venous flow must be avoided by giving special attention to the patient's position as well as placement of packing and retractors. In high-risk patients, either low-dose unfractionated heparin or low molecular heparin should be used as prophylaxis. Multiple controlled trials show that both are equally efficacious in preventing thromboembolism.

3. Prophylactic placement of vena cava filter. Randomized trials are lacking, but in longitudinal studies, filters have been shown to be more than 96% effective in preventing pulmonary embolism. Reasonable inidications at present would appear to be previous history of pulmonary embolus or proven deep venous thrombosis where the use of heparin is contraindicated.

STRESS ULCERATION AND GASTROINTESTINAL HEMORRHAGE

Stress bleeding was once a common postoperative complication, especially in the presence of sepsis or multiple organ failure, occurring in 20% of critically ill patients. Routine use of prophylaxis to maintain gastric pH above 4.5 has dramatically reduced the incidence of this dreaded complication. Antacid prophylaxis has now been largely replaced by H_2-receptor antagonists.

AIDS PROPHYLAXIS

The risk for health care workers of acquiring human immunodeficiency virus (HIV) infection from caring for infected patients is small. Skin puncture from needles or scalpels during surgery presents the most serious hazard. The estimated risk of transmission after hollow-bore needlestick is 0.3% for each incident.[4]

Because the HIV status of a patient may not be known before surgery, the Center for Disease Control (CDC) recommends that all patients be assumed infectious and it advises strict observance of universal precaution in handling blood and other bodily fluids. For example, the surgical team requires proper protective attire. Most surgeons now wear two pairs of gloves, protective eyewear, and special impermeable disposable gowns and masks. Sharp instruments are handled and disposed of according to protocol. Tissue retraction is performed with instruments as much as possible. If needle-stick or scalpel injury should occur accidentally, prophylactic treatment with zidovudine (AZT) is recommended.

REFERENCES

1. Goldman L, Caldera DL, Nussbaum SR, et al. Multifactorial index of cardiac risk in noncardiac surgical procedures. *N Engl J Med* 1977;297:845–850.
2. Zeldin RA. Assessing cardiac risk in patients who undergo noncardiac surgical procedures. *Can J Surg* 1984;27:402–404.
3. Pett SB Jr, Wernly JA. Respiratory function in surgical patients. Perioperative evaluation and management. *Surg Annu* 1988;20:311–329.
4. Fauci AS, Lane HC. Human immunodeficiency virus (HIV) disease: AIDS and related disorders. In: Fauci AS, et al, eds. *Harrison's Principles of Internal Medicine.* 15th ed. New York: McGraw Hill; 2001:1852–1913.

SELECTED READINGS

Clagett GP, Anderson FA Jr, Geerts W, et al. Prevention of venous thromboembolism. *Chest* 1998;114(5 Suppl):531S–560S.
Cook DJ, Reeve BK, Guyatt GH, et al. Stress ulcer prophylaxis in critically ill patients. Resolving discordant meta-analyses. *JAMA* 1996;275:308–314.
Eagle KA, Brundage BH, Chaitman BR, et al. Guidelines for perioperative cardiovascular evaluation for noncardiac surgery. Report of the American College of Cardiology/American Heart Association Task Force on Practice Guidelines (Committee on Perioperative Cardiovascular Evaluation for Noncardiac Surgery). *J Am Coll Cardiol* 1996;27:910–948.
MacKenzie CR, Charlson ME. Assessment of perioperative risk in the patient with diabetes mellitus. *Surg Gynecol Obstet* 1988;167:293–299.
Salem M, Tainsh RE Jr, Bromberg J, et al. Perioperative glucocorticoid coverage. A reassessment 42 years after emergence of a problem. *Ann Surg* 1994;219:416–425.
Zaloga GP. Early enteral nutritional support improves outcome: hypothesis or fact? *Crit Care Med* 1999;27:259–261.

Index

A

Abdominal esophagus
  blood supply of, 2
  lymphatic drainage of, 3
  perforation of, clinical presentation, 25
Abdominal pressure, precipitation of
    hernias by, 352
Abdominal trauma, 334–350
Abdominal wall, 351–362
Abscess
  anorectal, 305–307
  appendiceal, 317
  as a complication in hepatic injury
    treated nonoperatively, 343
  intraabdominal, 362–363
    management of, 364
  intraperitoneal, in Crohn's disease, 262
  liver, management of, 178–180
  pancreatic
    diagnosis of, 108
    treatment of, 113
  pelvic, transrectal drainage of, 364–365
  pericolic
    in diverticulitis, 283
    management of, 284–285
  perineal, conservative surgery for
    managing, 289
  retroperitoneal, 366–367
  splenic, 324
  subphrenic
    drainage of, 364
    after splenectomy, 330–331
Absorption
  in the gallbladder, 202–203
  in the large intestine, 247
  in the small intestine, 245–246
Absorptive surface, inadequate
  malabsorption syndrome due to, 255
  in bowel resection, 258
Acalculous cholecystitis (AC), investigations
    and treatment, 218–219
Acceleration-deceleration injury,
    abdominal, 334
Accessory spleen, 326
  identifying in open splenectomy, 327
Acetaminophen, as a cause of liver failure,
    166
Acetylcholine (ACh)
  triggering of acid secretion by, 43
  triggering of pepsin secretion by, 45
Achalasia
  clinical presentation of, 13–14

defined, 6
diagnosis and treatment of, 14
gastroesophageal reflux associated with,
  9–11
Achlorhydria, in VIPoma syndrome, 156
Acid infusion test, for evaluating chest pain,
  11
Acid-peptic disorders, 53–54, 56–69
Acid secretion
  abnormalities of, 51–55
  hypersecretion as a cause of peptic
    ulcers, 54
  hypersecretion in gastrinoma, 149
  mediation of, by gastrin, 138
  reducing, in esophagitis, 19–20
  regulation of, in the stomach, 41–45
    neural mechanisms for, 41–43
Acini, pancreatic, 91–92
ACTHoma, 159
Actinomycosis, 295
Acute cholecystitis, acalculous and
    calculous, 205–206
Acute respiratory distress syndrome
    (ARDS), in pancreatitis, 100
Acute variceal hemorrhage, management
    algorithm for, 171
Adaptive changes, renewal after small bowel
    resection, 258
Adenocarcinoma
  of the bile duct, 231–236
  esophageal
    diagnosing, 30
    incidence of, 28
  of the gallbladder, 231
  of the pancreas, 123–127
  risk of, in atrophic gastritis and
    pernicious anemia, 71
  of the small intestine, 296–297
Adenomas
  hepatic, 184–185
  parathyroid, 147
  pituitary, 147
Adenomatous polyps, 270–271
  gastric, 72
Adhesion formation, in peritonitis, 363–364
Adjuvant therapy
  for carcinoma of the stomach, 81
  for cholangiocarcinoma, 235
  See also Chemotherapy
Adrenal insufficiency, considerations arising
    from in abdominal surgery,
    371–372

Alanine aminotransferase (ALT), levels of,
    in cholangitis, 223
Alcohol
  cirrhosis induced by, 165
  pancreatitis induced by, 98–99
    chronic, 102
  portal hypertension and, 166–167
Alkaline phosphatase, elevation of
  in cholangitis, 223
  in obstructive jaundice, 208
  in sclerosing cholangitis, 228
Allergy, to milk, in chronic ulcerative
    colitis, 263
Alpha cells, of the islets of Langerhans, 93
Alpha-fetoprotein (AFP), levels of, in
    hepatocellular carcinoma, 187
Amebiasis, intestinal, identifying and
    treating, 295
Amebic abscess, liver, 178–180
American Association for the Surgery of
    Trauma, injury scale of, 342–343
American College of Surgeons, Advanced
    Trauma Life Support, on
    management of abdominal trauma
    injuries, 335
Amine precursor uptake, characteristic of
    endocrine cells of the pancreas and
    gastrointestinal tract, 146–147
Aminosalicylates, 288–289
Amoxicillin, for treating *Helicobacter pylori*
    infection, 68
Amyloidosis, in Crohn's disease, 263
Anal canal, anatomy of, 243–244
Anal fistula, following surgery for anorectal
    abscesses, 305
Anatomic distribution, in Crohn's disease,
    260
Anatomic relationships
  of the pancreas, 91
  of the spleen, 319–320
Anatomy
  of the abdominal wall, 351–352
  of the appendix, 311
  of the biliary tract, 198–202
  of the duodenum, 37–83
  of the esophagus, 1–5
  microscopic
    of the pancreas, 91–93
    of the stomach, 41–42
  of the pancreas, 89–93
  in paraesophageal hernia, 17
  of the peritoneum, 362–363

Growth of children with Crohn's disease, 262, 289

Growth factors, peptide, in the gastrointestinal tract, 160

Growth hormone releasing factor tumor (GRFoma), 159

H

Hamartomatous polyps, 296

Hamman's sign, in thoracic esophagus perforation, 25

Hartmann procedure, in diverticulitis of the colon, 284

Heartburn, 7
  as a symptom of esophageal disease, 11–13

Helicobacter pylori
  as a cause of peptic ulcer, 46, 51–53
  description of, 53–54
  detection of, 57–58, 68
  mucosa-associated lymphoid tissue tumors and, 81
  risk of gastric cancer with infection by, 71

Heller's myotomy, for achalasia treatment, 14–15

Hemangioma
  gastric, bleeding caused by, 70
  liver, 182–184
    treatment of, 182–184

Hematologic changes, after splenectomy, 330–332

Hematologic disorders, evaluating before surgery, 372

Hematoma
  classification of, 348–350
  duodenal, from blunt trauma, 337
  retroperitoneal, 366
    due to trauma, 348–350
    surgical management of, 348–350
  subcapsular, operative approach to, 346
  subphrenic, after splenectomy, 330

Hemobilia, as a complication in hepatic injury treated nonoperatively, 343

Hemoglobinopathies, 323

Hemophilia, surgery for patients with, 372

Hemorrhage
  in acute pancreatitis, 101
    from pseudocysts, 115
  in chronic ulcerative colitis, managing, 294
  as a complication in hepatic injury treated nonoperatively, 343
  in Crohn's disease, 262, 289
  gastrointestinal, in Meckel's diverticulum, 269
  after liver resection, 194
  recurrent variceal, prevention of, 174
  in ulcerative colitis, 264
  upper gastrointestinal
    acute pancreatitis as a cause of, 101
    peptic ulcer as a cause of, 63–65
  variceal, acute, 170–177

Hemorrhoid, 303–305

Hemorrhoidectomy, 305

Hepatic adenoma, 184

Hepatic artery
  anatomy of, 162–163

ligation of, in hepatocellular carcinoma, 194

substituted, identifying, 91

Hepatic iminodiacetic acid (HIDA) scanning, for diagnosing acute cholecystitis, 215–216

Hepatic injury, 342–347
  diagnosis of, 343
  management of, postoperative complications in, 347
  nonoperative treatment for, complications of, 343–346
  operative treatment of, 346–347

Hepatic surgery
  complications following resection, 347
  lobectomy, for hepatocarcinoma management, 190
  total hepatectomy, 194

Hepatitis, as a cause of fulminant liver failure, 166

Hepatitis B virus (HBV), as a cause of hepatocellular carcinoma, 187

Hepatobiliary complications, in acute pancreatitis, 101

Hepatobiliary manifestations, in Crohn's disease, 263

Hepatobiliary scintigraphy, 215–216

Hepatocellular carcinoma (HCC), 186–194
  metastasis in, 187
  pathogenesis of, 187
  prognosis in, after resection, 187
  surgical management of, 187–194

Hepatomegaly, in pancreatic neoplasms, 124

Hepatorenal syndrome (HRS), 166

Hernias
  inguinal or groin, 351–360
    surgery for, 354
    complications of, 356
  internal abdominal, 365–366
  paraesophageal, 17–19
  pathogenesis of, 351–352
  pelvic floor, 361–362

Hesselbach's triangle, direct inguinal hernia at, 352–353

Hiatal hernia, 17–25

Hill repair, in esophageal reflux management, 23

Histamine, role in acid secretion, 44

H$^+$K$^+$ATPase inhibitors, hypergastrinemia associated with, 55

Hodgkin's lymphoma, of the spleen, 324

Horizontal gastroplasty (HG), for morbid obesity, 86

Hormones
  defined, 46
  insulinotropic gut, circulating, 96
  motor function of the stomach controlled by, 49–50

Howell-Jolly bodies, postsplenectomy appearance of, 330

Howship-Romberg sign, 361–362

Human immunodeficiency virus (HIV) infection, prophylactic measures in surgery to avoid transmission of, 374

Humoral agents, in intestinal secretion, 246

Humoral mechanisms, for regulation of pancreatic enzyme secretion, 95

Humoral secretory products, of the stomach, list, 46

Hydatid cysts, 180–182

Hydrolases, lysosomal, synthesis by ribosomes of the pancreatic endoplasmic reticulum, 94

Hyperammonemia, in portal hypertension, 169

Hyperamylasemia, in acute pancreatitis, 107

Hyperbilirubinemia
  after liver resection, 194
  in obstructive jaundice, 208

Hypercalcemia, pancreatitis as a complication of, 99
  cell growth stimulated by, 138–139

Hypergastrinemia
  causes of, 54–55
  cell growth stimulated by, 138–139
  detection by radioimmunoassay, 58
  long-term effects of, 148
  risk of cancer in, 71–72
  after small bowel resection, 258

Hyperglycemia, in acute pancreatitis, 101

Hyperlipidemia, pancreatitis as a complication of, 99

Hyperparathyroidism, pancreatitis as a complication of, 99, 102

Hypersecretion
  of acid, in the stomach, 51
  of gastrin, in the stomach, 54–55

Hypersplenism
  partial splenectomy for managing, 329
  primary, 321
  secondary, 321–324

Hypertension
  association with obesity, 84
  portal, 166–170

Hyperthyroidism, managing, before elective surgery, 372

Hypertriglyceridemia, as a cause of pancreatitis, 98

Hypertrophic gastritis, risk of gastric cancer in, 72–74

Hypoalbuminemia, after liver resection, 194

Hypocalcemia, in acute pancreatitis, 101

Hypoglycemia
  effect of, on glucagon release, 97
  in hepatic resection, 347
  after liver resection, 194
  reactive, 68

Hypokalemia
  in gastric outlet obstruction, 66
  in VIPoma syndrome, 156

Hypoproteinemia, ascites in, 364

Hyposecretion
  of acid in the stomach, 53
  of gastrin, 55

Hypotension, of the lower esophageal sphincter, 7
  manometry for detecting, 19

Hypothyroidism
  constipation in, 257
  preoperative correction of, before surgery, 372

Hypovolemic phase, of pancreatitis, 99–100, 108–112

in pancreaticoduodectomy, 127
in postsplenectomy infection, 332
in primary peritonitis, 364
in pseudomyxoma peritonei, 366
in radiation enteritis requiring surgery, 257
in recurrent pyogenic cholangitis, 230
in shunt use, to prevent recurrent variceal hemorrhage, 174
in toxic colitis, 292
See also under individual clinical entities
Motilin, role in contraction of smooth muscle cells
of the small intestine, 246–247
of the stomach, 49
Motility
of the esophagus
disorders of, 13–15
disorders of, summary, 7
gastrointestinal smooth muscle, effect of gastrin-releasing peptide on, 143
intestinal, altered, diarrhea resulting from, 256
of the large intestine, 247
of the small intestine, 246–247
Motor function
disorders of, stomach, 55, 70
effects of gastrin, 139
of the gallbladder, 203
of the stomach, 48–51
Motor vehicle accidents
liver injury in, 342
retroperitoneal hematoma due to, 366
Mucocele, of the gallbladder, 208
Mucosa
esophageal, 2
factors protecting the gastric mucosa, 47–48
gastric, trophic action on the parietal cell, 44
primary defects of, malabsorption due to, 256
Mucosa-associated lymphoid tissue (MALT) lymph, gastric lymphoma arising from, 81
Mucosal restitution, defined, 48
Mucus, secretion of, regulation of, 45
Multiple cysts, congenital, 180
Multiple endocrine neoplasia type 1 (MEN-1) syndrome
apudomas occurring in, 147
association with VIPomas, 156
gastric carcinoma tumors associated with, 81
ruling out, in Zollinger-Ellison syndrome, 150–152
Musculature, colonic, and diverticulosis, 267
Musculoskeletal complications, in ulcerative colitis, 264
Musculoskeletal manifestations, of Crohn's disease, 263
Myc family of oncogenes, relationship with colon cancer, 271–272
Mycobacterium tuberculosis, inflammatory diseases of the small and large bowel in infection by, 294–295

Myeloproliferative disorders, splenectomy in, 324
Myocardial depressing factor (MDF), release from the pancreas, 100
Myocardial infarction
elective surgery, postponing after, 370
vasopressin as a cause of, 173
Myotomy, esophageal, for diffuse esophageal spasm treatment, 15

N

Napkin-ring carcinoma, 299
Necrosis
bowel, radiological signal of, 250
pancreatic, infected, 108
Necrotizing pancreatitis, surgical treatment of, 113–114
Neoplasms
of the biliary tract, 231–236
liver
benign, 182–185
primary malignant, 186–195
metastatic, to the liver, 194–195
pancreatic, 122–130
of the small intestine, 295–296
splenic, 324
See also Cancer; Carcinoma; Tumors
Nephrotic syndrome, postsplenectomy, primary peritonitis in, 364
Nerve supply
to the anal canal, 244
to the esophagus, 2–5
to the gallbladder, 200
to the liver, 164
to the rectum, 243
to the stomach, 39–41
to the visceral peritoneum, 362
Neurocrine mechanisms, in insulin release, 96
Neurocrine peptides, 137
Neurocrine secretions, of the stomach, 46
Neurologic disorders, constipation in, 257
Neuropeptide, life cycle of, 134
Neurotensin, 146
Neurotensinoma, 159
Neurotransmitters, of the gastric inhibitory tract, list, 135–136
Nifedipine, for diffuse esophageal spasm management, 15
Nissen fundoplication
contraindications to, in propulsive motility absence, 23
gastric emptying inhibition by, 50–51
in paraesophageal hernia management, 17–18
in reflux disorders, 21–22
Nitric oxide (NO)
role in swallowing, 2
Nocardiosis, 295
Non-Hodgkin's lymphoma
B-cell type, 81
splenic, 324
Nonlymphoid tumors, of the spleen, 324
Nonoperative treatment, of hepatic trauma, 343–346
Nonsteroidal anti-inflammatory drugs (NSAIDs)
as a cause of erosive gastritis, 53

as a cause of peptic ulcers, 54
inhibition of mucus and bicarbonate secretion by, 45
Nonsurgical management, of perforated esophagus, 26
Nutrition
absorption of nutrients in the small intestine, 246
in Crohn's disease, 288
defects in, correcting before surgery, 372–373
status of, in gastric outlet obstruction, 66

O

Obesity, morbid, 84–88
medical and surgical treatment for, 85
Obstruction
biliary, in chronic pancreatitis, 106
closed-loop, colonic, 253–254
colonic, 250–254
in diverticulitis of the colon, management of, 283–284
ductal, of the pancreas, 103
intestinal
in chronic pancreatitis, 106
constipation resulting from, 257
in Crohn's disease, 262
as an indication for surgery in Crohn's disease, 289
in mesenteric ischemia, 250
intrahepatic, portal hypertension caused by, 167
large bowel, 277–281
small bowel, 274–276
Obstructive jaundice, extrahepatic, 208, 220–223
Obturator hernias, 361–362
Octreotide
for managing carcinoid syndrome, 158
for managing dumping syndrome, 71
for managing fistulas of the small intestine, 282
for managing glucagonoma, 155
for managing symptoms of insulinoma, 153
receptors for, 143
Ocular complications, of ulcerative colitis, 264
Ocular manifestations, of Crohn's disease, 263
Ogilvie's syndrome, 254–255
Omentum
disorders of, 365
physiology of, 363
Omeprazole, for esophagitis management, 20
Open surgical approaches
to hernia repair, 354–356
splenectomy, technique of, 327–328
Operation, in small bowel obstruction, 276
Operative management
of acute mesenteric ischemia, 277–279
of chronic ulcerative colitis, 292–294
in insulinoma, 154–155
See also under individual clinical entities

Operative treatment
    abdominal exploration in
        Zollinger-Ellison syndrome,
        152–153
    in carcinoid syndrome, 158–159
    in colorectal cancer, 300–302
    of hepatic injuries, 346–347
    See also under individual clinical entities
Opsonins, production of, in the spleen, 321
Oral complications, of ulcerative colitis, 264
Oral contraceptives, association with
        hepatic adenoma, 184–185
Oral manifestations, of Crohn's disease, 263
Orchiectomy, in scrotal hernia repair, 360
Osmotic diarrhea, 256
Outcomes
    of acute mesenteric ischemia, 277
    in chronic pancreatitis, 122
    long-term
        after pancreaticoduodenectomy, 127
        of ulcer surgery, 67–69
    in resection of hilar cholangiocarcinoma,
        235
    of surgical therapy
        for liver metastasis in colorectal
            cancer, 195
        for necrotizing pancreatitis, 113
        for reflux disorders, 24
    See also under individual clinical entities
Oxyntic gland mucosa, gastrin as a growth
        regulator of, 138–139
Oxyntomodulin, structure and biological
        actions of, 142

P
p53 gene, mutations of, in colon cancer,
        274
Pacemaker, control of gastric motility by,
        48–49
Pain
    in acute cholecystitis, 217
    causes and management of, in chronic
        pancreatitis, 118
    control of, in acute pancreatitis, 112
    mediation of transmission of, by
        substance P, 144
    as a symptom
        of chronic ulcerative colitis, 290
        of pancreatitis, 100, 103–105
        of pancreatitis, acute, 106
        of peptic ulcer disease, 57
        of simple bowel obstruction, 249
        of small bowel obstruction, 274
Palliative therapy
    for carcinoid syndrome, 159
    for carcinoma of the stomach, 81
    for hepatocellular carcinoma, 194
    for malignant insulinoma, 155
    for managing glucagonoma, 155
    for VIPoma syndrome, 157
    for Zollinger-Ellison syndrome, 153
Pancreas, 89–131
    actions of gastrin-releasing peptide on,
        143
    arteries of, 91
    bicarbonate secretion by, 48
    bleeding from, 70
    cancer, TNM staging of, 123

disorders of, clinical management of,
        106–129
    embryology of, 89–90
    endocrine, 96–97
        defined, 89
        insufficiency of, in chronic
            pancreatitis, 105
    exocrine, 91–92
        defined, 89
        insufficiency of, in chronic pancreatitis
            105
        regulation of the secretions of, 94–96
    glucagon of, biological actions, 142
    injury to, 341–342
        in splenectomy, 332
        insulinomas of, 153
            neoplasms of, 124–127
    innervation of, 91
    neural mechanisms, for regulation of
        enzyme secretion in, 94–95
    pathophysiology of, 97–106
    physiology of, 93–97
Pancreatectomy
    distal, 119
    total, 119–122
        pancreatic neoplasm management,
            126–127
Pancreatic injury, classification of, 341–342
Pancreatic juice, composition of, 93
Pancreatic necrosis, diagnosis of, 108
Pancreatic neoplasm
    classification of, 122–123
    clinical presentation and diagnosis of, 124
    surgical management of, 126–129
Pancreaticoduodenal arteries, blood supply
        to the pancreatic head from, 91
Pancreaticoduodenectomy, 119
    mortality in, 127
    outcomes, long-term, following, 127
    for pancreatic injury management, 342
    pylorus-preserving, in pancreatic
        neoplasm management, 126–127
    in Zollinger-Ellison syndrome, 153
Pancreaticogastrostomy, 119
Pancreaticojejunostomy, end-to-side (DuVal
        procedure), for chronic pancreatitis,
        119–121
Pancreatic polypeptide (PP)
    cells secreting, of the islets of
        Langerhans, 93
    distribution of, 145
    family of, 145–146
    initiation of release of, by
        cholecystokinin, 140
    release of, 145–146
    secretion of, by apudomas, 148
Pancreatic resection, in chronic
        pancreatitis, 119
Pancreatitis
    acute, 97–101
        aspiration in, 112
        clinical management of, 106–115
        clinical presentation and diagnosis of,
            106
        complications of, 100–101etiology of,
            98–99
        general treatment for, 108–112
        grading of, severity of, 107–108

laboratory investigation of, 106–107
    surgical treatment for, 113–115
    as a complication of medication, 99
    chronic, 101–106
        clinical phases of, 99–100
        clinical presentation of, 115–122
        complications requiring surgery, 118
        endocrine and exocrine pancreas,
            insufficiency of in, 105
        etiology of, 102–103
        investigations of, 115
        outcomes in, 122
        pathogenesis of, 101–102
        surgical management of, 118–122
    necrotizing, 113
Pantaloon hernias, 359
Paracrine mechanisms, in insulin release,
        96
Paracrine peptides, 136–137
Paracrine secretion, 46
Paraduodenal hernia, 365–366
Paraesophageal hernia
    bleeding due to, 69
    clinical presentation and diagnosis of, 17
    pathophysiology of, 17
Parasitic infestation, intestinal
        inflammation caused by, 295
Parastomal hernias, 361
Parasympathetic innervation
    of the gastrointestinal system, 135
    of the small intestine, 240
Parenchymal disruption, in hepatic injuries,
        operative approaches to, 346–347
Parenteral nutrition
    in acute pancreatitis, 113
    complications of, 373
    perioperative, 373
Partial splenectomy, 329
Pathogenesis
    of chronic pancreatitis, 101–102
    of chronic ulcerative colitis, 263
    of colon polyps and colorectal cancer,
        270–274
    of Crohn's disease, 259–260
    of diverticular disease of the colon,
        267–268
    of hepatocellular carcinoma, 187
    of hernias, 351–352
    of portal hypertension, 166–168
    See also under individual clinical entities
Pathology
    of chronic ulcerative colitis, 264
    of Crohn's disease, 260–261
    of esophageal carcinoma, 28
    of stomach cancer, 75
    See also under individual clinical entities
Pathophysiology
    of the appendix, 312
    of the biliary tract, 203–212
    of the esophagus, 5–11
    of the liver, 165–170
    of the pancreas, 97–106
    of paraesophageal hernia, 17
    of the peritoneum, 363–365
    of the small and large intestines, 248–274
    of the spleen, 321–325
    of the stomach and duodenum, 51–56
    See also under individual clinical entities

Proteins
    digestion of, 245
    intracellular trafficking of, in the
        pancreas, 91–92
    synthesis of, in the liver, 164
Proctocolectomy, in toxic colitis
        unresponsive to medical
        management, 293
Proton-pump inhibitors, for esophagitis
        management, 19–20
Proto-oncogenes, alteration of, in colorectal
        cancer, 271–272
Proximal gastric vagotomy (PGV), for
        duodenal ulcer management, 58–59
    conditions for using, 62–63
Pruritus ani, 308
Pseudoaneurysm, as a complication of
        acute pancreatitis, 101
Pseudocysts
    in acute pancreatitis
        infection of, 100–101, 108
        treating hemorrhage of, 115–116
        treatment of, 114–115
    in chronic pancreatitis, 105
Pseudolymphoma, 75
Pseudomyxoma peritonei, 366
Pseudo-obstruction, colonic, 254–255
Pseudopolyps, in ulcerative colitis, 266,
        290–291
Psoas sign, in acute appendicitis, 313
Psychological factors
    in chronic ulcerative colitis, 263
    in Crohn's disease, 260
Puborectalis muscle, role of, in continence,
        247
Pulmonary complications, in splenectomy,
        330
Pulmonary function, evaluating, before
        abdominal surgery, 370
Pulsion diverticuli, motility disorders
        associated with, 15–17
Pyloric exclusion procedure, 338–340
Pyloric sphincter, 50–51
Pyloroplasty, after vagotomy, to prevent
        delayed gastric emptying, 51
Pyogenic cholangitis, recurrent, 209–212
    diagnosis and treatment of, 230
    mortality in, 230

R
Radiation injury
    gastrointestinal, 257–258
    obstruction of the small bowel, operative
        considerations, 276
Radiologic control, in variceal hemorrhage,
        173
Radiologic studies
    CT scan
        in acute appendicitis, 313
        in chronic ulcerative colitis evaluation,
            290
        in colorectal cancer, 300
        in Crohn's disease, 287
        in diverticulitis of the colon, 283
        in fistulas of the small intestine, 282
        in hepatocellular carcinoma, 187–189
        in large bowel obstruction, 280–281
        in liver abscess, 179

    in mesenteric ischemia, 277
    in sclerosing cholangitis evaluation,
        228
    in sigmoid volvulus, 281
    in variceal hemorrhage evaluation, 171
    plain x-ray
        for acute pancreatitis evaluation, 107
        for bowel obstruction evaluation, 251
        for chronic pancreatitis evaluation,
            115–117
        for diverticulitis of the colon
            evaluation, 283
        of duodenal retroperitoneal rupture,
            339
        for small bowel obstruction
            evaluation, 275
Radiologic testing, for perforated esophagus
        diagnosis, 25
Radionuclide imaging, ^{125}I-octreotide, to
        localize peptide-secreting tumors,
        159
Randomized clinical trials, of laparoscopic
        hernia repair, 356
Ranson criteria, for determining the
        severity of acute pancreatitis, 107
Ras family of oncogenes, relationship with
        colon cancer, 271–272
Raynaud's phenomenon, association with
        esophageal scleroderma, 6–7
Receptors
    for calcitonin gene-related peptide, 145
    for cholecystokinin, 140
    for gastric inhibitory polypeptide, 144
    for gastrin, 138
    for gastrin-releasing peptide, 143
    for glucagon, 142
    for pancreatic polypeptide, 146
    for secretin, 141
    for somatostatin, 143
    for substance P, 144
    for vasoactive intestinal polypeptide, 141
Rectal cancer, low-lying, surgical resection
        of, 302
Rectal prolapse (procidentia), 308–309
Rectum
    anatomy of, 242–243
    carcinoma of, 300
        operative treatment of, 302
    endarteritis at, from late radiation injury,
        257
    injury to, 348–350
    prolapse, 308
Recurrence
    of duodenal ulcer
        after proximal gastric vagotomy, 59
        after surgery, 67–69
    of inguinal hernias, 360
Red blood cells, diseases of, 323
Reflex control, of the gut, role of sensory
        innervation in, 136
Reflex pathways, in regulation of pancreatic
        enzyme secretion, 95
Reflux, minimizing, in esophagitis
        management, 19
Reflux theory, of pancreatitis initiation, 98
Regeneration, of the liver, 165
Regulation, of gastrointestinal peptides,
        133–135

Relationships, ancitornic, of the stomach,
        37
Renal disease
    correction of conditions associated with,
        before abdominal surgery, 371
    in liver failure, 166
Renal manifestations, in Crohn's disease,
        263
Repair, of incisional hernias, 360
Resection
    anterior, with suture fixation, in rectal
        prolapse, 309
    in bile duct tumor management, 233–235
    hepatic, in hepatocellular carcinoma,
        187–195
    liver, technique of, 190–194
    of a perforated esophagus, 27–28
    sacral, 302
Resistance, in portal hypertension, 167
Respiration, support of, in acute
        pancreatitis, 112
Respiratory disease, evaluating the risk
        from, in abdominal surgery, 370
Resuscitation
    electrolyte, in acute pancreatitis, 108–112
    in hepatic injury, 343
    in perforated peptic ulcer, 60–61
    in variceal hemorrhage, 171–172
    volume
        in acute pancreatitis, 108–112
        in hemorrhage from perforated peptic
            ulcer, 64
Reticuloendothelial system (RES), of the
        liver, function of, 165
Retinal pigment, congenital hypertrophy of,
        in familial adenomatous polyposis,
        270
Retrocecal appendicitis, 312
Retrohepatic caval injury, operative
        approach to, 347
Retroperitoneal rupture, of the duodenum,
        after traumatic injury, 337–340
Retroperitoneum, 366–367
Reynold's pentad, in cholangitis, 223–224
Right colon, carcinoma of, 296–299
    operative treatment, 302
Ripstein procedure, for rectal prolapse
        management, 309
Rough endoplasmic reticulum (RER)
    of pancreatic acini, 91–92
    synthesis of pancreatic proenzymes on,
        93–94
Roux-en-Y gastric bypass (RYGP), for
        morbid obesity, 85–87
Roux-en-Y hepaticojejunostomy
    in recurrent pyogenic cholangitis,
        230–231
    for repair of common bile duct injury,
        228
Rovsing sign, in acute appendicitis, 313
Rubber-band ligation, of hemorrhoids, 305

S
Salmonella typhi, infection by, 294
Salmon-Goodall rule, 307
Schistosomiasis, as a cause of portal
        hypertension, 166–167
Sciatic hernia, 362

Scleroderma, esophageal, 6–7
Sclerosing cholangitis, 209–211
    association with ulcerative colitis, 264
    diagnosis and management of, 228–229
    medical and surgical treatment for, 228
Sclerosis, of internal hemorrhoid, by
        phenol injection, 305
Sclerotherapy, endoscopic, to control acute
        hemorrhage, 172
Seat belt injuries, 335
Secretin, 140–141
    distribution of, 140
    family of
        gastrointestinal peptides of, 46
        regulation of bicarbonate secretion by
            release from the duodenum, 94
    release of, in the duodenum, 141
Secretin test, positive, in Zollinger-Ellison
        syndrome, 149, 159
Secretion
    altered, in the stomach, 51–53
    by apudomas, 147–148
        biliary, stimulation of, by secretin, 141
    by carcinoid tumors, 157
    by the colon, of bicarbonate and
        potassium, 247
    by insulinoma, 153
    of mucus by the gallbladder, 202
    in the pancreas, 93–94
    by the small intestine, 246
    by VIPomas, 156
Secretory block theory, of pancreatitis
        initiation, 98
Secretory diarrhea, 256
Secretory disorders, of the stomach and
        duodenum, 51–55
Sections, of the esophagus, 1–5
Segmental anatomy, of the liver, 162
Segmentectomy, liver, 190
Selective total gastric vagotomy, 58–59
Sengstaken-Blakemore tube, to control
        bleeding, 172–173
Sensory nervous system, of the stomach,
        40, 48
Sepsis
    in acute pancreatitis, 100
        diagnosis of, 108
    after liver resection, 194
    in operative treatment of liver injury,
        347
    postsplenectomy, 326, 332
Serotonin, association of
    with carcinoid tumors, 157
    with chronic pancreatitis, 105
Shigella pathogens, infection by, 294
Short bowel syndrome, 258
Shouldice herniorrhaphy, 355–357
    advantages of, 360
Shunts, to prevent recurrent bleeding in
        variceal hemorrhage, 174
Sickle-cell anemia, 323
Sigmoid colon, in diverticular disease of the
        colon, 264
Sigmoidoscopic reduction, of sigmoid
        volvulus, 281
Sigmoid volvulus, 253–254, 281
Signet-ring cells, association with
        carcinoma, 75–76

Simple obstruction
    colonic, 250–253
    small bowel, 249
Skin diseases
    association with Crohn's disease, 262–263
    association with ulcerative colitis, 264
Skin pigmentation, in Peutz-Jeghers
        syndrome, 295
Sleep apnea, in obese individuals, 84
Sliding hernia, 359
    defined, 353
    hiatal, 18–25
Small cell lung cancer, bombesin as a
        growth factor in, 160
Small intestine
    anatomy of, 239–241
    benign neoplasms of, 295–296
    bleeding from, 70
    blunt trauma injury to, diagnosis of, 347
    diverticula of, 268–270
    embryology of, 239
    fistulas of, 282
    injury to, from blunt trauma, 347–348
    metastasis to, 296
    obstruction of, in Meckel's diverticulum,
        269
    physiology of, 244–247
    resection, consequences of, 258
Smoking, as a risk factor
    for Crohn's disease, 259
    for postoperative, pulmonary
        complications, 370
Sodium, absorption of, in the small
        intestine, 245–246
Solids, gastric emptying of, 50
Solitary cysts, liver, 180
Somatostatin
    biological actions of, 143–144
    distribution of, 143
    inhibition of intrapancreatic neurons by,
        94
    roles of, in the stomach, 45–46
    secretion of
        from the delta cells of the islets, 96,
            143–144
        stimulation by gastrin, 139
Somatostatinoma, 157
Spasm, esophageal, diffuse, 14–15
Spherocytosis, hereditary, 323
Sphincter of Oddi (choledochal sphincter)
    anatomy of, 198–199
    physiology of, 203
Sphincteroplasty, 119
Sphincterotomy, technique of, 222
Sphincters
    lower esophageal, 1–4
        abnormalities of, 7–11
        defective, antireflux surgery in the
            presence of, 20
        hypertensive, 9
    pyloric, 50–51
    upper esophageal, 1–3
        abnormalities of, 5
Spigelian hernias, 361
Spleen, 319–333
    clinical disorders of, 326–332
    metastasis to, 324
    pathophysiology of, 321–325

physiology of, 321
relationship with the stomach, 37
surgical anatomy of, 319–321
traumatic injury to, grading, 325
Splenectomy, 326–332
    infection following, mortality of, 332
    surgical technique in, 327–329
Splenic artery, blood supply to the pancreas
        from, 91
Splenic cysts, 324
Splenomegaly
    portal hypertension as a cause of, 169,
        321
    sequestrative, 323–324
Splenorrhaphy, to manage intraoperative
        splenic injury, 330
Squamous cell carcinoma, esophageal,
        incidence of, 28
Staging
    of colorectal cancer, 302–303
    of esophageal carcinoma, 28–29
    of gastric cancer, 77
    TNM, of pancreatic cancer, 123
    See also Classification; Grading
Steatorrhea, in Crohn's disease, 286–287
Steering wheel injury, retroperitoneal
        rupture of the duodenum resulting
        from, 337–338
Stenting, in managing unresectable bile
        duct tumors, 235
Steroid therapy
    contraindication to, in amebic colitis,
        295
    for Crohn's disease management, 289
Stomach, 37–83
    benign neoplasms of, 72–75
    carcinoma of
        clinical presentation of, 77
        pathology of, 75
        staging of, 77
        surgical treatment of, 77–78
        survival after surgery, 79
        TNM classification of, 78
    clinical disorders of, 56–81
    herniated, in paraesophageal hernia,
        17–18
    motor disorders of
        medical treatment for, 70
        surgical management of, 70
    pathophysiology of, 51–56
    physiology of, 41–51
    resection of, in esophageal carcinoma
        surgery, 31
Strangulated obstruction, 249–250
    of the small bowel, 275
Strasberg's classification, of laparoscopic
        injuries to the biliary tract, 226–228
Stress ulcer, after liver resection, 194
Strictures, biliary, due to injury, 225–228
String sign, in Crohn's colitis, 288
Submucosa, small vessels of, late radiation
        injury to, 257
Subphrenic hematoma, after splenectomy,
        330
Substance P (SP), 144–145
    distribution of, 144
    of the esophageal nerve supply C-fibers,
        3

ISBN 0-387-00721-0

EAN

9 780387 007212 >